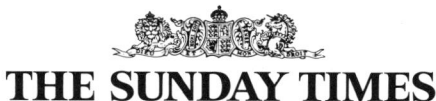

NEW BOOK OF BODY MAINTENANCE

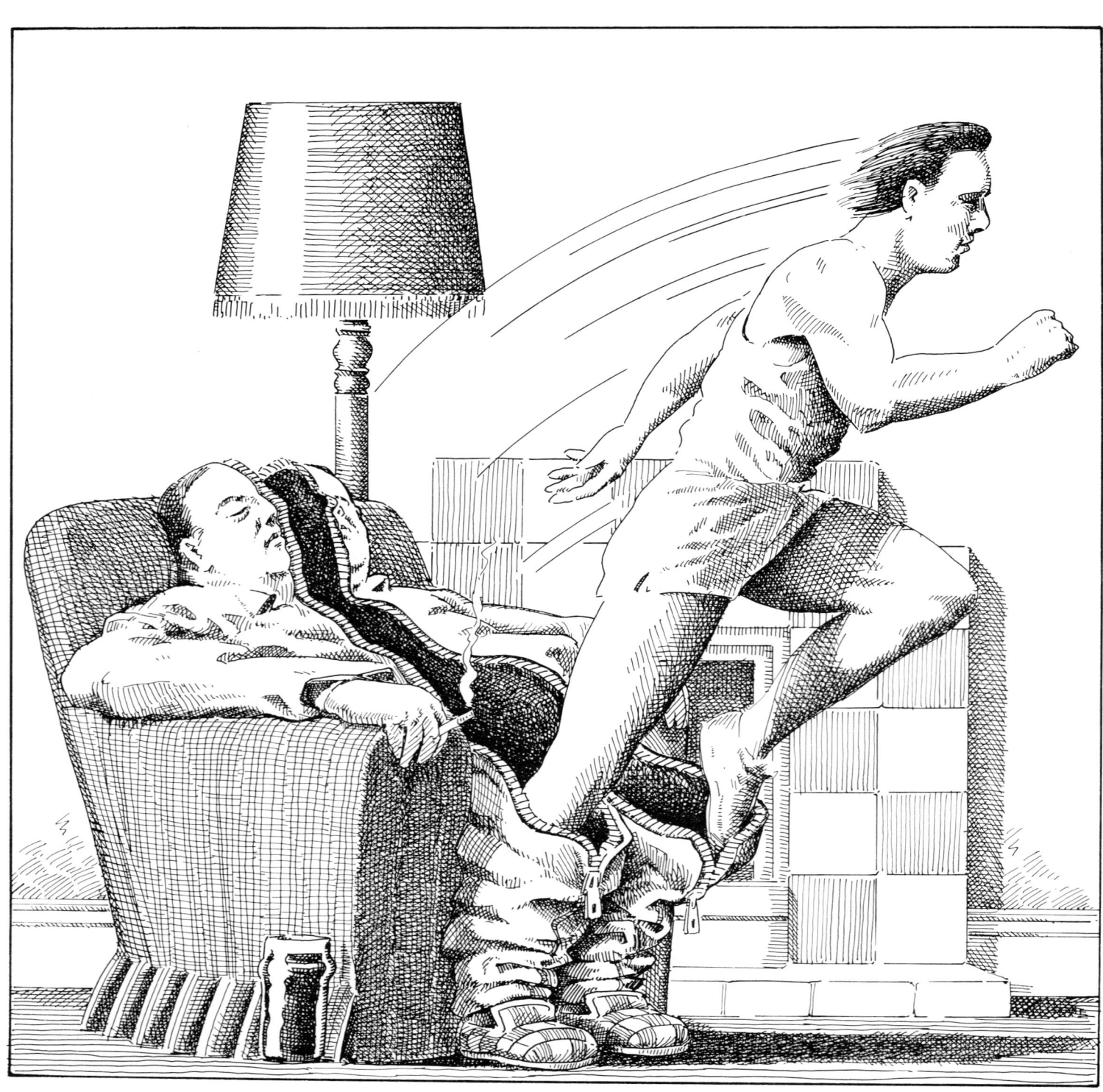

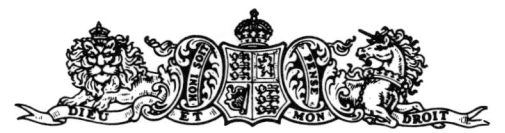

THE SUNDAY TIMES
NEW BOOK OF BODY MAINTENANCE

EDITED BY OLIVER GILLIE, CELIA HADDON AND DERRIK MERCER

MERMAID BOOKS   LONDON

The Sunday Times Book of Body Maintenance
first published June 1978 © The Sunday Times Magazine

This revised edition first published in Great Britain in Mermaid Books by Michael Joseph Ltd
44 Bedford Square, London WC1
1982
© The Sunday Times 1982

All Rights Reserved. No part of this publication
may be reproduced, stored in a retrieval system,
or transmitted in any form or by any means, electronic,
mechanical, photocopying, recording or otherwise,
without the prior permission of the Copyright owner

Limp edition ISBN 0 7181 2193 7
Cased edition ISBN 0 7181 2209 7

Typeset by Rowland Phototypesetting Ltd
Bury St Edmunds, Suffolk
Printed in Great Britain by
Jolly & Barber Ltd, Rugby
Bound by Dorstel Press Ltd, Harlow

Editors
OLIVER GILLIE
CELIA HADDON
DERRIK MERCER

Art Editor
CLIVE CROOK

Additional contributors
MARGARET ASHWELL   CAROLINE CONRAN
ROSEMARY ATKINS   NORMAN HARRIS
MICHAEL BATEMAN   TONY OSMAN

Many medical experts and organizations have acted as consultants during the preparation of this book and its predecessor; they are credited in the acknowledgements on pages 8–9. Photographers and artists are credited at the end of the book on page 237.

Oliver Gillie is Medical Correspondent of the *Sunday Times* and recently won the award for Specialist Writer of the Year in the National Press Awards. Other books include *The Living Cell*, *How to Stop Smoking*, *Who Do You Think You Are?* and *The Sunday Times Guide to the World's Best Food* (co-editor).

Celia Haddon is a freelance author and journalist who was formerly on the staff of the *Sunday Times*. Other books include *The Limits of Sex*.

Derrik Mercer is Associate Editor (Channel 4) of *Independent Television News* and was formerly Managing Editor (News) of the *Sunday Times*. Other books include *The Sunday Times Book of the Countryside* (co-editor).

Clive Crook is art editor of the *Sunday Times Magazine* and *Sunday Magazine*. He also designed *The Sunday Times Book of the Countryside*.

Contents

Acknowledgements 8–9

Foreword 9

Introduction 10

1: Pregnancy and Childhood 12
Pregnancy/Childbirth/The Early Years/Accidents

2: Exercise 40
The Joys of Fitness/Health Checks/Aerobic Exercise/Indoor Exercise/Sport

3: Stress and Relaxation 66
Stress/Relaxation/Headaches/Depression/Suicide

4: Diet 76
Nutrition/Slimming

5: Maintaining the Bodywork 106
The Back/The Feet/The Hair/The Skin/The Joints/The Eyes/The Ears/The Teeth

6: The Major Hazards 128
Smoking/Heart Disease/Cancer/Drug Dependence/Alcoholism

7: Staying Healthy at Work and Play 154
Colds and Flu/Hazards at Work/Preventing Infections/Rules of Hygiene/Allergies

8: Sex and Health 169
A Happy Sex Life/Menstruation/Contraception/Sexual Infections/The Menopause/Age and Sex

9: Holiday Health 186
Vaccinations/The Journey/When You Arrive

10: A Healthy Old Age 192
Starting to Live/Conserve Health and Fitness/Checklist of Symptoms

EMERGENCY 206
Alphabetical Guide to Emergencies/When to Call the Doctor

Appendix One: Good Food 216
Appendix Two: Your National Health Service Rights 230
Appendix Three: Further Information 232
Picture Acknowledgements 237
Index 238

Acknowledgements

This book began life as an eight-part series in the *Sunday Times Magazine*. That was in 1976 and since then the original material has been greatly expanded and revised to appear as books in both Britain and the United States. Now it is published again, extensively revised with many new subjects added and many more expanded as well as updated. However, the guiding principle behind the book not only remains constant but is also today far more widely accepted than when we began: it is that most of us can improve our health more by changing our lifestyles than by relying upon the wonders of medical science.

We are grateful to the many reviewers and specialist bodies who have commented favourably upon our attempts to present the latest medical thinking in simple and dispassionate laymen's terms. We have tried to avoid sensationalism, although some conclusions *are* alarming: the needless suffering caused by smoking, the manifest dangers of unfitness and so on. However, medical knowledge is rarely a question of absolute truth; much is inevitably a matter of opinion or interpretation. In such matters we, as journalists, are indebted to the many medical experts who have helped us compile this book and its predecessors. Sometimes they provided much of the original material, sometimes they read our draft manuscripts to check that our layman's language was not achieved at the expense of accuracy. But if any errors have survived the processes of checking and double-checking, the blame does not rest with the individuals and organizations whose help we acknowledge below. Not even this distinguished panel of consultants could ensure that every reader will agree with every word in the book. And responsibility for any opinions expressed within a book naturally rests with its authors rather than its advisers.

Margaret Ashwell, who advised us on slimming, is in fact a medical specialist rather than a journalist. A member of the scientific staff of the Medical Research Council, she was previously research officer for the *Which? Slimming Guide* and as Margaret Allen wrote *The Joy of Slimming*. The other contributors, acknowledged on page 5, are past and present journalists on the staff of the *Sunday Times*.

Among individuals who helped us in the preparation of the original volume of this book were Dr Hugh Jolly, head of the paediatric department, Charing Cross Hospital, London; Mr Geoffrey Chamberlain, FRCS, consultant obstetrician, Queen Charlotte's Hospital, London; Dr R. W. D. Turner, Senior Research Fellow in Preventive Cardiology, University of Edinburgh; Professor J. N. Morris, Department of Community Health, London School of Hygiene and Tropical Medicine, University of London; Dr Mervyn Davies, Department of Environmental Physiology, London School of Hygiene and Tropical Medicine, University of London; Dr Beric Wright, executive director of the BUPA medical centre, London; Dr Malcolm Carruthers, director of Clinical Laboratory Services, Maudsley Hospital, London; Dr Stanley Taylor, consultant cardiologist, General Infirmary, Leeds; Dr J. D. G. Troup, consultant physician, Department of Rheumatology and Rehabilitation, Royal Free Hospital, London, and Senior Research Fellow, Department of Orthopaedic Surgery, University of Liverpool; Mr Jonathan Hazell, FRCS, of the Royal National Institute for the Deaf; Mr Barrie Jay, FRCS, consultant ophthalmic surgeon, Moorfields Eye Hospital, London; Mr Arthur Swallow, lecturer at the London Foot Hospital; Dr Ian Caldwell, consultant dermatologist, Jersey General Hospital; Dr Ian Davies, director of Department of Periodontology, Royal Dental Hospital of London; Professor Charles Fletcher, formerly Professor of Clinical Epidemiology, Royal Postgraduate Medical School, University of London; Professor T. Symington, director of the Chester Beatty Research Institute, London; the honorary medical secretary of the British League against Rheumatism; Surgeon Vice-Admiral Sir Dick Caldwell, then executive director of the Medical Council on Alcoholism; Dr Leonard McEwen, formerly Senior Lecturer in Pharmacology, St Mary's Hospital Medical School, London; Dr. D. A. J. Tyrrell, head of the Clinical Research Centre's Division of Communicable Diseases; Dr Marcia Wilkinson, director of the Regional Neurological Unit, Eastern Hospital, London; Mr James Hamilton, assistant secretary in TUC social insurance and industrial welfare department; Dr Harry Levitt, of the BUPA medical centre, London; Dr J. K. Oates, consultant venereologist, Westminster Hospital, London; Dr Tony Wisdom, consultant venereologist at Queen Mary's Hospital for the East End, London; Dr Anthony Turner, Senior Overseas Medical Officer, British Airways; Sir Ferguson Anderson, Professor of Geriatric Medicine, Glasgow University; J. F. G. Coles, secretary of the St John Ambulance Association; Mr E. W. Shepard of the Department of Health and Social Security; Dr Peter Abrahams, lecturer in anatomy, Middlesex Hospital Medical School, London; and Mrs Elspeth Maclean director of Home and Leisure Safety, Royal Society for the Prevention of Accidents.

Many of these individuals or their organizations have helped us again to ensure that the accuracy which was praised upon the earlier volume's publication was maintained. In addition we are indebted to Dr Malcolm Whitehead, lecturer of the Department of Obstetrics, King's College Hospital Medical School, London; Professor Malcolm Laker of the Institute of Psychiatry; the Rev David Evans of the Samaritans; Dr Hugh Gough-Thomas, executive director of the Medical Council on Alcoholism; Dr Alan Maryon-Davies of the Health Education Council; Ian Williams, field officer of British Red Cross; Professor K. V. Mortimer, Royal Dental Hospital of London; Mr Yehudi Gordon, obstetrician, Royal Free Hospital, London; Sheila Kitzinger, author and expert on childbirth; Steve Karmy, audiological scientist, Bilsom International; Janet Balaskas and Meloma Huxley, experts on yoga exercises for childbirth.

Among organizations who helped us were the Department of Health and Social Security; the Health Education Council; the Consumers' Association; the Family Planning Association; the Samaritans; the Arthritis and Rheumatism Council; Back Pain Association; The Migraine Trust; the Institute for the Study of Drug Dependence; MIND;

Foreword

Royal Society for the Prevention of Accidents; the Pre-Retirement Association; Age Concern England; the British Red Cross; British Rheumatism and Arthritis Association; Health and Safety Executive.

We are also grateful to several publishers for allowing us to reproduce material from their books. The weight tables for babies are taken from *Babyhood*, by Penelope Leach, pages 184–7, copyright Penelope Leach 1975 and reprinted by permission of Penguin Books Ltd. The noise table in the section Hazards at Work (Chapter 7) is also reprinted by permission of Penguin Books Ltd; it is taken from *Noise*, by Rupert Taylor, pages 55–6, copyright Rupert Taylor 1970. The advice on choosing shoes is printed by permission of the Consumers Association, from the May 1973 issue of *Which?* Crown Publishers Inc., Her Majesty's Stationery Office, Churchill Livingstone, and the Michigan Heart Association also gave us permission to reproduce material as indicated in full elsewhere in this book.

This book has been through so many lives that many other people have contributed to one stage or another: the staff of the *Sunday Times Magazine*, for instance, who worked on the series which was to provide the launching-pad for the books. We are grateful to two editors of the *Sunday Times*, Harold Evans and Frank Giles, for giving their blessing to the projects. For this edition Annette Smith provided invaluable secretarial assistance.

by Dr Keith Taylor, Director-General of the Health Education Council

Prevention and health: everybody's business, the title of a booklet the Department of Health and Social Services published in 1976, emphasized the need for people to think and talk about the place of prevention in the long-term developments of health services, and how much these will depend on the attitude and actions of the individual about his or her own health. In order to have an attitude or to take action, knowledge is needed, and *The Sunday Times Book of Body Maintenance* provides this in good measure and in a clearly illustrated and very assimilable form. It is wholly different in content and style from those home doctoring books so popular in the nineteenth century, which served a useful function when the diagnostic and especially the therapeutic capabilities of medical professionals were by today's standards rudimentary. It provides very effectively messages about health education for individuals and families. The information is enhanced by relevant facts of anatomy, physiology and pathology, illustrated in an original and eye-catching way. In consequence, though not intended to be a layperson's text of body structure and function, it fulfils its function very successfully.

This second edition, *The Sunday Times New Book of Body Maintenance*, incorporates changes, some reflecting new knowledge, some a new and more appropriate emphasis. The preventive aspects of medicine are woven into the fabric of a healthy lifestyle to create an attractive and easily understood pattern. Clearly, the potential for improving the quality of our lives with regard to health is enormous, since so many diseases depend on individual behaviour.

I favour particularly the section on food and dietary recommendations. It is to be hoped that all of the factors which contribute to our choices of food will in time cease to be in conflict and will assist us in adopting healthier eating habits. The section which deals with keeping fit in old age is excellent and should be widely read by health professionals, as well as by adults of all ages.

This book deserves wide readership. It should be in every home and no health education unit should be without it. It is a useful contribution to an increasingly consumerist society and may help to bring the achievement of the World Health Organization's 'health for all by the year 2000' a little nearer.

Keith Taylor
May 1982

Introduction

This book promises no miracle cures, but its message is an optimistic one: there is abundant evidence that our health can be improved as much in the future as it has over the past hundred years. Its inspiration is the increasing belief of medical scientists that our hopes of living longer and living better depend more upon ourselves than any technical or pharmaceutical wonders now being developed in laboratories. Only charlatans guarantee good health, and we do not propose to join their number, but we can outline a lifestyle which according to the best available information should keep you fit and improve your health.

This declaration of intent was written in 1978 when the predecessor to this volume was first published. It was then pioneering a revolution in attitudes towards health. To an astonishing degree yesterday's revolution has become today's conventional wisdom. Streets and parks are full of runners, supermarkets full of shoppers seeking 'low-fat' produce. And people who have altered their lifestyles can draw fresh encouragement from the American experience. There, where the changes in personal habits such as smoking, diet and exercise have been greater than in any other Western country, there has been a 30 per cent fall in deaths from heart disease over the last decade.

This book is a body owner's manual for the care and maintenance of the only body you will ever have; however remarkable the achievements of transplant surgeons, there is no likelihood of a trade-in after, say, forty-five years. That prevention is better than cure, nobody would dispute. But it is not easy to put into practice. So much recent research seems not only very confusing but also opposed to traditional beliefs. Foods such as milk and eggs, which we have been brought up to believe were 'good', are in some cases now labelled 'bad' if eaten in more than moderate quantities. Many fundamental aspects of modern life – cities, cars, television, lifts – now have their detractors. Yet it is clearly impractical nonsense to pine for a rural heaven where somehow disease would be unknown; it is how human beings cope with modern life that matters. This book is dedicated to no single theory and offers few medical 'truths'. We have attempted to present a simple and undogmatic assessment of current medical thinking about all the prime problems of physical health. It is a layman's guide not to what doctors can do for our health but to what we can do to help ourselves.

However, concentrating on illness and what *not* to do would be a depressing way to live. Life is to be enjoyed rather than just grimly survived. We have therefore tried to present a positive attitude to food, exercise, stress and general health. By learning how to maintain the body in good running order, life in any case becomes more enjoyable, as well as lasting longer. This consoling, even cheering, thought marks a fundamental change from the world of medicine fifty or a hundred years ago.

A century ago four babies out of ten born in England and Wales failed to survive to adulthood. Little boys who reached their first birthday could expect to live until they were just forty-eight. Their sisters were luckier: if they survived their first hazardous year of life they would live on average until they were fifty. Today, the expectation of life *from birth* is 69.2 for men and 75.6 for women. The population of the United Kingdom has doubled while the birth-rate has halved. From the maternity ward to the geriatric wing, new skills and equipment are enabling lives to be saved that once would have been irretrievably lost. Vaccination programmes have made children largely immune from illnesses which once claimed thousands.

Today there are new problems. Sometimes they are consequences of past successes; the conquest of disease has greatly increased the numbers of people who now survive not merely into their fifties but into their seventies and beyond. Other problems stem from scientific or chemical processes which were unknown at the turn of the century, such as radiation. Most common of all, though, are illnesses which were comparatively rare fifty years ago, notably heart disease and cancer. There are, inevitably, many variations as people grow older, but add all the deaths together and you find that two in three are caused by heart disease, cancer and strokes. To some extent these, too, are a consequence of ageing populations: the incidence of each increases with age. Increasingly, however, they are claiming younger and younger victims. Heart disease is now a middle-age problem, while cancer is a major killer even in childhood. Age alone cannot therefore be their cause; it can only increase their likelihood. If this gives hope that

The Class Distinctions of Disease
The table below gives the increased or decreased risk – in percentage terms – of a man from each of five social classes dying from certain causes. The particular work he does is not the main contributory factor as similar differences of risk exist for wives of men in these categories. Diet and lifestyle are major influences

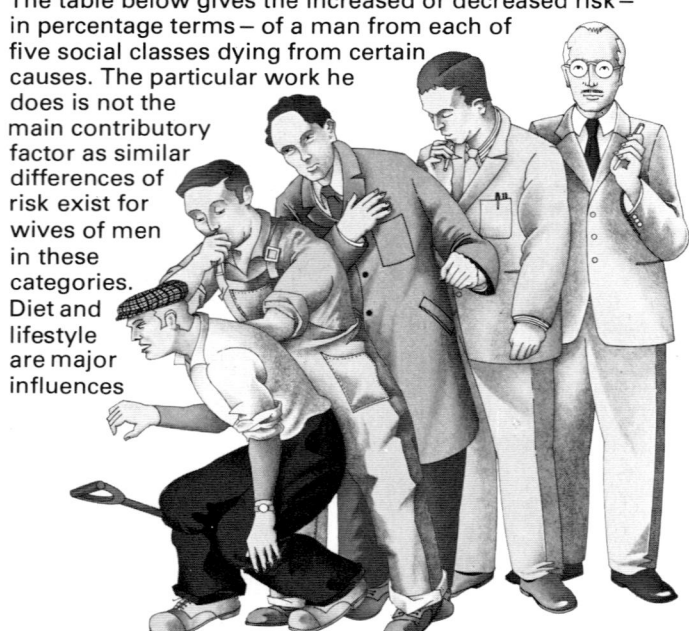

Cause of Death	Unskilled	Semi-skilled	Skilled	Managerial	Professional
Tuberculosis	+85	+ 8	− 4	−46	−60
Stomach Cancer	+63	+14	+ 1	−37	−51
Lung Cancer	+48	+ 4	+ 7	−28	−37
Coronary Disease	+12	− 4	+ 6	− 5	− 2
Bronchitis	+94	+16	− 3	−50	−72
Duodenal Ulcer	+73	+ 7	− 4	−25	−52

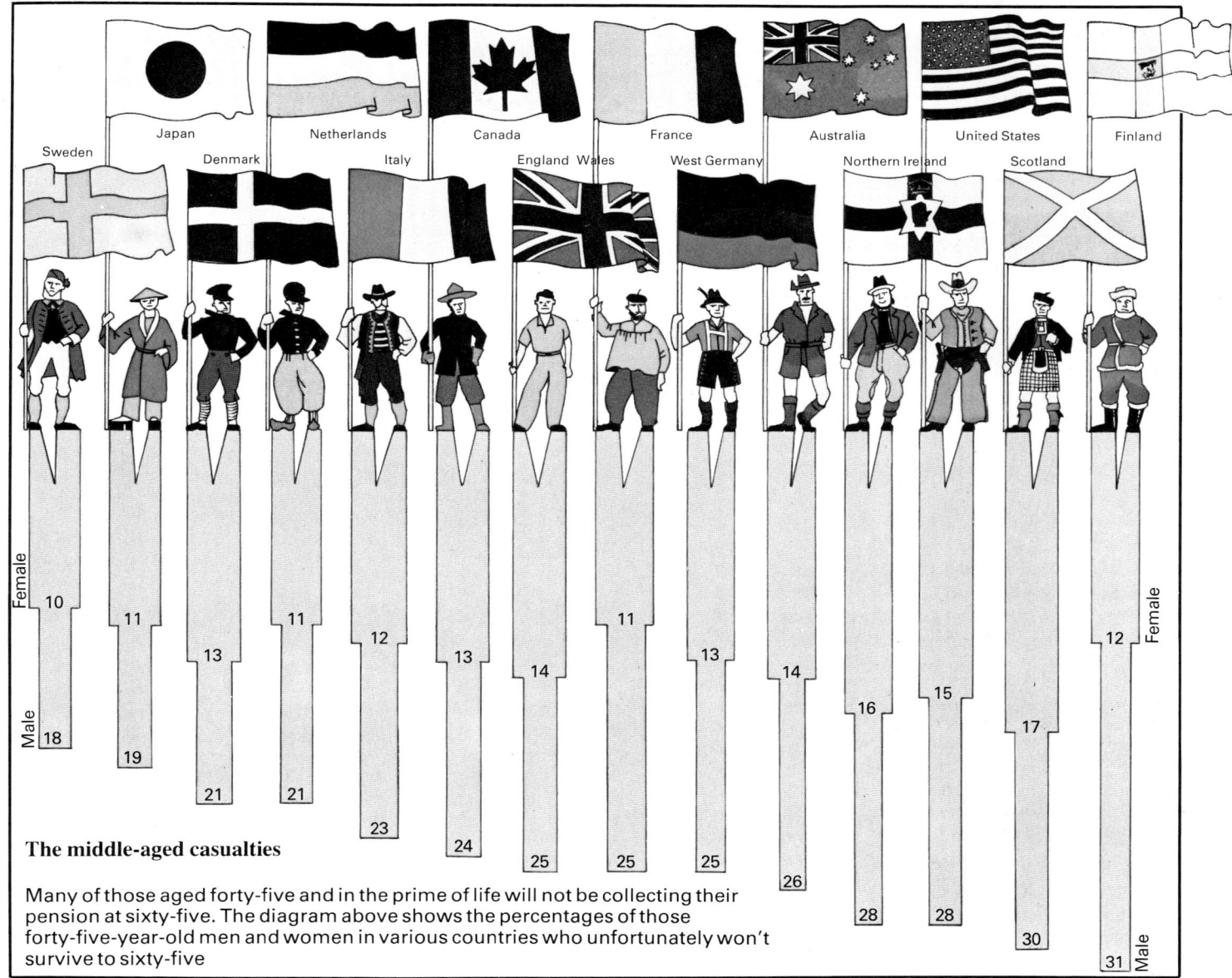

The middle-aged casualties

Many of those aged forty-five and in the prime of life will not be collecting their pension at sixty-five. The diagram above shows the percentages of those forty-five-year-old men and women in various countries who unfortunately won't survive to sixty-five

these modern killers may be prevented or averted, it is not the sole ground for optimism. Why should death-rates vary so dramatically from country to country? What can explain the difference within countries between regions and income groups? The existence of such differences shows clearly that illness and death are caused by factors other than some intrinsic failing in the human body.

Genetic or climatic factors might contribute to international differences but not to those within nations. Nor would climatic factors alone explain the differences between the health of, say, Japanese people living in Japan and Japanese immigrants in the United States. Economic differences go some way towards explaining variations in health between income groups but cannot be the major cause of health differences between broadly comparable countries. Environmental factors, such as differing occupational hazards, have a direct relationship to health differences between income groups. But they cannot explain the similar differences which exist between the non-working wives of different income groups. Health services also vary in their quality and availability. Sweden's low infant-mortality rate, for instance, is largely attributed to the excellence of their hospital care. No nation is so advanced in medical knowledge, however, for this to be the dominant factor. Nor could it explain variations within a country. This leaves one other potential variable: lifestyles.

Lifestyles have received increasing attention from doctors and medical scientists in recent years. To some extent this is a response to the elusive search for cures to non-infectious diseases such as heart disease, cancer and strokes. If they cannot be cured, how can they be prevented? What is their cause? Why are they rampant today yet more rare eighty years ago? Why are they more common in some countries than others? Why are some occupations more vulnerable than others? The detective work involved in this medical quest is known as epidemiology. Its disciples are increasingly singling out the lifestyle of the Western world, notably our diet and lack of exercise, as the most likely root-cause of our problems.

The evidence is advanced in detail elsewhere in this book but it does mean that we have it in our power to influence our own health and that of our family. But this book is neither a substitute for your family doctor nor an encyclopedia of medical knowledge; whole volumes have been written about individual sections of this book, and we have scarcely ventured into mental health. There will also inevitably be some generalizations in a book of this kind that do not apply to some individuals. If in doubt, see a doctor.

1: PREGNANCY AND CHILDHOOD

Pregnancy

Birth is a time of great hope but also a time of crisis. A good birth is the best start there is for a healthy, happy life ahead. A distressing birth may take months or even years for mother and baby to overcome. Each new baby is a miracle. The newborn baby has already survived the most difficult period of life: something like a third of babies are lost in the first two months following conception, many so early that a woman does not even know she has miscarried.

The most important single thing a woman can do to obtain the best outcome of her pregnancy is to ensure a healthy body. This means aiming at a new lifestyle in which you take more care of yourself. It means a new way of looking at things because you now have a big stake in the future. The new lifestyle involves giving up some things like smoking, and limiting alcohol, but it also has an important positive side: you must now take care to eat well and to take exercise.

CONCEPTION AND FERTILITY

With the accumulation of more knowledge about pregnancy a new idea is emerging – that a man and a woman should plan ahead to make sure that conception occurs just at the right moment. This pre-conceptual care has already started in the United States. The idea is to bear as healthy a child as possible by making sure that conditions are right from the beginning.

Pre-conceptual care is based upon two principles. The first principle is that a healthy sperm and a healthy female ovum make for a healthy baby. The second is that the foetus in the womb is vulnerable from the very start. Even before the woman realizes she is pregnant, the foetus can be affected by what she eats and drinks, or her general bodily condition, so it is as well to adopt a healthy lifestyle before attempting conception.

Pre-conceptual care, by increasing the health of the parents, also promotes fertility. This forward planning may be particularly advantageous for older couples because fertility diminishes with age. Here are several suggestions for those who want to maximize their fertility and give their baby the best start.

1. Would-be mothers should check with their doctor that they have had rubella (German measles) or been immunized against it. If you have not been immunized against it, have it done at least two months before coming off the pill, or ensure that other means of contraception are working well, because the vaccine can damage the foetus. If you are uncertain whether you have been immunized against rubella, you can ask your doctor to arrange to have you tested.
2. The woman should stop taking the contraceptive pill from three to five months before trying to conceive. During these months the couple should use barrier methods of contraception – either the sheath or the diaphragm. Women often take some time to conceive after ceasing the pill, so you are probably not wasting time. The five-month gap helps the hormonal system to settle down before conception, and the body to replace vitamins and minerals whose levels are reduced while on the pill.
3. Stop smoking and drinking alcohol. Both may harm the sperm or the fertilized egg.
4. If either partner is on drugs prescribed by the family doctor, ask him if you could safely stop taking them. We still do not know exactly which drugs may or may not affect the sperm or the fertilized egg. To be absolutely on the safe side, both partners should stop taking non-prescription drugs like aspirin and other painkillers. Do not smoke cannabis. Pot smoking makes even young men produce malformed sperm, like those from a man in his seventies.
5. The couple should change to a healthy diet (see pages 14–15 and Chapter 4). Avoid tinned or cooked meats, or meats containing preservatives. Avoid tinned foods generally, since tins may be sealed with lead.

A new organization called Foresight (see Appendix Three) now exists in Britain to help parents plan ahead for conception. Foresight suggests that you ask your doctor to give you a thorough medical overhaul before trying for a baby. Antenatal clinics automatically give pregnant mothers tests for venereal disease and diabetes (indicated by sugar in the urine), but Foresight suggests that these tests should be done before becoming pregnant so that any problem can, as far as possible, be corrected first.

INFERTILITY
After the age of thirty, a woman's fertility declines, and there is likely to be a delay in conceiving. But, if you have

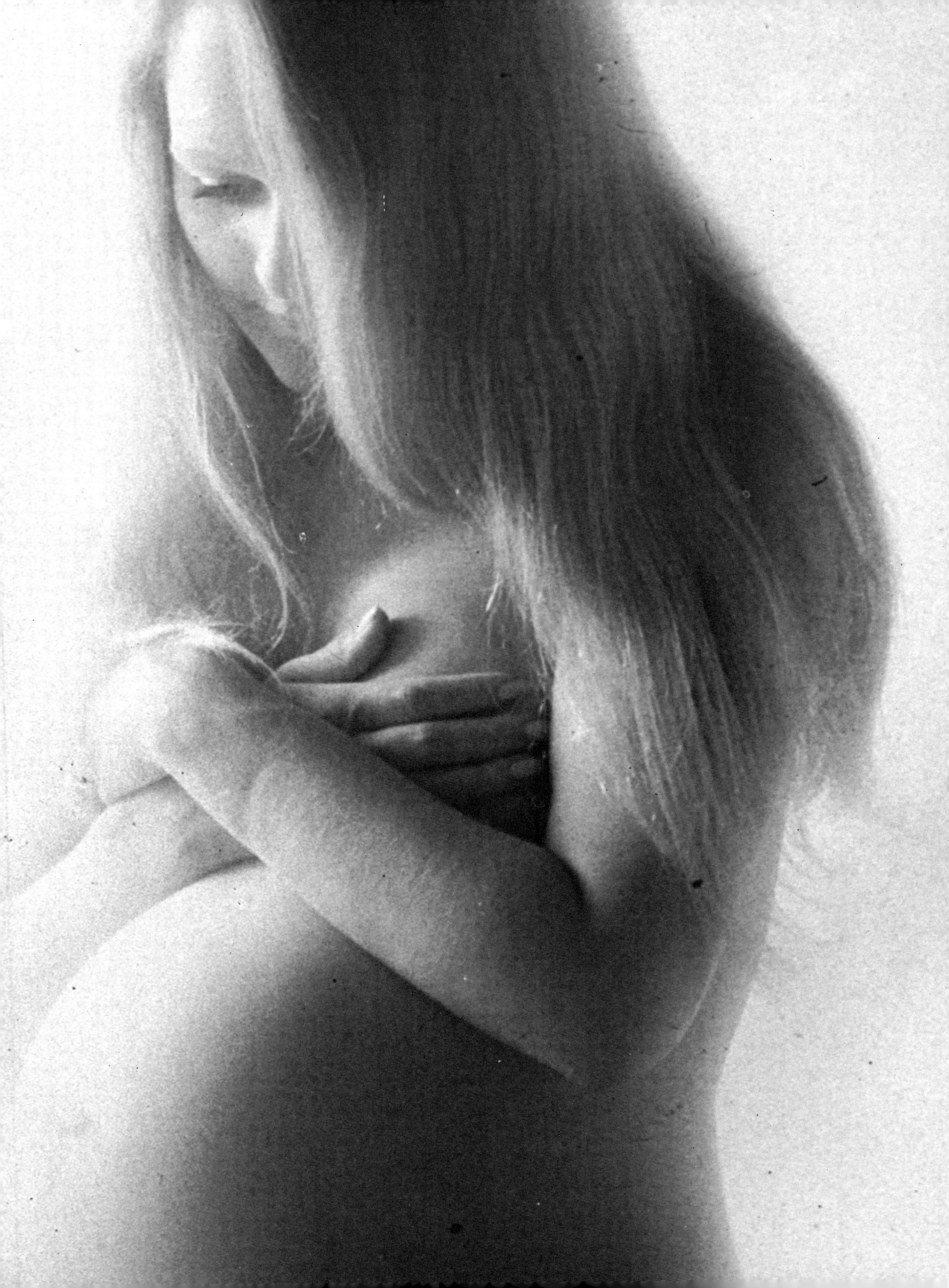

still failed to get pregnant after a year of trying, it is time to seek help. You will need to start with your family doctor. The National Health Service is not very well organized to deal with fertility difficulties and arrangements vary from area to area. Do not let your family doctor simply tell you to go away and keep trying. Insist upon referral to a specialist.

Some areas have sub-fertility clinics which deal with the couple together. In other places, the woman is referred to a gynaecologist while the man is treated by a urologist. Sometimes the man is offered no treatment at all, even though in four out of ten couples the fertility problem lies with the husband. Insist patiently but firmly upon tests for him too. Help, advice and support is forthcoming from the National Association for the Childless (see Appendix Three).

SIGNS OF PREGNANCY

The first sign of pregnancy is often a missed or scanty menstrual period. However, even before this some women notice a heaviness of the breasts, slight nausea early in the mornings and increased frequency of urination. Other symptoms are an increased vaginal discharge, feeling more tired than usual and having a peculiar taste in the mouth. A pregnancy test may be done on a sample of urine from eight days after the last period should have ended. The test may be done by your own doctor, by a local family planning clinic, a commercial testing service, or with a kit bought from the chemist.

HOW TO TAKE CARE DURING PREGNANCY

The most critical stage in the development of a baby – the formation of the spinal cord and brain – is complete by the time a woman notices that her last menstrual period is two weeks overdue and she is no more than six weeks pregnant. This is why good diet and every care should be observed before conception. But the following six to eight weeks of pregnancy are almost as equally crucial. During this time, eyes, ears and limbs are being formed. By the end of the twelfth week of pregnancy the baby is about 1 inch long and its shape has been decided.

A baby inherits from parents the genes which decide eye and hair colour, blood-group and body chemistry. But the hereditary process sometimes makes mistakes and then the growing baby is usually miscarried. The majority of miscarried babies have abnormal numbers of chromosomes – the minute strings of DNA which carry the inherited genes.

It is usually impossible to determine why a baby is born malformed after a normal pregnancy – the cause of eight out of ten birth malformations is still unknown. The cause is sometimes hereditary, but more often it is some factor in the environment as yet unidentified. Infectious diseases, drugs, toxic chemicals such as pesticides, or perhaps some deficiency in the diet of the mother are recognized causes of birth malformation. In the majority of cases there is nothing she could have done to prevent it. However, there are many things that a woman should know and do if she is to have the best chance of giving birth to a healthy baby.

You may well find it impossible to follow all the guidelines which we suggest here in order to give your baby the best chance. Or you may have 'broken' one or more of the guidelines before you knew you were pregnant. *Do not worry too much*. It is always worth remembering that many pregnancies turn out well even when a woman has ignored all the best advice. If you have not done some of the things we recommend here, it is quite understandable that you should be concerned, but the past cannot be changed. There is a lot you can do from now on to get into good condition, *whatever stage you are at* – concentrate on that.

The chances of anything going wrong in an individual case as a result of one individual act – taking aspirins or tranquillizers, for example – are too small to be calculated. Indeed, these drugs may be harmless in normal circumstances – no one is certain. Good nutrition may help to prevent damage from some drugs. Nevertheless, the consensus of medical opinion is that drugs should always be avoided in pregnancy where possible. These and other precautions are therefore worth taking. We are simply presenting current medical thinking so that women can decide for themselves what, if anything, they should or should not do.

If you really want a baby and things seem to have gone wrong, there are a few circumstances when an abortion might be the best recourse. Termination of pregnancy may be seriously considered when a mother has German measles in the first three months of pregnancy, or when a doctor diagnoses some defect such as Down's syndrome (mongolism) or spina bifida (see pages 21–2), but the decision can only be taken by the parents themselves. There are few other circumstances when an abortion might reasonably be considered to be the best course of action on medical grounds alone.

THE PREGNANT DIET

It is common sense to eat well in pregnancy. There is mounting scientific evidence to show that women on poor diets are more likely to have malformed babies than women on normal diets. Women suffering from malnutrition in Third World countries do have babies who are underweight and who may as a result suffer a permanent intellectual disadvantage. Apart from smoking and poverty, the major identifiable cause of premature births in Western countries is poor diet; and attempting to reduce weight around the time of conception and during pregnancy may also cause premature birth or abnormalities.

Premature birth is a major cause of death in the first month of life. Advances in medicine allow most of those premature babies who survive to develop perfectly normally, but prematurity is still a major cause of cerebral palsy and is also associated with an increased risk of epilepsy, blindness, deafness and mental handicap. As many as a quarter of pregnant mothers might be at risk from inadequate diet judging by the experience in Canada, where nutritional counselling of women by the Montreal Diet Dispensary reduced the number of premature births by a third. Check the recommended diet below to see if you are eating properly.

One survey, made by Professor R. W. Smithells of Leeds University, suggests that a shortage of folic acid – one of the B vitamins – may play a part in causing two of the commonest birth abnormalities: spina bifida and anencephaly. Further support for the theory comes from the observation that drugs which interfere with the normal action of folic acid in the body may cause human malformations. According to another theory, chemicals called nitrites and nitrosa-

PREGNANCY/PREGNANCY AND CHILDHOOD

> **A RECOMMENDED DAILY DIET**
>
> 1. A pint of milk – or 4 oz (50 g) cheese – for protein and calcium. Fresh semi-skimmed milk provides just as much protein and calcium but is less fattening. Cheese is by far the richest and most readily available source of calcium, which is necessary for the growing bones of the baby. Alternative sources of protein and calcium for women who do not like milk or cheese are soya beans, other soya products, small fish eaten bones and all, and cereals.
> 2. A portion of meat, fish or an egg to provide protein, iron and B vitamins. (Alternatives: soya products and whole cereals.)
> 3. A helping of root or raw green vegetables to provide vitamin C and folic acid.
> 4. Fruit, frozen orange juice or potatoes to provide further vitamin C.
> 5. Bread to provide energy and vitamins – preferably wholemeal bread, which will prevent constipation. Alternatively, eat a bran or wholemeal breakfast food to avoid constipation. Beans, lentils and oats (eaten as muesli or porridge or in other ways) are also excellent sources of protein and roughage.
> 6. Plenty of water – about a pint – in addition to tea and coffee in normal amounts.
> 7. Eat liver or an oily fish (e.g., herrings, mackerel, sardines) once a week for vitamins A and D. For those who do not like fish, margarine and eggs are good sources of vitamins A and D. (Butter and milk products are poor sources of D.) Carrots and dark green vegetables are good sources of A. White fish once a week for iodine.

mines, present in preserved meats such as ham, corned beef and frankfurters, may have an association with spina bifida and anencephaly, so some people would say it is safer to avoid these during pregnancy.

For you and your baby
1. Always choose fresh foods in preference to processed or tinned foods; bread to biscuits. Never eat mouldy food.
2. Eat well; never diet in pregnancy. However, you can avoid unnecessary weight gain by cutting down on empty calories: biscuits, sugar, jam, confectionery and sweetened drinks. Always prefer bread and potatoes because these are valuable sources of nutrients and protein as well as energy. Eat as much of these as you wish.
3. Only take vitamin tablets under doctor's instructions. Extra vitamins should not be necessary for a normal woman observing a proper diet.

Vegetarians: There is no reason why a woman should not have a vegetarian diet in pregnancy, but special knowledge is then advantageous. For example, soya products are advisable as an extra source of iron and seaweed as an extra source of iodine. Advice can be obtained from The Vegetarian Society, 53 Marloes Road, London W8.

MORNING SICKNESS
Women who suffer sickness and vomiting during pregnancy are most at risk nutritionally because they may find that tea and biscuits are all that they can keep down. If they are able to substitute milk and bread or dry toast, their intake of essential nutrients will be much improved. Another trick is to eat cold foods. Not all women feel nauseous on rising; some find that the early evening, when everyone else is having a large meal, is their worst time to eat. For these women, a good breakfast is the best answer.

INDIGESTION AND HEARTBURN
Indigestion and heartburn, the regurgitation of acid from the stomach causing a burning pain in the chest, is a common problem in pregnancy. A number of simple measures help to avoid it. Eat smaller and more frequent meals. Examine your diet and try to avoid those foods – different for everyone – which seem to cause heartburn, and eat alternatives with the same nutritional value. If you suffer from indigestion or heartburn in bed, raise the head end by four to six inches. This helps prevent acid from being regurgitated. Milk is a natural antacid and can be a great help in stopping indigestion. If you do not like milk, try any of the proprietary antacids available from your chemist.

IRON TABLETS
Iron tablets are given to most women in pregnancy to prevent anaemia. But, if they cause constipation or bowel upsets, try taking them with the main meal of the day. If they still cause problems, it is generally medically acceptable not to take them, as long as you ensure that your blood is being monitored regularly for anaemia.

TEETH
A woman's teeth often suffer in pregnancy because calcium is absorbed from them to make the baby's bones. They will suffer less if you ensure there are no untreated spots of decay. Dental treatment is free in the UK in pregnancy and until the baby is one year old. So make sure you have a check-up early in pregnancy, and make sure you go for another routine check-up after the baby is born (see also section on Teeth, pages 124–7).

SLEEP, RELAXATION AND STRESS
Stress may cause miscarriages and premature births, although it is difficult to measure stress accurately, or even be certain that different people mean the same thing when they use the word. However, it makes sense to slow down during pregnancy and to learn to relax – particularly if you feel tense and worried. Relaxation and preparation-for-childbirth classes are often run by hospitals, local authorities and charities (see Appendix Three). Avoid unnecessary stress or strenuous work during pregnancy if you possibly can. If you have to move house, do it in planned, easy stages.

Try to get all the sleep you feel you need. This will be about eight hours every night and you will probably need an additional period of rest during the day, especially in the later months. Remember your body is working harder than usual feeding the baby, and you have extra weight to carry around. Relaxation is helpful so that you have time to think about the future. Try to avoid any unnecessary new projects at this time. (For more information on relaxation and sleep, see pages 69–71.)

If your pregnancy is proceeding normally and you do not have any special problems (check with your doctor), then there is no reason why you should not carry on doing most of the things you usually do, including travelling and many sports, provided you feel comfortable and confident while doing them. You may find that you become uncomfortable on long journeys and it is a good idea to stop and move around after an hour or two. Avoid having your legs crossed for long periods, because this slows the circulation of the blood.

If children are conceived and born in close succession it puts a much greater stress on the mother, both during pregnancy and afterwards. A two-year gap between births usually gives a mother the chance to recover fully and give the next baby the best chance, but a gap of four years is probably ideal, enabling each child to have a lot of attention while small. A longer gap also has the advantage of avoiding the more extreme rivalry and competition between children that can develop in brothers and sisters born close together.

TOBACCO

The greatest precaution a woman can take by herself to ensure the best outcome of her pregnancy is to give up smoking, if she has not already done so before she started to try and become pregnant. Husbands should also stop smoking because a woman who is sitting in a smoke-filled room absorbs smoke in the air which is in turn passed to the baby. The babies of mothers who smoke are low in weight at birth, and Professor Neville Butler of Bristol University has calculated that some 1,500 babies die in Britain every year as a direct result of mothers' smoking. Babies whose mothers smoke have on average fewer cells in their bodies and brains, and so they have a smaller size and weight, and lower intelligence, than would otherwise have been the case.

Ideally, a mother should also not smoke during the first year of the baby's life. Babies whose mothers smoke are more frequently admitted to hospital with chest infections in the first year of life than those whose mothers do not smoke, according to research by doctors at the Hadassah University in Israel. It is still not clear whether the cause of the baby's chest infections is the cigarette smoke or the germs coughed by the mother, who is more prone to chest infection as a result of smoking.

ALCOHOL

The Royal College of Psychiatrists suggests that women should not drink at all in pregnancy. The college says, 'Even very moderate social drinking may be associated with decreased birthweight and an increased risk of spontaneous abortion.' This advice comes down on the safe side, as any official advice must. The evidence is of course difficult to interpret, because women who drink may also have lives which are different in other ways from women who do not, and it is not easy to separate out all such factors. However, there is no doubt that heavy drinking in pregnancy can cause birth malformations, particularly affecting the head, and mental retardation. These malformations appear to be caused by alcohol itself rather than any particular alcoholic drink. Mineral water with a slice of lemon, orange and tomato juice are the safe drinks to go for. But there may be no harm in a shandy (beer and lemonade) or a light beer such as pale ale or a light lager taken simply for refreshment. Avoid all spirits, wines and strong beers.

SEX

Women used to be advised to avoid sexual intercourse for six weeks before and six weeks after birth. Today it is accepted that a pregnant woman may have intercourse throughout pregnancy as long as it is comfortable and enjoyable and there is no pain in the vagina or abdomen. Sex should be avoided if there is any bleeding from the vagina or if intercourse causes any blood, as there is then a danger of infection of the womb. Once the waters have broken, birth is imminent and intercourse is not advisable because of the danger of infection.

Intercourse in the conventional 'missionary position' with the man on top becomes awkward once the womb begins to enlarge, and the man must avoid putting his whole weight on it. Other positions are generally preferable. For example, the woman may be on top or the couple may lie on their sides with the man behind. Making love with what Sheila Kitzinger (author of *The Experience of Childbirth*) calls 'careful tenderness' may help a couple's relationship to develop and increase their awareness of the baby. However, some women are naturally frightened about intercourse during pregnancy. There is no danger that intercourse will cause a miscarriage under normal circumstances. But if a woman has had repeated miscarriages it may be advisable to abstain from sex in later pregnancy.

As mentioned before, when planning a pregnancy it is best to change from the contraceptive pill to a mechanical method of contraception such as the diaphragm or condom for at least three months before attempting to conceive. If a woman becomes pregnant with an intra-uterine device (IUD) in position, then it is wise to consult a doctor with a view to its removal, but there is a risk of miscarriage if this is done. If the pregnancy is wanted, it may be better to leave it in position.

INFECTION

If a pregnant woman catches a virus infection which enters the blood-stream, there is a chance that the virus will cross the placenta and infect the baby. The baby's body is much less able to resist this attack than an adult's because the immune defences are not yet properly developed, and the virus may interfere with the delicate time-sequence of development.

German measles (rubella) causes defects in up to 50 per cent of babies if the mother catches the infection for the first time during the first three months of pregnancy. There is a slight risk in the fourth or fifth month. Affected babies may be born with damage to the heart, cataract and other eye abnormalities, deafness in varying degree, mental retardation, brain damage or delayed growth; and this depressing list is not complete. About 250 babies are born each year in the UK with malformations caused by German measles. But vaccination against the disease is now available and should be done well before starting a pregnancy.

If a mother gets a mild infection of German measles during pregnancy it is unlikely to spread to the baby if she has already been vaccinated or previously had the disease. Doctors therefore recommend that teenage girls are vaccinated. Vaccination against German measles or use of other live vaccines should be avoided during pregnancy, because the live viruses in these vaccines can infect and damage the growing baby.

Cytomegalo virus (CMV) is another common virus infec-

PREGNANCY/**PREGNANCY AND CHILDHOOD**

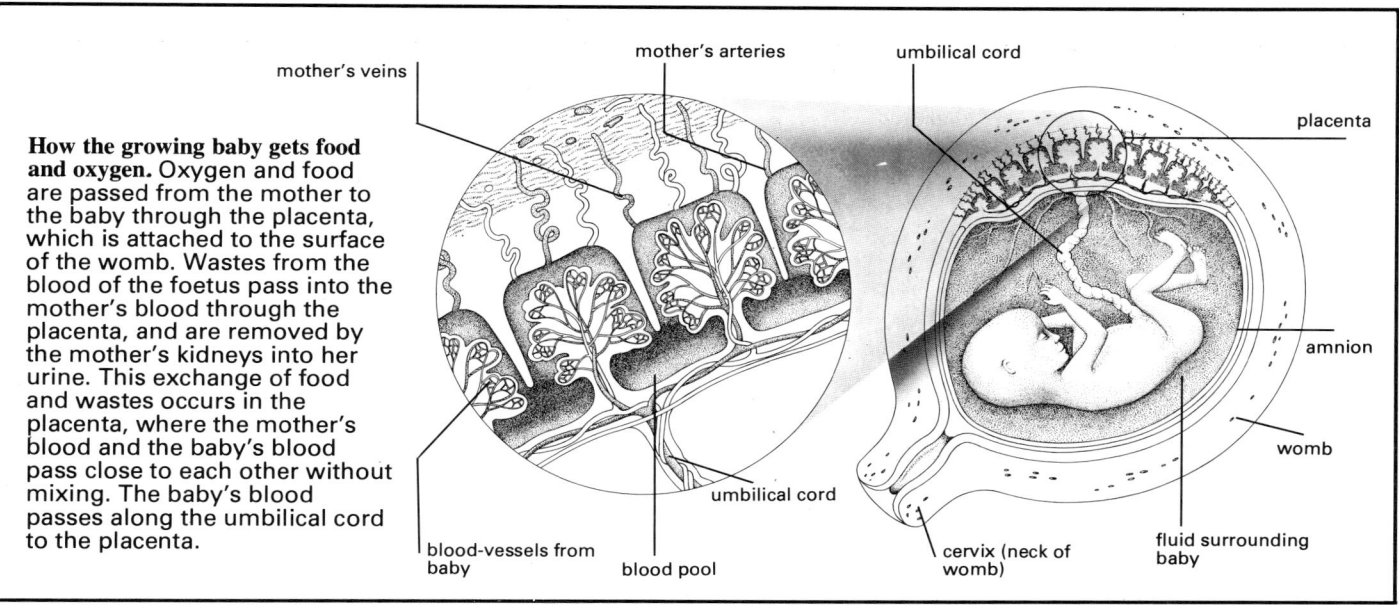

How the growing baby gets food and oxygen. Oxygen and food are passed from the mother to the baby through the placenta, which is attached to the surface of the womb. Wastes from the blood of the foetus pass into the mother's blood through the placenta, and are removed by the mother's kidneys into her urine. This exchange of food and wastes occurs in the placenta, where the mother's blood and the baby's blood pass close to each other without mixing. The baby's blood passes along the umbilical cord to the placenta.

tion which may cause some 800 malformations a year. However, it causes scarcely any recognizable symptoms in adults and a pregnant woman is therefore unlikely to notice anything unusual. CMV may cause low birth-weight, prematurity, deafness or mental retardation similar to the results of German measles infection.

CMV is spread from one adult to another by close personal contact, and sexual intercourse. Babies and children spread it in their urine. Particular attention to hygiene – handwashing, for example – should help to avoid infection. Both husband and wife should also avoid intercourse with other partners during pregnancy. At present, no vaccine is available against CMV.

Herpes virus, infection of the vagina or cervix (see pages 180–1), may be transmitted to the baby during delivery, and if the baby is infected the virus will damage or kill it. Women with herpes are also more likely to suffer miscarriage. Herpes is difficult to treat. If you have had an attack in the past, inform your obstetrician. If tests show it is still active, then it will be advisable to deliver the baby by Caesarian.

Influenza infection during pregnancy can, in rare cases, also cause malformations. Since the influenza virus does not usually enter the blood and does not normally reach the baby, it may be that damage results from the high temperature which often occurs in influenza. Aspirin, which is of course often taken for flu and colds, has been suspected as a possible cause of malformation when women take it during pregnancy. However, there is no really convincing evidence that it is a hazard. So should a pregnant woman take aspirin when she has flu? Doctors disagree. But the sensible solution is to take aspirin for illness which causes a rise in temperature, but not for minor colds and headaches.

Other virus infections such as **mumps** and **chickenpox** are also suspected of causing occasional birth defects, and **syphilis** remains an important cause of malformations, responsible in Britain for some fifty cases a year.

Toxoplasma, a parasite found in raw meat and animal droppings, is also responsible for some fifty malformations a year. These include eye defects, brain damage and mental retardation. Women may avoid the disease by not eating raw or rare meat and avoiding contact with animal droppings, particularly cat litter, during pregnancy. A woman who has always kept animals is likely to have been exposed to the disease and be resistant. The main point to watch is that this is not the moment to start keeping a cat for the first time. There is no vaccine against toxoplasma, and it is therefore a good idea to encourage young girls to play with cats so that they can develop immunity to the parasite before there is any chance of pregnancy.

Pregnant women should take care to wash fastidiously after gardening or use gloves, because animal droppings are so common in soil. As with other attacks on the foetus, damage is most likely to be sustained within the first three months of pregnancy and so some people think it best to farm out cats with friends during that period.

PRESCRIPTION DRUGS

Eight out of ten women in the UK take at least one prescribed drug other than iron when they are pregnant, and six out of ten take non-prescribed drugs, according to an estimate made by Professor John Forfar of Edinburgh University. The widely accepted advice that women should not take drugs in pregnancy is not, apparently, widely followed. Professor R. S. Illingworth, Professor of Child Health at Sheffield University, says, 'The best advice that one can offer to any pregnant woman is that she should take a medicine only when absolutely necessary – and that is rare.'

Although all new drugs must be tested on pregnant animals before they are passed by the Committee on Safety of Medicines, this can never guarantee that they are completely safe in human pregnancy. It is well established that a drug which does not cause malformations in animals can still cause human malformations. In any case, there are thousands of drugs on the market which are just beginning to be reviewed by the UK Committee on Safety of Medicines. They were given licences as of right when new legislation was passed after the thalidomide tragedy and have not been subjected to the rigorous tests demanded

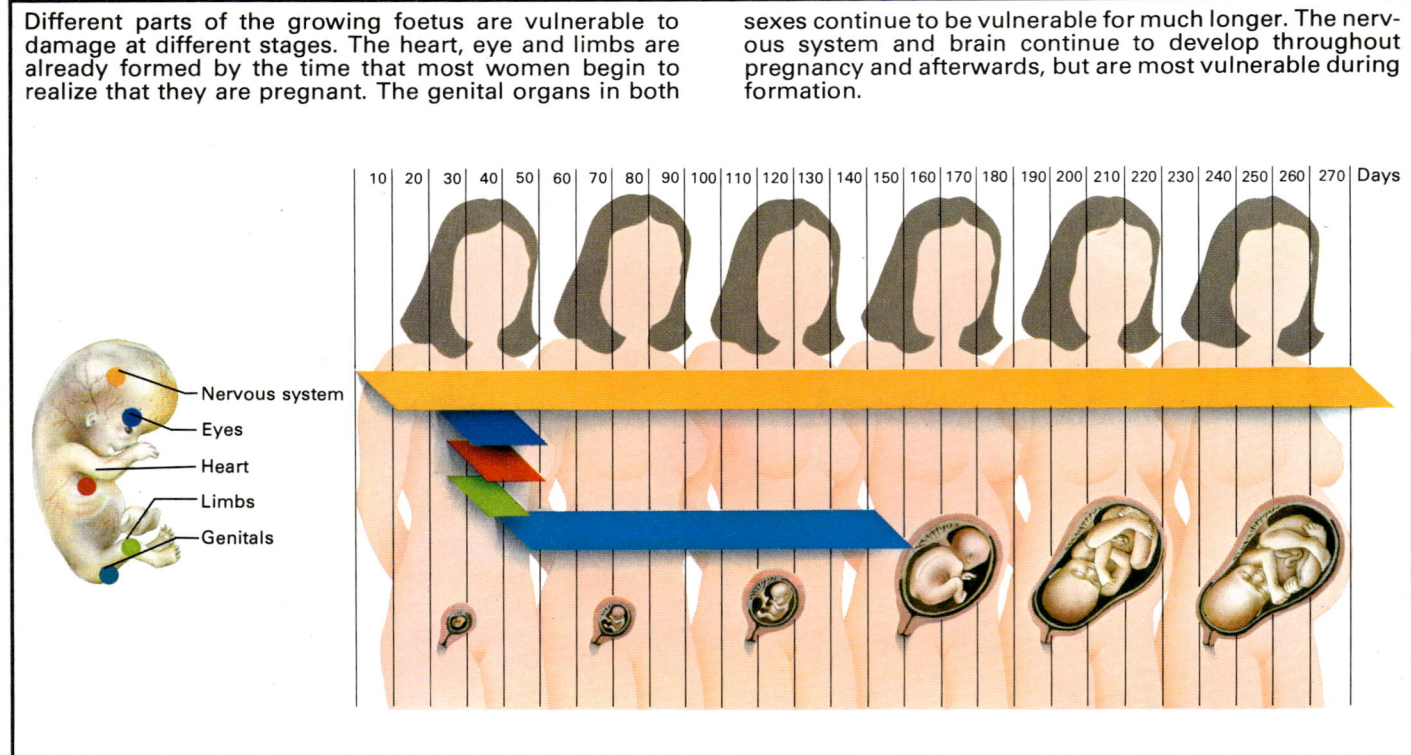

Different parts of the growing foetus are vulnerable to damage at different stages. The heart, eye and limbs are already formed by the time that most women begin to realize that they are pregnant. The genital organs in both sexes continue to be vulnerable for much longer. The nervous system and brain continue to develop throughout pregnancy and afterwards, but are most vulnerable during formation.

now of new drugs. The committee is now beginning to investigate these drugs but its work will take years to complete. In other countries the position is similar.

There is a long list of drugs known to be associated with abnormalities, although it is often unclear whether the drugs actually cause the abnormality or are just indirectly involved. Tetracycline, for instance, is an antibiotic drug widely used to treat infections ranging from pneumonia to cystitis. It is sold under at least a dozen different tradenames and is best avoided during pregnancy because it may interfere with the growth of the baby's bones and discolour the baby's primary teeth.

Barbiturate drugs and phenytoin – a drug given to epileptic women to prevent convulsions – have also been suspected of causing birth defects such as cleft lip or palate or mental retardation. However, following two studies, one in the USA and one in Finland, it was discovered that the birth of abnormal babies to epileptic mothers was unrelated to drugs. It seems that a mother who suffers from epilepsy is twice as likely to have an abnormal baby whether or not she takes drugs. It would therefore be quite wrong for epileptic women not to take the drugs which help to control their illness. In any case, epileptic mothers still have excellent prospects of having a normal baby.

Illegal drugs such as LSD, cannabis and heroin should all be avoided in pregnancy if for no other reason than that they may have harmful effects on the baby.

The following additional effects of drugs in pregnancy are known or suspected: certain sex hormones may cause masculinization of the foetus and an increase in bone-age. Certain anti-thyroid drugs may cause the infant to develop goitre – a swelling of the thyroid gland in the neck. Certain drugs given against cancer, leukaemia and severe psoriasis may cause abnormal development of the skull and abortion. Blood anti-coagulants may cause bleeding of the baby in the womb with subsequent abnormalities or death.

Sulfonamide antibiotics, used to treat many common infections, may cause pigment to be deposited in the nervous system which may possibly cause mental retardation. Some drugs used to treat blood pressure are believed to cause bowel spasm or pneumonia in babies after birth. Even anti-histamine, used to treat motion sickness and allergies, has been implicated as a cause of malformations; but there is no proof. Tranquillizers such as Librium and Valium have been suspected of causing birth defects but there is no hard evidence against them.

If you want to start a family and are on regular drug treatment, check with your doctor whether it might be better to wait; if you become unexpectedly pregnant while undergoing drug treatment, also consult your doctor.

NON-PRESCRIPTION DRUGS

Aspirin in large doses may cause a baby to bleed in the womb, which may in turn cause local abnormalities such as irregular development of limbs or fingers. Regular consumption of large quantities of aspirin during pregnancy has been found in Australia to be associated with stillbirths, low birth-weight and bleeding after birth, but not with abnormalities. The tendency to bleed of babies whose mothers take a lot of aspirin is a direct result of aspirin interfering with the normal clotting process. Many patent headache-tablets contain aspirin, which is usually listed in the contents under the scientific name acetylsalicylic acid. An occasional aspirin need be no cause for worry, but do not dose yourself with them regularly: see your doctor.

Some dentists recommend that pregnant women take fluoride tablets to give a baby good teeth. However, later research suggests that fluoride does not cross the placenta and get into the baby – so the exercise is pointless.

Well-tried, mild herbal teas such as mint are probably quite harmless in pregnancy. And raspberry leaf tea is traditionally recommended as bringing about an easy labour. However, scientific knowledge of herbs is very patchy and side-effects are not well documented. So, like drugs, most medicinal herbs and herbal preparations are best avoided in pregnancy.

Vitamin tablets should not be taken unless specifically suggested by a doctor or nutritionist. Vitamin A, for example, is known to cause malformations when given in excessive amounts to pregnant animals.

OPERATIONS AND X-RAYS

Non-urgent medical operations and X-ray examinations of the abdomen should be avoided if there is a possibility of pregnancy. Dentistry involving general anaesthetics should also be avoided if at all possible. If dental treatment with anaesthetic is absolutely necessary, for example for an extraction, then it is best done in a hospital.

All the commonly used anaesthetics can cause spontaneous abortion or abnormal development in animals, and are a recognized hazard early in pregnancy for women who work in operating rooms, where they may be exposed to small doses of escaped gases. X-rays of pregnant women may increase the risk of the baby getting leukaemia in later life and can also induce mutations in the sex cells (ovary or testis) of both mother and baby. However, the risks are very small.

Routine pregnancy tests are not possible until eight days after the last menstrual period is due to have ended. So it can be difficult for the doctor definitely to exclude pregnancy before a decision is taken to operate, and in any case a woman may easily become pregnant while waiting for an operation. It makes sense to take stringent precautions against pregnancy at such a time.

Pregnant women and new-born babies are often X-rayed unnecessarily. According to a survey by the radiation protection committee of the British Institute of Radiology, in some hospitals, up to one-third of pregnancies are X-rayed. The survey, published in the *Lancet* in February 1976, shows that two unidentified but major British hospitals X-ray 34 per cent of pregnant women; whereas another major UK hospital X-rays only 9 per cent of women. Dr J. H. E. Carmichael and Dr R. J. Berry, who published the survey, say these high figures 'show a disturbing situation', and that current practice is 'not acceptable'.

CHEMICALS

Some hair dyes are now suspected of being a possible cause of cancer. Hair dyes are absorbed through the scalp into the blood and may reach the growing baby, which is probably more sensitive to cancer-causing chemicals than the adult. So it is advisable not to dye the hair during pregnancy. However, it is probably quite safe to bleach the hair, which is a quite different process.

Women in certain jobs are exposed to chemicals which may cause birth abnormalities, when exposure occurs in the first three months. For example, ethylene thiourea, used until recently in the rubber industry, has been found to cause birth abnormalities as well as cancer in rats. In many industries, women may be unknowingly at risk from chemicals which they breathe in or absorb through their skin or from chemicals on food eaten on the factory floor. A pregnant woman who has a job which exposes her to chemicals in a laboratory or in industry and who has had a miscarriage might consider changing her work.

EXERCISE IN PREGNANCY

It is important to continue with normal exercise in pregnancy provided you feel well and comfortable. Pregnancy is a natural state, not an illness, so you should not treat yourself like an invalid. It is a good idea to keep going with a sport if you have one. However, you have to make allowances for a change in the balance of your body, for feeling less competitive and for being less able to make quick bursts of energy.

This means that you may prefer long walks which require a steady energy output rather than tennis or jogging. Certain types of exercise such as horse riding are sometimes advised against in pregnancy because of the danger of falls. However, there is no reason why an experienced horsewoman should not continue to ride so long as she chooses a quiet horse and does not take risks. But remember that later in pregnancy the weight of the womb alters the balance of the body – so be cautious.

Swimming is a particularly good form of exercise in pregnancy because the water supports the weight of the womb, providing relief, while the limbs move freely. Cycling is also good exercise for a similar reason. The abdomen is held rigid while only the legs move. For extra comfort it is possible to obtain a gynaecological saddle which is specially designed for comfort in pregnancy. Dance is another type of exercise which may also specially appeal in pregnancy because it can be either soothing or stimulating, according to type.

Whatever exercise you choose to do, learn to move your body so that you make room for the baby. When the abdomen begins to grow large avoid bending too much at the waist. And avoid exercises that put a sudden strain on the abdominal muscles, which are already stretched by pregnancy.

EXERCISE FOR BIRTH

Special exercises during pregnancy can help to develop habits of good posture which will ease the last months of pregnancy, when the baby becomes heavier. These exercises also help prepare for the birth. Various different types are available (see Appendix Three) and it is a good idea to join a local class such as those run by the National Childbirth Trust.

Particularly interesting is a new set of yoga exercises specially designed for pregnant women by Meloma Huxley, and Janet and Arthur Balaskas. If you have done yoga already then this is obviously the right thing for you, but it is not necessary to have done any yoga before to enjoy these exercises and benefit from them. They are designed to stretch the muscles and tissues of the pelvic area and so to ease the passage of the baby. They are also designed to strengthen the muscles involved in kneeling and squatting so that these positions, which are often more comfortable, can be adopted by women in childbirth. Because we sit in chairs instead of squatting, the muscles of the pelvis, so important in childbirth, are stiff, as are ankles, knees and hip joints. The exercises given below are taken from a book by Janet and Arthur Balaskas called *New Life* (see Appendix Three), which should be referred to by those who want to go beyond the most basic stage.

PREGNANCY AND CHILDHOOD/PREGNANCY

EXERCISE IN PREGNANCY

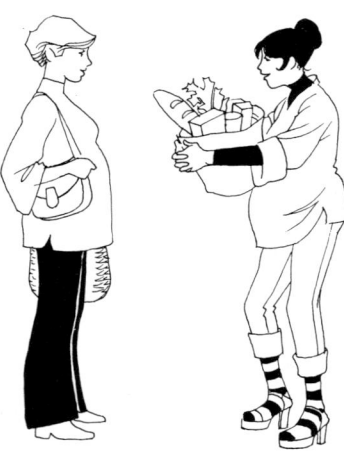

Good posture (*left*) is very important. Don't sag (*right*). Keep weight evenly between the heels and the balls of the feet, use abdomen and buttock muscles, and walk tall.

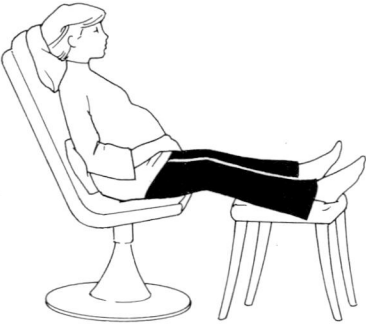

Sitting: support the back and head to avoid strain. Use little cushions at small of back and neck. Whenever possible, rest with legs raised and fully supported. A bean-bag cushion provides excellent support, but be sure to get on and off it on hands and knees.

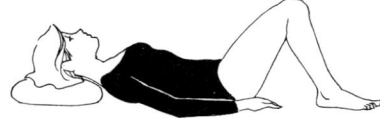

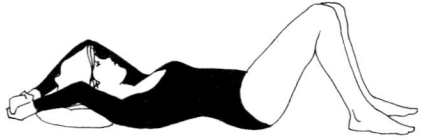 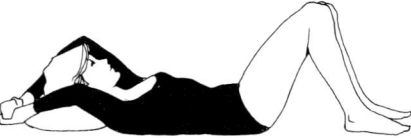

Lie on back as above. Press back against floor and pull knees up with hands. Tighten buttock muscles, then relax. Repeat five times.

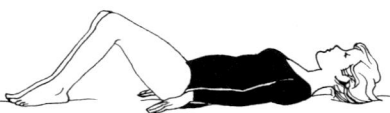 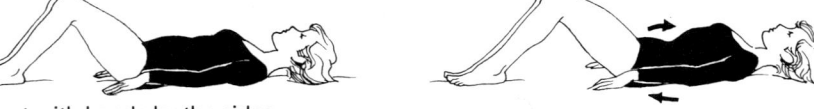

With hands above head (*left*) arch the back, then press back against floor and pull up on pelvis at the same time. Feel rotation of the pelvis. Relax. Repeat five times.

Repeat with hands by the sides.

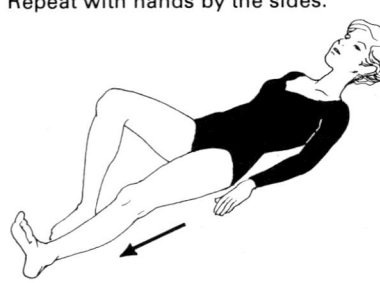 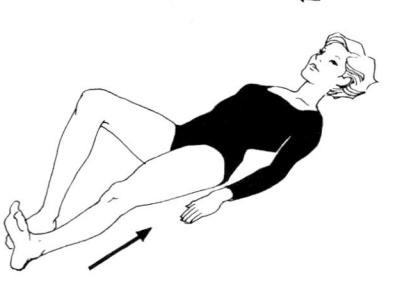

Lie on back with left leg straight and right bent. Keeping left leg straight, use your hips to slide the leg up and down, using waist muscles. Repeat five times with each leg.

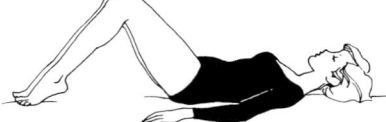 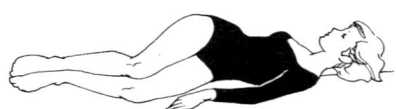

Lie on your back with knees bent and heels raised. Keeping shoulders flat and knees together, gently roll knees to the left as far as is comfortably possible. This will raise your right hip, and you will feel a turning movement at your waist. Return to original position and repeat five times for each side.

The tailor pose

Sit on the floor against a wall with the soles of your feet touching each other and close to the body, and knees apart. Now, using your hands, gently put pressure on your knees and move them towards the floor. It doesn't matter if they are nowhere near the floor at first; gradually you will develop more flexibility.

At first you will probably feel some pain on the inside of the thighs. Massage this tight painful place with your fingers. Do the exercise for one minute at first and build up to five minutes. Practise the position when reading, watching TV or spending time with friends. This exercise stretches the inner thigh muscles and opens the pelvis.

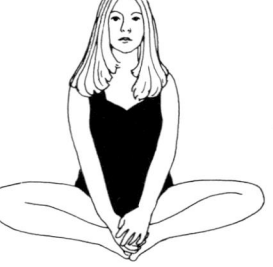

Squatting

Stand with feet about 18 inches apart and toes turned outward. Bend your knees keeping them apart, until you can put your hands on the ground in front of you. Let your heels come off the ground, if this is easier, then rock back and forth from toes to heels. Hold on to a door handle or table to support yourself. Make sure you do not let your ankles collapse inwards and that your knees turn outwards. If you find this very difficult, use a low stool or a pile of books to sit on at first until you can manage it unaided. Try to do this for five minutes a day.

The squatting position has long been recommended by doctors as a more natural position to use when emptying the bowels during pregnancy. Put a small box or stool in front of the lavatory to stand on so that you can squat. This position is said to reduce the chances of piles developing – piles are a frequent accompaniment to pregnancy.

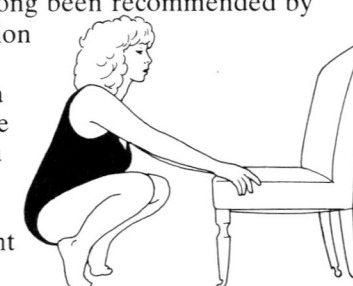

*Diagram based on the illustrations in *Your Body and your Figure*, published by Churchill Livingstone, Edinburgh.

The frog pose
With your knees on the floor, comfortably apart, sit down between your heels. Use a cushion between your feet for extra comfort, if you wish. After a minute, lean forward and rest on your elbows, or, if you wish, lean onto a bed or chair. Hold the position for a minute, building up to five or ten minutes with practice. This position opens the pelvis and flexes muscles in legs and ankles. It is also a very comfortable position in pregnancy and labour because it relieves backache.

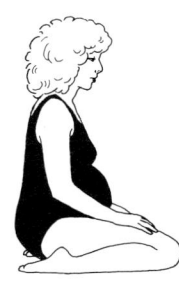

All-fours position
Another way to relieve backache is to go on all-fours with knees apart, legs and arms at right angles to the body. As a variation of this, arch your back a little and tuck your tail in. Practise rotating your hips in a circle and enjoy the relaxing feeling.

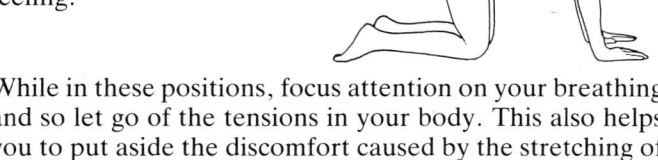

While in these positions, focus attention on your breathing and so let go of the tensions in your body. This also helps you to put aside the discomfort caused by the stretching of muscles and sinews. This practice in concentrating on breathing will help when you have labour contractions.

DOWN'S SYNDROME AND SPINA BIFIDA

DOWN'S SYNDROME (MONGOLISM)
Down's syndrome is the commonest cause of severe mental retardation in the UK. About one in five hundred babies is born with Down's syndrome, but a mother aged forty-five is about a hundred times more likely to have a Down's baby than a mother aged sixteen. In women under thirty the incidence of Down's births is less than one in a thousand, but in women over forty-five it is one in sixty. Most obstetricians recommend that all women over forty, or sometimes over thirty-five, who are pregnant should have a test so that a Down's baby may be aborted if the parents wish.

In this test, called amniocentesis, a needle is inserted into the womb to withdraw a sample of fluid which contains cells from the baby. These cells can be grown in the laboratory and used to identify a baby with Down's syndrome. Down's syndrome is caused by the chance inheritance of an extra small chromosome – the tiny strand of DNA which carries the genes determining heredity. This extra small chromosome can be seen in dividing cells under a microscope. Amniocentesis is usually done at sixteen to eighteen weeks from the start of pregnancy.

As a result of some mistake, the extra small chromosome is not eliminated from the egg when it divides before fertilization and the presence of the chromosome in every cell of the body interferes with normal development. It is not known why the extra chromosome is not eliminated from the egg, and at present there are no special measures a woman can take – other than amniocentesis – to avoid a Down's baby. Down's syndrome is not usually inherited, but occasionally it can be. Special tests can identify parents who carry the factor for the rare hereditary form when this is suspected.

Rarely, amniocentesis itself may cause a baby to miscarry, and may even cause damage to the baby if the needle is not correctly placed, so it is not a procedure to be undertaken lightly. Cells obtained by amniocentesis can be used to tell the sex of the baby, which may sometimes be important, for example, to avoid inherited defects which are sex-linked – that is, show up only in boys. But it would involve an unjustified risk to use amniocentesis simply in order to have advanced knowledge of a baby's sex. More than twenty-five different rare inherited conditions can be identified by amniocentesis.

SPINA BIFIDA
Two other common birth malformations are spina bifida and anencephaly. They are both defects of the formation of the nervous system, and affect between one and two babies per thousand births in England and Wales. The incidence is higher in the north of England, Scotland and Northern Ireland. The spinal cord and brain are formed in the growing embryo by folding of a sheet of tissue to form a tube – the neural tube – which closes up at the top end to form the brain and closes at the bottom to form the end of the spinal cord. When the bottom end fails to close properly, the baby may develop with an open spine – spina bifida – which interferes with nervous control of the lower limbs and the nervous reflexes controlling the bladder. When the top end of the neural tube fails to form a complete brain – anencephaly – the baby usually dies shortly after birth.

Babies with spina bifida vary greatly in the degree of their affliction. Some develop hydrocephalus – swelling of the head as a result of accumulation of fluid – but this can often be controlled by inserting a plastic tube (shunt) which allows the excess fluid to drain back into the body. Others are born with a deformed spine which together with partial paralysis of the legs makes walking difficult, or sometimes impossible.

Although a small proportion of spina bifida babies – perhaps one or two in ten – may have a normal life, the majority are confined to wheel-chairs and spend most of their lives in institutions. As a result, some paediatricians do not think that it is right to take extraordinary surgical measures to keep them alive, and only operate on those spina bifida babies who are mildly affected.

A women who has had one spina bifida or anencephalic baby has a one in twenty chance of having another; a woman who has had two spina bifida or anencephalic babies has a one in ten chance of having another. However, the condition is not inherited in any simple way. A susceptibility to having babies with defects of the spinal cord or brain may be inherited but it is only a susceptibility, and doctors are searching for a factor in the environment which may cause the condition. Suspicion focused a few years ago on the eating of green potatoes or potatoes affected by blight fungus. However, women who avoid potatoes scrupulously throughout pregnancy can still have spina bifida babies, and most experts now think that the potato theory is totally mistaken.

PREGNANCY AND CHILDHOOD/PREGNANCY

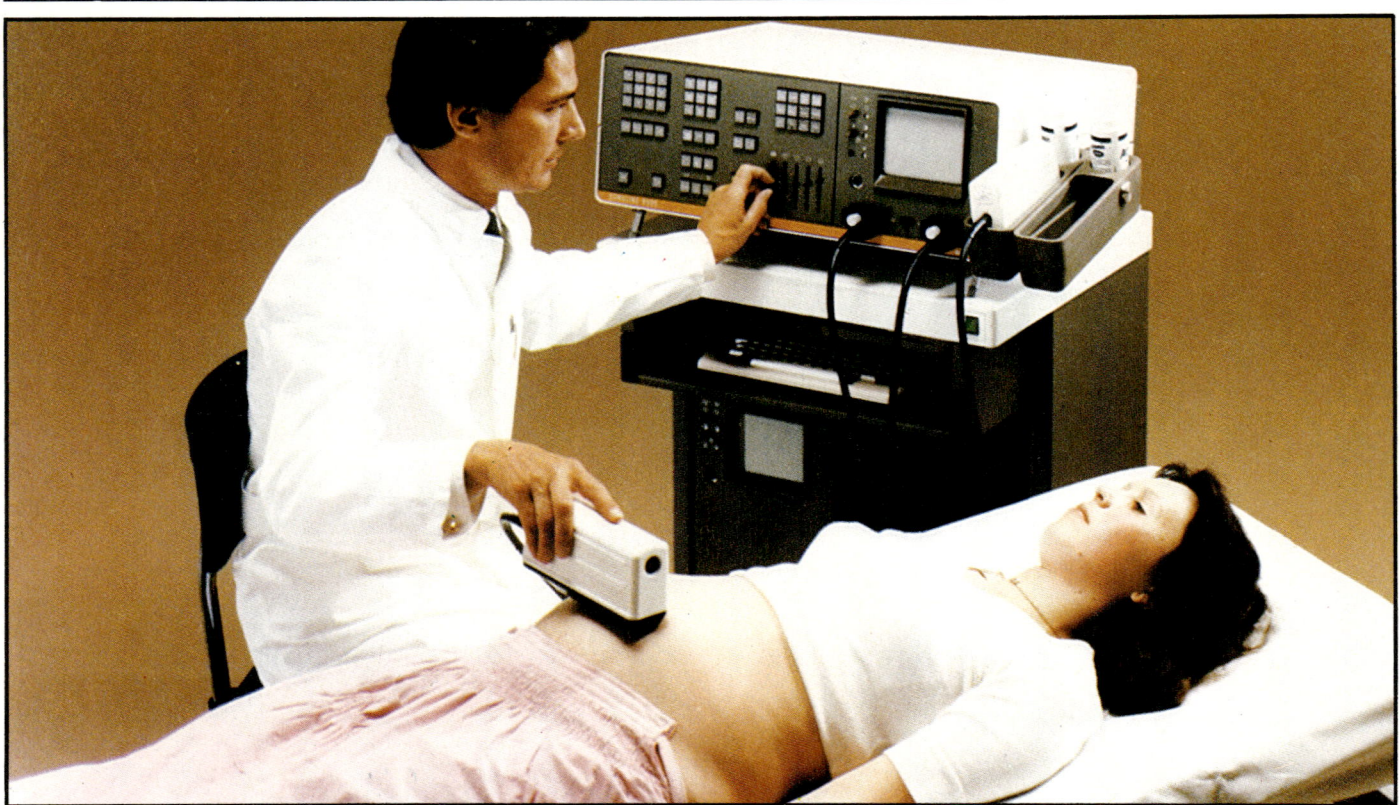

Distance between the two 'x's = 30 mm (crown, left; rump, right) – foetus is approximately nine weeks old.

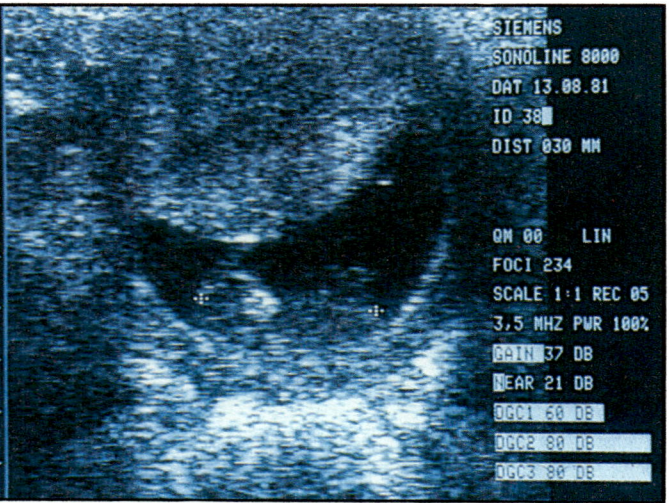

An ultra-sound test (top) enables doctors to monitor a pregnancy and establish what stage it has reached – even, on occasions, to tell whether a birth will be twins. The 'picture' shows the location of the foetus and placenta while alerting doctors to any problems

Mothers who have had a spina bifida baby have been found to have lower than normal amounts of certain vitamins in their blood. It has recently been concluded from several studies that giving women who have had a spina bifida baby supplements of vitamins for some weeks *before conception* dramatically reduces the chances of the next baby suffering from the defect. The most important of these vitamins is probably folic acid, which is obtained from liver, dark green vegetables such as spinach, broccoli, spring greens, and whole cereals, wheatgerm, eggs, tomatoes, lettuce and oranges.

A high risk of spina bifida can be determined by a blood test on the mother at sixteen to eighteen weeks of pregnancy. This detects α-fetoprotein – a substance which leaks out of the baby's nervous system if it is damaged and enters the mother's blood-stream. If this test is positive, an amniocentesis test (see Down's syndrome) must be done to confirm the diagnosis.

ANTENATAL CARE

Antenatal care is important because doctors can detect a number of problems at an early stage when it is still possible to correct them. In Britain, a woman may choose whether to go to hospital for antenatal care or to get it from a GP obstetrician who may or may not be her usual GP. If she chooses a new GP obstetrician, she can return to her own

GP afterwards if she wishes. If you want to have your baby at home (see below) you should preferably choose a GP who is prepared to supervise a home delivery.

Under a recent UK law, you are entitled to time off work to attend a doctor or clinic for antenatal care. So do not worry about any loss of pay. You have this right regardless of how long you have worked for your present employer. Just let them know when you are going and get your appointment card stamped in case your employer wishes to see it.

One of the most important advances in medical care has been the use of ultrasound to measure the growth of the baby. If the baby is not growing properly it may be because it is not getting sufficient nutrition from the mother's body. In that case it may be advisable to induce the baby prematurely. Doctors also check the mother's blood for anaemia which may be corrected by iron tablets, and watch her blood pressure and weight. These and other tests may give warning of problems to come.

However, the mother herself is probably the best monitor of the baby's condition. She can feel the baby moving inside – vigorous movement is a good sign. After twenty-eight weeks of pregnancy the baby should be making a minimum of ten noticeable movements a day. If the baby is not moving as much as this, or if the mother notices a marked decrease in the frequency of the baby's movements, then she should consult her doctor. On the right we give a checklist of warning signals you should look out for; consult your doctor if you notice any of them.

WARNING SIGNALS IN PREGNANCY

If you have any of the following symptoms consult your doctor as soon as possible:

Bleeding from the vagina.

Severe or continuous nausea and vomiting.

Continuing or severe headache.

Swelling or puffiness of the face or hands, or marked swelling of the feet or ankles.

Blurring of vision or spots before the eyes.

Pain or burning on passing urine.

Chills and fever.

Sharp or continuous abdominal pain.

Sudden gush of water from the vagina before the baby is due.

Marked reduction in baby's movements.

Childbirth

A mother usually knows instinctively the importance (and difficulty) of the birth she is expecting. But for the world around her it is commonplace – just another baby. Parents often have to argue to have their special needs and interests understood. Expert though doctors and maternity services are in saving life, their understanding of emotional needs has too often been dismal. So what can a prospective mother and father do for themselves?

HOME OR HOSPITAL?

There is pressure on women to have their babies in hospital. Hospital is the safest place if there are complications, but not necessarily safer for an ordinary delivery. Home has advantages which can never be provided by a hospital. The atmosphere is more informal, a mother can eat the food she likes, be surrounded by her friends and children and listen to her favourite music. However, to have your baby at home you will probably have to be extremely determined.

If there is any suggestion that the birth may be complicated, then the baby *should* be born in hospital. If you score two or less on the risk chart, you might reasonably plan to have your baby at home, although other special circumstances may make a hospital birth advisable in individual cases. Any change in your health later in pregnancy may also make it necessary to revise plans and have the baby in hospital.

Risk chart
Score for each category which includes you. If the total is two or less, you are among the 70 per cent of women who have a low risk of complications.

Unmarried (single, divorced or stable union)	1
More than 30 years old	1
Under 20 years old	1
Previous baby died before or after birth	2
Three or more miscarriages	2
Previous Caesarean delivery	1
Previous malformed child	1
First baby	1
Kidney or heart disease	4
High blood pressure in repeated tests	2
Diabetes	4
Anaemia	1
Rhesus blood complication possible	3
Height less than 62 inches	1

CHILDBIRTH CLASSES

Some classes in hospitals simply provide information while others involve active preparation for the birth. Active preparation has been found to help women use fewer drugs during delivery and give a better chance of a spontaneous birth without the use of forceps. Although it is difficult to prove, this probably benefits the baby; certainly many women find it more satisfying. (See Appendix Three for details about classes.)

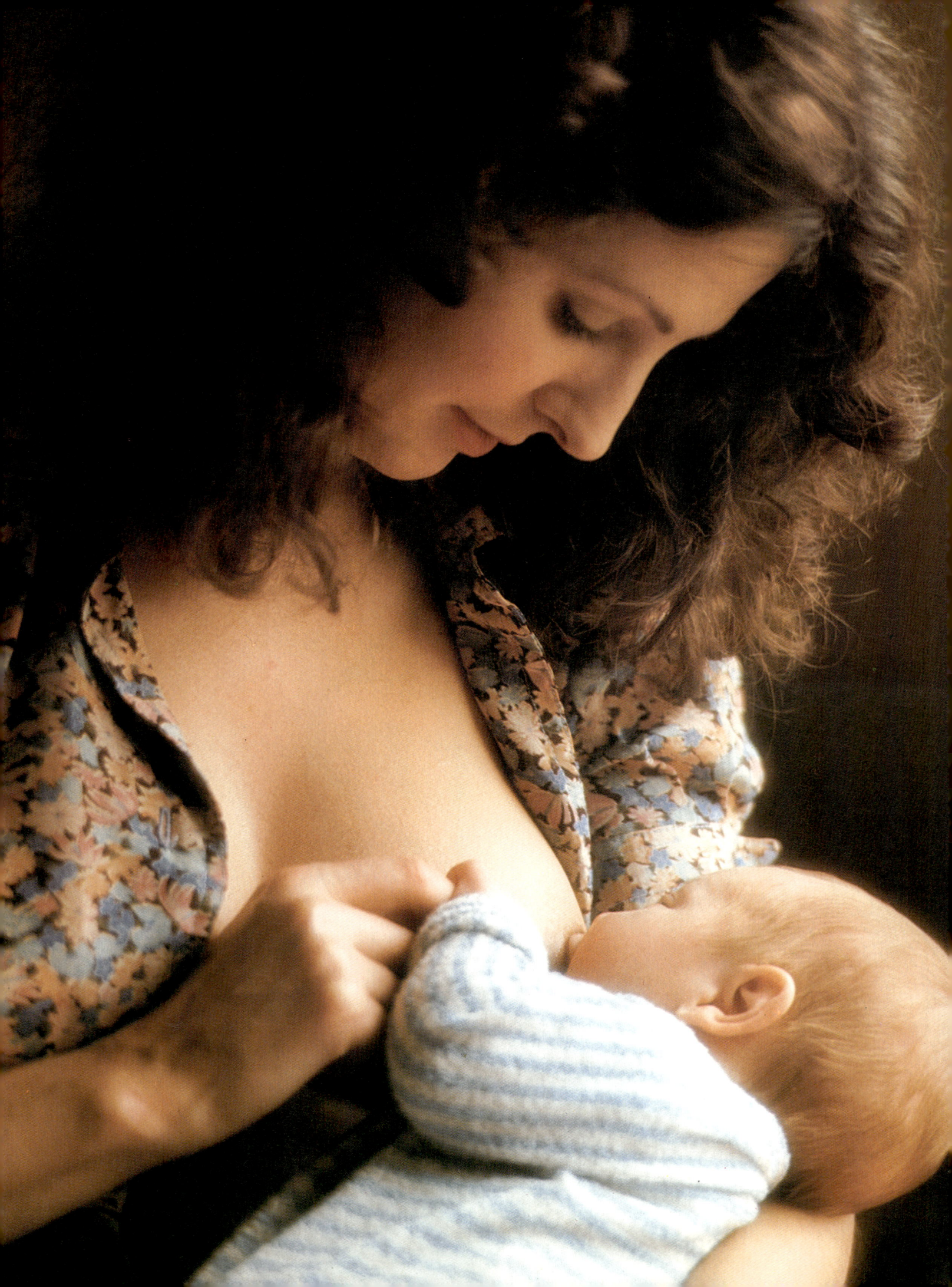

THE FATHER'S PRESENCE

If you want your husband or a friend to be with you during the birth, arrange this with your doctor and the hospital authorities well in advance. In the UK it is official Department of Health policy to allow fathers to be present where possible, but the ultimate decision rests with hospital staff on duty at the time. Fathers are often asked to leave while examinations are made and decisions taken about what will happen next. If a wife does not mind, there is no reason why the father should not be there during examinations. He may be able to calm his wife if the doctor has to report poor progress, or be able to arbitrate if a decision has to be made about induction. Sometimes fathers are soothed into believing that nothing much is happening and find that the baby is born while they are sent home for a nap or out for a meal. It is best to wait around and take quick snacks in the hospital. Sharing in the birth not only helps the mother at the time but can be a bonding memory for ever.

INDUCTION

There has been a major debate within the medical profession on the ethics and safety of induced childbirth. Induction is not necessary simply because a woman has reached the date at which the baby is expected or gone a week or two beyond it. It is difficult for a doctor to know precisely when a baby is due and a mother's dates are often not reliable, especially if she has been on the pill. If a baby is induced there is a risk that it may be premature. If the baby has to be induced – and sometimes it is necessary – then it is reasonable to expect the doctor to discuss the reasons with the mother and to consider waiting to see if circumstances change.

ANAESTHETICS

Some hospitals make epidurals – local anaesthetics applied in the space next to the spinal cord – available to any woman who wants one. But some hospitals do not have an obstetric anaesthetist, or the anaesthetist is only available in office hours, which means that if you want an epidural the baby will be induced. An epidural is more likely to prevent a woman from fully participating, because full sensation is lost from the waist down. It can also, rarely, cause side-effects such as severe headache or constipation for some days afterwards; but it does provide complete relief of pain in the majority of cases. Many women complain that they are given unwanted anaesthetics – injections or gas – which make them dopey. It is often difficult to refuse an injection, but the staff have no right to give them against your will. If they do, then technically they are assaulting you and could be liable to the complaint procedures outlined in Appendix Two.

POSITION

Women in labour usually find it uncomfortable to lie on their back for any length of time, and it can be bad for the baby because it may interfere with the supply of blood to the womb. However, women in some hospitals are still told to lie on their backs because this is most convenient for medical staff. You should not normally be asked to lie on your back for more than five to ten minutes. Many women lie on their sides but there is no reason why a woman should not sit up supported by pillows with her legs bent – or squat on the floor, stand, kneel, be on all fours, or walk about so long as it is comfortable.

CUTTING THE VAGINA

It has become common to make a cut at the entrance to the vagina – episiotomy – to get the baby out quickly. Sometimes this is necessary when the baby is in distress, or to prevent an awkward tear. Sometimes it is done simply out of routine. Episiotomy cuts must be sewn up and the repair is not always satisfactory. It is worth telling your consultant and midwife that you would prefer not to have an episiotomy if it can be avoided.

LEBOYER DELIVERY

The French doctor Frederick Leboyer (see Appendix Three) suggests that the emotional well-being of the baby is overlooked in the modern atmosphere of the delivery room with its bright lights and noise. He says lights should be low, the baby should be put on the mother's stomach after it is born and the cord cut only after it has stopped pulsating. Some obstetricians are prepared to use some of Leboyer's methods on request.

FEEDING THE BABY

If delivery is normal, there is no reason why the baby should not be put immediately to the breast – before it is cleaned and wrapped – if the mother wishes. The sooner the baby is put to the breast the better, because this stimulates the flow of milk and assists the delivery of the afterbirth. Many midwives appreciate this now and are willing to do so if the mother asks. The baby should not get cold – the mother's skin is hot after the exertions of the delivery – and this is the natural place for the baby. If necessary a blanket can be thrown over mother and baby. Research shows that the vital bond between mother and child is formed most easily in the first few hours after birth, and that delay in giving a mother her baby can affect their relationship for years.

The Early Years

Few activities are as natural as bringing up children, yet few responsibilities can sometimes appear so daunting. Newborn infants have always been frail and vulnerable. A century ago parents had many children but did not expect them all to live to adulthood; parents today, in the Western world especially, have fewer children but greater expectations. And their optimism is largely justified. Childbirth is safer, while improvements in housing, sanitary standards and immunization have virtually eradicated diseases which once claimed tens of thousands of young lives.

The advance of medical knowledge has thus saved countless lives and eased the pain of countless more. But it has also produced a welter of research and conflicting theories about child-care which can bemuse as much as enlighten. The trend towards smaller families has intensified parental unease. Today's new parents are likely to have been children in small families with little experience of babies or children. Unfamiliarity breeds uncertainty, so no wonder

PREGNANCY AND CHILDHOOD/THE EARLY YEARS

they join the millions of readers of Dr Spock and other child-care specialists.

Nor are books the only source of expertise available to parents today. Special child-care clinics help to monitor children's health and development on an almost weekly basis through the early years. Health visitors operating through these clinics, or even visiting the home, not only help to ensure that health problems are identified and tackled at an early stage but also act as a general source of information to worried parents. The best and most experienced of parents will need such medical advice from time to time, advice based on knowledge about hundreds of babies. However, parents should not be overawed by their new responsibilities. People have been bringing up children for thousands of years in far less propitious circumstances than today. And it is significant that the experts themselves urge parents to trust more to their instincts. Dr Spock regarded his advice as 'common sense' while Britain's Health Education Council has published a pamphlet for parents entitled *You know more than you think you do*.

For instance, your instinct will tell you to cuddle your child and your instinct will be right. The sensation of touch is the only message from the outside world which is comprehensible to a baby: he* understands being held close and the touch of another skin. He needs human contact as spontaneously and freely and nakedly as the temperature permits. Physically and emotionally, baby needs cuddling and crooning and cooing and talking. It gives him a feeling of love and security that will be etched into his personality. And a secure child has an increased chance of becoming a healthy adult.

This book's concern for child development is restricted to matters of physical health, with the emphasis, as throughout the book, on what can be done to prevent illness and promote good health. More general guides to child development are listed in Appendix Three. We have divided this section into three age groups – the first six months; from six months to five years; and the early school years – but in many cases the detailed advice on topics such as diet and teeth overlap from one section to another. One piece of common sense that all parents surely know is that children cannot be divided into neat little categories. Children are individuals and they develop differently.

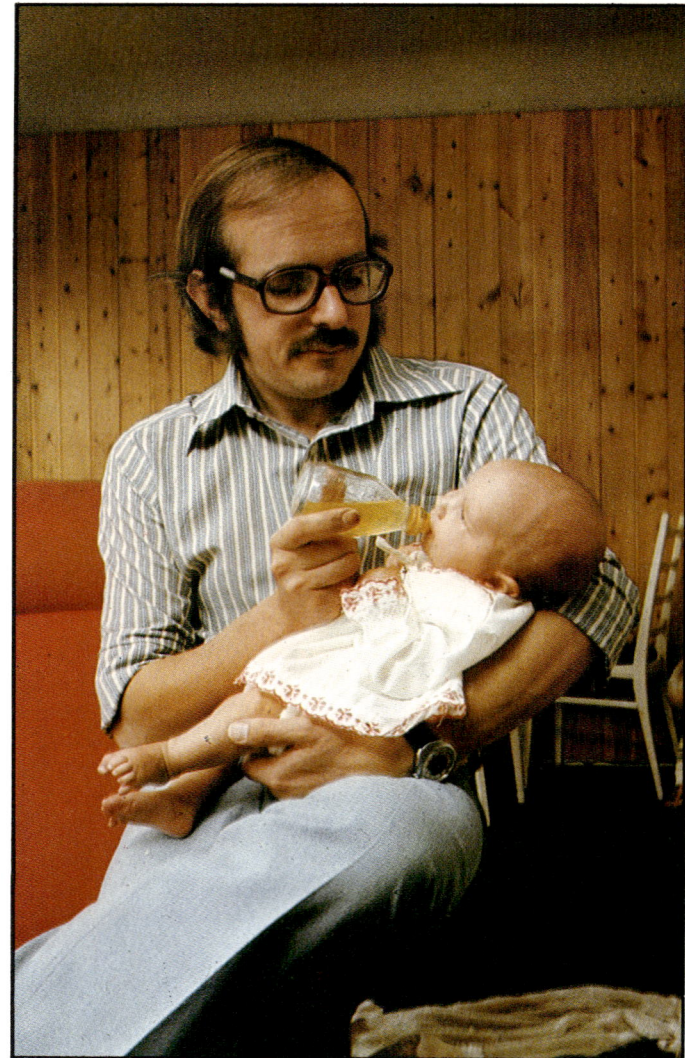

Increasingly, baby care is a shared family role, which is good for both parents as well as the child

BUT WHAT ABOUT THE MOTHER?

Baby may come first but, before we discuss the care of the child, let's spare a few thoughts about the mother. Parenthood changes lives more than marriage nowadays. While elation, fulfilment and a sense of achievement are feelings frequently associated with motherhood so, too, are exhaustion, depression and a feeling of being trapped. The early months of disturbed nights impose a great strain on parents – however marvellous the baby.

Mothers should find time to look after themselves as well as the baby. Exercises help restore the figure (as well as morale), while short trips out of the house diminish the feeling of being a slave to the family. Forget about keeping the house spotlessly clean. It is more important to rest and relax when you can. It is also more important to find time to spend with your partner. Try to understand each other's feelings. Fathers can help mothers by sharing some of the burdens of parenthood which means coping with nappies as well as walking the pram; mothers can help their partners by making it clear that they don't always take second place to the new arrival.

Parenthood is a time of changed relationships with everyone – your partner, your own parents and with your own image of yourself. It would therefore be surprising if at times tensions did not arise. Try to be patient and understanding; don't forget the good things about parenthood and don't forget sex. Gentle lovemaking can be resumed when it feels comfortable, although if in doubt wait until the post-natal check at about six weeks.

If depression is severe or persistent, you should seek medical help. Post-natal depression is not inevitable but it is a recognized state and doctors are experienced in helping a woman through it. But talk also to other mothers. The National Childbirth Trust runs a network of post-natal support groups which can put you in touch with other mothers who have often experienced – and overcome – problems that may seem overwhelming to you. Many localities also have mother-and-toddler groups which again offer companionship, a chance to get out of the house and also an opportunity for your child to make friends. It could be easier than you think to start one up yourself – try advertising in your doctor's surgery, library or church hall.

---

*No male chauvinism is intended: 'he' the baby helps us to differentiate the baby from 'she' the mother.

THE FIRST SIX MONTHS

FEEDING

Babies have been 'designed' to live on human milk. Cows' milk was likewise intended for calves, not young humans. Breast-feeding is therefore the ideal way to feed young babies. The mixture is right, which is not guaranteed when a harassed mother makes up a bottle; the quantity is usually right, since milk is normally produced on a demand-and-supply basis which only a few women fail to achieve if they wish to breast-feed; and by every test, breast-feeding protects a child from disease, since the human milk carries antibodies against infection at a time when the child has not yet developed his own. Breast-feeding is particularly advisable for mothers travelling to, or living in, warm countries because it gives positive protection against gastro-enteritis, which can be extremely serious in young infants.

Breast-feeding has other advantages, too. These range from a lower incidence of nappy rash to fewer cot deaths (where children are found inexplicably and suddenly dead), although nobody really knows why this should be so. Even when children cease to be children it has been suggested that some illnesses are less common among those who were breast-fed than those who were bottle-fed. Such future protection could also stem from the fact that breast-fed babies are much less likely to be overfed and overweight. Mother's milk is thus the best by far, and the longer you can continue breast-feeding the better. Even a short period – the first two weeks or a month – is invaluable.

Although breast-feeding is the ideal, some mothers will produce insufficient milk and have no option but to bottle-feed from the earliest days. For a variety of reasons many others will switch to bottle-feeding during baby's first months. They should not worry about its adequacy. Modern formulae are available which are much closer to human milk than they used to be; baby will receive all the nutrition he needs for healthy development. The bottle must be clean and sterilized, of course, and the mixture made *precisely* in accordance with the instructions on the packet or tin. Making it stronger is making it worse rather than better. It not only leads to overfeeding and overweight but may overload the baby's body with sodium, which can have serious consequences. Never add salt, since this can harm a baby's kidneys, and never add sugar: you will only give the baby a taste for sweet food which will lead to tooth decay.

But, whether breast-feeding or bottle-feeding, do consult your doctor or health visitor about whether or not to add any extra vitamins. Breast milk may contain insufficient vitamin D, fresh cows' milk insufficient vitamins C and D. Powdered formulae usually contain all the necessary vitamins.

One routine part of a baby's visit to a child health clinic is to be weighed. The only feeding problem which afflicts children, short of food poisoning, is a shortage of good food. It is a common, desperate problem in many parts of the world. In the more affluent Western countries, feeding problems have a different character. Doctors here are increasingly more worried about babies being overweight than underweight. The two graphs on these pages show average weight-gain for the first year of life. As you can see, this can vary considerably depending on the size of the child, and no baby has yet been born whose weight will increase at such constant average rates. In real life, babies' weights go up at varying rates, sometimes spurting, sometimes slowing. Weight *is* important if your child appears to be exceptionally heavy or light but parents should not be too obsessive about it. Whether it concerns sleeping, feeding, teething or anything else, babies are individuals and as such will vary from one another.

You can help avoid overfeeding by sticking to milk alone for the first few months. Opinions vary about the best time to introduce mixed feeding (with solids as well as milk) but it is probably best to make the change gradually between the fourth and sixth month. Babies have survived and thrived on any number of different diets (and theories) so do not be dogmatic about right and wrong times. Be flexible and introduce mixed feeding gradually. It is not a competition with targets to be achieved by this or that date. But do not start too early: milk supplies all a baby's nutritional needs in the first few months in the most easily digestible form. Adding solids or cereals too soon will lead to overweight; adding cereals may also lead to digestion difficulties in later life, so vegetables, meat, fish and cheese should form the most important elements of a baby's mixed diet. This should certainly be introduced by about six months, because baby will then need the extra iron in egg yolks, vegetables and meat that milk alone cannot supply.

Indeed, one sign that baby is ready for mixed feeding is

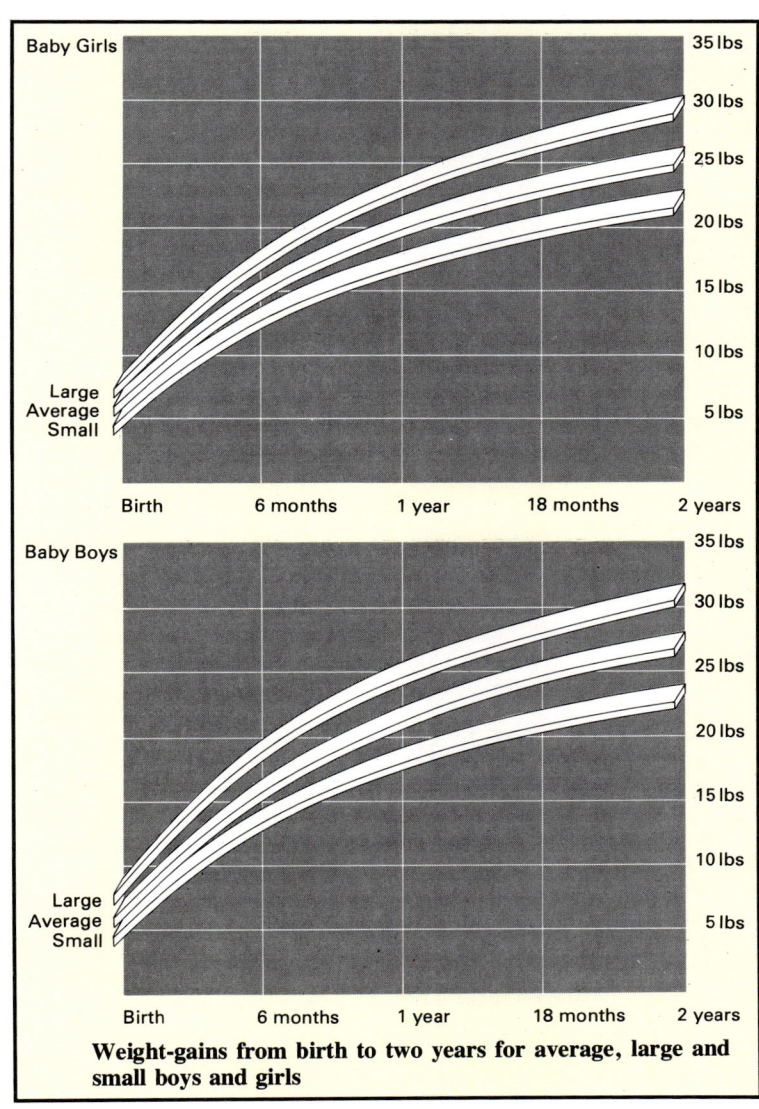

Weight-gains from birth to two years for average, large and small boys and girls

when he still seems hungry after a good milk feed, but if in doubt talk to your health visitor. Introduce solids very gradually: just a teaspoonful is enough at first. And 'solids' is perhaps a misleading description. Baby's food must be mashed or sieved so that there are no lumps. It is necessary neither to buy nor to prepare special baby food. Quite often you can adapt parts of the family meal. There are many tins or jars of baby food on the market but make sure baby has some fresh foods.

The Health Education Council has recommended ten rules or hints for feeding babies:

Do
*give your baby a variety of foods for a variety of tastes
*mash or sieve all your baby's food at first
*feed at your baby's pace rather than yours
*give extra water, especially in hot weather
*let baby feed himself, however messy at first.

Don't
*add salt or sugar to feeds
*give cereal at more than one meal a day
*give your baby food that is too hot
*give sweet foods or drinks between meals
*leave your baby alone when eating.

Feeding-time is also important because it satisfies baby's needs for comfort as well as food. It is impossible not to hold a baby close while breast-feeding, of course, but if bottle-feeding try to make sure you also cuddle baby closely. Feeding is a deeply emotional activity to a child. When he feels hungry, he feels distress: he is quite unable to reason that, 'It's all right, I'll get enough food in due course.' All he can do is to express his distress by shrieking. If mother comes quickly to feed him, he feels secure and happy. He associates mother as food provider with mother as source of love. It is part of learning to love.

Mother, too, can associate food with love and this can lead to a dangerous trap. A child who is not hungry at one mealtime will not want to eat much. The statement seems banal but, as feeding her own baby is an emotional experience for the mother, she may feel rejected if her child declines food for which he has no appetite. She may then attempt to persuade him to take more food which will probably make him cross and possibly make him sick. It is never right to quarrel with a child about his food. Healthy normal children do not starve themselves, so try not to worry. Accept that baby will sometimes be more or less hungry than usual and that some children, like some grown-ups, have smaller appetites than others. But consult your doctor if loss of appetite persists for several days and you are at all uneasy. Never worry if a child misses one meal: he will usually make up for it at the next.

CRYING
Crying is part – a large part – of a baby's language. It is used neither to annoy nor to exercise his lungs; it is used to say something. It is the baby's form of vocal communication. It can reflect a yearning for physical contact or play as well as hunger or distress. A mother's natural reaction is to pick baby up and cuddle him. This is the proper reaction. Her only problem is to work out whether baby is thirsty, hungry, too hot, too cold, frightened, lonely or bored. But she soon learns to distinguish between the different cries, which means baby has successfully communicated his feelings.

There is a school of thought which argues that mothers who rush to their babies as soon as they cry will 'spoil' them. But psychological research shows the contrary: babies who are left to cry for a long time become more difficult and tearful children. So again the mother's instinct is right. The cry should not be ignored and mothers should not worry about whether they are doing the 'right' thing by comforting their crying child.

A worried mother – worried for any reason – can transmit her worry to the child and trigger another problem. Her emotional state, whether it be worry, tension or unhappiness, may even be enough to set the child crying again. A tense, unhappy mother will also find it difficult to comfort the baby and this will only make her more tense. It is all too easy for a potentially disastrous cycle to begin this way and it is all too common for new mothers to be tense and worried. They have so much to do and so little time. If mothers do feel run down, then for their sake and their baby's they should seek help from their doctor or health visitor, or try and find someone who can help to give them an occasional break.

PLAYING
Playing is a vital aspect of learning and growing up. Parents often think that children can only play when they are six months or older. By this they tend to mean play with toys or romp around a room. But play begins – or should begin – in the very earliest days. A baby who strokes his mother's breast during feeding is playing and learning to use his hands; a baby lying on the floor and kicking his legs is playing and learning to exercise his body; a baby watching and later touching a mobile strung across his cot is similarly playing and learning. As baby grows older his play becomes more ambitious, so much so that you have to think constantly about safety. He does then begin to play with toys but often will gain as much fun through an improvised toy as one bought expensively in the shops. Play helps to develop control of the body, including sight and hearing as well as muscular co-ordination and other physical skills. It is therefore an integral part of a child's physical development. It is also an opportunity for parents to talk to their children as they play with them. Baby will not understand the words but he needs to hear the noise of the human voice. The more a baby hears words, the more readily he will learn to use them himself. So do not be shy or self-conscious: talk and sing to your baby often. It should be as natural and spontaneous as smiling.

DAILY ROUTINE
Mothers should not make themselves anxious by fretting unduly about a daily routine. Babies do not work like clockwork. How much they eat and how much they sleep will vary enormously from one baby to another, right from the earliest days. Feeding has already been discussed. Sleeping should be even less of a problem, at least for the baby. Babies will sleep for as long or as little as they need. Parents of wakeful children should try consoling themselves with the knowledge that there is some evidence that babies who need the least sleep are on average brighter children. The only other essential part of any baby's day is playing. A daily bath is useful but not essential; high standards of general hygiene *are* essential.

EYESIGHT

The first six months of life are crucial in the development of eyesight. Vision is not fully developed before three months, which means that eyes are very vulnerable throughout this period. Any sign of damage or infection should be reported to the doctor immediately. It is only as a baby's eyes develop that he begins to align the eyes together and see properly. During the first six months he begins to develop binocular vision, which means using both eyes together to see objects in depth. Until he manages this, he may look a little cross-eyed or have a 'wandering eye'. But if a baby over three months old still squints and looks cross-eyed, the cause is usually some fault in learning how to interpret depth. He should be seen promptly by a doctor or eye specialist. At this stage, steps can be taken to rectify squints so it is important not to delay. If you are worrying unnecessarily, the doctor will not mind; if there is some cause to worry, he will welcome the opportunity of dealing with the squint at the best time. Early detection is vital.

STAGES OF GROWTH

Babies develop at such different rates that it is impossible to suggest states or stages of development which should be reached at specific ages. A very wide range is 'normal'. But it is natural for parents to worry if a child seems slow in certain skills. Parents should always be alert to any problem which may need medical help but generally they should regard 'stages of development' as no more than useful or interesting guidelines. Not only do babies vary so greatly but the child who is first to reach one given stage may not necessarily be the first to reach another. There is certainly no guarantee that he will grow up into the most intelligent or most agile or most successful of any group of babies. Many an early developer has been overtaken by a late starter.

Ultimately it does not really matter that much if baby smiles at six or eight weeks, crawls at seven or nine months and so on. But if you think your child's development is way outside the norm, consult your doctor. These are some approximate milestones in the first months of life:

1. Most babies *smile* at around six weeks, rarely more than a week earlier or more than four weeks later.
2. Most babies *sit up* by around six months but they will not be able to hold themselves in this position for very long or be particularly manoeuvrable – this comes one to three months later.
3. Most babies will be *rolling over* from stomach to back by six months. Rolling the other way comes one to four weeks later.
4. Most babies cut their first *teeth* – the lower central incisor – at six months. By the time he is a year old he will have six incisors; they may come regularly or in sudden bursts. (See below for further information on young teeth.)
5. Most babies will *crawl* at around nine months and *walk* on their own at some time between twelve and eighteen months. A few babies omit the crawling stage altogether. Babies begin to pull themselves to their feet to *stand up* at around seven months. But variations are huge in all three skills.
6. Most babies will *speak* two or three words when they are one year old and be able to construct simple sentences one year later. But they will be 'vocalizing' much earlier.

Between six and nine months they will make sounds like 'ma' or 'pa' or 'da', which thrills their parents but does not mean they have understood these common abbreviations for mother and father. (See below for further information on speech and hearing.)

7. Most babies will be able to use their hands to grasp, pull and push when *playing* by the time they are one year old. Skills such as using building-bricks develop in the following year.

FROM SIX MONTHS TO FIVE YEARS

DIET

By six months 'feeds' become 'meals' which are taken more or less at adult times – breakfast, lunch and tea. By a year the times remain the same but the meals are taken with the rest of the family – an important part of any child's social development. The child will also then start eating 'normal' – meaning adult – food. The habits established then are likely to remain for the rest of his life.

Children learn marvellously quickly about food from their parents, but this can also mean they learn the wrong habits and values. Children are more impressed by what their parents do than what they say. If parents start the day on a cup of coffee and a piece of buttered toast, there is no point in their extolling to their six- or seven-year-old the virtues of starting the day with a 'proper' breakfast. Childhood can be a fine opportunity for the parents to develop good dietary habits for their own benefit as well as their children's. Just what this involves in terms both of what we eat and how we cook is spelled out in Chapter 4, it is never too late – or too early – to start.

Generally, what is good for adults is good for children. So fresh foods are better than convenience foods, although tired and harassed mothers are bound to use some convenience meals. This will do no harm but they should not become the corner-stone of anyone's diet. One particular way in which parents can help their children is to keep them away from sugar and sweets; both are attractive to children but reduce their appetite for nutritious food and have the distinct disadvantage of rotting the teeth.

TEETH

Good teeth start in infancy and an alarming number of not-so-good ones finish there. In the United Kingdom, two million milk-teeth (as children's first teeth are known) are so rotten each year that they have to be removed by dentists. The rot that literally sets in then also continues because the bacteria which are consuming the milk-teeth can attack the 'adult' teeth already developing in the jaw. Two terrible statistics result. British dentists remove 10 *tons* (about 50,000 kilogrammes) of teeth a year because they have been improperly cared for; about one-third of all people in the UK over the age of sixteen have no teeth of their own left. If you want your child to be among the other two-thirds, restrict sugar and sweets as mentioned above and explained further in the section on teeth later in this book. Eating only at mealtimes has a double value. It is better nutritionally and better for the teeth. Anything eaten between meals tends to be sugary, and sugar is the breeding-ground for the bacteria which form the acids that

PREGNANCY AND CHILDHOOD/THE EARLY YEARS

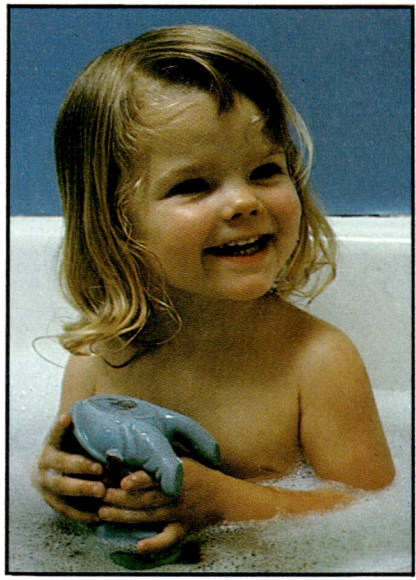
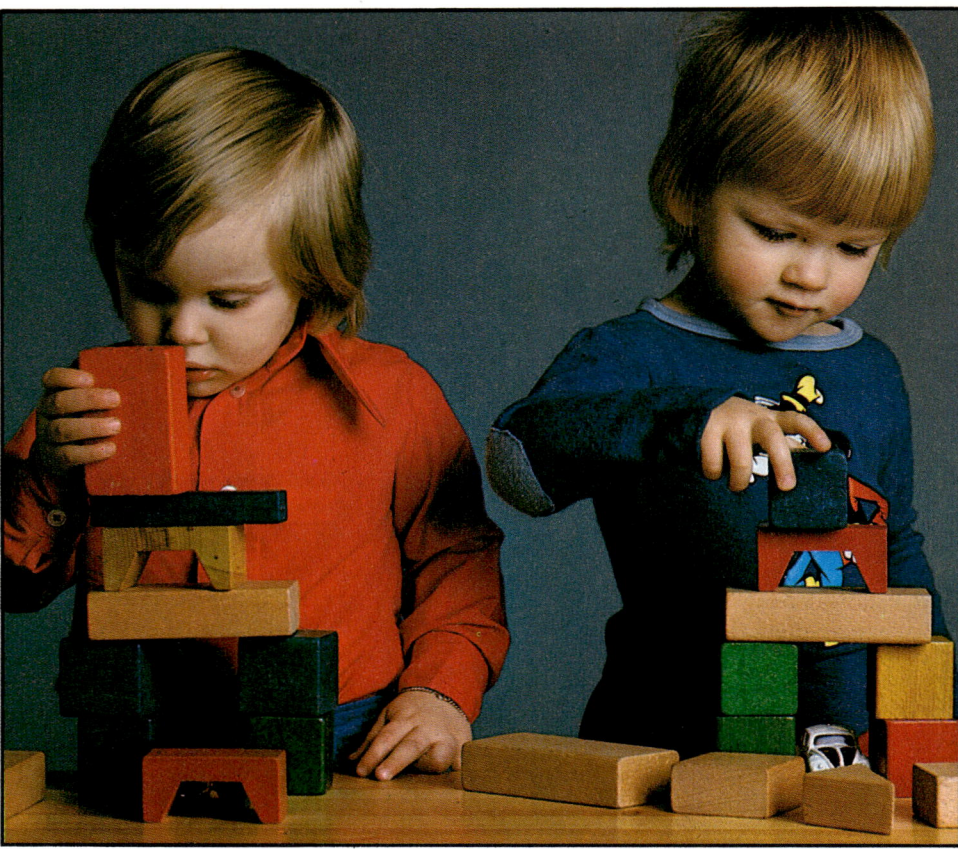

Through play children learn physical co-ordination as well as how to relate to the outside world. Often, simple improvised games with water and building bricks prove as popular – and beneficial – as those with more elaborate and expensive toys

rot teeth. If sweets are to be eaten, have them at the end of meals.

You can also help your child's teeth by trying to brush as soon as the first milk-tooth appears. It does not matter particularly at this stage whether you brush up and down or side to side or, as dentists eventually recommend, in small circular movements. From the age of three or four, children can start brushing their own teeth but you should still supervise this. By nine or ten you will not need to supervise, but make sure they do not start skipping it. Whatever the age, teeth should be cleaned at least twice a day.

The British Dental Association recommends the use of fluoride toothpastes. These are particularly valuable for children because the fluoride can be incorporated into the teeth as they are growing during the first ten years of life. This is one reason why toothbrushing must become part of the daily routine from the earliest possible days. You can increase the protection by using fluoride tablets, available from chemists. With luck, the tooth-preserving habits of a lifetime will be established in childhood.

EYESIGHT AND HEARING

Whereas teeth usually start life in good condition and are then destroyed by their owners, eyes and ears, or rather sight and hearing, may be poor from the start. If your child holds toys unusually close or far away when playing, get expert advice. And if a child does not seem to notice what you say when he cannot see you, also consult a doctor.

Either or both of these defects may show up clearly when a child starts going to school. A child who wants to sit at the front of the class may be short-sighted, and teachers who report that 'he doesn't listen to anything' may really be describing a child whose hearing is bad, possibly because there is wax in his ears. However, it may be more serious.

Poor hearing should be detected as soon as possible because it will affect the development of a child's ability to talk. An experienced doctor can sometimes detect the problem from the more limited vocalizing and babbling of a six-month-old baby with hearing difficulties. A baby can use a hearing aid from the age of about six months and this will help him develop better speech than he otherwise would. But this is something on which parents will need specialist guidance.

If a child squints – one eye going repeatedly into a corner – then he should be seen by a specialist. If parents or close relatives have squints, the child should have a routine eye test between two and a half and three years; if any irregularity is observed, tests may be repeated at six-monthly intervals. Ideally, every child should have their eyes tested between three and five, before going to school. If nothing is wrong, another examination is not necessary for perhaps two years and at two-yearly intervals afterwards.

SPEECH

Speech – the deliberate use of words in original sentences – is a unique human achievement. Other animals can learn a very limited version of the human language in signs and symbols, but none can match human skill and sensitivity. Yet simply because speech is our best means of communication, we sometimes forget just what an achievement it is and expect too much of our children.

Children develop the ability to talk, like they develop every other ability, at their own rates, and a very wide range is 'normal'. A child will *on average* be able to use a few words, singly but with meaning, between twelve and eighteen months. Some time between the second and third year he will manage to put sentences together and hold simple conversations. By about five he will have a mastery of the technique of the spoken language.

You can help your child to speak if you remember how he learns. Speaking can be learned only by imitation, so the parent should take every opportunity of talking to a child. But a child has limitations. He can deal with short, simple sentences only. The advantage of this kind of sentence is that every word is part of the simple message. 'Don't take that' is simple. 'You know you shouldn't touch my knitting' is so complicated that the child will gain virtually nothing from the words, although the *tone* will convey the message of exasperation.

For the same reason, you should speak slowly to a child. As he has no language of his own at this stage, what he is really doing is learning a foreign language. And we all know how difficult it is to pick out individual words from the rapid flow of a foreign language.

Children do not say much that is of riveting interest at first. We are fascinated by their first words but tend afterwards to let them chatter on without paying much attention. But if we want to help them learn the skills of speech and communication, we must help them by listening, by answering them in sentences they can follow, and eventually by correcting their grammar and pronunciation. The art of correction is delicate. If you are too ready to correct, conversation grinds to a halt. It is difficult, even for an adult, to continue conversations that are interspersed with sentences like, 'You mean sausage, dear. Now what were you saying?' On the other hand, a child can easily develop bad speech habits that can take root. This is obviously a risk if you continue to allow very bad pronunciation. But it also happens if you continue to allow them to use a pronunciation or phrase which you find amusing; children are very willing to entertain you with what eventually becomes fossilized baby-talk. Simply because a child is not fluent we are sometimes tempted to finish his sentences for him. But to do his talking for him handicaps his learning. This problem can also arise if there is an elder brother or sister who is over-ready to show off their expertise.

The importance of speech makes it inevitable that parents worry over apparent delays and difficulties in mastering this essential art of communication. Usually a late start is not serious; children, as we have said before, vary as greatly in mastering the ability to speak as they do in all other abilities. Some problems such as stuttering or lisping are often temporary. If not, speech therapy can 'cure' many children and improve all of them. However, sometimes speech difficulties are symptoms of deafness or the result of a genuine disorder. So if in any doubt, consult your doctor and seek specialist advice.

For all children, however, a mastery of words – spoken and written – is of absolutely fundamental importance. Parents can help by talking to their children from the first weeks of life. They can do this by discussing picture stories when the children are young, by reading books with words as they grow up, by listening to what a child is trying to say and by encouraging them as well as correcting mistakes. By promoting a child's ability to talk and developing the vocabulary you will also be preparing the ground for learning to read. Children's books have improved out of all recognition in the last decade; if you doubt it, go and look round your local library. Reading to your children is a marvellous bonding experience for the family, while making books a habit when a child is young will enhance the rest of his or her life.

FITNESS

Baby will be crawling or even walking by around his first birthday. Movement is obviously another crucial skill. It is important for a child's psychological as well as physical development, so try not to worry, induce fear or interfere. This is the way a child finds out about the world, and children are much more sensible and safe than parents often credit. They explore cautiously, extending their range bit by bit. But they are as rattled by cries of 'Look out!' and 'Be careful!' as you would be when driving a car. They will also learn from the occasional bump and bruise, but innate caution and relatively tough skins cannot preclude every hazard. Childhood accidents are a major source of injury and even death. Children need protection from some hazards both inside and outside the home (see the next section in this chapter).

Later in this book we devote much of a chapter to the message that the health of the adult greatly depends on getting enough exercise. This habit is almost certainly born young and, unfortunately, in some children it dies young too. Parents should do what they can to get a child to be active. Babies will vary as to when they start crawling or walking, but consult the doctor if your baby seems particularly late starting. It may well be nothing, but it does no harm to ask. As children grow older they should be encouraged to use their own feet for getting about. Do not take them by car to places they can reach under their own toddler power. A four-year-old can walk a couple of miles on a shopping expedition; a nine-year-old can cycle ten miles (but should for safety reasons be accompanied by a parent and avoid main roads); an eleven-year-old can go on lengthy camping expeditions. Schools, too, will help to keep them active with organized sports.

FEET

If a child is to enjoy moving on his own two feet, these must be kept sound and undeformed. A growing foot needs as much freedom as possible. Let your child go barefoot as much as possible and remember that tight socks (or tight stretch-suits) can be as harmful as tight shoes. Pram shoes should also be avoided. When a child begins to walk the bones of the feet are only partially formed. The feet are thus still 'soft', which is why they can be deformed by tight shoes. When your child does have to wear shoes, therefore, make sure they are comfortable and fit well. Shoes are outgrown so quickly at this age that fit matters far more than quality. *Never* buy children's shoes from a shop that asks you the size: children's feet should be remeasured every time. In Britain, major libraries, child welfare clinics and the Health Education Council can supply lists of approved shoe-shops for children.

These are six points to look for when buying shoes:

1. Shoes should be fitted to leave 2–2½ sizes (about ¾ inch or 18 mm) growing room between the end of the longest toe and the end of the shoe.
2. Shoes must fit firmly at the heel.
3. Shoes should have an adjustable fastening for a firm fit round the instep.
4. Shoes must be wide enough to allow toes to move.
5. Shoes should be able to bend as the foot bends.
6. The shape of a shoe should fit the natural shape of the foot. And socks should be big enough to give a loose easy fit at the toes.

PREGNANCY AND CHILDHOOD/THE EARLY YEARS

VACCINATION

Vaccination or immunization has played an essential part in the decline in infectious diseases over the last fifty years. Some have declined to such an extent that immunization is no longer carried out on all children – smallpox, for example. In Western countries the risks from whooping cough may not be much greater than the risks of side-effects such as brain damage from the vaccination itself. This is now being hotly debated within the medical profession and whooping cough vaccination is no longer routine in Sweden and Germany. However, British health authorities believe that the benefits outweigh the risks. A recent investigation in Britain has found that the whooping cough vaccine causes severe brain damage in from one per hundred thousand to one per fifty thousand children. This has to be balanced against the risk of the disease itself causing death in tiny babies, damage to the lungs or to the brain. Whooping cough is excluded from the list below because of the current controversy; it is very much a matter for parents to decide themselves in conjunction with their family doctor. Vaccination against whooping cough does give valuable protection for people living in overcrowded conditions and in countries outside Europe, North America and Australasia where the disease is much more common. But one unfortunate effect of the whooping cough debate has been a decline in the number of children being vaccinated against other infectious diseases. It cannot be stressed too much that this is unwise: where vaccination is safe, it is preventive medicine at its simplest and best. The ages for different vaccinations are only approximate and are sometimes varied by individual doctors. For further information on infectious diseases generally – their prevention and treatment – see Chapter 7.

6 to 12 months: *Diphtheria/tetanus, polio.* The best reaction is usually achieved if the first dose is delayed until the baby is six months old. Repeat doses are given first after an interval of six to eight weeks and then again after a further interval of four to six months.

1 to 2 years: *Measles.* This should not be given within three weeks of any other live vaccine. Delay to the age of two years will reduce the risk of an occasional severe reaction.

5 years or school entry: *Diphtheria/tetanus, polio.* Repeat vaccinations may sometimes be given earlier at around three years to children attending nursery school.

10 to 13 years: *Tuberculosis (BCG)* for all children who show no natural immunity to tuberculosis after testing and *rubella (German measles)* for girls. All girls are advised to have the latter, even if they have had German measles once, in order to avoid the risks of catching it during pregnancy. The vaccination is not advised, however, within three weeks of the BCG vaccination.

15 to 19 years: *Tetanus and polio.* Repeat or booster vaccinations.

OFF TO SCHOOL

The change in a child's life when he starts school is enormous. Unless he has been going to playschool or a nursery, this may be the first time he has spent a day, regularly, away from home and parents. Playschool or nursery is obviously a good way of acclimatizing himself to the change as well as a good way of learning sociability and other early educational skills. But if a child has not had this opportunity, his parents should help him to prepare for his first days at school.

Whatever the parents think of their own schooldays, they should emphasize the pleasures of school when they tell him about it. Stress the adventure. Tell him what a big grown-up boy he has become. Do not say things like, 'At last, I'm free to get on with something.' It may be a relief to have the child away from home all day but the child need not know this. It certainly will not help him adjust to his new life.

This life will be much more energetic than he is used to, so he will need plenty of sleep; the household day may need to be slightly rearranged to fit in with the school hours. Sleep is important not merely because you do not want your child to be sleepy at school but because of fundamental health reasons. A child short of sleep may grow more slowly than he should and is more likely to be underweight. There are no firm rules for bedtimes, however. If a child is bright and willing to get up in the morning, he is getting enough sleep; if he is still tired in the morning, then he is not getting enough sleep. But as a rough guide, a child between five and seven should be in bed by seven o'clock during term-time and the child between eight and eleven in bed by eight o'clock.

The new demands of school also make proper diet and feeding especially important. Children, even more than the rest of us, need a good meal to start the day. Breakfast should include wholemeal cereal and some fruit. One egg, grilled bacon or some fish can be valuable, but not even small children should eat too many eggs or too much meat (see Chapter 4). Baked beans on toast or grilled tomatoes are a quick alternative. If they want some toast and marmalade or jam too, so much the better. They should not be encouraged to bolt their food, which means that they (and their cook) must get on the move at a suitably early hour in the morning.

Many children eat their midday meal during term-time at school and there is a tradition of not liking school food. It obviously will not be as good as home cooking but they should be encouraged to eat it, especially as it has to sustain a child throughout the afternoon. If possible, try and call at the school to see what they are eating. Parents tend to believe that it is a sound, solid meal crammed with vitamins and protein, perhaps counteracting any shortcomings in their own meals. Nowadays, with economies causing cuts in the school-meal service, this belief may be false. Indeed, in many places school meals are being dropped altogether. Packed lunches are therefore increasingly an alternative to traditional school meals. Try to prepare a balanced packed lunch with fruit and yoghurt rather than cakes or biscuits. Vary the fillings of sandwiches, too, using cheese, fish pastes and cold meats rather than jam.

Children usually want something to eat when they get home from school. If they do have anything, it should be light enough not to spoil their appetite for the main evening meal an hour or so later. Everybody should have three proper meals a day for their health's sake; they are more likely to do so if the habit starts young.

Hygienic behaviour, to use a euphemistic phrase, is also a habit which should be started young. Children should wash their hands after going to the lavatory and before eating food. If they are told the reason and supervised carefully, the habit will take root.

Young children generally do not need to be told to take exercise, as any parent will testify. But as they reach adolescence young people, girls probably more frequently than boys, sometimes decide that sport and exercise in general is not for them. It is not glamorous enough, they say, or it may even 'spoil' their developing glamour by making them too muscular. It is difficult for adults to influence adolescents very effectively, but any success in getting them to realize that exercise, on the contrary, makes them more attractive (as well as generally fitter) will pay dividends in later life. It helps to imbue healthy habits if the parents appear to be speaking from experience and practising what they preach.

WHAT PARENTS SHOULD NOT DO

A child learns a lot from his parents – for good or ill. Smoking is the most obvious bad example. It may be that a baby does not learn to smoke from watching his parents but it is not safe to rely on even that. From the age of a few months the child will accept the idea that smoking is something that adults normally do – like walking and talking – and therefore admirable and to be imitated. If you do not smoke, your child is much less likely to take up smoking himself, and you will also be protecting him in the early months by not polluting the atmosphere in which he must breathe.

A parent can also introduce a child to heavy drinking if this again seems to be normal adult behaviour. The children of alcoholics are more likely to become alcoholics themselves. This is not an inherited trait but an imitated one. The most constant examples to a child are its parents, however caring or careless they may prove to be. Older children should be introduced to alcohol gradually. Learning to cope with alcohol is a long way from learning to roll over from stomach to back, but it is all part of the development from baby to adulthood.

Accidents

Accidents are the commonest cause of death in children and cause more deaths in under-fifteens than the next two causes of death combined – respiratory diseases and cancer. About one out of every eighty children has an accident each year requiring admission to hospital, and as many as one in six children attends a hospital casualty department each year. Many of these children are left with severe disabilities.

Much more could be done by government, local authorities and parents to prevent many of these accidents from happening. Many people do not realize that there is greater danger to a young child of dying in the home or garden than there is of dying on the roads. The first step in prevention is to recognize the source of danger.

In 1979 almost as many children in Britain under five died from falls in the home (20) as died from injuries sustained as passengers in motor cars (22). And more children died from choking or suffocation (166) than all those who died on the roads (92). Burns, fires and scalds killed 69 children under five, 21 were killed by drowning while poisoning killed 10, electrocution killed 2. And 65 children were murdered or battered to the extent that they died of their injuries, although this is generally accepted to be an underestimate.

Children under one year old are especially liable to choke or suffocate on food, toys or small objects such as buttons, beads or coins. These should be kept out of the children's reach, and infants' food should not contain lumps until they are old enough to chew properly. Babies suck until about six months of age, when they gradually learn to chew. Ideally, infants should be given only liquid food or smooth spoon food until six months of age. They can then be introduced slowly to soft solid foods until they have all their chewing teeth and are able to manage most things, although it is still wise not to give infants anything which is at all tough.

Around the age of one year old, when children become mobile, they begin to find all sorts of things on the floor and on tables which they could not reach before which could choke, poison or suffocate them – beware particularly of plastic bags. And at this age they begin to be able to reach hot pans on stoves or teapots on the table. Burns and scalds are two of the commonest causes of moderate to severe injury in children. Also the child, still uncertain and inexpert in movement, is likely to pull over his high chair, or fall from furniture. Fractures and concussion are another common cause of moderate to severe injury, and each year around six infants tragically drown while left unattended *in a bath*.

By the age of three or four, the child is exploring more on his own and begins to discover where the bleach, turpentine, paraffin – and the nail-polish remover – have been hidden, unless they are out of reach. The fact that these substances do not taste nice seems to make no difference. The child discovers things hidden in the garden shed or may fall in the lily pond; or has learnt to switch on an electric socket and may start a fire by poking paper into the heater, or by fiddling with the pilot-light on the cooker.

By the time the child gets to school age, the dangers change again. Falls from trees and walls are a danger, especially for boys, while girls are more prone to burns and scalding accidents in the home. However, road accidents then become the greatest danger, causing the deaths of some 600 children a year and injuries to 45,000 more. A child has a one in twenty chance of being involved in a road accident before the age of fifteen.

It is no good trying to insulate children totally from danger. They must be exposed to dangers before they can learn to avoid them. But exposure to danger must be made in a carefully calculated way at an age when a child is fully able to understand it.

HOW TO AVOID ACCIDENTS

IN THE HOME

Heating: Radiant electric fires can give an inquisitive child who grasps the element a terrible burn, or may ignite inflammable clothing or furniture when placed too close. In small rooms, radiant fires should be at a high level attached to a wall. Alternatively, use a convector heater or place the radiant heater in a fireplace surrounded by a childproof guard attached to the wall. If you buy a paraffin heater

PREGNANCY AND CHILDHOOD/ACCIDENTS

make sure it is one of the self-extinguishing kind which goes out when tilted to an angle of 45 degrees. Do not use gas or oil heaters in small unventilated rooms. Get any old gas appliances inspected by the gas authority.

Kitchen: Pilot-lights on a cooker are a potential danger. Choose a cooker without pilot-lights, and use an electric lighter for the gas. Keep the lighter on a high shelf. Use a guard around the cooker to prevent pans being pulled off. Always turn handles in, use the rings at the back whenever possible and if you are buying new pans, try to get short-handled ones. Keep a small fire-extinguisher near the cooker to deal with burning fat. Always put teapots and hot pans well out of reach of children. Keep matches out of reach, and instruct children in the dangers of fire by means of outdoor camp-fires. Only buy electric gadgets, including fires, which say they conform to British Standards. Never keep cleaning materials, soap powders, bleach, paints or paraffin under the sink or at floor level.

Living room and bedroom: Falls from furniture are a real danger. Never leave a small baby propped up unattended or out of reach on a chair. The baby may wriggle and fall off the chair or get into some awkward position where he may be smothered. Arrange furniture as far as possible so that it does not enable young children to climb high. Bunk-beds require special care since every year children are killed or injured through falling out while asleep. Make sure that the guards are used to make it as difficult as possible to fall out, and remove any furniture the child might collide with on the way down. Make sure that the floor beside the bunks is covered with a soft rug. Do not give pillows to babies under twelve months, since they may cause suffocation: at least twenty children died this way in 1979. Beware of projections on cots which may catch children's clothing so that they may hang. Never tie anything such as a dummy on a cord around a child's neck.

Windows: Make sure that children cannot open windows more than 100 mm (about 4 inches). Fittings designed to make windows burglar-proof are often suitable for preventing windows from being opened too far by children inside the house, and the window can still be opened wide on a hot day when adults are in the room. Use safety glass.

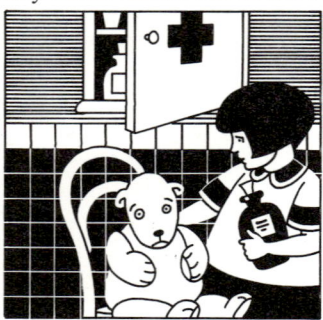

Bathrooms: Locks which can be opened from the outside with a screwdriver or by a string-push are a great advantage in case of emergency. Apart from the danger of infants drowning if left unattended, the greatest risks are posed by medicines. The photograph on page 36 shows how much like sweets drugs can appear.

This is why medicines should always be locked in a cupboard or childproof medicine cabinet. Do not take tablets in front of the children because this encourages them to imitate you. Never encourage children to think of drugs as sweets in order to get them to take them. If your children need medicine, ask the doctor not to provide it in the form of a sweet flavoured syrup. Children sometimes drink the whole bottle because they like it and believe that a whole bottle may do them more good. It may of course be necessary to use a syrup to get your child to take essential medicine, but try an ordinary formulation first. Flush old

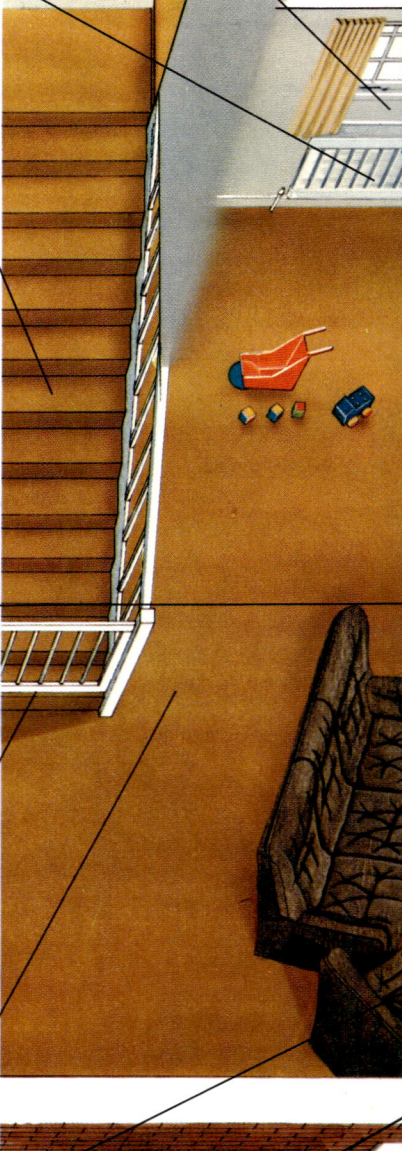

How to make your home childproof: 23 ways of cutting the

Radiators: very hot radiators present an obvious hazard to adventuring young hands. Consult central heating specialists to see if your system can be adapted to lower temperatures

Windows: safety-catch stop children opening them sufficien to be able to fall out. Essential, of course for upstairs windows but desirable downstairs, too.

Stairways: should be well-lit with a light-switch at top and bottom. The banisters should be firm, the stairs unobstructed. Nothing flammable should be stored underneath the stairs in case of fire.

Shelving: must be securely fixed to walls, preferably with rounded edges and ends to avoid sharp, dangerous corners. From the safety point of view this is the prime consideration but to protect adult property, such as books and records, it's often better to keep all shelving high and out of a child's reach.

Safety gate: keeps crawling youngsters safely downstairs (or upstairs). Ideally have one at both top and bottom of the stairs.

Flooring: fitted carpets are ideal because they lessen the chance of children slipping. If carpets or rugs are not fitted, make sure they are laid – and preferably fixed – on non-polished floors.

Toys: give big toys to small children so that they cannot swallow small items like beads or marbles.

Electric appliances: kee flex short without 'joins' and where possib out of children's reach. Don't allow it to run under carpets and if possible run only one appliance per point No bare wire, obviously.

ACCIDENTS/**PREGNANCY AND CHILDHOOD**

accidents in the home

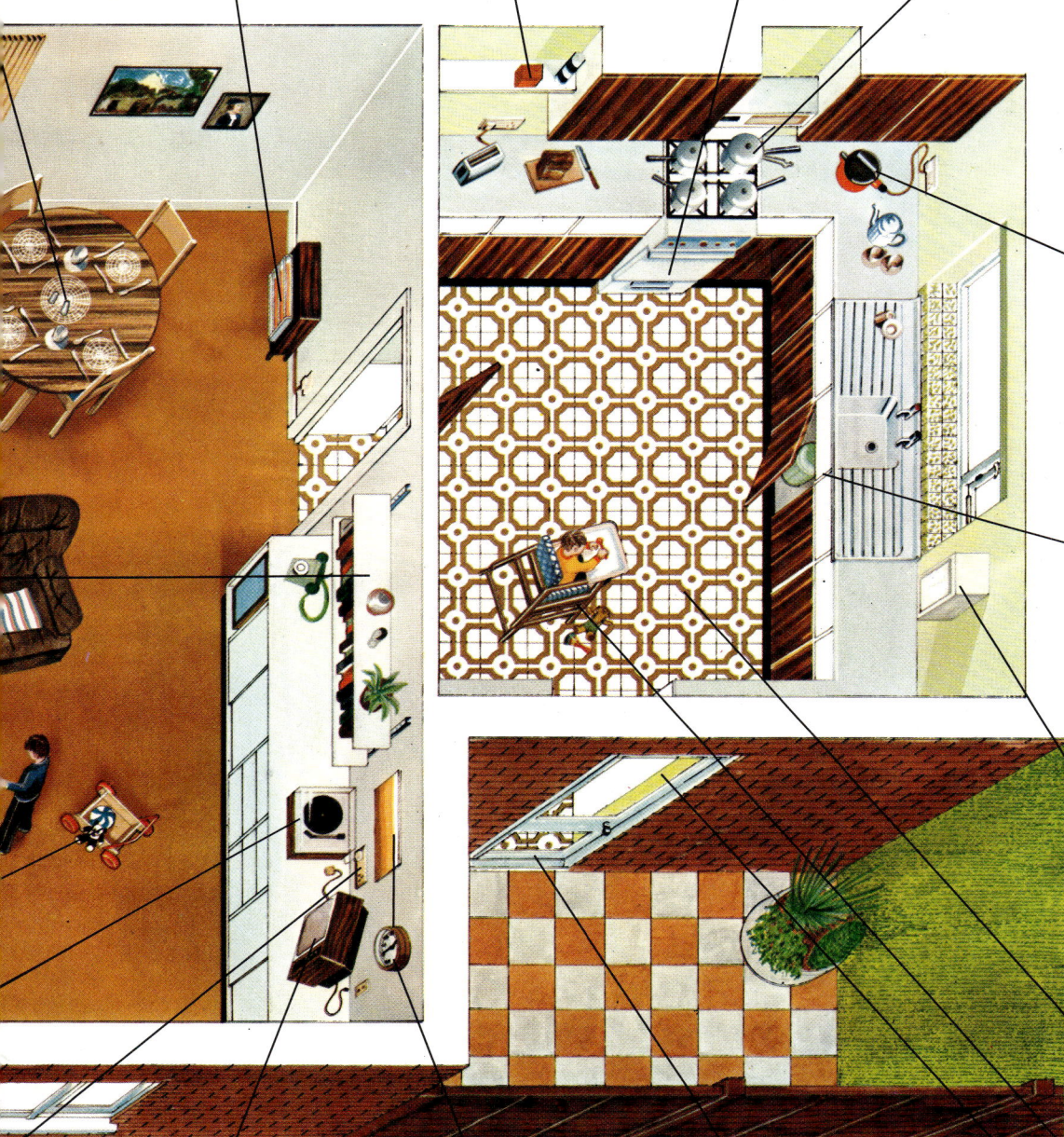

Dining table: keep hot drinks from the edge. If you can manage without a tablecloth this will lessen the chance of a child tugging the cloth – and all that rests on it – off the table to the floor.

Fire: by law all gas and electric fires must have fixed guards. With youngsters fit an additional one. Open solid fuel fires should also have a guard secured to the fireplace surround.

Matches: should always be kept out of children's reach in a high cupboard or on a high shelf.

Cooker: turn handles of saucepans to the side if cooker has a worktop on each side. If not, prevent children from pulling over pots and pans by fitting a cooker guard.

Chip pan: never leave pan unattended when cooking chips. In the event of fire never use water, always smother with a damp cloth.

Kettle: flex for all electric equipment should be kept short, but especially for electric kettles. Hook it up if necessary to make it less likely that a child can pull a kettle off a kitchen worktop and pour boiling water all over him or herself.

Storage under sink: keep bleach and other poisonous cleaning agents away from children by putting these items in a high cupboard. Turps, paint and other DIY materials should, where possible, be kept in a lockable outside shed.

First-aid cabinet: useful to keep in the kitchen since this is where many accidents happen and where children are more likely to be under surveillance. Must be lockable. Don't also use it to store foodstuffs.

Flooring: non-slip flooring such as vinyl or cork is particularly important in a kitchen where people carry hot food and liquids. Use non-slip polishes, too, but keep floor clean; wipe up spilt liquids at once.

Chairs: children should always be secured by a safety harness when in a high chair.

Plants: should be of the modern shuttered design. If worried about particularly inquisitive children, 'dummy' or blind plugs can be bought to the tempting holes.

Television: disconnect the plug when the set is not being used.

Clock and mirror: locate these on a wall away from the fireplace so that children don't stand or climb near a fire to see them.

Doorways: should be well-lit with switches conveniently placed. Avoid gloom, glare or shadows. 'Sink' the doormat wherever possible.

Doors: glass in all doors, including French windows or patio doors, should be made of laminated or tempered glass.

35

PREGNANCY AND CHILDHOOD/ACCIDENTS

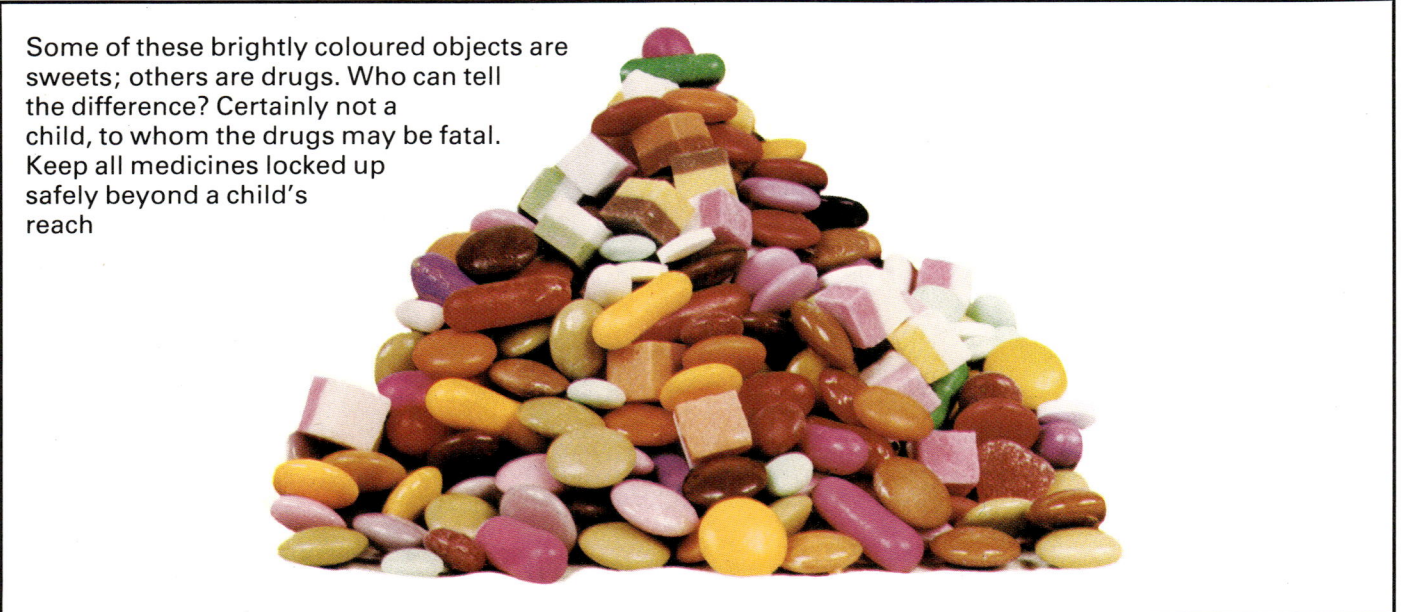

Some of these brightly coloured objects are sweets; others are drugs. Who can tell the difference? Certainly not a child, to whom the drugs may be fatal. Keep all medicines locked up safely beyond a child's reach

drugs down the lavatory. However, everyone, regardless of age, should use medicines properly. Follow the Medicines Code:

1. Always read directions carefully and give or take the exact dose recommended.
2. Never give a medicine which has been prescribed for you to someone else who seems to have a similar ailment.
3. Never 'borrow' medicines that seem to be the same as yours.
4. Never take or give medicines in the dark.
5. While taking a medicine prescribed by your doctor do not take any other medicine before seeking his advice.
6. Do not hoard surplus medicines or drugs that have passed their expiry date. But never put unused medicines in the dustbin or on a fire; return them to your pharmacy and ask the pharmacist to destroy them for you.
7. Keep all medicines out of the reach of children; store medicines in a lockable, childproof cabinet.
8. If you are advised not to drive, drink or operate machinery while taking drugs, don't.
9. If you are pregnant, ask your doctor or chemist about any medicines you take.
10. Tell the doctor about any side-effects.

IN THE PLAYGROUND

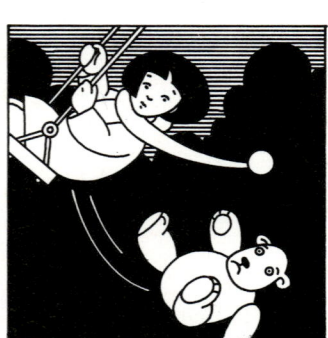

Although playgrounds have dangers, they are much safer for children than playing on the street, and provide children with invaluable training in the judgement of moving objects. Three-quarters of playground accidents analysed by *Which?*, the British Consumers' Association magazine, involved children under six. It is therefore unwise to let children of this age play unless supervised by an adult. Swings, roundabouts, slides and climbing-frames all need careful watching. *Which?* found that playgrounds with a supervisor in attendance were much safer, probably because the supervisor controls dangerous use of equipment. Risks could be cut by improvements in equipment – particularly by providing impact-absorbing swings, placing climbing-frames on sand or rubber tiles which will help to break a fall, and improving the design of moving equipment so that fingers or whole limbs cannot be trapped.

IN THE GARDEN

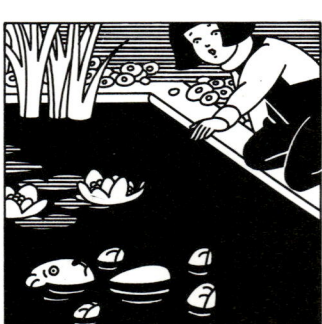

The garden shed is a fascinating place full of mysteries for children. Chemicals used in the garden, however, are much more dangerous than most of those in your bathroom cupboard. Garden chemicals should therefore be kept under lock and key. Never transfer garden chemicals to old lemonade or whisky bottles, as this has proved a death-trap not only for children. The lily-pond is another potential source of danger, and should be fenced off if young children are allowed to play unsupervised in the garden. Special care needs to be taken with lawn mowers, especially powered ones: do not let children play around you while you are mowing.

Gardens are full of poisonous plants, and so children must be taught never to eat anything from the garden without being told that it is all right. Their attention should be brought to brightly coloured berries, and they should be told that these are not good to eat. The message can be reinforced by fairy tales such as Snow White, which includes descriptions of poisoning. Snow White went into a coma after eating a poisoned apple and only awoke after receiving the attentions of the prince; nowadays a doctor has to suffice.

The most common and most hazardous garden plant is the lovely laburnum, whose attractive yellow blossoms turn into little pods resembling small pea-pods. Children love to play with them in shop and kitchen games. Deadly nightshade is another dangerous plant; it is closely related to the tomato and the potato but the small berries, which

ACCIDENTS/PREGNANCY AND CHILDHOOD

Poisons in the country.

The fruits that grow in the country and by the roadside can look mouth-wateringly attractive — especially to children at play during the summer holidays. But many are also extremely dangerous and, if eaten, can cause serious illness or even death. The variety of poisons is startling, and for some there is no known antidote. One man has died after eating a cupful of apple pips which, like those of some other fruits, contain elements of prussic acid. Often the most serious hazard is the least likely. The foxglove, for instance, has such a nasty taste that if children eat a little they spit it out quickly. Poisoning is much more likely to result from less toxic but more 'attractive' and edible plants such as the seven illustrated here. Wild fungi looking like mushrooms can also be poisonous, so beware. If in doubt, leave it alone; if poisonous plants *have* been eaten, consult a doctor.

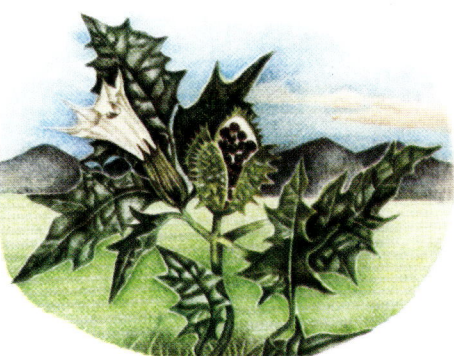

1. *Thorn apple.* Thrives in hot, dry summers on waste ground, releasing poisonous black seeds when ripe. Causes dry skin and mouth, dilated pupils, delirium.

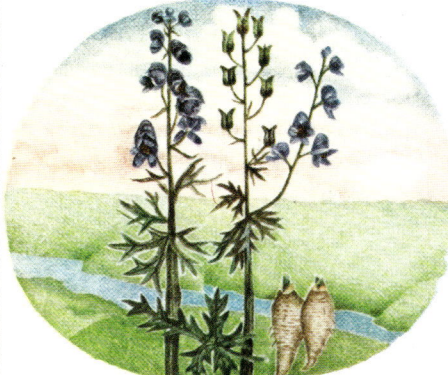

2. *Monkshood.* The most dangerous British plant although less common than some. The roots have been mistaken for horseradish but they contain the poison aconite.

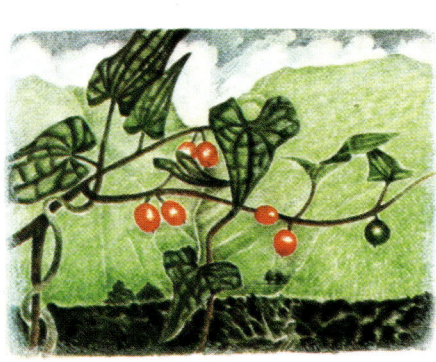

3. *Black Bryony.* Very common in hedgerows, twining around other plants. Produces clusters of deadly bright scarlet berries. White bryony is less common but also very dangerous.

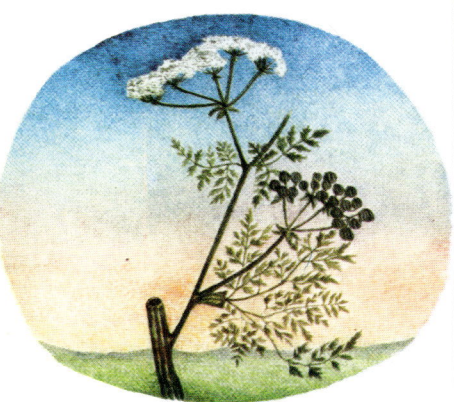

4. *Hemlock.* The leaves have been mistaken for parsley and the seeds for anise, a kitchen herb. The hollow stalks also make dangerously ideal pea-shooters.

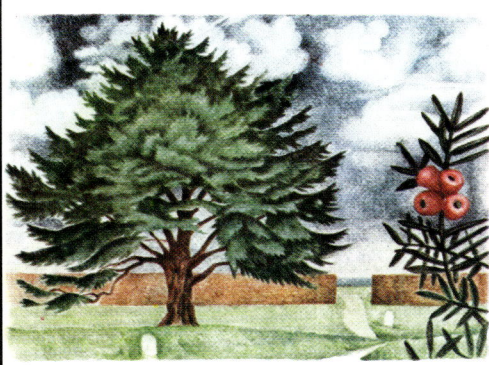

5. *Yew.* The most deadly tree. Its brilliant red berries contain seeds which can cause death from heart failure. Survival after poisoning is uncommon.

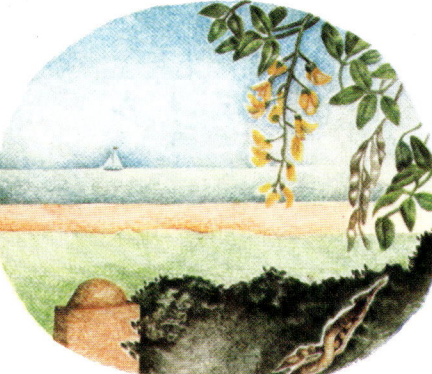

6. *Laburnum.* Commonest cause of plant poisoning in Britain. The fruit pods contain brown seeds which can cause vomiting, convulsions, coma and even death.

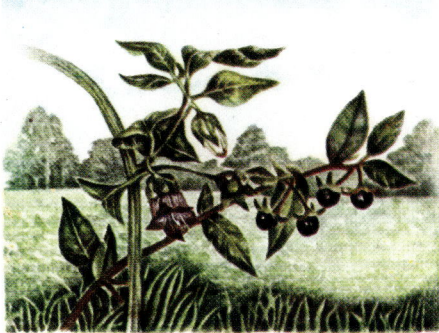

7. *Deadly nightshade.* The glossy black cherries attract children. Usually twenty to thirty cherries will cause death, but children have died after eating only two or three.

resemble tiny tomatoes, are highly poisonous. Watch out also for the giant hogweed and its smaller relatives belonging to the family *Umbelliferae*; its large hollow stems make very effective pea-shooters. However, the plant irritates the skin, producing unpleasant weals and a rash.

Country children often have a lore of their own which may not be known to parents who are city bred. They know that they can eat the young buds of the hawthorn, the early leaves on the beech tree or the young sucker roots of the wild rose, and other wild food which is harmless. But be careful if you are searching for wild food. It needs special attention: always be sure your children learn from someone who is really knowledgeable in country ways.

IN THE CAR

Every year ten thousand children are injured and seventy-five killed while travelling in cars. To safeguard children, provide them with the appropriate seat or harness for their age. Babies under one year old should be in a carrycot held secure by straps attached to the rear seat of the car. Young children between approximately nine months and four and a half years should be belted into a special safety seat in the back of the car. Children of school age should sit in child harnesses in the back of the car.

Never let a child travel in the front of a car. Even if you are wearing a seat belt yourself, it would be impossible to protect a baby in a crash if you were carrying the infant in your arms in the front seat. It is now illegal to travel in the front seat without wearing seat belts (unless receiving medical dispensation) and it is always preferable for a child to use safety systems designed for their size and weight rather than adapt to adult systems. So the safest place for a child is undoubtedly in the back seat with the appropriate child restraints. (One side-benefit of these restraints, especially the car seats for toddlers, is that by enabling a child to see out of the window they reduce the chances of travel sickness.)

ON THE ROAD

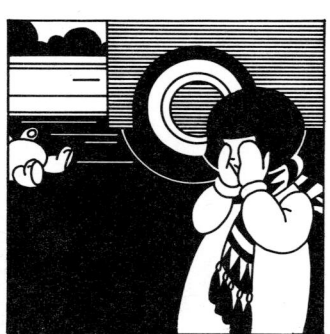

Parents often greatly underestimate the difficulties children have in learning to cross the road safely. Children under seven years old, and many older children, cannot be expected to be able to deal with all the circumstances which may arise when crossing a road. Children under five may not be able to fasten their coat buttons and talk at the same time – they need all their concentration to do one task. Older children often have the same problem when faced with crossing the road. Dr Stina Sandels, director of the Institute for Child Development Research in Stockholm, and a leading authority on children and traffic, says, 'We have seen six to seven year olds who are unable to cross the road and watch out at the same time but who instead try to look first and then walk.' Young children are not able to divide their attention.

The flow of traffic is variable and may change suddenly so that it becomes extremely difficult for children to follow what is happening and deduce when it is safe to cross. Adults generally find it safest to cross the road at junctions. However, Dr Sandels's research has found that children often find it more confusing at junctions, and prefer to cross on straight stretches. The situation at road junctions is too complicated for children's understanding of traffic, and they seem to realize it. Children only see the traffic from their own egocentric point of view, and do not usually learn to understand what a driver may do next until they are teenagers.

The basic problem children have, according to Dr Sandels, is developing insight into what is happening on the road. They do not see the quick glance to right and left which adults make, so they cannot imitate it. They are too small to look over the tops of cars and grasp the traffic situation. Most children are naturally cautious of dangers they are able to appreciate, but they must be taught to appreciate the special dangers of traffic.

Children must be taught much more than just how to cross the road. They should be taught from an early age never to play in traffic areas such as car parks, garage exits, pavements of busy roads or streets. They must be taught not to play beside cars and never to hang on to moving vehicles.

Point out to children the features of traffic which are important. Get them to look at cars which are near and distant, approaching and receding, and at the same time to listen to the noise they make. Point out traffic-lights and explain what they do.

Always walk beside your children when crossing the road. Never call to a child to cross the road, but cross over to the child. If you drop a child off from a car, put the child down on the side where the child is going. Teach your children to walk on the inside of the pavement, so that they do not stumble into the gutter with the chance of hitting a passing car.

Teach your children the Green Cross Code, which has now replaced the old-fashioned kerb drill:

A. First find a safe place to cross.
B. Stand on the pavement near the kerb.
C. Look all round for traffic and listen.
D. If traffic is coming, let it pass. Look all round again.
E. When there is no traffic near, walk straight across the road.
F. Keep looking and listening for traffic while you cross.

Also teach them to choose a place where drivers can see them. Or in crowded parking conditions to check first that there is no one at the wheel of the cars they must pass between, and then to walk out until they can see if anything is coming.

If your children must come home from school in the dark, provide them with reflective material on their coats or reflective discs which hang from coat pockets and advise them to pull down their hoods (if they wear them) when crossing the road, so that they can see properly. Tell them that policemen will always help them to cross the road. Never threaten them with the police, which will destroy their confidence in seeking help in traffic.

The problems posed by traffic are intensified when cycling. Not only do you require knowledge of traffic but also the ability to handle a bike safely. As a general rule, children under the age of nine should never be allowed out on the road alone. Make sure a child has the right size bike and that it is adjusted and maintained properly. Go cycling with your children so that they can learn from you the techniques of passing parked cars, navigating roundabouts or traffic junctions and hand signals. Teach children to ride in single file; encourage your child to go in for the cycling proficiency test; and teach young children to watch out for people when cycling on pavements. And remember, when driving, that children need extra care and caution: give them extra room when passing and be careful when opening doors. Give them the help you would like others to give your children.

IN THE WATER

Water is fun – but it is also dangerous. A baby can drown in very shallow water (even a bath) and every year children drown in places like canals, ponds, swimming pools and the sea. Adults are vulnerable, too. In all, about a thousand people drown each year in Britain – most of them in inland waters or close to the shore.

At the waterside keep an eye on young children all the time. Make sure they wear inflatable arm bands. Don't let them play by themselves with inflatable dinghies or mattresses since these can be swept out to sea by the tide. If older children want to learn canoeing or other water sports,

ACCIDENTS/**PREGNANCY AND CHILDHOOD**

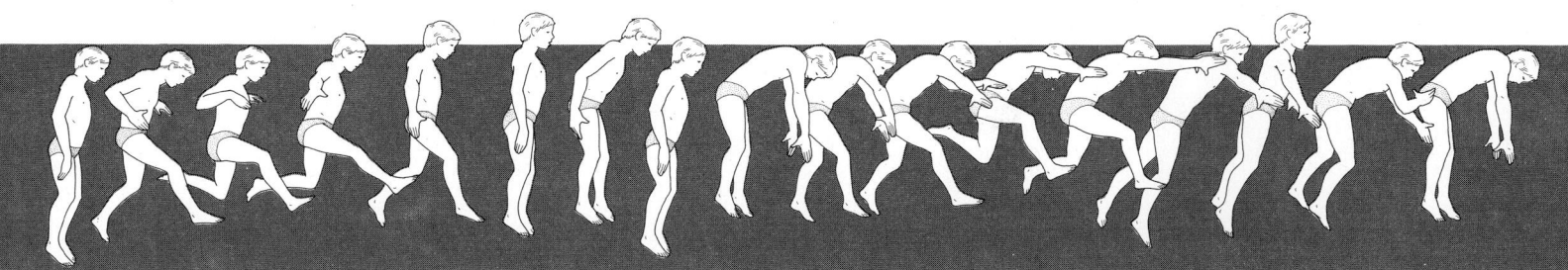

High-buoyancy float: Hold your breath under water only as long as is comfortable, then breathe out steadily through your nose as you follow the arm and leg movements to raise your head out of the water. The arms come up the body, out to the sides and down, and the legs make a simultaneous scissor movement. As the mouth clears the surface of the water, take a quick breath (only one or the rhythm will be lost) and then let your body sink back to the vertical rest position, moving your arms away from your body slightly to stabilize yourself and ensure that you don't sink too fast. Repeat as you like, but *don't* leave it to the last moment before taking a breath.

Low-buoyancy float: Everyone should try to master both techniques before concentrating on the one which feels most comfortable, but this is perhaps the easiest and most relaxing. The body hangs over in the water, arms and legs hanging vertically and neck completely relaxed. To take a breath, cross your arms in front of your body and then sweep them round in a leisurely wide arc, rather like a breast stroke. This, combined with a scissor movement with the legs and breathing out steadily through the nose, lifts the head out of the water. Take a quick breath, then allow the body to return to hanging position. Keep all movement relaxed and slow.

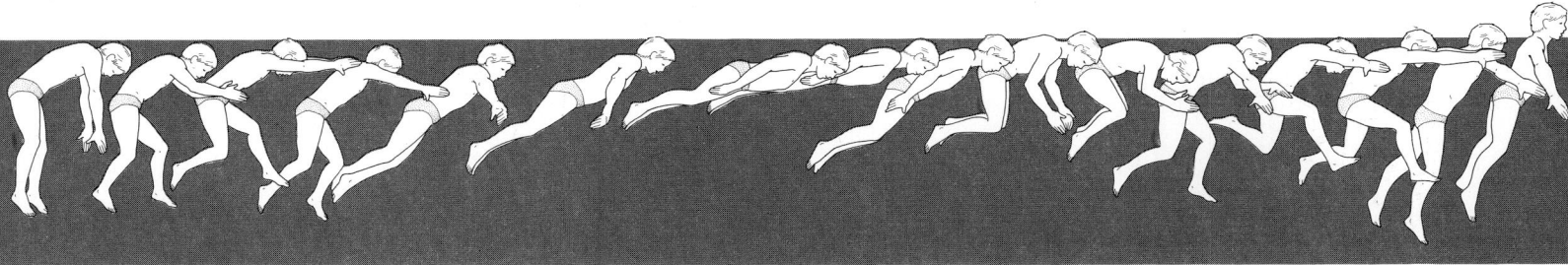

Travel stroke: The high- and low-buoyancy-float positions may be very relaxing but they won't actually get you anywhere. It is possible, however, to incorporate the positions with a travel stroke as shown above, in this case using the low-buoyancy float with the travel stroke. Take up the low-buoyancy position. When you have set up a rhythm of breathing and hanging, start the travel stroke. After taking a breath, instead of relaxing completely, keep your head down and perform a slow breast-stroke arm movement and a scissor kick with the legs, pulling your body horizontally through the water. As you finish the movements, let your body continue horizontally for as far as possible, keeping hands by your sides and feet together. As you slow down and need to take a breath, bring your legs down to the vertical position and your arms across the body to perform the arm movement and scissor kick needed to bring your head out of the water so you can get a breath. Repeat as necessary.
Note: In America it is sometimes claimed that 90 per cent of drownings could be avoided if people knew these techniques. That is not accepted in Britain, and it would be unwise to regard bobbing as a substitute for the many other excellent safety measures that are taught. People in boats or canoes should always wear life-jackets.

be sure they wear life-jackets. But be sure, too, that they can swim. One unfortunate casualty of local authority spending cuts has often been swimming lessons, but it is still usually possible to find lessons available at swimming pools.

If you do get into difficulty, try not to panic. Thrashing about usually makes matters worse. The technique shown in the illustrations is known in America as 'drown-proofing', although this is perhaps too optimistic in its implication. It cannot be guaranteed to save you, especially in the cold waters of the North Sea, but it will give you more confidence if you do get into difficulty, and conserve your energy while you wait for help or swim slowly to the shore.

'Drown-proofing' or 'bobbing' uses very little energy and in warm water you can bob confidently for an hour or more. When instructors first tested the technique in Britain, they were unsure what length of time to set for exam certificates, so they told children to continue for as long as they could. Some dropped out after an hour; others went on all day, being fed from the side of a pool. After fourteen hours they were called out. To find your buoyancy level, hold your breath and sink gently in a vertical position. Highly buoyant people will float with the water level between nose and chin; the less buoyant will find the level at their foreheads.

2: EXERCISE

The Joys of Fitness

Fitness is good for you. There are few other statements about our health which can be made with equal certainty. So why is unfitness an increasing problem in Western countries? To a considerable degree it is a direct result of our way of life. We ride to work in cars, buses or trains; we use escalators or lifts rather than stairs; we sit down most of the day not only in offices but on many factory production-lines; we rely more and more on mechanization and automation; most of us cease to play any sport when we leave school; we spend more time watching television than on any other leisure activity; and too often the walking, gardening and do-it-yourself work around the house we do cannot make up for it. No wonder so many of us are so unfit.

Unfitness is easier to recognize than fitness is to define. However, organic fitness is generally taken to mean a body free from disease and infirmity – in other words, basic health – while dynamic fitness is the ability to move vigorously and live energetically. Dynamic fitness, to which this chapter is devoted, has several components: the efficiency of heart circulation, muscular strength and endurance, balance, flexibility, co-ordination and agility.

WHY FITNESS MATTERS:
TEN BENEFITS OF REGULAR AND ADEQUATE EXERCISE

The people most in need of exercise tend to be those who least feel like taking it. Yet there are clear physiological benefits to strengthen the resolve.

We list below ten benefits of regular and adequate exercise that have been observed and established with various degrees of certainty, although individuals differ in response within each category of benefit. They illustrate the message that exercise should be taken for its own sake because it is beneficial and makes sense in itself, quite apart from any possibility of the prevention of a heart attack. 'Regular adequate exercise' is described in detail on page 46.

1. Exercise is of general benefit because it helps maintain the cardiovascular system, muscles and joints in good working order. Moderate physical demands can therefore be met without excessive physical effort so that activities are not limited by an unnecessarily low physical condition.
2. The 'training effects' of vigorous aerobic exercise (also known as large-muscle, dynamic activity, see pages 46–52) are greater efficiency of circulation, particularly in the heart and working muscles, and of oxygen transport and use around the body. Less effort is required of heart and lungs to provide the muscles with oxygen. Exercise improves blood-supply of the heart muscle itself and of the peripheral muscles. Higher levels of physical activity have been shown to be strongly associated with a lower incidence of coronary heart disease; regular vigorous exercise may therefore reduce the likelihood of death or disability due to heart attack.
3. More generally, physical activity increases muscle strength, the strength of joints, their flexibility and mobility, the strength of tendons and muscle attachments. The improved strength of the postural muscles may also help to prevent or ease low back pain (see pages 106–12 for more about back pain).
4. This all contributes to greater physical endurance and less fatigue. Increased physical capacity enables an individual not only to accomplish daily tasks more comfortably but also to extend their range of activities. The quality of life can thus be enriched and the sense of well-being enhanced.
5. Exercise involves the expenditure of calories and thus counteracts obesity. The stimulating effect of regular exercise on the metabolism may lead to even greater weight-loss.
6. Exercise improves a wide range of physiological functions, e.g. lowering the level of blood-fats, of triglycerides, and more doubtfully of cholesterol; it raises the level of protective high-density 'lipoproteins'.
7. Physical activity helps to counteract stress and channel aggressive drives. For many people it also helps with sleep.
8. Exercise improves posture, appearance, self-image.
9. Mild hypertension (high blood pressure) may also be reduced by regular exercise.
10. The general benefits of exercise are particularly important as a preparation for a healthy retirement and for those already in their later years. The physical capacity of elderly people can be improved with training, despite the decline of some muscular systems. Fitness in old age can help avoid or delay the need for institutional care which causes too much anguish to individuals and families (as well as cost to the state).

Actress Bo Derek (opposite), star of *10*, and Tarzan's Jane of the 1980s, scores top marks as she jogs for fitness as well as beauty

*This section does not cover exercise for children or the elderly, since this is discussed in Chapters 1 and 10.

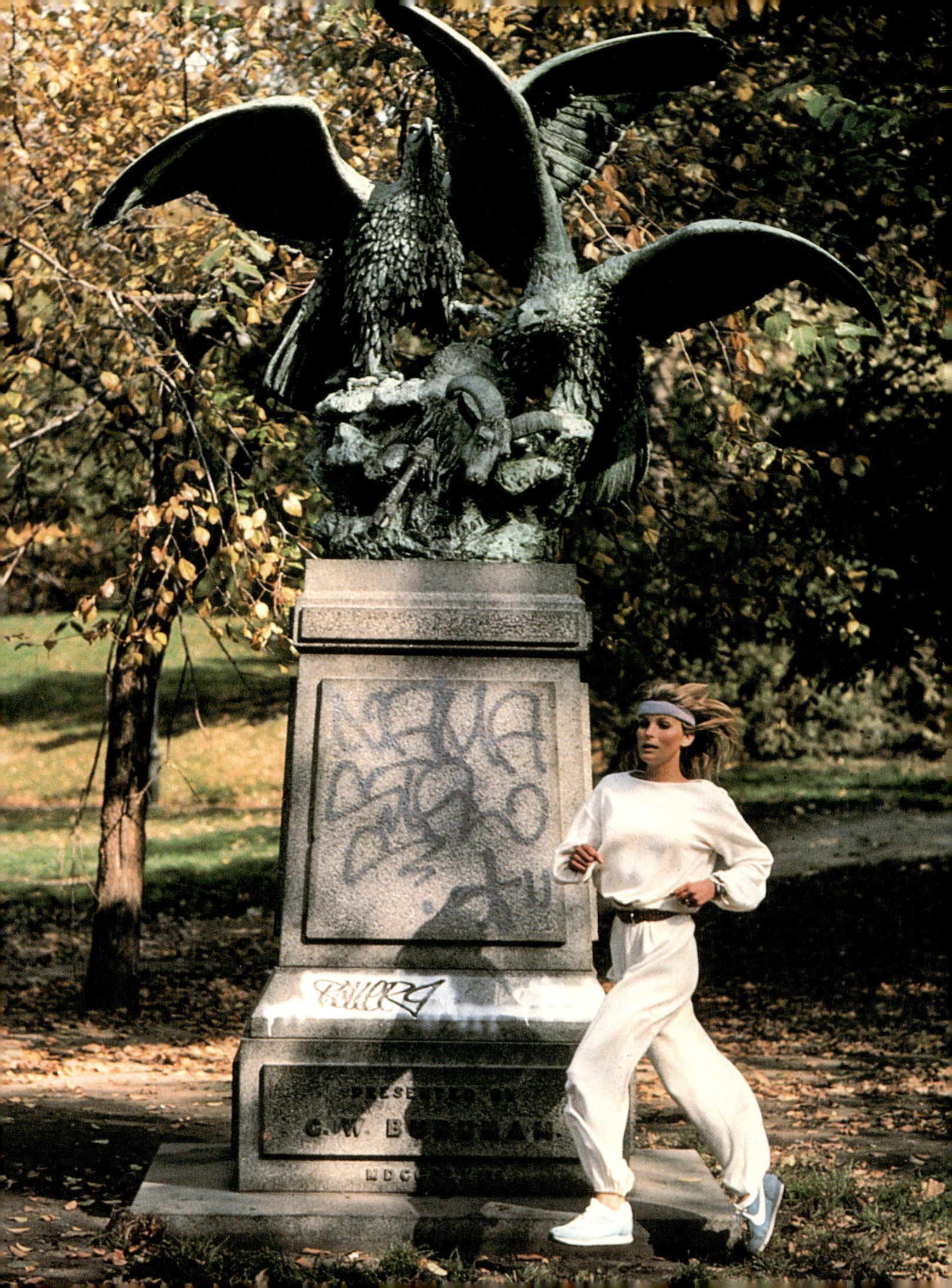

EXERCISE/THE JOYS OF FITNESS

LIVING LONGER
Exercise is no elixir of life. Fitness can guarantee neither good health nor a long life, but it does make both more likely. Life is prolonged primarily through the effect of dynamic exercise on the heart and circulation. There is the secondary effect of helping to reduce weight and this, too, may ultimately benefit the heart. The consequences of inactivity are that the body deteriorates as the key organs weaken. It is *unfitness*, therefore, that shortens life.

Heart disease is the biggest single killer illness in the Western world. In Britain it is responsible for a third of all deaths in men under seventy. Anything that can lessen the chance of such heart disease, therefore, has a dramatic effect on the prospects for life and health. Numerous research projects have now shown that people in light or sedentary jobs are more likely to suffer and die from coronary heart disease than people in jobs involving substantial physical activity. Other surveys have since indicated that exercise in leisure time may help to achieve the same beneficial effect as a physically active job.

One of the most significant surveys has been undertaken by Professor J. N. Morris, of the University of London and Britain's Medical Research Council. This studied the daily lives of almost eighteen thousand British civil servants engaged in sedentary or very light work between the years 1968 and 1970. The survey sampled the physical activity undertaken in their spare time, and the results suggest that people taking vigorous exercise are significantly less likely to suffer from coronary heart disease. By 'vigorous exercise' Professor Morris meant high-energy exercise equivalent potentially to heavy industrial work. The form of the exercise in practice varied from swimming and hill-climbing to brisk walking and heavy gardening.

LIVING BETTER
For many people the fact that they enjoy exercise and feel the better for it, plus (if they think of it) the possibility of a longer life, will be reason enough for exercise. There are other benefits than longevity, however.

Losing weight: Most people calculate how far you have to walk to lose ten pounds and conclude that exercise cannot help much in slimming. But nobody becomes fat overnight, so it is unrealistic to expect to become slim overnight. In fact recent research which has included exercise as well as dietary measures in weight-control programmes, plus the results of studies of metabolic consequences of exercise for overweight people, suggests that exercise should now be regarded as an integral part of programmes to counter obesity. The increased energy expended during a two-mile walk, for instance, may be small, but in the long-term it is highly significant if it becomes a daily habit. The effect of exercise on the metabolism has now been shown to be even greater, since it seems that exercise raises the metabolic rate and leads to the loss of far more weight than would have been predicted for the actual exercise undertaken. Thus a previously inactive person walking an extra four miles a day, even at the slow pace of two miles per hour, would lose twenty pounds over the year assuming no change in diet. Combining exercise with dieting is even more effective.

Gaining vigour: The effects of exercise on the heart, circulation and muscles mean that you will have more vigour. If you have to run for a bus, or walk briskly, or climb some stairs, you are not so likely to get out of breath. You will be less tired at the end of a normal day. You will have energy left over to undertake fresh activities. You will be more lively, and life will seem more fun. These are subjective feelings, but they are none the less real for many people, and thus the greatest incentive of all of physical fitness. The improved flow of blood to the skin tones it up, so you may *look* better, too.

Coping with stress: Healthiness in body traditionally has been associated with healthiness in mind. It sounds like puritan propaganda but greater vigour does enable people to accomplish their daily tasks with less strain. Many people also report sleeping better at night if exercising regularly. This contributes to a calmness or psychological resilience in the face of stress which is difficult to measure but which is generally reckoned by doctors to be one of the greatest benefits of physical fitness. It is also possible that physical activity is a way of channelling aggressive drives.

TYPES OF EXERCISE
The two broad types of exercise are *isometric* and *dynamic* exercise. Isometric exercise involves substantial muscle contraction without any body movement – for instance, weight-lifting; dynamic exercise is repeated muscle contraction achieved through movement. Isometric exercises are useful for developing the strength of particular muscle groups, although they are not recommended for people suffering from heart disease or high blood pressure. It is dynamic exercise which most improves general physical fitness and health and may protect against heart disease.

Dynamic exercise offers many routes to fitness. We will look at three broad approaches to dynamic exercise: aerobic activities, such as running; indoor exercises; and sport. What they have in common is that each involves some degree of body movement. Each type of exercise has its advantages, but aerobic exercise is the most important component in any fitness programme because it improves muscular efficiency – and the heart is the most important muscle of all. Aerobic or cardiovascular exercise means sustained rhythmic activity that involves large muscle groups (particularly the legs) and increases the amount of oxygen processed by the body in a given time. Thus working muscles are made more efficient, the pulse rate lowered and heart disease is less likely. (Nutrition, smoking and stress are also associated with heart disease, however, as we discuss elsewhere in this book.)

While it is therefore important to incorporate some form of aerobic activity in any exercise programme, it is also essential to find an activity that you enjoy. Otherwise you are unlikely to practise it sufficiently regularly to achieve its potential benefits. Whatever activity is pursued, do not neglect the possibilities for improved fitness through simple changes in your everyday life. Putting more effort into your gardening, using stairs rather than lifts and, above all, walking can significantly improve overall fitness. Increased walking often provides the essential first step in any fitness programme for a previously inactive person and is particularly suitable for older people.

WHO CAN EXERCISE?
Pretty well anyone can get fitter. Neither a late start nor a low starting-point will completely deny the benefits of physical fitness. Indeed, a low base offers most individuals a greater potential for improvement. You may never run a

THE JOYS OF FITNESS/EXERCISE

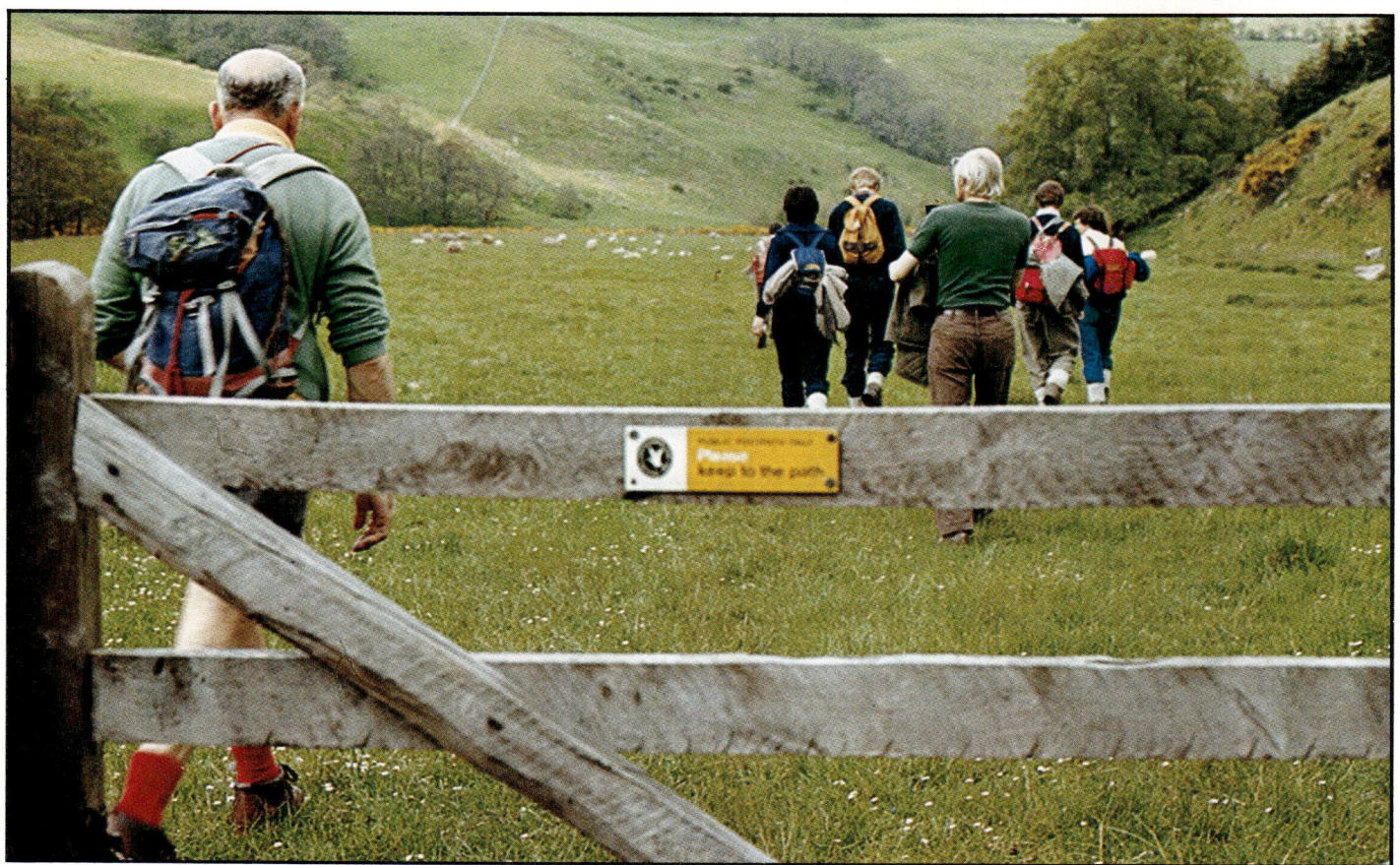

Walking: a route to fitness that is accessible to all ages and may be enjoyed in beautiful surroundings

four- or five-minute mile, but what matters is coming close to your own body's potential. Exercise is necessary to prevent physical atrophy. In other words, the long-term health hazards of *not* exercising exceed the short-term risks associated with a planned fitness programme. But before starting a fitness programme you should be sensible and satisfy yourself that, although out of condition and unfit, the exercise will not cause you undue distress. Do you need a medical examination? This is what the Royal College of Physicians and the British Cardiac Society say:

Most people do not need a medical examination before starting an exercising programme. There are no risks in regular dynamic exercise as long as the programme begins gently and only gradually increases in vigour. Older persons, the obese, and those with a history of cardiovascular disease or symptoms, should first consult their doctor. Those who develop unexpected symptoms during exercise (like getting too easily out of breath, for example, or dizziness or palpitations) should also seek medical advice.

This is an essentially reassuring message so long as people follow the advice to begin gently and only gradually increase the vigour of an exercise programme. But it does no harm to be more specific in interpreting such generalized advice. It is therefore sensible to consult your doctor about exercise if:

*you are over forty-five and have been inactive
*you are overweight (see pages 88–105)
*you have ever had high blood pressure or heart trouble
*you suffer from back or joint pains
*you have chest trouble such as asthma or bronchitis
*you are recovering from an illness or operation.

Some American authors have devised elaborate self-testing methods for assessing fitness which involve either monitoring the pulse rate after exercise or measuring the distance covered in set times. These have come under criticism from several leading British physiologists who argue that these are not only too discouraging but too demanding for people who have not taken any physical exercise for twenty years or more. However, some simple tests can be useful – if only to convince people that they are not as fit as they like to imagine! See page 48 for two such tests.

To sum up: always take exercise cautiously, especially at first, and only gradually increase its intensity. But do not confuse sensible caution with steering clear of exercise altogether. Even ailing bodies can be strengthened by careful, progressive exercise. Be patient: do not expect miracles overnight. Aching limbs will precede radiant health, but if you persist you will soon feel better. Some people like to set themselves targets, but unfit people should beware of pushing themselves too hard. You should, for instance, be able to talk when taking exercise such as jogging. It does not have to hurt to do you good; simply walking more often is a start on the road to fitness.

WHEN TO EXERCISE

Sometimes the form of the exercise dictates the time you can practise it. Many sports, for instance, cannot be pursued at night. But the only times not to exercise vigorously are when you are ill or in the hour or so after a meal. Whatever generations of army physical instructors may say, there is no medical merit in the early dawn. Exercise at the time of day that best suits you.

Health checks

The health check is a standard element in the American way of medicine. An electrocardiogram (ECG) test on the heart has come to be a routine precursor to exercise for middle-aged Americans. Most British doctors think such checks are necessary only for people over fifty or with a history of cardiovascular trouble. Nevertheless, the demand for screening tests is steadily growing in Britain, although expense restricts them largely to the private sector of health care.

If everyone was observant about changes in their health and did not hesitate to ask their own doctor when they were worried about something, health screening checks would not be necessary. Usually nothing can be found to be wrong, and after screening a person can go away with relief of their immediate anxiety. Nevertheless, among those who are screened there is more undiagnosed disease than might be expected, although most of it is minor. Screening services can also identify those people who are at high risk of developing certain diseases, particularly those caused by smoking and excessive drinking, and give precautionary advice.

Screening has, however, been criticized because disease often cannot be detected by scientific tests before a person has noticed symptoms themselves. And even when disease is detected early it is not always possible to do anything to prevent it from worsening.

The most important part of a check-up, when you talk to the doctor about your health and he asks you questions, is your previous history. More than 50 per cent of internal illnesses are picked up by doctors on the basis of the history alone, 20 per cent are picked up by physical examination and the remainder by laboratory tests.

Choose a doctor or clinic which is prepared to spend time with you. A thorough check-up should take about an hour. Some of the tests may be done by nurse practitioners, but the final physical examination and interview should be with a doctor. Tell the doctor anything which is worrying you, even if you are afraid he may think it is silly.

The most valuable tests are for high blood pressure, certain hearing and vision defects and perhaps cancer of the cervix of breast (see pages 142–6). Testing of people over sixty for hearing and vision, poor nutrition and difficulty in walking is especially worthwhile.

Ears.

Almost 50 per cent of men and women over sixty-five are deaf to some degree. In a proportion, this can be cured by simply syringeing the ears to remove wax. For others, specialist advice, an operation or hearing aids can improve hearing and bring a new interest in life. The screening of old people, and of people in noisy jobs, for deafness is badly needed; in older people deafness is as common as poor sight.

Heart.

Electrocardiograms (ECGs) sensitively record every beat of the heart and if it misses a beat, or a beat is irregular, then the machine records it. Even so, between 25 and 50 per cent of those who suffer from angina – an early symptom of heart disease – have normal ECGs. Although some heart disease can be detected it is not possible even with the most elaborate tests to be certain that someone's heart is in good condition. And it is not until heart disease has progressed a long way that it can be detected by screening tests. This is

Eyes.

If you cannot read a number plate at twenty-five yards, or a telephone directory at nineteen inches, you may need glasses. Anyone who has reached the age of forty-five without needing glasses should get their eyes checked, because sight fails increasingly with age. Check-ups every two or three years afterwards are advisable.

One in ten blind people have lost their vision as a result of *glaucoma*, a disease which causes a rise of pressure in the eyeball. The increased pressure flattens the small blood-vessels in the back of the eye, cutting off the blood-supply to the light-sensitive retina which then dies. People who have a relative who has suffered from glaucoma, and people over fifty-five are most at risk of getting the disease.

Glaucoma can be treated effectively if caught early before too much damage is done. Danger symptoms include the following: pain in the eye; occasional bouts of blurred vision occurring in dull light, large rainbow rings round a clear bright light, and loss of the ability to see an object, at the edge of the field of vision, which is not being looked at directly. If you have these symptoms seek an early eye examination.

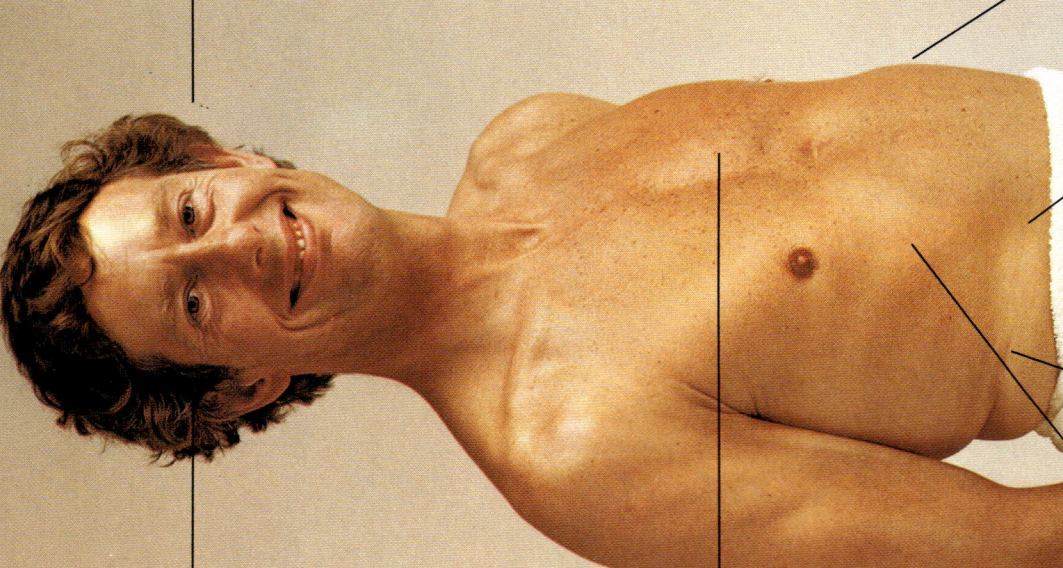

Weight.

Being overweight is the easiest condition to screen for since it simply means weighing someone. It is associated with an increased risk of death from diabetes, blood-vessel disease, stroke, pneumonia and diseases of the digestive system. More details on all these problems can be found elsewhere in this book.

Blood pressure.

A few people who suffer high blood pressure complain of headaches, dizziness or palpitations but most complain of no symptoms, so the condition is not likely to be discovered unless someone has their blood pressure measured. High blood pressure has serious consequences if left untreated, and so screening for blood pressure is the most rewarding of all the standard health checks. (See Chapter 6 for further details of how to avoid and treat high blood pressure.)

Urine.

Tests may detect kidney disease, diabetes or infection. However, kidney disease is not commonly enough detected to make the test useful for health screening. A test for sugar in the urine may provide a useful early warning of diabetes, but the disease cannot always be treated effectively until it progresses to the point where the patient begins to be bothered by other symptoms which would bring him to consult a doctor.

Women's problems.

Annual health checks are often regarded as a largely male preserve. This is not in fact so. Most private organizations offering such services welcome female as well as male customers. And there are some tests which are only applicable for women, of course, most notably the highly desirable checks for cancer of the cervix and breast, subjects covered in Chapter 6.

Lungs.

Mass radiography has proved useful in detecting tuberculosis, but so far has not proved useful in detecting lung cancer. By the time a lung cancer is detectable on an X-ray it is usually so large that the chances of effective treatment are no better than they are for people whose cancers are picked up in the normal way by their own doctor. Dr Victor Hawthorne of Glasgow University picked up about 200 lung cancers out of nearly a million people X-rayed. Despite being picked up early they did no better than other lung cancer patients.

But a newly established test of lung volume pioneered by Professor Charles Fletcher at Hammersmith Hospital, London, can detect early lung damage which is the first stage in the development of chronic bronchitis. This test could be used as part of a campaign to persuade people not to smoke. However, identifying the people at risk – smokers – is not the problem. The problem is to persuade them to give the habit up.

Liver.

Blood-tests may detect early liver disease. The most frequent cause is drinking too much alcohol; a new test can pick up early damage to the liver and indicate those people who are drinking more than they should.

Rectum.

Bleeding from the rectum is often neglected because people blame it on piles. Bleeding from the rectum should always be investigated because it can also be a sign of rectal cancer. Rectal cancer has excellent prospects of cure if caught early. Piles should in any case be treated, because if neglected they can cause anaemia simply through persistent loss of blood. Tests are also available for hidden blood in the stools, which may be a sign of cancer higher up the bowel. However, these tests are not yet considered sufficiently reliable for use on people who have no symptoms. In older people any major changes in bowel habit should be reported to the doctor.

Aerobic Exercise

The term 'aerobics' was invented by an American fitness expert called Dr Kenneth Cooper, who as much as anyone else is responsible for the jogging craze. It is christened 'aerobic' because it is exercise which needs a lot of air, or rather oxygen. Not only needs it, as indeed one needs oxygen all the time, but demands it as a matter of urgency, requiring possibly more than the body can get. It might have been better to call it cardiovascular exercise since this is the area of its effect, but aerobic is the name which caught the public imagination.

Aerobic exercise is the jogger running one or two miles at sustained speed, rather than the sprinter who runs a hundred metres – a task achieved on his body's store of oxygen and energy. Aerobic exercise has three characteristics:

1. It must involve large muscle groups of the body, such as the legs, in rhythmic contractions.
2. It must be performed continuously for at least twenty minutes.
3. It must be vigorous enough to engage the whole body.

During such rhythmic, sustained and vigorous exercise your pulse rate and breathing will be more rapid, because you are using oxygen at a faster rate to supply the hard-working muscles.

The ultimate consequence of this training effect is to improve the efficiency of the cardiovascular system and working muscles, thus strengthening the heart, improving the circulation and increasing the muscles' ability to utilize oxygen.

To achieve this training effect it is generally agreed that 'regular and adequate exercise' means exercise at least three times a week for between twenty and thirty minutes. It also raises the heartbeat or pulse rate to around 70 per cent of its maximum.

The easiest place to count your pulse or heart rate is the radial artery in the wrist. Turn your palm to face you, move your second and third finger along the thumb side of your wrist until you feel a steady pulsation, then count the number of pulsations.

It is also simple enough to work out your 'pulse rate goal'. The maximum individual heart rate declines steadily with age from about 200 at twenty years of age to 160 at sixty – sex differences are less important. The much-respected US Stanford University Heart Disease Prevention Program thus suggests these pulse-rate goals:

Age 20–29: 138–142 beats per minute
Age 30–39: 130–134 beats per minute
Age 40–49: 122–126 beats per minute
Age 50–59: 113–117 beats per minute
Age 60–69: 105–109 beats per minute

But pulse rate goals or targets should not be interpreted so zealously that exercise loses its sense of enjoyment. Similarly the amount of exercise needed by individuals will vary. If obesity is a problem, as well as general unfitness, it

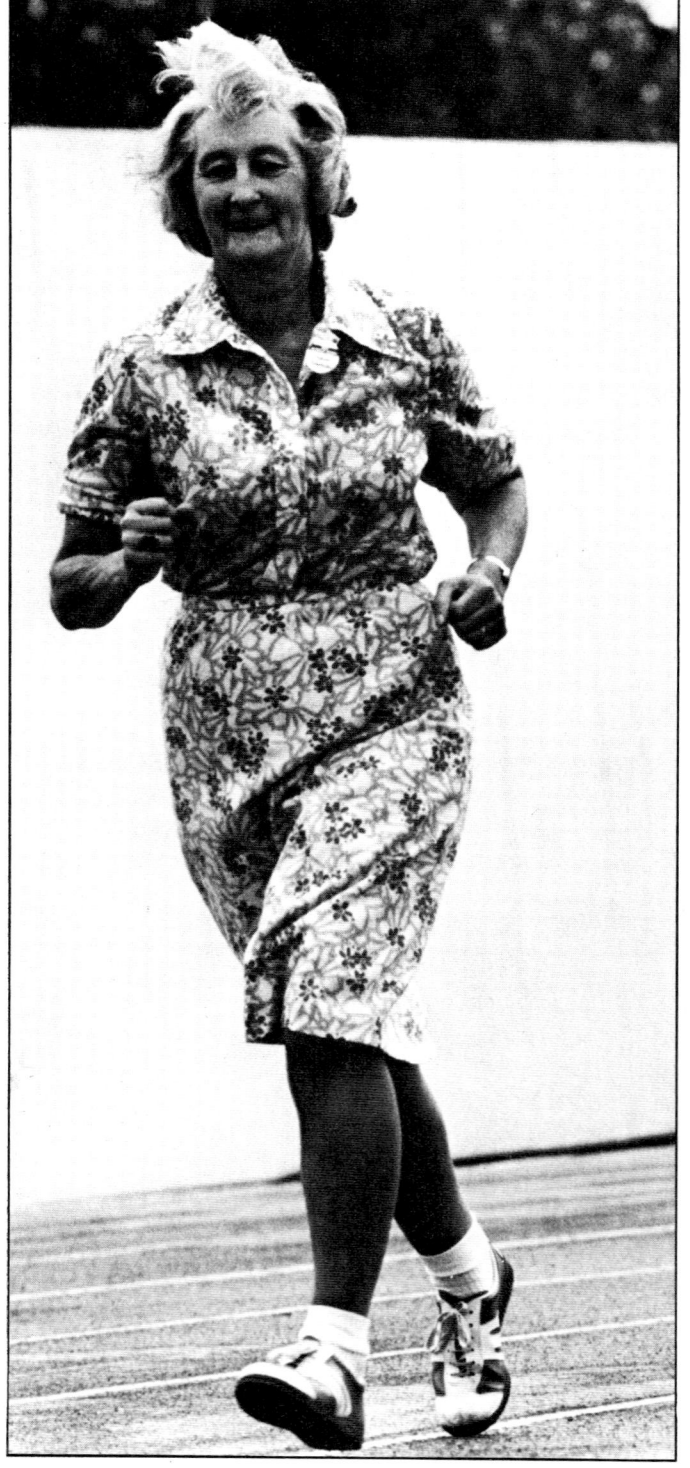

is likely that some form of exercise will be required more frequently than three times a week.

As an example of how ordinary people can take up 'vigorous' or aerobic exercise and as a demonstration of improved efficiency and well-being, we offer two case histories from a dozen middle-aged people whom we tested over a nine-month period which began and ended with tests on a treadmill ECG (electrocardiogram).

Sylvia Baynham
Aged fifty-seven when tested, housewife and part-time library assistant. After raising a family she 'had taken no real exercise for twenty-five years. I had never felt *un*-fit',

but walking up stairs was hard work and she was aware that flab meant she was a bit overweight. On the initial treadmill ECG test she accomplished the fourth of a maximum seven stages. The ECG showed some irregularity, so she started a modified fitness programme. Within three months, the irregularity of the ECG pattern had been abolished and her exercises no longer needed to be restricted:

I'll always remember that first time on the treadmill, the last couple of minutes were agony – and I only got to stage four! So I was delighted that on my second session I reached the same stage without too much effort, and this accomplished just by running up and down stairs each day. I chose this method of exercise because I hate the cold, and the thought of going for a walk or run in the winter just meant I would never exercise. Now, I can exercise whenever I have fifteen minutes to spare without changing into special clothes.

The stair-climbing routine consists of choosing a flight of ten stairs (in her case, ten of a flight of thirteen) and going up them five times to a minute, i.e., five times up, five times down. A doddle, perhaps, for just one minute, but fairly demanding when it involves – as it soon did for Mrs Baynham – fifty flights in ten minutes:

People have asked me if I get bored, and ask what I think about. In fact I don't really have much time to think, I'm too busy counting my trips, and as to being bored – well, surely if it is boring, it's worth it for such a short time to get fit. I'm glad I started exercising, for I am now fitter, I walk better and I don't get out of breath so quickly. Psychologically it has also done me good; I was the oldest of the group by about six years and, having stayed the course, this has done wonders for my morale.

Alan Thurgood
Aged forty-two when tested, businessman. Until five years previously, he had taken regular exercise and was once 'ridiculously fit'. As a competitor in orienteering, he remembered that 'when fresh, one found the check-points more easily'. For a business executive like himself, he reasoned, this must indicate that physical fitness enhances mental efficiency. Mr Thurgood, described by the officiating doctor as 'well motivated' – despite being overweight at nearly 200 pounds – did well in the treadmill test to accomplish the maximum stage, number seven.

Running became his principal form of exercise. At his holiday cottage near the coast, a round of golf was either preceded or followed by some running. Other people might not wish to chain themselves to time-and-distance goals, but Alan Thurgood is evidently one of the variety for whom this is the only way to take exercise:

I need motivation and incentive. Initially it was very encouraging to see the medical results, which were good, but then I had to set other incentives. This I did by planning a new circuit each month, immediately running it very hard and setting a time; then having as my objective to run it in the same time with reasonable ease by the end of the month. New circuits are one way to avoid boredom. Another way is to have company, and chat. Or to have a race with the other fellow, with handicaps. Above all, to make it enjoyable you have to make it a habit; if you're doing it regularly it's enjoyable, less often and it's hard work.

By the end of the programme Alan Thurgood was, he says, enjoying his cigars and his beer more; and he had lost weight (ten pounds) and was once again taking up orienteering and squash. His test figures indicated, according to

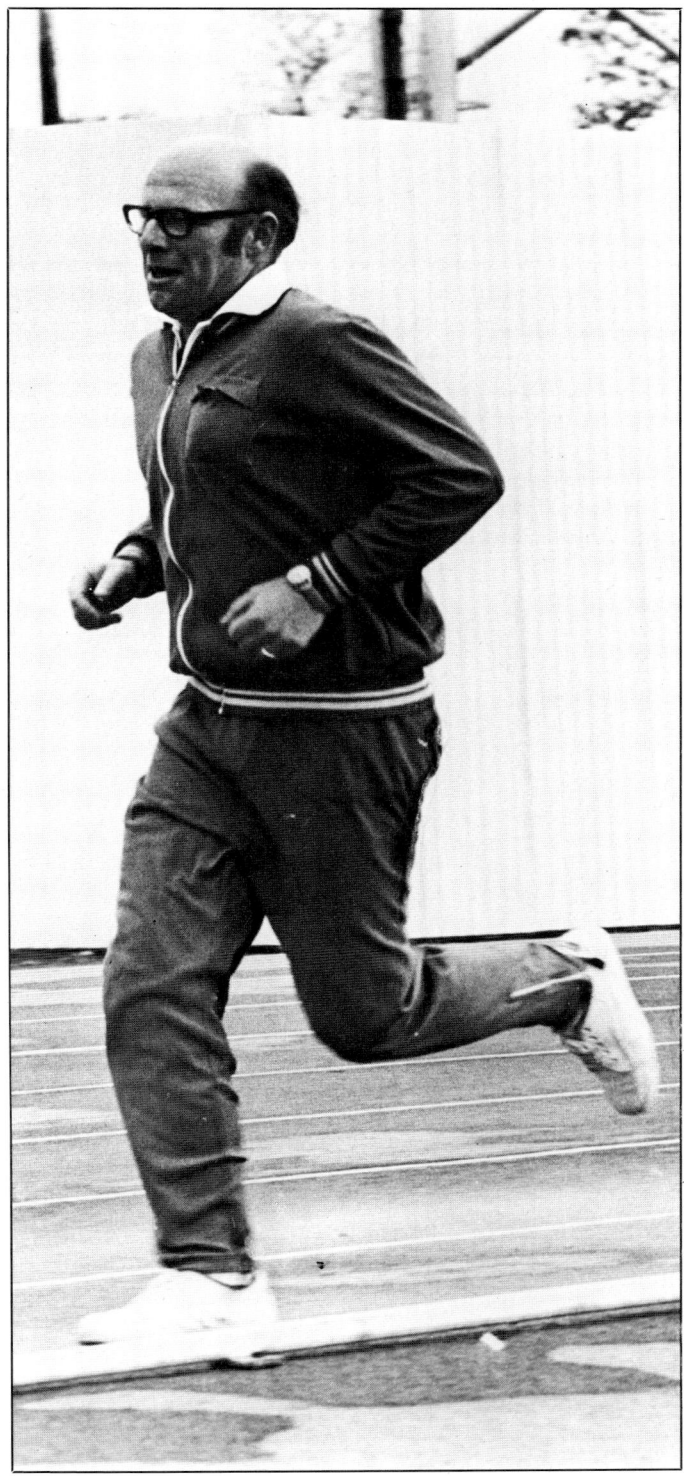

the doctor, 'the unmasking of a true athletic heart which had been starting to go to seed'.

The figures overleaf show the generally improved performance of these two candidates when, nine months after the first test, they exercised on the ECG treadmill to the same level they had initially achieved.

Improvement was achieved by all the twelve people whom we tested. Amongst all of them, heart rate at the highest exercise load averaged out at 160 in the first test, and in the second the average was 142. And the figures after one minute's recovery showed a drop from an average of 123 to an average of 94.

What this means is that all twelve people were, as a result

EXERCISE/AEROBIC EXERCISE

Heart-Rate: Beats/min	Sylvia Baynham		Alan Thurgood	
	Before	After	Before	After
At rest	77	82	64	40
During Exercise				
Stage 1	110	95	78	48
Stage 2	125	105	87	62
Stage 3	138	123	100	75
Stage 4	155	148	112	86
Stage 5	—	—	132	110
Stage 6	—	—	160	120
Stage 7	—	—	168	140
Recovery after Exercise				
Minutes 1	130	100	123	78
Minutes 3	92	80	98	55
Minutes 5	95	84	87	45
Weight (Kilos)	68.5	67.5	89.1	81.7

of the programme, doing the same exercise more economically at less stress. But this was not all. There were also interesting results in tests for the level of cholesterol, the substance which, in increased amounts, is associated with coronary heart disease. Some evidence for the effect of exercise seems to be indicated when all the candidates showed an obvious decrease in cholesterol level, almost invariably *without* any alteration to diet.

Additionally, there were of course the less tangible benefits connected with a sense of well-being, which all the subjects said they experienced. For example: 'I'm getting more value from sleep – even with less sleep, there's more benefit . . . I am at a period in my life which does tend to cause depression, and I've been feeling much less depressed, much more cheerful. . . . At the end of a long flight, I no longer suffer from the pilot's chronic complaint of backache. . . .'

The attractions of vigorous or aerobic exercise are that (a) improvements in fitness can be monitored; (b) activities can be pursued by individuals, unlike most competitive sports; (c) activities are intensive and therefore improve fitness quickly.

Simply taking your own pulse rate one and five minutes after exercise will give you an indication of improvement. Many people like or need this encouragement; people such as Alan Thurgood like to set themselves goals. And many like elaborately structured fitness programmes such as those offered by Dr Kenneth Cooper in his various aerobics books (see Appendix Three). Dr Cooper took the basic activities for individuals such as walking, running, swimming and cycling, and worked out point-scores according to the distance covered in different times. Choose whatever activity you like, do it as often or as little as you like, says Dr Cooper, just so long as you score 30 points a week for men or 24 points for women. This will mean that you will have exercised at sufficient intensity to have raised your pulse or heart rate to beneficial levels.

FITNESS TESTS

Before commencing any of the most popular aerobic activities you may wish to check your own fitness. As explained on page 43, most people will *not* require formal medical check-ups before starting an exercise programme. But here are two simple guides to your degree of fitness – or unfitness.

1. The walk test: If you can walk three miles comfortably (or alternately walk and run) in forty-five minutes, then you are fit enough to start running. If you can't pass the test, walk three miles a day until you can.

2. The step test: Step up and down briskly onto a chair or bench, alternating your leading foot. A fit person under fifty should be able to hold a conversation without being too short of breath after three minutes of stepping; a reasonably fit over-fifty-year-old should manage this after two minutes. (NB: always stop this test as soon as you feel too tired to go on.)

RUNNING

Running is the most natural form of aerobic exercise and the one which is generally regarded as the most beneficial. To run and not to raise the pulse rate is physically impossible. Jogging, which is basically slow running, may have begun as a fashionable craze but for vast numbers of people it has become a way of life. Not only do film stars and politicians do it but so do tens of thousands of men and women all over the country. A decade ago the city jogger would invariably attract stares and often supposedly witty comments; nowadays he (or, increasingly, she) is so commonplace a sight that nobody pays any attention. Fun runs have become family days out; marathons have become mass participation sports: nearly a hundred thousand people requested entry forms for the 1982 London marathon.

You do not need to run the 26 miles 385 yards of a marathon to gain the benefits of running, however. Three runs a week of around twenty minutes will be sufficient to achieve the cardiovascular improvement described earlier. Indeed, at the beginning, it is best to limit yourself to such a programme. Get used to the exercise gradually. As the muscles, joints and ligaments become accustomed to the exercise, they will be better able to handle more frequent or longer runs. Many people find it helps to run at a regular time of day but one of the reasons for running's popularity is that it is an individual sport. You can run at a time of day that suits yourself; you do not need special equipment; you do not require team-mates or opponents as in so many sports; and you do not need special coaching. The joy of jogging – subject to the safety precautions outlined on page 43 – is that virtually anyone can do it anywhere or any time.

Many, probably most, joggers are not people who were renowned athletes during schooldays. They begin running usually as a simple way of getting fit. The more they run, of course, the greater their stamina becomes and the greater the benefit to their heart and circulation. But what begins as a means to achieve greater fitness often becomes pleasurable in itself. What was once an effort of will-power (particularly in winter) becomes something to look forward to. You feel better mentally as well as physically, since running sheds tension as well as pounds. It is worth remembering this because the first steps after years of unfitness may not be so joyous. One consolation of unfitness is that the scope for improvement is greater, however. So remember that, too, as you get ready to run.

WHAT TO WEAR

One attraction of running is that it needs so little equipment. Track suits may look good and to the extent that they boost morale they may help. But they are not essential.

AEROBIC EXERCISE/EXERCISE

WARMING UP FOR A RUN
1. Stand facing a wall that is approximately three feet away. Lean forward and place palms of hands against the wall. Keep heels firmly on the floor and slowly bend elbows until you feel strain in the backs of the legs. Hold the position for twenty or thirty seconds. Repeat.
2. Lie on back with knees slightly bent, then sit up by tucking in the chin and curling the body up from the floor. Arms can be stretched out over the head or – what is more difficult – locked behind the head. Sit up fifteen times in order to strengthen stomach muscles.
3. Lie on back with legs straight and arms at sides. Keep legs together and lift them until they are over your head and parallel with the ground. Hold position for twenty seconds. Try and touch floor behind head with your toes if you can, but back sufferers should tackle this exercise with caution.
4. Stand arm's length from wall with left hand on wall for support. Grasp right ankle with right hand and pull foot back until the heel touches buttocks. Lean forward from waist as you lift. Hold for twenty to thirty seconds and then repeat exercise with other hand and foot.
5. Sit on floor with one leg extended straight ahead. The upper part of other leg should be at right angles to body, but the heel should be close to buttocks. Slowly slide hands down extended leg and touch foot. Hold position for twenty to thirty seconds, then slowly lean back and rest elbows on floor. Repeat with other leg extended.
6. Sit on floor and spread legs straight at about twice shoulder width. Rest left hand on left thigh and grasp inside of right foot with right hand. Keep back straight and slowly straighten right leg until it is about 45 degrees from floor. Hold for twenty to thirty seconds and then repeat with other leg.

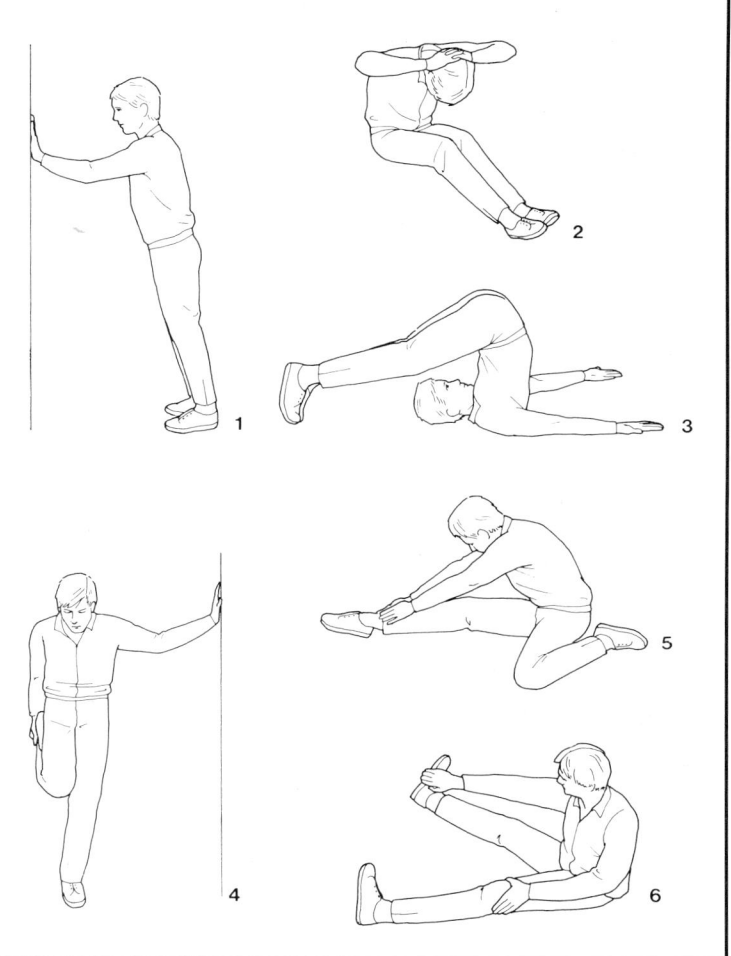

Clothes need only be comfortable, reasonably loose and suitable for the time of year. In summer shorts or cut-off jeans and a T-shirt or vest will be enough. Light colours reflect the sun's rays so they are preferable in the summer. Winter jogging does require warmer clothing obviously, but you will need fewer clothes than temperatures might suggest. This is because running generates lots of body heat and too much heat leads to exhaustion. If it is very cold, several layers of light clothing are better than one or two thick layers because they help trap the heat – and because a layer can be discarded if, as often happens, you start out cold and end up hot. Hats are useful in extremes of heat or cold but the only crucial items upon which it is worth spending money are shoes.

Plimsolls are okay to start with but regular jogging requires something sturdier; after all, each shoe lands on the ground some eight hundred times a mile. The running boom has resulted in a proliferation of 'training' shoes in everything from chain-stores to specialist sports shops. The price range is equally diverse but here are some points to look out for:

*soles should be firm but thickly cushioned
*the shoe should be flexible, especially at the ball of the foot
*the heel must be stable and wide, but not so high that it cuts the skin
*avoid shoes with interior stitching that can cause blistering
*if you wear socks, be sure to wear them when trying on new shoes
*choose a shoe with good arch support
*avoid shoes with plastic linings
*break in any new shoes gradually before going on a long run in them.

The importance of shoes is that they are the first line of defence against blisters, sore feet and aching ankles and knees. But better to run – for a time – in ordinary shoes than not to run at all.

WHEN TO RUN
With sensible clothing you can run at almost any time during the year. You can run by day, although avoid hours of extreme heat. You can run by night, although ideally wear reflective clothing or sashes of the kind sold at cycling shops. There are only two basic rules:

1. Don't run within two hours after a meal.
2. Don't run vigorously in the early stages of your exercise programme; build up strength gradually.

WHERE TO RUN
Another attraction of running or jogging is that you can begin at your own front door. You certainly do not need a running track – and in any case for most people running in circles takes away much of the fun. It's more fun to run in parks or along towpaths and to some extent it is easier on the feet than running along pavements. But it's fun to work out your own routes and to vary them to give variety. Even familiar local streets can take on a fresh look as you jog

EXERCISE/AEROBIC EXERCISE

around on a fine summer morning. If you are a road runner, take particular care and stick to pavements wherever possible. The individual nature of running is for many people an intrinsic part of its appeal. However, if you would rather have company, track down one of the many jogging groups which have been formed recently – see Appendix Three for details.

PREPARING TO RUN

Although running is an ideal activity for improving cardiovascular fitness, it does little to promote suppleness or joint mobility (see table, page 63). This has two consequences. First, you should try to combine running with some keep-fit exercises such as those on pages 54–7; you could, for instance, do the exercises on days that you don't run. Second, you should do a few such exercises in order to warm up *before* you run.

Some runners warm up simply by starting off very slowly. But five minutes or so of preliminary stretching exercises offer greater benefit since they will help prepare the joints and muscles for the exertions to come. Stretching increases in importance as you get older since muscles become more prone to tightening – and therefore injury – with age. Ideally, you should also use the stretching exercises *after* you have finished your run since this will lessen the chances of stiffness.

Grade 1 of the keep-fit exercises in this book (see pages 54–5) would help to get the circulation going and stretch some muscles, but there are a number of exercises designed more specifically for runners – see panel.* On all exercises *stretch slowly* and avoid sudden, jerky movements; take things easily at first. Do not over-stretch.

ON YOUR RUN

Unlike many sports – tennis or golf, for instance – running is a natural activity that does not require special skills. Athletes may need coaching to develop particular attributes (e.g., stamina or speed) but running for fitness requires only that you run naturally. The guidelines below may help, but they are not to be regarded as absolute rules; as with most of this section, they will soon become second nature.

1. **Don't** worry about the length of your stride; just run at what seems a comfortable pace and the stride will follow naturally.
2. **Don't** lean too far forward; keep in an upright position with body straight and head up. Don't look at your feet.
3. **Don't** run on your toes; try to land on your heel, then roll foot forward before pushing off again with the ball of the foot.
4. **Don't** worry about what your arms are doing; elbows should be slightly bent but relaxed. Shake arms from time to time to prevent tightness in shoulders.
5. **Don't** try to breathe only through the nose; gulp in as much air as you need through the mouth.
6. **Don't** – as has been said here before – try to run too fast, too long or too often too soon. You will gradually build up stamina so that speed and distance can be increased. Time spent running is in any case more important than distance covered but, initially, don't think about speed and don't worry if you have to walk now and then; most new joggers do.
7. **Don't**, above all, forget that running is supposed to be fun. So don't fret unduly about these or any other guidelines. There is no mystique in running.

A fun run in California, where the jogging boom really began in the 1970s

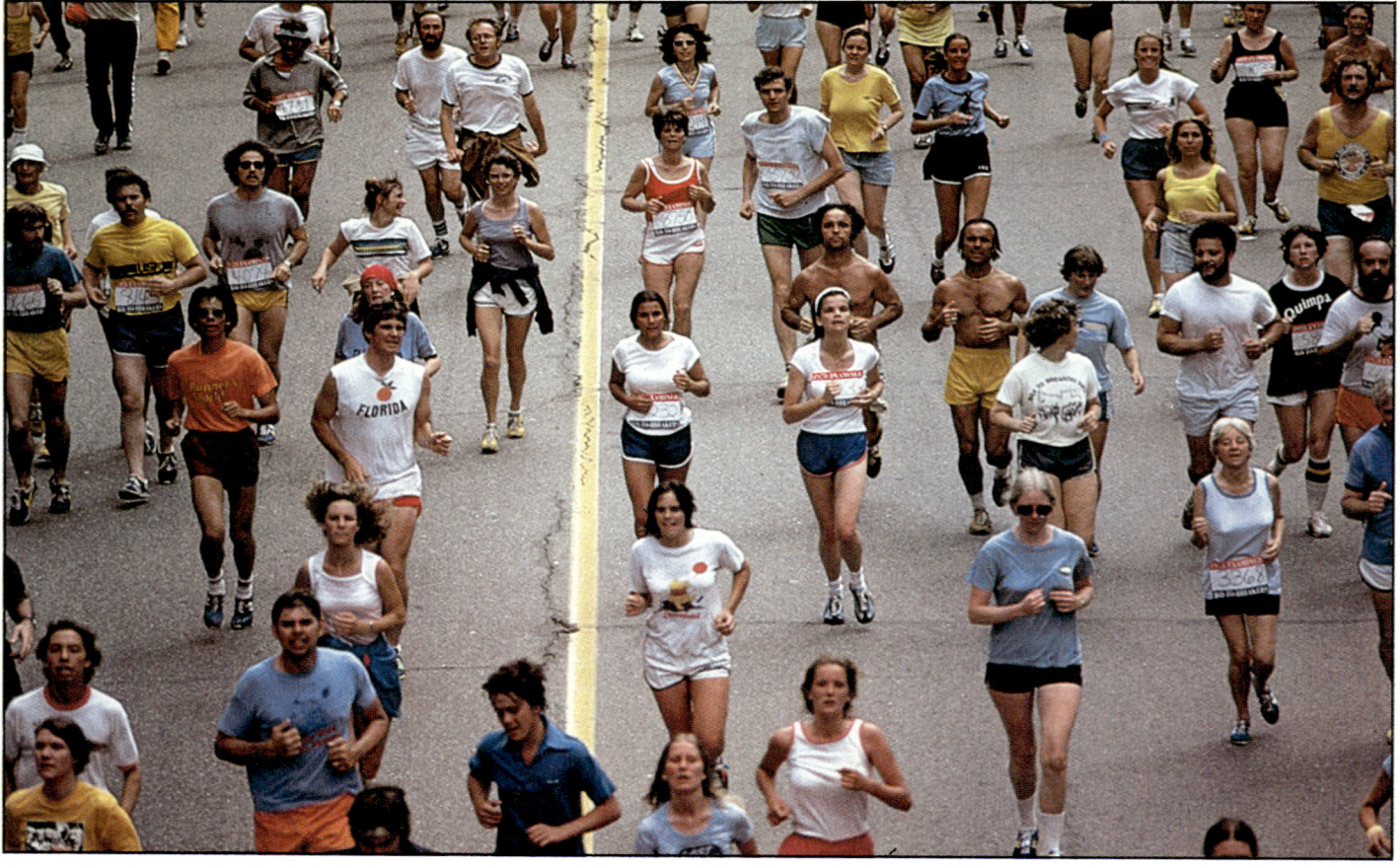

*Adapted from handbook on running prepared by US President's Council on Physical Fitness and Sports.

Running becomes addictive for many people. Yesterday's weekend jogger thus becomes tomorrow's marathon competitor. If you are tempted to run competitively, there are plenty of clubs and specialist books detailing training programmes – see Appendix Three for examples. But in running for fitness you are not aiming to beat anyone: you should aim simply at improving your own performance since that indicates greater fitness.

AFTER YOUR RUN

Stretching after a run (see warm-up exercises) helps ward off soreness and muscle injuries. Always cool down gradually by either tackling these exercises again or walking for a while (or both). Don't stop too suddenly and don't eat within twenty minutes of finishing a run. A hot bath will soothe away some of the soreness that is inevitable when you start subjecting your body to exercise after years of inactivity.

WOMEN AND RUNNING

In 1964, for the first time, women were allowed to race 800 metres in the Olympic Games; anything further was regarded as excessive or in some way unfeminine. In 1984, women at the Los Angeles Olympics will be competing in a marathon. This symbolizes the revolution in what is now accepted as within women's physical capacities.

Britain's Joyce Smith in fact personifies the dramatic change in women's running. She was first chosen to run for her country in 1960 and four years later was running at the Tokyo Olympics in the 800 metres. In 1982, at the age of forty-four, she won the women's race in the London Marathon for the second year in succession – at a record time of just under 2½ hours. And she has her sights set firmly on the Los Angeles Olympic Marathon in 1984.

The barriers are also coming down at humbler levels as more and more women take up jogging. There is every reason for them to do so since women stand to gain the same benefits from exercise as men. But many women still feel more inhibited and more self-conscious than men about running in public – a legacy, no doubt, of an education system that generally puts less emphasis on physical exercise for girls than it does for boys.

Nevertheless, women should take heart not only from the example of others but also from a growing body of evidence suggesting their suitability for exercise. Women may be slower generally than men, but there are indications that they do not tire so easily. Some running coaches also claim to have detected a more natural running style in women than men.

Women who want to run should follow the same guidelines as set out above, although there are naturally a few problems which are peculiar to their sex: notably period pains and pregnancy. Women have been running in great numbers for too short a time for the evidence to be conclusive but so far it appears that period pains are eased by running. And while pregnancy is not thought to be a good time to start running, most doctors think it is perfectly safe for women with normal pregnancies to continue running if they have previously done so regularly.

In one area the boom in women's running is an unqualified boon and that is clothing. Good sports shops will now stock running shorts made specifically for women as well as that true sign of our fitness-conscious times – the jogger's bra.

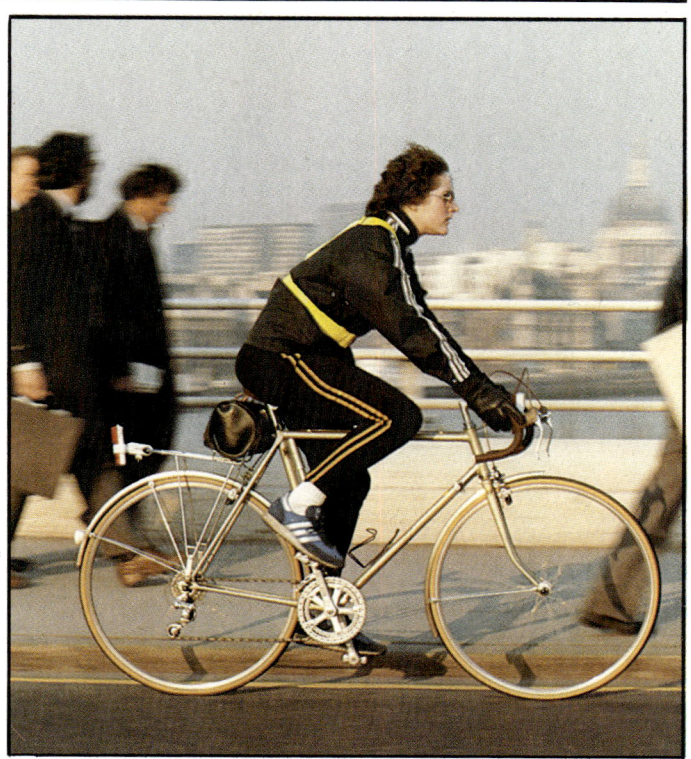

Cycling to work saves money – and aids fitness at the same time

CYCLING

Cycling is another of the basic aerobic activities featured in the books of Dr Kenneth Cooper. It is excellent exercise for the heart and leg muscles because of its regular and rhythmic nature. Cycling also has other attractions: it can be an activity for all the family (subject to road-safety care) and it can be a cheaper way of getting to work or the shops. However, you usually have to push harder for longer than is necessary to achieve the equivalent physical gains from running.

This is largely because exercise needs to be continuous if the full cardiovascular benefits are to be achieved in as little as twenty minutes. Most cyclists inevitably find themselves slowed down, and often stopped, by traffic; they therefore need to add distance in order to compensate for such delays and stoppages. Cycling in towns can also be dangerous: be sure you know the Highway Code and wear some reflective clothing at night. Better still, check to see if any bike paths have been created in local parks: ask the council or at cycle shops or clubs.

Many older people find it easier to take up cycling again than to contemplate running; again, the economic attractions of cycling give a twofold benefit from such exercise. Since cycling involves less strain on the feet than running, it can be tackled more readily by people with feet or joint problems. In two respects, however, cycling involves the same guidelines as those discussed earlier for running.

First, you should begin gradually. Don't try to go too far, too fast, too soon: let your stamina develop slowly. Second, cycling does little to enhance suppleness or the strength of muscles other than those in the legs. Ideally, therefore, cycling should be combined with other activities such as the keep-fit exercises on pages 54–7.

EXERCISE/AEROBIC EXERCISE

SWIMMING

Swimming comes close to being the ideal form of exercise. It is excellent for promoting stamina, strength and suppleness. It is also particularly suitable for older people or anyone suffering from back problems or arthritis. This is because the water helps take the weight away from joints such as the hips and knees. Swimming is therefore one of the few sports where it is not necessarily a handicap to be overweight.

One should perhaps mention a further 'advantage' of swimming which is so fundamental that it often goes unstated – it can save your life.

The crawl stroke is the most effective for full cardiovascular benefits because it is the most arduous, although other strokes such as backstroke, the butterfly and breaststroke greatly aid mobility and develop additional muscles. Coaching lessons are available at many public swimming pools and these may be worth considering since an improved style will increase ability to swim for longer periods. Efficient breathing is the way to being able to swim well. However, initially, most people find that they soon get out of breath and stop to float on their backs or tread water for a while – and this is one of the great drawbacks associated with swimming as a sole form of exercise.

In order to improve the condition of the heart and muscles you need to swim continuously for at least ten minutes, preferably using the crawl. Anyone starting swimming after years of inactivity would, of course, be no more able to achieve this target than he or she would be able to run non-stop for ten or fifteen minutes straightaway. Nor should they try to do so. Someone who normally swims only during the summer holidays should build up stamina as gradually as we have urged novice joggers and cyclists to do. However, swimmers face two particular difficulties.

First, technique matters more with swimming than it does for the two previous aerobic activities. Many people, for instance, are uncertain about how and when to breathe during the crawl. Another problem is wasting too much energy kicking the legs. The effect of such problems is that you tire too quickly and don't spend long enough swimming.

Second, there is the social nature of the swimming pool itself. A lot of time supposedly spent swimming is in fact spent splashing around. And many pools are too crowded to enable people to swim for any distance or time without interruption; the recent development of so-called leisure pools, with their slides and wave machines, has added to this problem.

Nevertheless, it would be wrong to emphasize difficulties at the expense of the great potential gains to be achieved from swimming. Everyone should be able to swim, but if you're basically a social swimmer make sure you complement your swimming with other forms of exercise that provide the continuous arduous exercise your heart and muscles need. The keep-fit exercises described on pages 54–7 should also be followed in order to enhance mobility and flexibility of *all* joints, thus promoting all-round physical fitness.

'Leisure pools' offer fun for all the family and provide an easy introduction to physical activity. But conventional pools are better for the more concentrated swimming necessary to improve fitness

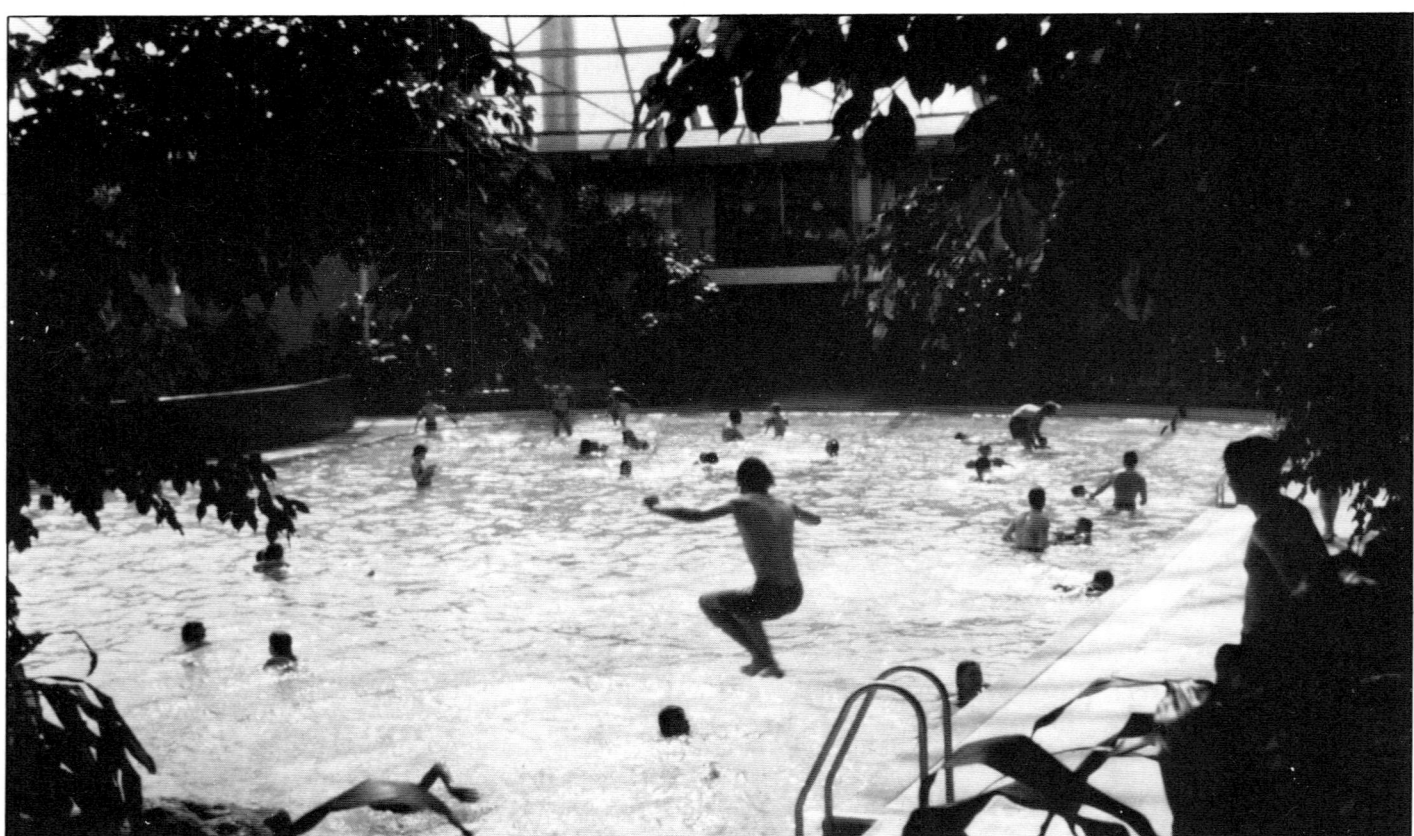

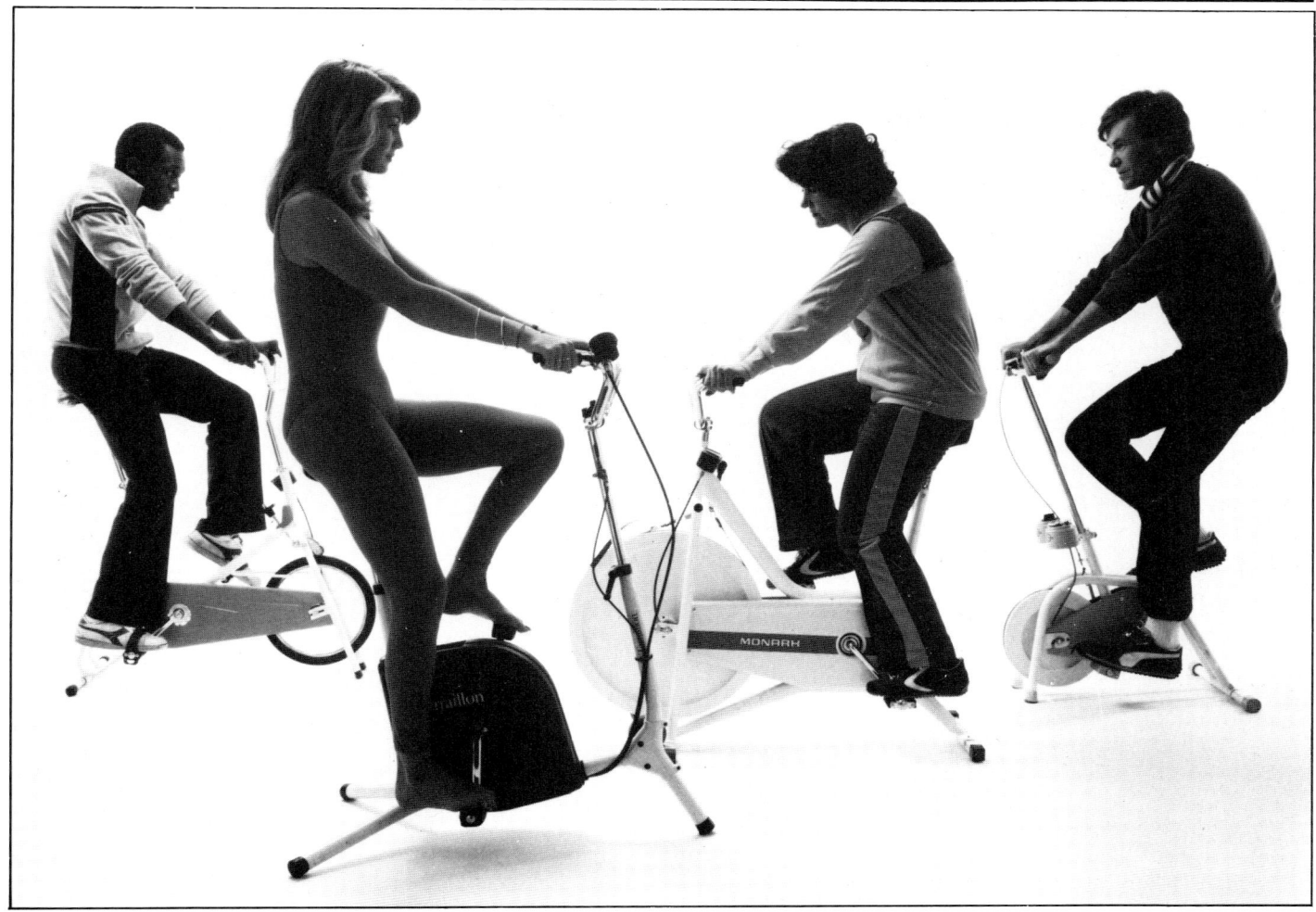

Exercise bikes get you nowhere – except towards fitness without being rained on

Indoor Exercise

Newspapers and magazines regularly advertise other aids to fitness. 'Ten minutes daily,' the advertisements say, 'is all you need to get fit' – provided the ten minutes is spent using the advertised rowing machine or indoor bicycle or bar-bell and weights, or chest expander.

There are times when indoor exercise *is* an attraction. And half an hour's vigorous cycling on a machine would train your heart and muscles to the same extent as thirty minutes spent cycling in the open air – possibly more so, since 'real' cycling involves stops for traffic. But no equipment can ever be a substitute for human effort – especially for really unfit people. Exercise bikes still have to be pedalled, rowing machines still have to be rowed.

The disadvantages of exercise machines is that they are rarely cheap and more likely to be boring. Pedalling an exercise bike on a winter's day may seem more attractive than going outside in the cold, but cycling along a country lane is more likely to tempt people into exercise on warmer days. However, some people find it convenient because they can watch TV, listen to music, or babysit at the same time.

The only thing that matters is that people maintain their exercise. If exercise bikes or rowing machines help people to do this, then good luck to them. Possibly the money spent on a 'home gymnasium' may influence their determination. All they should beware of is thinking that machines will make anything easy; they should be especially wary of all claims for the magical slimming properties of any machines.

Not all indoor exercise is dependent upon machines, however. Keep-fit exercises (or calisthenics, as they are sometimes known) require no equipment whatsoever. Yoga, like keep-fit exercises, can be practised individually at home but many people prefer the companionship and encouragement offered through courses run by local sports centres or gymnasiums.

The last few years have seen a great increase in the number of such centres. If you are lucky enough to live near a sports centre run by a local authority, you will usually find a great array of exercise activities available at far lower prices than charged by commercial gymnasiums or health clubs. Council-run centres are also more accustomed to the needs of families so that, at the best of them, babies and toddlers can be left at a crèche while their parents exercise.

EXERCISE/INDOOR EXERCISE

KEEP-FIT EXERCISES

The convenience of keep-fit exercises has always been among their strongest attractions. No special clothing or equipment is required. They are usually done indoors, so the weather outside is irrelevant. You do not need to rely on other people turning up as in most competitive sports. You do not waste time travelling to the sports centre. Nobody (other than your family, perhaps) will laugh at your early puffing efforts. They can be done at any time of the day (or indeed night) except in the hour after a meal.

The advantages of keep-fit exercises are their concentration and variety. You not only waste no time travelling or dressing but you are also benefiting every minute you are exercising. Yet that is also a drawback of such exercise: you benefit *only* when you are doing a particular exercise. Activity is not normally sufficiently sustained to have the optimum effect on the heart and circulation. Make the most of these limbering-up exercises by moving quickly from one activity to another, with running in place to develop stamina. Keep-fit exercises are perhaps best deployed as an addition to a general exercise programme. They certainly develop greater mobility than, say, running, which otherwise is 'good' cardiovascular exercise. Another attraction of this form of exercise is that it is programmed to incorporate a complete range of physical activities for not only different muscle groups but also all levels of fitness – or unfitness.

The *Body Maintenance* exercises fulfil these objectives. There is a less demanding *Grade 1*, which is essentially to get you up and down stairs without all that huffing and puffing; *Grade 2* will at least make it possible for you to run for a bus without feeling that what you need instead is an ambulance; and *Grade 3*, if you keep it up for any length of time, should get you back to near the fitness of your youth. Whatever your grade, the exercises only take a few minutes. What matters is to practise them *every day*.

These exercises were first devised for the average man or woman by Captain Simon Cook and Sergeant Tony Toms of the Royal Marines. Such origins should remind us that, although the exercises may be a speedy way towards fitness, they will not necessarily be easy – especially for the very unfit. But do not be scared: the exercises were devised for ordinary mortals who want to climb stairs rather than scale cliffs.

Be sure to follow the instructions for each exercise carefully. People who suffer from back pain should take particular care, and perhaps consider alternative forms of exercise. The number of repeats specified is only a guide. You can do more or less, according to what level of fitness you are aiming for or indeed to what you can manage. Stick to one grade if you like, or graduate from one to another. Aim to improve your performance in terms of skill and speed as well as number. Forgetting it 'just for one day' makes it easier to forget for another day as well. The more you demand of yourself, the more you will benefit and the more enjoyable the exercises themselves will become.

Grade 1: A Loosening-Up Course to Start

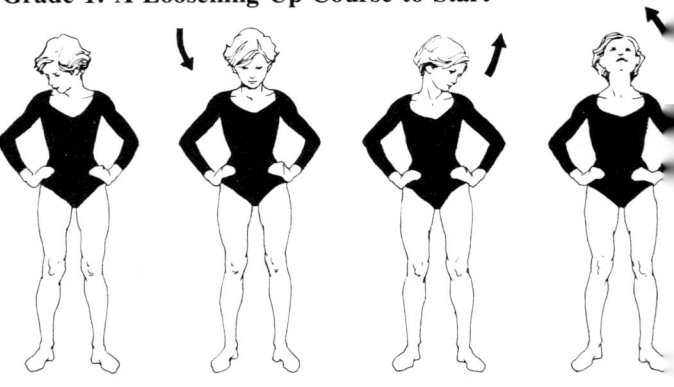

1. *Head-circling.* Stand erect, feet comfortably apart, hands on hips. Pull chin in, circle head 10 times in one direction, then 10 times in the other direction.

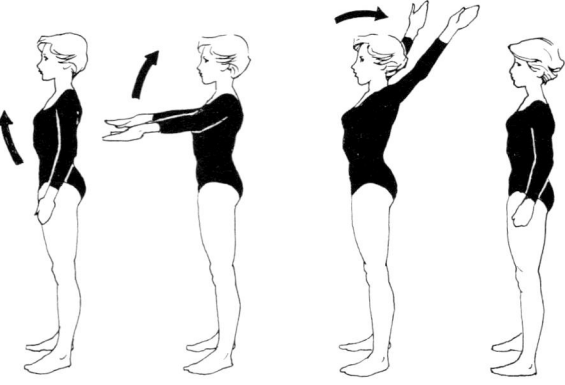

2. *Arm-circling.* Stand erect, feet apart. Circle both arms simultaneously like propellers 10 times, then 10 times in reverse direction.

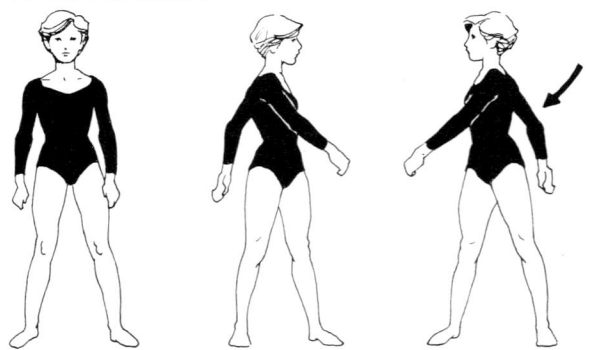

3. *Trunk-twisting.* Stand erect, feet apart, arms loosely by sides. Turn trunk and head to left and then to right. Repeat this whole movement left and right 10 times.

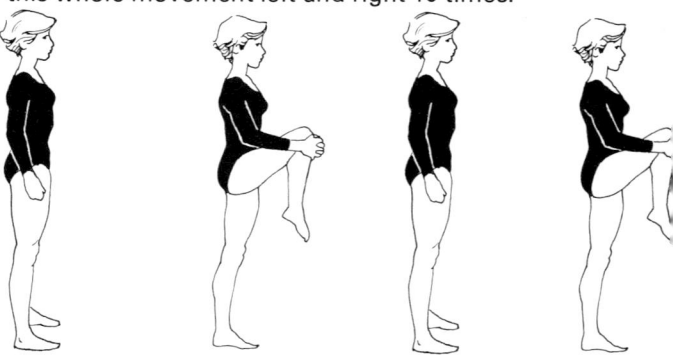

4. *Knee-clasping.* Stand erect, feet apart. Bend one knee upwards and pull it vigorously into your chest with both hands. Same with other knee, and repeat 10 times with each knee.

INDOOR EXERCISE/**EXERCISE**

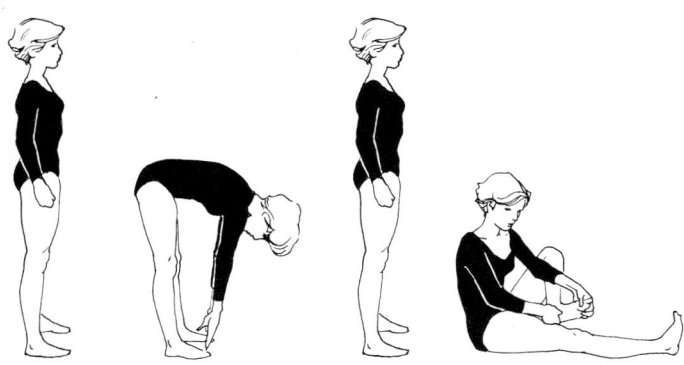

5. *Toe-touching.* Stand erect, feet apart. Bend down to touch toes, keeping legs straight if possible. Return to upright position, repeat 10 times.

6. *Ankle-rotating.* Sit on floor with one leg straight. Bend other leg over the straight leg, hold the foot of the bent leg, and turn ankle full circle. 10 times each ankle.

Grade 2: Getting in Trim the Easy Way

For men. This is for bodies fit enough for stronger exercises. Warm up first with thirty seconds on each of the Grade 1 exercises.

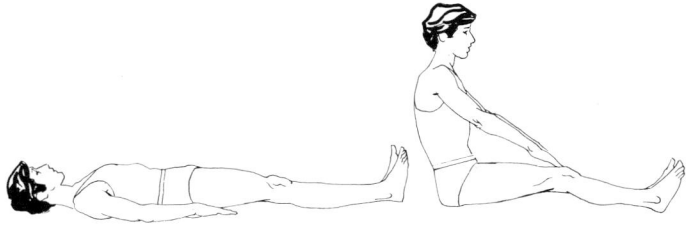

1. *Sit-ups.* Lie on back with a comfortable cushion for the head. Rise without use of arms to near-sitting position. Hands must touch knee-caps. Return to lying position. Repeat 15 times.

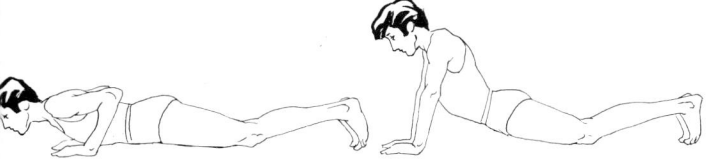

2. *Half push-ups.* Lie facing floor. With palms flat, push up till arms are straight, lower trunk remaining on floor. Return to lying flat and repeat 10 times. (This may be uncomfortable for anyone with back pain. An alternative is to do a few push-ups using knees as the fulcrum – starting with the knees bent.)

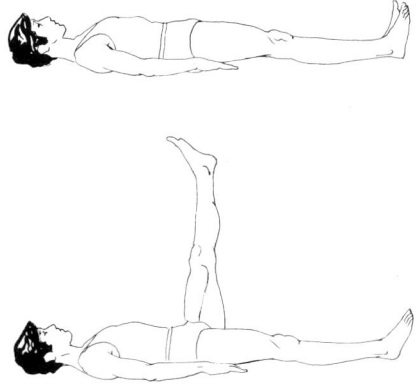

3. *Leg-raising.* Lie on back and raise each leg alternately to the vertical. 20 times each leg.

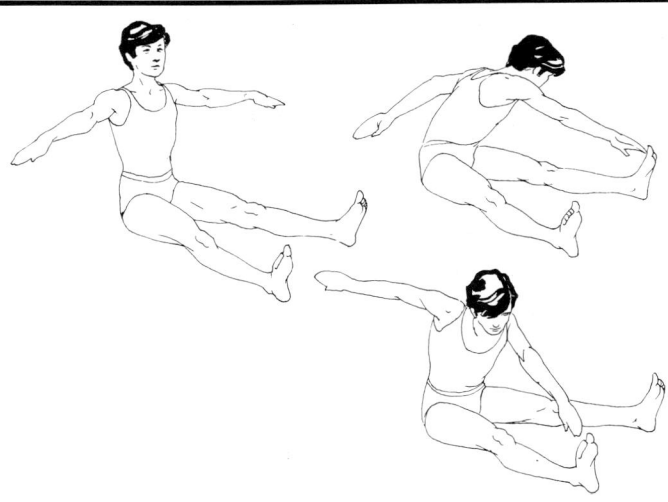

4. *Sitting toe-touching.* Sit with legs straight and apart, stretch right hand to touch left toe then left hand to right toe. Repeat whole movement 30 times rhythmically.

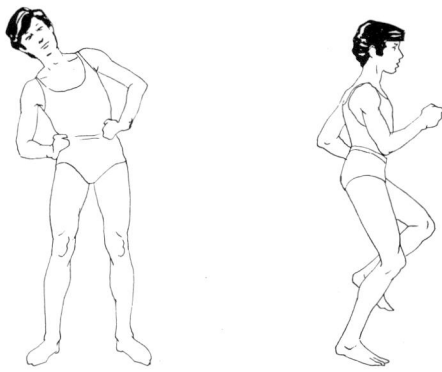

5. *Side-bending.* Stand with feet comfortably apart, hands on hips. Bend body from waist, reaching down as far as you can, first on left side, then on right. 20 times each side.

6. *Spot-running.* Run on spot counting a pace each time the right foot touches the floor. 100 paces or one minute.

For women. These exercises can help posture and to some extent flatten the tummy and reduce the waist, but they are not an alternative to a diet for the overweight. Warm up first with 30 seconds of each Grade 1 exercise.

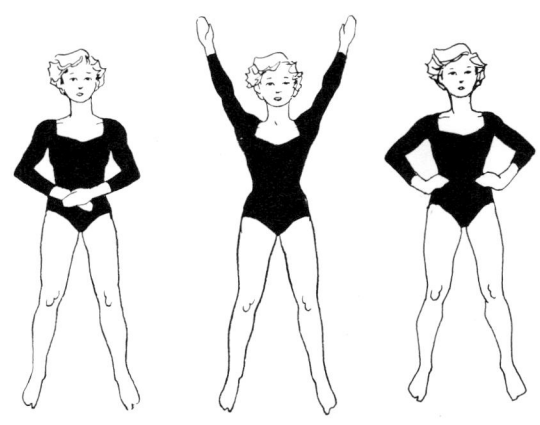

1. *Arm-raising.* Stand with feet comfortably apart, cross wrists over stomach. Keeping arms straight, swing them upwards and outwards and return. 20 times.

EXERCISE/INDOOR EXERCISE

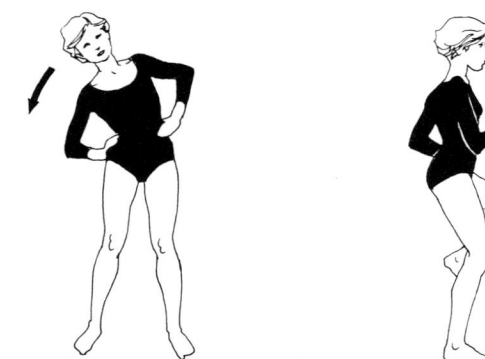

2. *Side-bending.* Stand with feet comfortably apart, hands on hips. Bend body from waist, reaching down as far as you can, first on left side, then on right. 15 times each side.

3. *Spot-running.* Run on spot, counting as right foot touches floor. 40 paces.

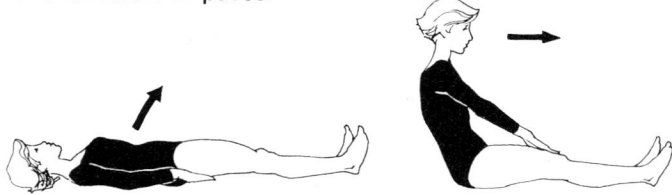

4. *Sit-ups.* Lie on back with a comfortable cushion for the head. Rise without use of arms to near-sitting position. Hands must touch knee-caps. Return to lying. Repeat 15 times.

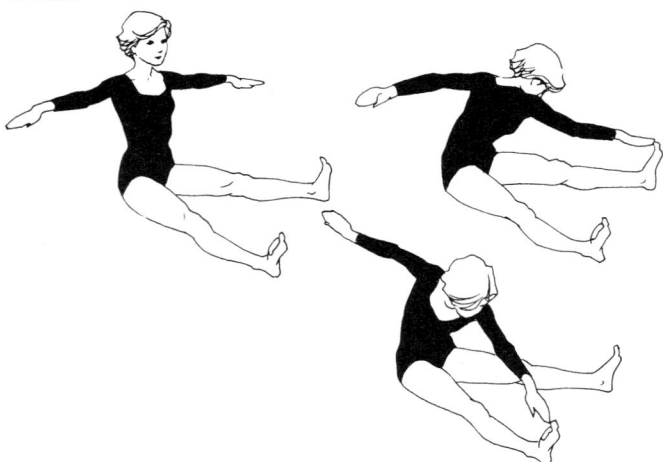

5. *Sitting toe-touching.* Sit with legs straight and apart, stretch right hand to touch left toe, then left hand to right toe. Repeat whole movement 10 times rhythmically.

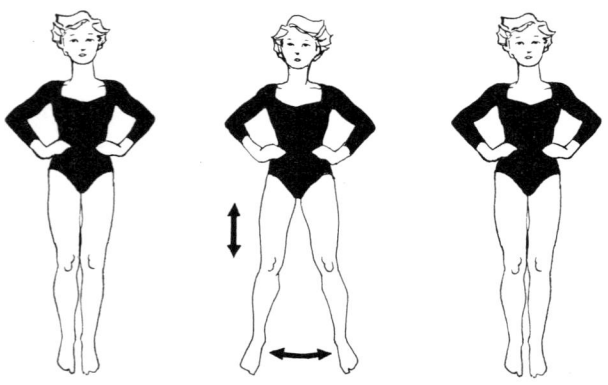

6. *Astride-jumps.* With hands on hips, jump feet apart and then together again, repeating whole movement 30 times rhythmically.

Grade 3: Bursting with Health

For men. Once you have attained this level without too much discomfort you can say you are giving your body a thorough servicing. Warm up first with thirty seconds of each Grade 1 exercise.

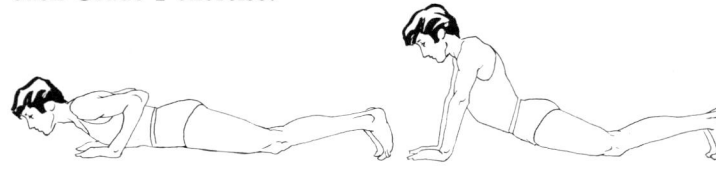

1. *Half push-ups.* Lie facing floor. With palms flat, push up till arms are straight, lower trunk remaining on floor. Return to lying flat. Do as many as you can up to 20 times. NB: back-pain sufferers should see the cautionary note under the first exercise in Grade 2 for men.

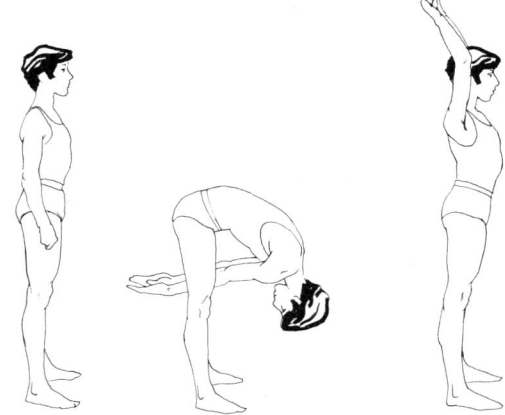

2. *Dorsal swing.* Stand with feet wide part, hands by your sides with back twelve inches away from wall. Touch wall between legs, then swing up to touch wall above head. 20 times.

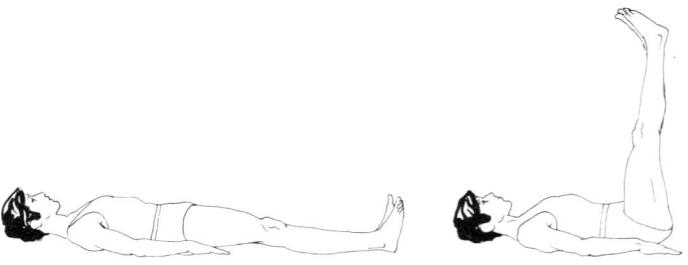

3. *Leg-raising.* Lie on back. Raise both legs to the vertical, then lower them slowly to floor. 15 times.

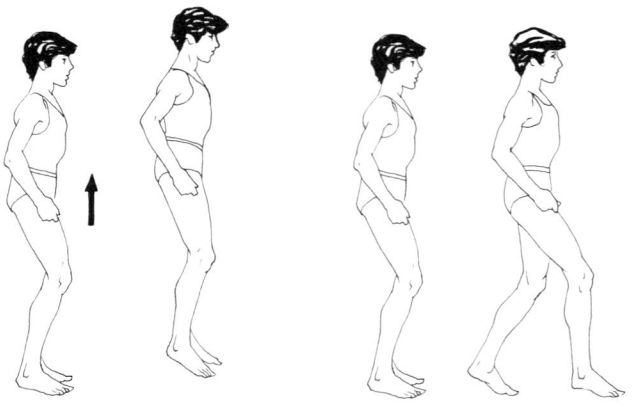

4. *Skip-jumps.* Stand with feet together, hands by sides. Spring up and down off the balls of your feet, 30 times. Repeat 30 times more, skipping with one foot forwards, other backwards alternately.

INDOOR EXERCISE/EXERCISE

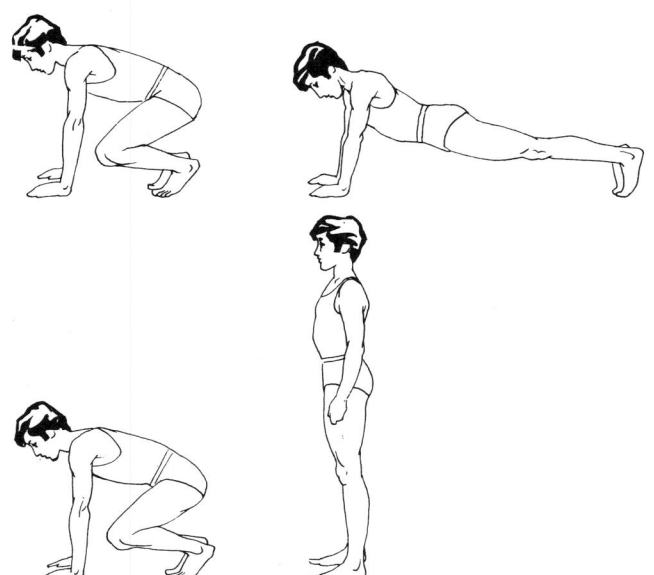

5. *Burpees.* From standing, crouch with hands on floor, then shoot legs backwards to the push-up position. Return to crouch and then stand up. This is one 'burpee'. Repeat 15 times.

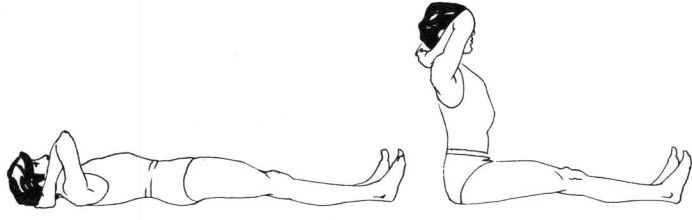

6. *Sit-ups.* Lie on back. Sit up to vertical position, bending knees if necessary. 30 times.

For women: This grade should be attempted only after six weeks of daily Grade 2 exercises. Warm up first with twenty seconds of each Grade 1 exercise.

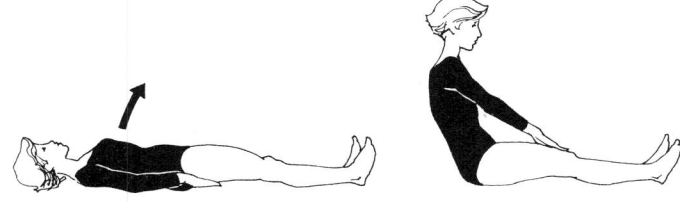

1. *Sit-ups.* Lie on back, rise without use of arms to near-sitting position. Hands must touch knee-caps. Return to lying. 20 times.

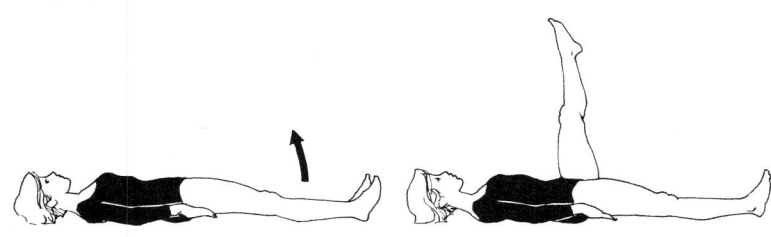

2. *Leg-raising.* Lie on back. Raise both legs to the vertical, then lower them slowly (to count of ten) to floor. 10 times.

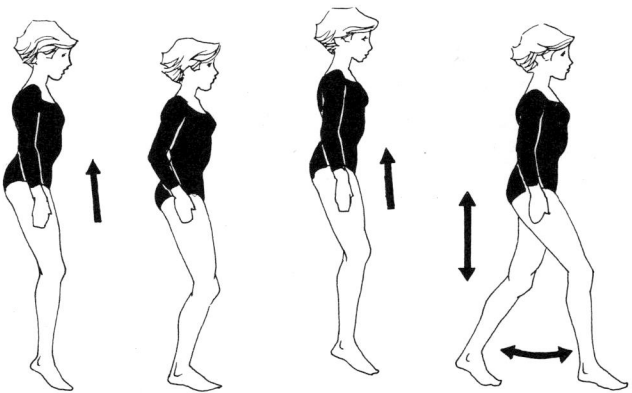

3. *Skip-jumps.* Stand with feet together, arms by sides. Spring up and down off the balls of your feet, 30 times. Repeat 30 times more, skipping with one foot forwards other backwards alternately.

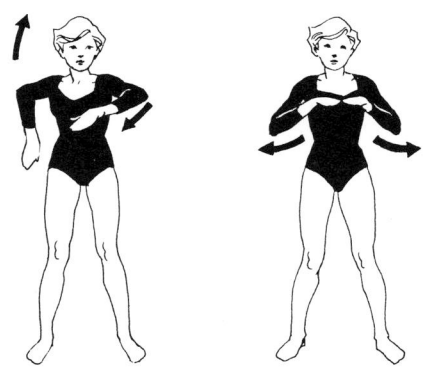

4. *Free-standing swim.* Stand with feet comfortably apart and with your arms 'swim' the crawl, breast-stroke and back-stroke. 20 of each stroke.

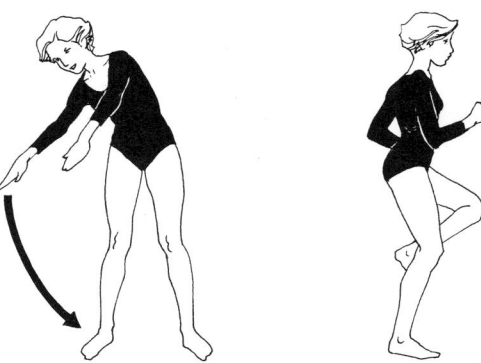

5. *Trunk-rotating.* Stand with feet comfortably apart, arms stretched up above head. Make a circle with arms and trunk, brushing floor with hands in front at lowest point of movement. 10 times to left, 10 times to right.

6. *Spot-running.* Run on spot for one minute.

EXERCISE/INDOOR EXERCISE

YOGA

Yoga is a pleasant and absorbing way for people of all ages to get fit and stay healthy. Britain is already the world's largest centre for yoga study outside India, but the subject is still widely misunderstood as suitable only for mystics or contortionists.

WHAT IS YOGA?

The word 'yoga' means union or communication. Yoga is a pragmatic science evolved over thousands of years which deals with the physical, moral, mental and spiritual well-being of man. The traditional path to a mastery of yoga is the Eight Limbs of Yoga first described by Patanjali in about 200 BC.

The first two 'limbs', Yama (moral commandments) and Niyama (purification through discipline), control passions and emotions. There are at least two hundred Asanas (postures) which keep the body healthy and strong. The next two stages, Pranayama (rhythmic control of the breath) and Pratyahara (freeing the mind from the senses), are known as the inner quests. Dharana (concentration), Dhyana (meditation) and Samadhi (a state of super-consciousness brought about by deep meditation) finally

OUR LESSON EXPLAINED

The nineteen positions demonstrated by Maxine Tobias, one of the Inner London Education Authority yoga teachers, can be performed by nearly every novice yoga student within three months of starting weekly classes. Beginners can expect to find postures like these taught in one-hour classes all over Britain, and to feel increasingly relaxed and revitalized after each session. Yoga is not a competitive activity. By working intelligently, a person hampered by stiff joints and weak muscles can derive as much benefit as someone who finds the postures easier to perform. The movements and final positions are precise and require instruction. The diagram below indicates the three major categories of pose and the time devoted to each in a one-hour session. The numbers refer to the postures demonstrated by Ms Tobias. These individual postures bear their original Sanskrit names and a brief description of their effects.

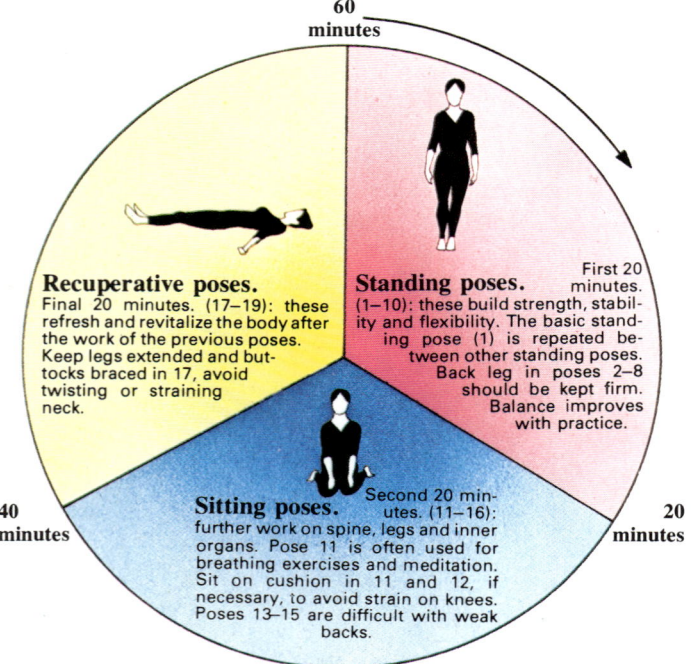

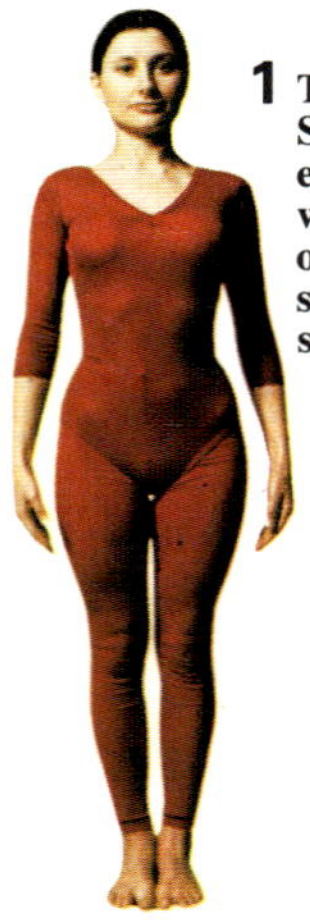

1 TADASANA. Standing erect and with weight evenly on both feet; straightens spine.

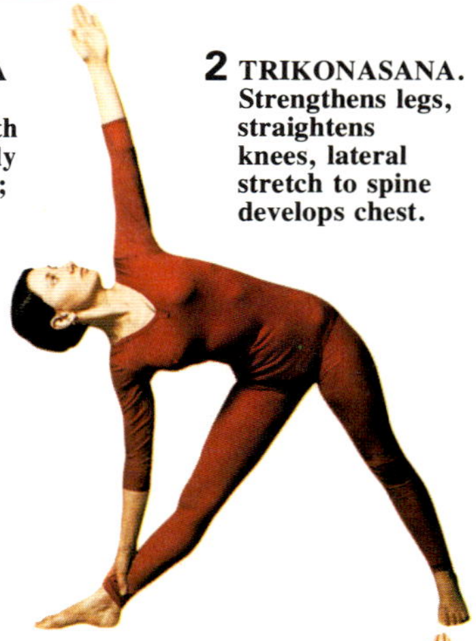

2 TRIKONASANA. Strengthens legs, straightens knees, lateral stretch to spine develops chest.

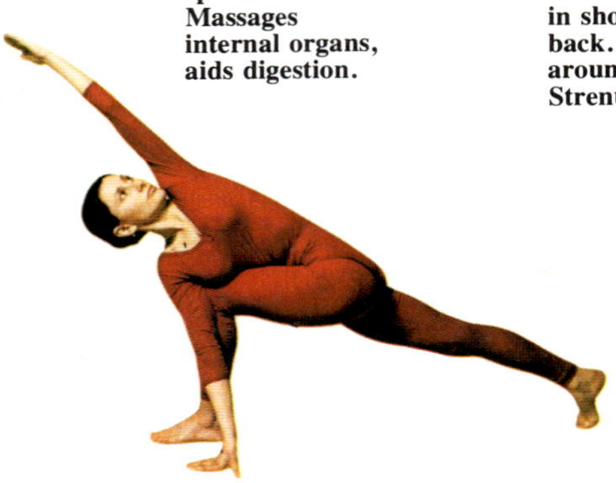

6 PARIVRTTA PARSVAKONASANA. More intense spinal twist. Massages internal organs, aids digestion.

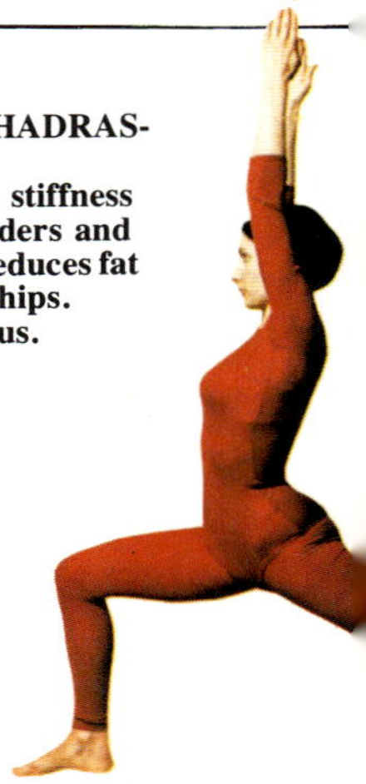

7 VIRABHADRASANA 1. Relieves stiffness in shoulders and back. Reduces fat around hips. Strenuous.

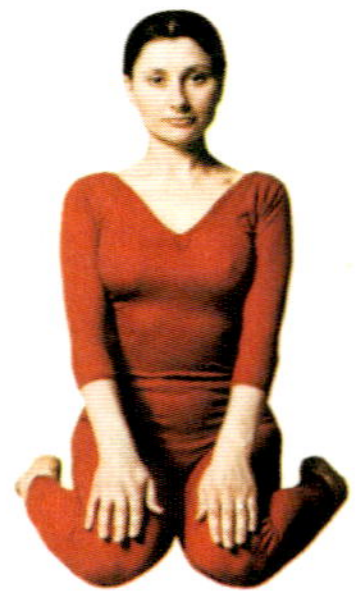

11 VIRASANA. Rests legs after standing poses. Good for knees, corrects flat feet.

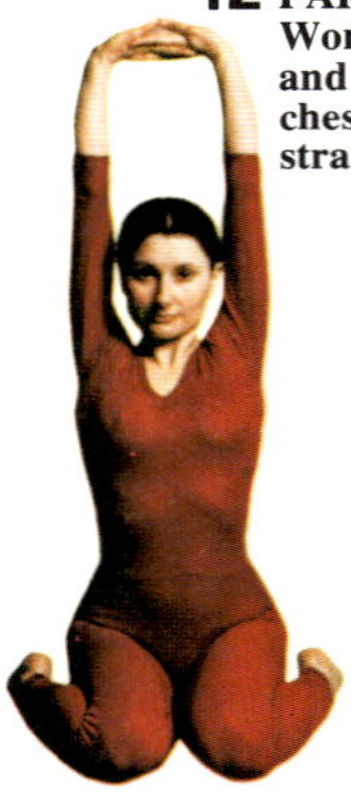

12 PARVATASANA. Works shoulders and develops chest. Keep spine straight.

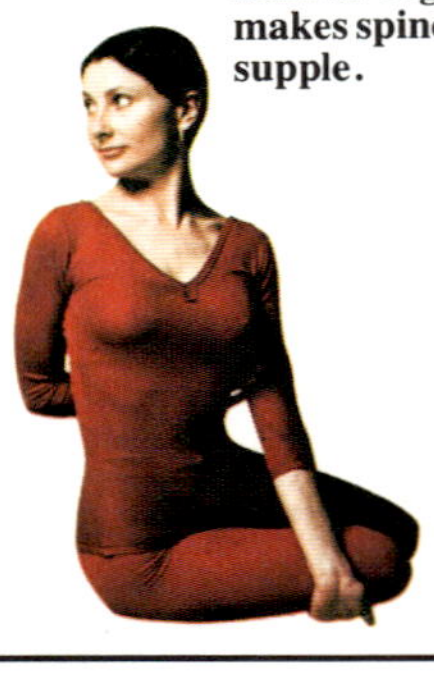

16 BHARADVAJASANA. Gentle twist on dorsal and lumbar region makes spine more supple.

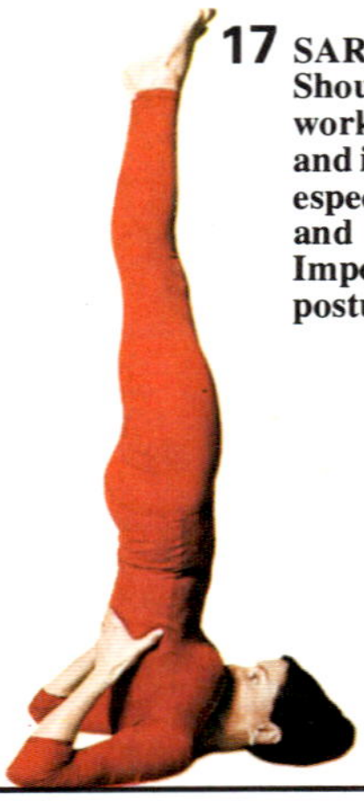

17 SARVANGASANA. Shoulder stand works on glands and inner organs, especially heart and liver. Important posture.

Recuperative poses. Final 20 minutes. (17–19): these refresh and revitalize the body after the work of the previous poses. Keep legs extended and buttocks braced in 17, avoid twisting or straining neck.

Standing poses. First 20 minutes. (1–10): these build strength, stability and flexibility. The basic standing pose (1) is repeated between other standing poses. Back leg in poses 2–8 should be kept firm. Balance improves with practice.

Sitting poses. Second 20 minutes. (11–16): further work on spine, legs and inner organs. Pose 11 is often used for breathing exercises and meditation. Sit on cushion in 11 and 12, if necessary, to avoid strain on knees. Poses 13–15 are difficult with weak backs.

3 PARSVAKONASANA. Tones legs, develops chest, reduces fat around hips, relieves sciatica and constipation.

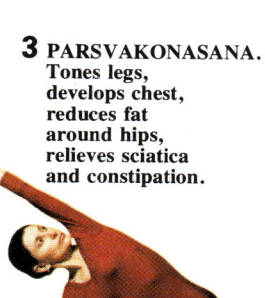

4 PARSVOTTANASANA. Works hip-joints, spine and wrists. Corrects rounded shoulders. Keep head relaxed.

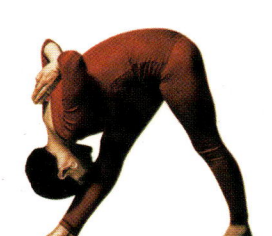

5 PARIVRTTA TRIKONASANA. Gentle spinal twist. Tones thigh, calf and hamstring muscles.

8 VIRABHADRASANA II. Strengthens leg and back muscles. Tones abdominal organs.

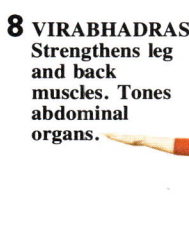

9 UTTANASANA. Extends legs and spine, tones inner organs, rests heart and brain.

10 VRKSASANA. Tones leg muscles and develops balance and poise.

13 DANDASANA. Sitting at right-angle on perineum, strengthens back muscles and straightens spine.

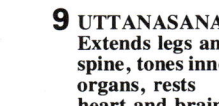

14 NAVASANA Tones kidneys. Strengthens abdominal muscles. Strenuous.

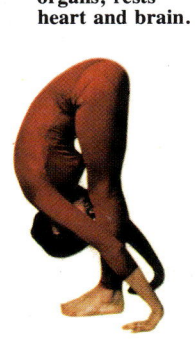

15 ARDHA NAVASANA. Works on liver, gall-bladder and spleen. Strengthens abdominal muscles.

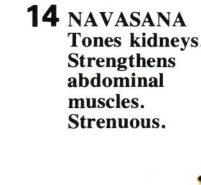

18 HALASANA. Further extension in spine. Preparation for forward bending poses. Chair under feet may help.

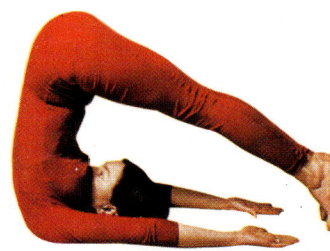

19 SAVASANA. Important to end with 10-minute relaxation in corpse pose. With breathing exercises, calms brain activity. Beginners apt to fall asleep, but pose should be reinvigorating.

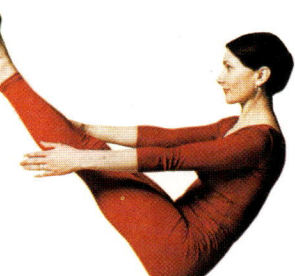

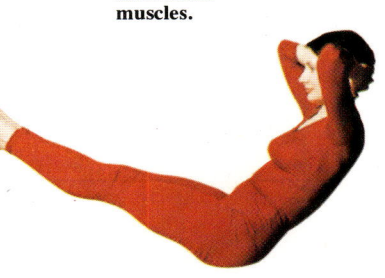

DOS AND DON'TS

1. **Do** continue to breathe normally through the nose in the postures and accentuate the exhalation slightly.
2. **Do** wear unrestricting clothes and remember to exercise both sides of the body.
3. **Do** attend classes to learn the above postures correctly.
4. **Do not** strain; stay in position as long as is comfortable.
5. **Do not** expect to achieve all the positions at once. Daily practice produces improvement.
6. **Do not** attempt yoga postures before consulting a doctor if you are more than three months pregnant, or have any medical problems.

EXERCISE/INDOOR EXERCISE

allow the yogi to realize his self. Yoga has several branches or divisions, but in the West students largely concentrate on Hatha Yoga, an approach concerned primarily with bodily posture – the Asanas. The relaxation and physical benefits achieved from practising even just once a week are a sufficient reward for many beginners, and quickly become apparent.

HOW DOES YOGA AFFECT DIET?
The only special dietary rule to observe when taking up Hatha Yoga is always to practise on an empty stomach. It is not advisable or comfortable to perform postures within about four hours of having eaten, but you need not change your diet in any way. Those who become serious yoga followers do usually lose the taste for meat, and often stop or cut down on tobacco and alcohol. These measures are also good for health as described elsewhere in this book. One of the classic yoga texts, the *Hatha Yoga Pradipika of Svatmarama*, says, 'The yogi should take a nourishing and sweet food mixed with milk. It should be pleasing to the senses and nutritive.'

WILL YOGA AFFECT MY HEALTH?
Considerable claims are made for the medical benefits of correctly practised postures. The medical profession remains divided over some of the wilder claims, which include alleviating appendicitis and ulcers, but supports the general notion that the physical postures, like other exercises, can be useful preventive medicine and that particular postures may help to relieve certain medical complaints such as backache, constipation, insomnia and flat feet.

The calm, relaxing effects of yoga are accepted as a valuable antidote to urban stress and strain. Serious ailments should not, however, be treated with yoga unless medical advice has been given and a qualified teacher consulted. It is also all too easy to damage muscles, joints and the spine without proper supervision.

If you suffer from heart trouble, dizziness or back disorders, you should never take up yoga, or any other strenuous activity, without consulting a doctor. Women should not perform all the postures during menstruation, for the last six months of pregnancy or for three months after giving birth.

Charles T. Kuntzleman and the editors of the US *Consumer Guide* in their book *Rating the Exercises* produced an eight-point summary of yoga's most frequently claimed benefits for general health and fitness. It is:

1. Yoga can improve flexibility and grace.
2. Yoga does not improve endurance or stamina.
3. Yoga is probably a good way to release tension and stress.
4. Yoga does not maintain proper circulation (although it may be helpful in reducing high blood pressure).
5. Yoga does not improve the strength of the vital organs and glands.
6. Yoga may improve the firmness and strength of selected muscles and muscle groups.
7. Yoga does not produce a taut, smooth skin.
8. Yoga makes only a meagre contribution to weight control.

Yoga alone is therefore an inadequate programme for diet control or physical fitness. This is firstly because it expends too few calories to have a significant effect on overall weight. Secondly, it does not have the beneficial effects on the heart and lung – the so-called cardiovascular exercise – that stem from such activities as running, swimming, cycling or walking. Use these activities therefore to build up your endurance (and the consequent heart-lung training effect) and use yoga for its beneficial effects on flexibility and for general lessening of stress and tension.

WHERE CAN I LEARN?
Most local authorities now offer yoga classes in their adult education programmes. Courses for beginners usually start in September. The size of class fluctuates from about fifteen to thirty. Teaching standards and styles vary. If your local authority does not provide classes, ask at a local sports club or health-food shop. Local newspapers and publications such as *Yoga Today* and *Time Out* often carry advertisements, but students should ensure that teachers are qualified. Private classes can often be arranged with local-authority yoga teachers, which allow for more detailed personal attention. These are far more expensive, of course.

WHAT EQUIPMENT WILL I NEED?
Yoga demands extensive stretching of the body and it is therefore most comfortable to wear loose clothing. T-shirts and footless tights, cotton trousers or shorts, are ideal. Avoid clothing that has buttons, belts or buckles. Try to find a clear patch of floor-space in a quiet, clean, airy room where you can practise regularly without interruption. The only equipment necessary is a folded blanket used for the sitting and recuperative postures. It can be instructive to observe yourself in a mirror, but it must be perpendicular to the floor and full-length to be of benefit.

THE IYENGAR METHOD
Many yoga students in Britain follow a method developed by the Indian yogi and guru, B. K. S. Iyengar. He began teaching in India in 1936 and has subjected the practice of yoga to detailed examination, which he continues at his institute. One of his first pupils in the West was Yehudi

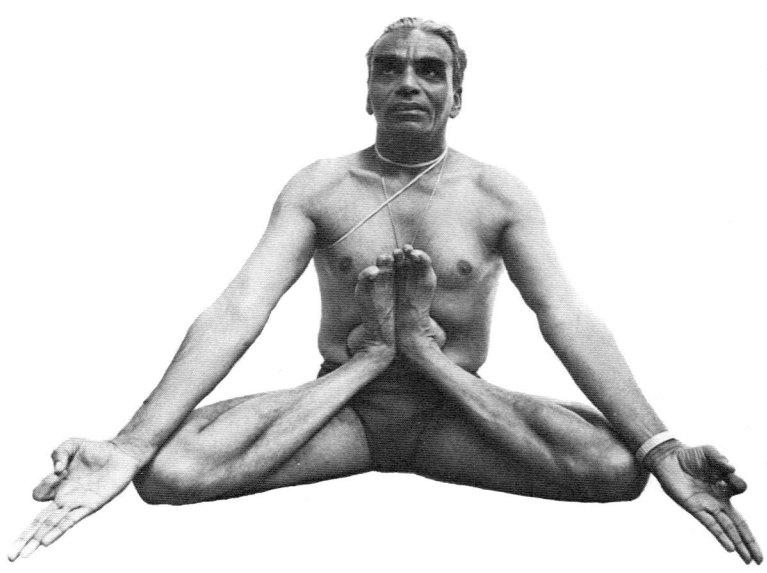

The doyen of yoga students, B. K. S. Iyengar, demonstrates an advanced posture at his Institute

Menuhin, who describes the Iyengar method as 'a technique ideally suited to prevent physical and mental illness and to protect the body generally, developing an inevitable sense of self-reliance and assurance'. The beginner first learns the Asanas (postures) before being led on to Pranayama (control of breath). Iyengar is an advocate of an integrated approach to yoga, known as Astanga or Raja yoga. Although the goal remains the same, there are other paths of yoga, each with a different emphasis, such as Bhakti, Jnana and Kundalini yoga.

HOME GYMNASIUM

Exercise bikes and rowing machines are the most popular types of home-exercise equipment. They are both forms of the dynamic exercise to which we have devoted most of this chapter. They both use rhythmic large-muscular movements so that the heart and circulation work in the same way as they would for 'real' cycling or rowing.

The attraction of exercise machines is their convenience. You can continue to exercise through the worst of the winter weather; you can even exercise while watching television. If you don't mind the boredom, therefore, such machines do offer a route to fitness, albeit an expensive one.

The effectiveness of an exercise bike depends upon something called the resistance device. This enables you to make the cycling easier or harder, according to your degree of fitness. Set the resistance device on the minimum setting and the pedals turn freely; set it on maximum and you have to pedal very hard indeed to turn them at all.

By delicately adjusting the resistance device so that the bike appears to require the same pressure each time you use it, your state of fitness will steadily be improved. Without such resistance devices exercise bikes will not enable you to develop your fitness. More sophisticated (and therefore costlier) machines also have speedometers and distance meters which, together with a graduated resistance device, enable people to monitor their fitness programme more precisely. The more expensive rowing machines are similarly capable of adjustment as you become progressively fitter.

For beginners the advice for exercise machines is just the same as that for any aerobic exercise: start slowly and build up gradually. Warm up with some keep-fit exercises since these will not only lessen the possibility of muscle strain while on the machine but provide the extra mobility or suppleness required for overall fitness. Exercise equipment can also fulfil a valuable role in maintaining fitness. If you are a keen cyclist, for instance, an exercise bicycle is valuable when bad weather or dark evenings make it difficult to train. Similarly with rowing machines, although these cannot approximate so closely to real rowing.

ISOMETRIC EXERCISE

This develops strength and 'bulks up' particular muscles, whereas *dynamic* exercise improves overall physical fitness and the cardiovascular system in particular. Isometric exercise will help you look more like Mr Universe but it will not by itself bring the benefits to general health offered by dynamic exercise. If you wish to pursue a programme of

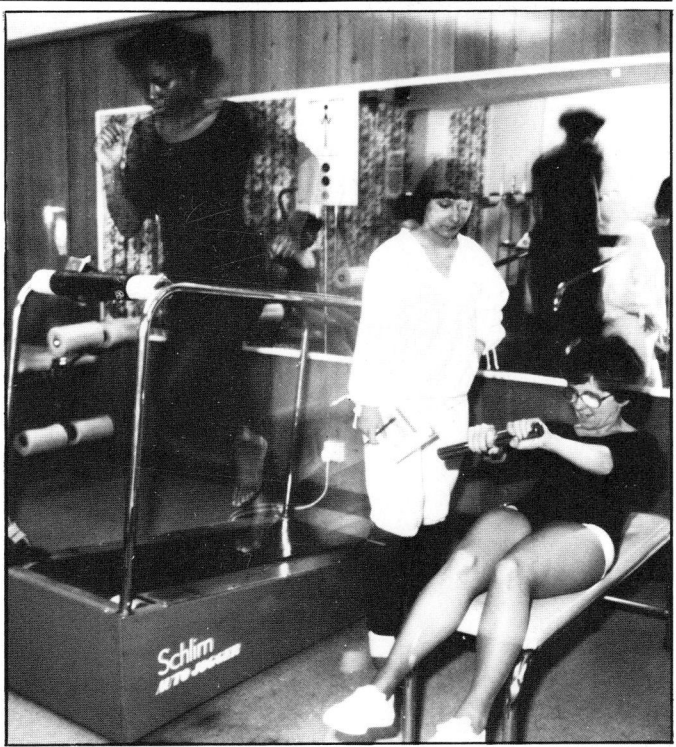

Running the treadmill: more and more health clubs, such as this one in Birmingham, are offering equipment to promote aerobic fitness

isometric exercise, take care not to overtax your strength. Dynamic exercise can lead to strains but in general it is self-limiting. With weights such as bar-bells, you can easily hurt yourself: always start with small weights and only gradually increase the weights.

Before looking, briefly, at the role of weight-lifting in an overall fitness programme it is worth emphasizing that weights are not the only form of isometric exercise. Indeed, pure isometric exercise requires no equipment whatsoever. What it involves is simply maximum muscle contraction against an immovable object. In an office, for instance, hold both sides of a typewriter and press inwards as hard as possible as if trying to get the hands to meet. Hold for five seconds and that counts as isometric exercise of the arm and chest muscles.

Isometric exercise is thus intensive development of the strength and bulk of particular muscles. Programmes of such exercises are offered in various book – the Charles Atlas 'dynamic tension' programme which has promised to turn generations of seven-stone weaklings into husky heroes is no more than a form of isometric exercise. Such exercises can be performed for almost any muscle, but should never involve muscle contraction for longer than a few seconds. They are very effective in developing strength but do nothing for suppleness or stamina.

Weight-*training* has a similarly restricted benefit and should also be approached with some caution. It is not to be confused with weight-lifting, however. Weight-training has more modest ambitions. Women, in particular, might be reassured that a weight-training programme will not result in rippling muscles in their shoulders and thighs. Weight-training is best regarded as part of an overall fitness programme once you have attained a good level of fitness through dynamic exercise. What it offers is a way of maintaining and developing fitness. The weights involved are quite light since the emphasis is more on the number of lifts than the actual load carried. Weight-training can be adapted to the needs of different kinds of sportsmen or sportswomen who will want to improve particular strengths. It can be done at home but, initially at least, it is probably best done under the skilled supervision of a gymnasium or sports centre.

OTHER ROUTES TO FITNESS

HEALTH CLUBS

Private health clubs and gymnasiums are booming as people become more fitness-conscious. A good local-authority sports centre may well offer a cheaper way to fitness but not everybody will have access to such a centre. Some private gymnasiums are also better equipped than local-authority establishments. And paying money seems to help some people persist in their fitness programme.

Problem number one, however, is how to choose between the many clubs and gymnasiums which now exist in or around the bigger cities. Their style can range from the spartan to the exotic. In one sense, the trimmings do matter because a gym has to be sufficiently attractive to lure you there regularly. But more important is the range of equipment on offer and the quality of supervision.

If a gymnasium devotes most time to weight-training or body-building, it will do little to promote the dynamic fitness which is best for general health. What you want is an all-round fitness programme that improves the heart and circulation, increases mobility and enhances strength. Exercise bikes – and enough of them – are therefore more important than bar-bells. You also want a gymnasium with instructors capable of devising a programme for your degree of unfitness. Instructors should also be present to monitor and encourage you. Assessing the instructors is always difficult. You can ask about their qualifications but a better idea might be to ask some existing members for their views. If possible, try out a gym on a short-trial basis before committing yourself to a major investment. And always check to establish any additional costs for specific courses.

Some gymnasiums and health clubs run introductory group courses for activities such as keep-fit exercises or yoga. Sometimes, too, these are tailored for particular age groups: special keep-fit classes are often run for people over sixty, for instance. These courses are ideal for beginners since they will feel less self-conscious than when venturing alone into a club where everyone else seems fitter and apparently knows how to use all the equipment.

DANCE

Anyone who doubts that dancing can be regarded as exercise clearly has not danced for some time. Whether the music is rock or old-time, dancing offers excellent exercise for everyone from their teens to old age. For retired people, dancing is particularly appealing since it combines exercise with a social life. (Loneliness is one of the great trials of old age; dancing provides a means of meeting members of the opposite sex after the death of a life partner.)

Not all dancing need be done in pairs, however. In recent years there has been a growth in popularity of dance classes designed specifically as a means of fitness. One-hour lessons take people through some basic dance movements that stretch a wide range of muscles. The music helps you sustain the exercise in a more continuous – and therefore more beneficial – way than is normal for simple keep-fit exercises. Such dance classes are sometimes run by gyms or organizations like the YMCA, but more often they are run privately by specialist groups or teachers. Most are aimed at women. Look in local papers or ask at community associations.

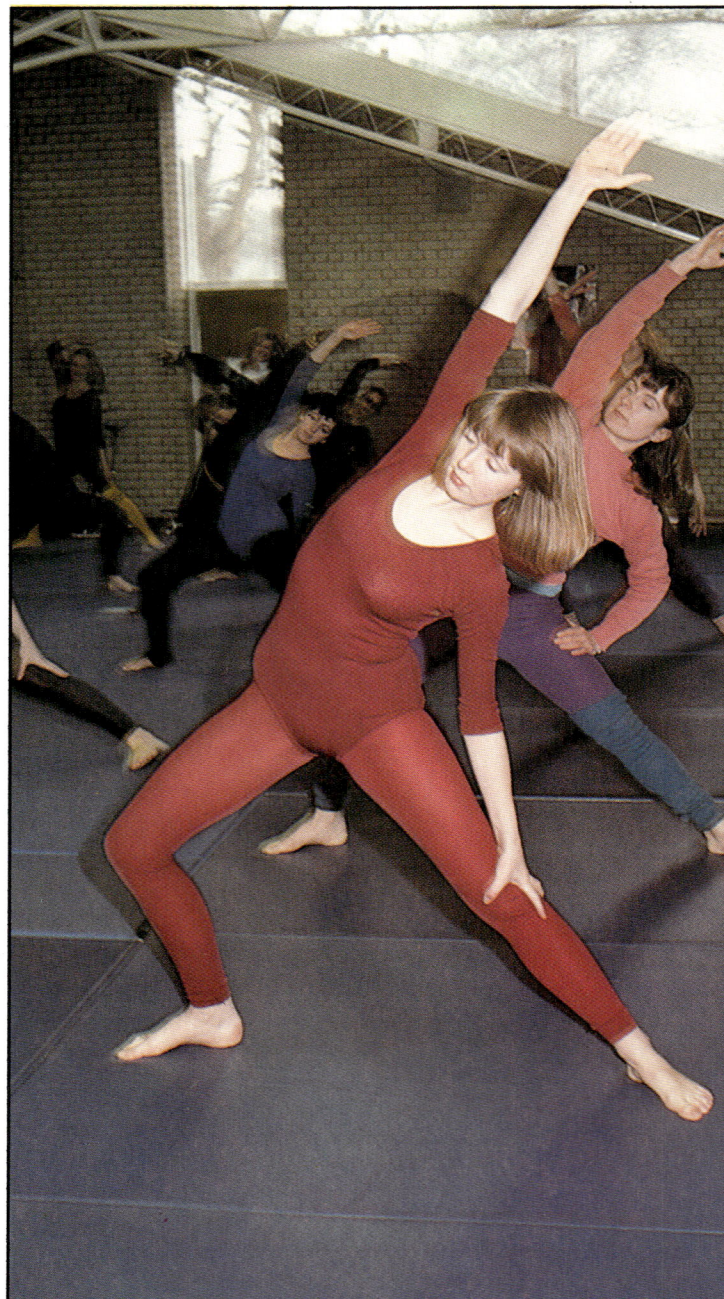

Organized dance classes provide excellent exercise for all ages

Sport

All exercise may be good for you but different types of exercise affect the body in different ways. The jogger who pounds round the local park, for instance, will have more stamina than the gymnast – who has flexibility and suppleness of body. One of the attractions of keep-fit exercises such as those mentioned above is that they are structured to improve all-round fitness. But toe-touching hardly has the intrinsic appeal of participatory sport.

Some people will use exercises or jogging simply to achieve sufficient fitness to take part in their favourite sports; others will hope that sport itself will get and keep them fit. It all depends, of course, on the sport they wish to pursue, and on their own state of fitness. In the tables that follow, we have rated sixty-four sports and other activities for their differing physical effects on the human body.

The tables are adapted from the findings of an International Committee on the Standardization of Physical Fitness Tests. Medical experts from thirty-seven countries were represented on this committee, whose research provided the basis of a minutely detailed textbook, *International Guide to Fitness and Health*, published by Crown Publishers Inc. of New York. Some British doctors believe their American counterparts underestimate the potential for fitness in activities such as gardening and DIY. We have therefore included a few of the domestic and non-sporting activities contained in the *International Guide*'s tables in order to provide a comparison of their fitness potential with some of the most popular sports.

THE FITNESS RATINGS OF SPORT
A. General Endurance
B. Muscular Strength
C. Mobility of Joints

The potential effect of each activity in each category is indicated by three ratings:
1. great effect (***)
2. moderate effect (**)
3. little or no effect (*)

The table shows the differences between sports. The common denominator, though, is pleasure. And because sports are a social pleasure, and doing well at them is part of this pleasure, there is a greater chance that you will not only keep at them but also train for them. This makes it far more likely that you will reach and maintain a healthy level of fitness. You can get fit through sport, therefore, but do not expect to do so with one weekly game of squash or tennis. Nor should you expect much pleasure if you are too unfit to enjoy a sport. Some sports demand a reasonable level of fitness *before* you take them up – basketball, for instance. Even hill-walking needs a rudimentary fitness. If you are unfit, then choose a sport where you can select your own level of exertion – solo canoeing or swimming, for instance – and can thereby do more to improve your own level of physical fitness.

(Adapted from *International Guide to Fitness and Health*, by Leonard A. Larson and Herbert Mickelman (c) 1973 by Leonard A. Larson and Herbert Mickelman; used by permission of Crown Publishers Inc. The full guide contains additional activities and categories such as 'Skills' and 'Neuro-Muscular Relaxation' which we felt were more subjective)

		General Endurance	Muscular Strength	Mobility
1.	Archery	*	**	*
2.	Badminton	**	**	**
3.	Baseball	*	*	**
4.	Basketball	***	**	**
5.	Billiards	*	*	*
6.	Bowling (American)	*	*	*
7.	Boxing	***	***	*
8.	Canoeing	**	***	*
9.	Climbing stairs	**	**	***
10.	Cricket	*	*	**
11.	Croquet	*	*	*
12.	Curling	*	*	**
13.	Cycling (Speed)	***	**	*
14.	Dancing	**	*	*
15.	Darts	*	*	*
16.	Digging in Garden	**	***	**
17.	Driving	*	*	*
18.	Fencing	*	**	***
19.	Fishing	*	*	*
20.	Football (American)	**	**	**
21.	Football (Soccer)	**	**	**
22.	Golf	*	*	**
23.	Gymnastics	*	**	**
24.	Hiking	**	**	*
25.	Hockey	**	**	*
26.	Horse Riding	**	*	*
27.	Housework	*	*	**
28.	Hunting	**	*	*
29.	Ice-hockey	**	**	*
30.	Jogging in place	**	*	*
31.	Judo	*	**	**
32.	Jumping (Ski)	*	**	**
33.	Karate	*	**	**
34.	Kayaking	**	***	**
35.	Lacrosse	**	**	**
36.	Mountain climbing	***	**	**
37.	Mowing lawn	*	**	*
38.	Orienteering	**	**	*
39.	Rowing	***	***	*
40.	Rugby	**	**	**
41.	Running (Sub-maximal)	***	**	*
42.	Sailing	*	**	**
43.	Sawing	**	***	*
44.	Scuba diving	**	*	**
45.	Sculling	***	***	**
46.	Shooting	*	*	*
47.	Skating (Ice)	**	**	*
48.	Skating (Roller)	**	**	*
49.	Skin-diving	***	**	**
50.	Skiing (Cross-country)	***	***	**
51.	Skiing (Downhill)	**	**	*
52.	Snooker	*	*	*
53.	Squash	**	**	***
54.	Surfing	*	**	**
55.	Swimming (Sub-maximal)	***	***	***
56.	Table tennis	*	*	**
57.	Tennis	**	**	**
58.	Volleyball	*	*	**
59.	Walking briskly (over 1 hr.)	**	*	*
60.	Washing/polishing car	*	**	**
61.	Water polo	***	**	**
62.	Water skiing	**	**	*
63.	Weight lifting	*	***	*
64.	Wrestling	**	**	**

EXERCISE/SPORT

TEAM GAMES
Team games are rarely the best way to get fit, although, sadly, often all that is learned at school. The unfit are left lagging far behind their fitter colleagues or the ball or both. Even the fittest only participate in many team games for short periods of time. Stop-watch checks on soccer players, for instance, have shown that the very best players in the most 'active' midfield positions rarely possess the ball for more than three minutes of a ninety-minute match. But at least they will be running for most of the remaining eighty-seven minutes, unlike cricketers of whom only two out of twenty-two will usually be competing actively at any one time. Some people, however, like the camaraderie of teams, which may give them an incentive to train regularly.

Such training is necessary because most team games involve bursts of sudden activity which make great demands on the heart and circulation. In addition to a high degree of general fitness, sports also require high performance from certain groups of muscles. To improve your game, you can thus work out exercises or training programmes tailored to your particular needs. But these are only suitable once you have achieved a good level of overall fitness.

Although we have cautioned against team games as a *means* to fitness, this does not mean that all such sports can be rated equally. In general, games with large numbers of participants are less good than those where fewer people are involved. Basketball, for instance, offers more continuous activity and a wider range of muscular movements for all its players than does soccer – although the basketball player is sometimes withdrawn for rest periods not available in football.

Sometimes, too, the same sport makes greatly differing demands on fitness according to where you play. An American survey once showed that a woman playing hockey as a half-back or midfield player ran half a mile more in a sixty-minute game than a forward in the same match. The forward, however, probably needs greater speed. Cricket is the game where standards of fitness probably differ most. To bowl fast for any length of time requires considerable fitness; to be a slip-fielder stretches concentration rather than muscles. However, variations such as these enable people to continue playing sports they enjoy for many years. As speed declines a footballer, for instance, can use his skill and experience in a different position just as a fast bowler learns to substitute variety of delivery for sheer pace.

COMPETITIVE SPORTS
Some people need the spur of competition to provide the motivation for their exercise. But if competition implies the desire to win, they should prepare themselves for disappointment as they grow older, or at least seek their opponents solely from their contemporaries. Otherwise the inevitable decline in strength and speed as you grow older becomes increasingly the difference between success and failure. Ball games between individuals are generally better for fitness than team games, but they still depend on the ability of *both* players to sustain the action. The spasmodically explosive nature of sports such as squash can lead to strains on muscles and joints, however.

Squash is perhaps the best ball game for keeping less good players on the move – but you do need to be moderately fit. Aim to improve your fitness through running or swimming before starting to play squash – and remember the safety checks outlined on page 43. But assuming that you have this minimum degree of general fitness, squash offers many attractions – always assuming, too, that you can find somewhere to play the game.

First, squash allows a greater margin of error than, say, tennis, which means that less good people can keep the game going for longer. Second, this more continuous activity is the key to cardiovascular improvement. It therefore follows that squash is more likely to have a beneficial effect on the heart and circulation, although this is less assured than the effects of a pure aerobic programme such as running.

Tennis requires greater precision than squash and is thus less likely to engender continuous activity among novices. Ironically, rallies are also likely to be short if you or your opponent is very good. Nevertheless, tennis offers simple and usually accessible exercise that *helps* improve fitness while being inadequate in itself to achieve it. Tennis (along with other racket sports such as squash and **badminton**) also improves the strength and mobility of the playing arm. The beneficial effects on muscular strength of the legs depend upon the intensity with which the game is played. Badminton offers much the same advantages and disadvantages as tennis apart from being more of a year-round sport.

MIDDLE-AGED SPORTS*
There are only two special rules for the middle-aged and they apply whether the seeker-after-fitness is bent on sport, jogging or morning exercises:

Golf is not enough in itself to achieve fitness but it is an enjoyable sport that can be played by men and women of most ages

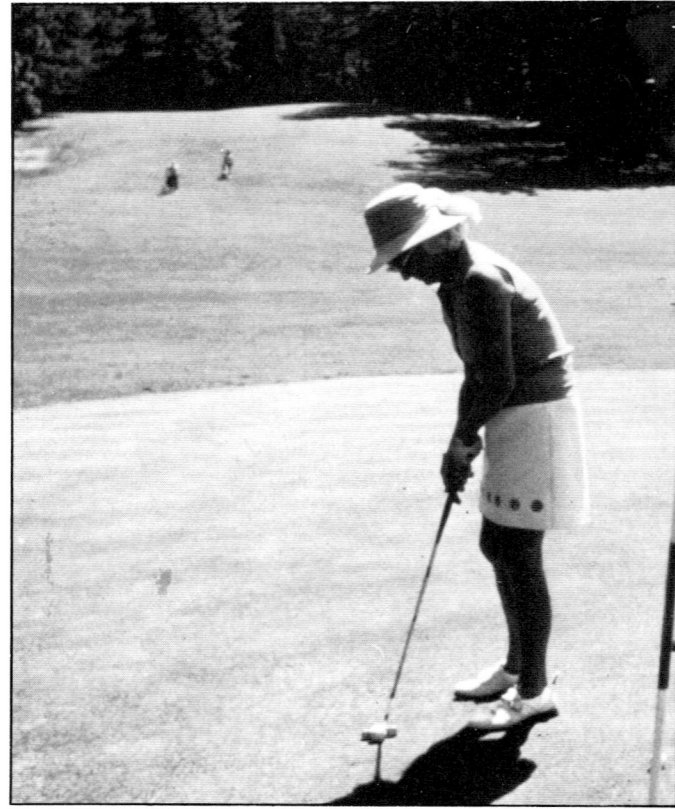

*For exercise in old age, see pages 198–200

SPORT/EXERCISE

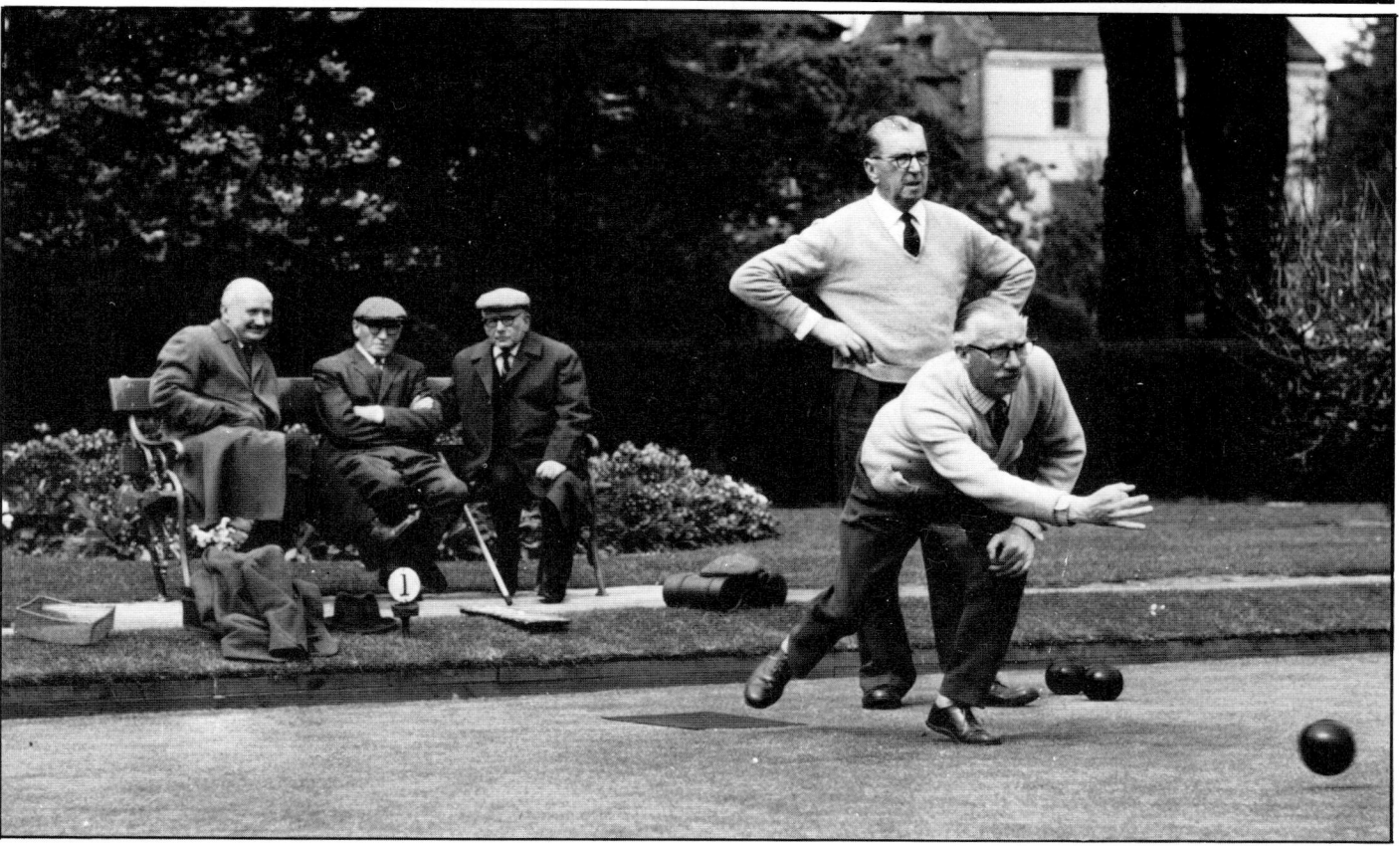

Bowls is identified as a sport for the elderly, although the champions are younger. It won't get you fit but the companionship and fresh air can certainly do you good

1. Do take things cautiously. You cannot erase years of neglect with a sudden bout of furious activity. Running too fast too soon can lead at the least to strained muscles and joints, as we have noted.
2. Exercise within the 'heartbeat' range for your age described earlier is harmless enough, but the main thing is to be sensible about yourself. Use your common sense, therefore, but do also read the general safety check outlined earlier in this chapter (page 43).

Many sports clubs have special classes, competitions or sections for the over-forties, -fifties and even over-sixties. Choosing a sport is very much a matter of individual preference; there is no universal best-buy offering the maximum health benefit for the minimum exertion. But generally the best sports for middle-aged people are those where the level of activity is determined by themselves rather than by opponents who may be much better (or much worse) than them. Likely sports in this category include swimming and solo rowing or canoeing. Golf, bowls and rambling offer gentler exercise but good recreation. Badminton, tennis and – for fitter middle-aged people – squash are the most popular competitive sports.

Golf is not, of course, a sport solely for the middle-aged. In fact, players like Jack Nicklaus are regarded as veterans on the professional circuit by the time they have reached their fortieth birthday. But it can be sufficiently gentle to be maintained well into the retirement years. An average golfer walks about four miles during his 18-hole round. This activity is no doubt 'good' for you but it is not enough to get you fit in the sense that we have described fitness in this chapter. The heartbeat is at no point raised sufficiently to achieve the improvement to the heart and circulation which is at the root of general fitness. However, the walking doesn't do any harm, particularly if you carry your clubs and walk briskly, and the golf swing improves the mobility of shoulders and trunk. It may also help you relax – if the pursuit of a good round doesn't become too obsessive.

SPORTS FOR THE FAMILY
Most of the sports featured in our tables can be played by men and women. There is only one strictly female sport – netball; and only two – boxing and ice-hockey – which are normally confined to men. Women have far fewer 'active recreations' than men and have traditionally been more reluctant than men to take up organized sport in their middle age. There is no reason why this should be so and many sports report increasing female participation, just as more and more women are taking up jogging (see page 51). But if women do still feel shy or ungainly, they should consider keep-fit exercises or keep-fit classes.

Sport is often regarded as an enemy of family life. The husband and father who spends the weekdays at work disappears for long stretches of the weekend to play football or cricket. Some sports, however, are ideal for all the family. Swimming in the local baths or leisure centre, country walking, cycling, tennis, badminton, canoeing and orienteering, for instance, offer opportunities for families to play together at weekends or during their holidays. The children, and perhaps their parents, will learn new skills; the parents will certainly improve their fitness; and the families will stay together.

3: STRESS AND RELAXATION

Stress

Everybody is under stress. Adam and Eve in the Garden of Eden were under stress. Yet most medical experts agree that there is more stress in our lives today than ever before. Driving a car, for instance, or travelling by plane produces a stress that our ancestors did not have to cope with. More than ever before, we need a strategy to deal with the hidden strains and pressures of life.

Every week most of us face stress in our daily lives. We run for and miss that bus or train that will take us to work. We face worrying tax demands and bills; the mortgage, the bank overdraft, the rent or some other financial anxiety nags at us. We work with people we don't really like, or we have the occasional quarrel with our husband, wife, boss or colleague. All these experiences, which are the normal wear and tear of living, are stressful.

Then there are the more serious strains. If a parent, a partner or a close friend dies, the bereavement takes its toll of our mental and physical health. Divorces, court cases, accidents, or an illness in the family are all major strains. Oddly enough, success can be stressful, too. Promotion, starting a new job, more responsibility, all take their toll.

For some people these stresses will be relatively easy to live through. We all know people whose response-rate is low. They are able to deal with panics without getting fussed. Their attitude to life is easygoing, relaxed and, indeed, they are often very enjoyable people to have around. For others, stress piles up. Under the strain of events, they feel 'nervy', anxious, or always on the go.

When we are upset by the strains and stresses of life, most of us suffer minor disorders, like headaches, insomnia, indigestion, diarrhoea, or just general aches and pains. Stress, indeed, has been linked with conditions like migraine, asthma and ulcers. Even more serious disorders like hypertension or high blood pressure, and coronary heart disease, many doctors believe, are more likely to occur in people under a great deal of stress. Proving this link is extraordinarily difficult. But what has been proved is that a stressful event definitely has its effect on the health of human beings. An American, Dr Richard Rahe, did a careful study of some two thousand five hundred naval officers and men. He looked at their lives, and in particular whether there had been any major changes in the last six months. Then he checked their health in the following six months.

He found that those men who had experienced events that changed their life pattern were more likely to become

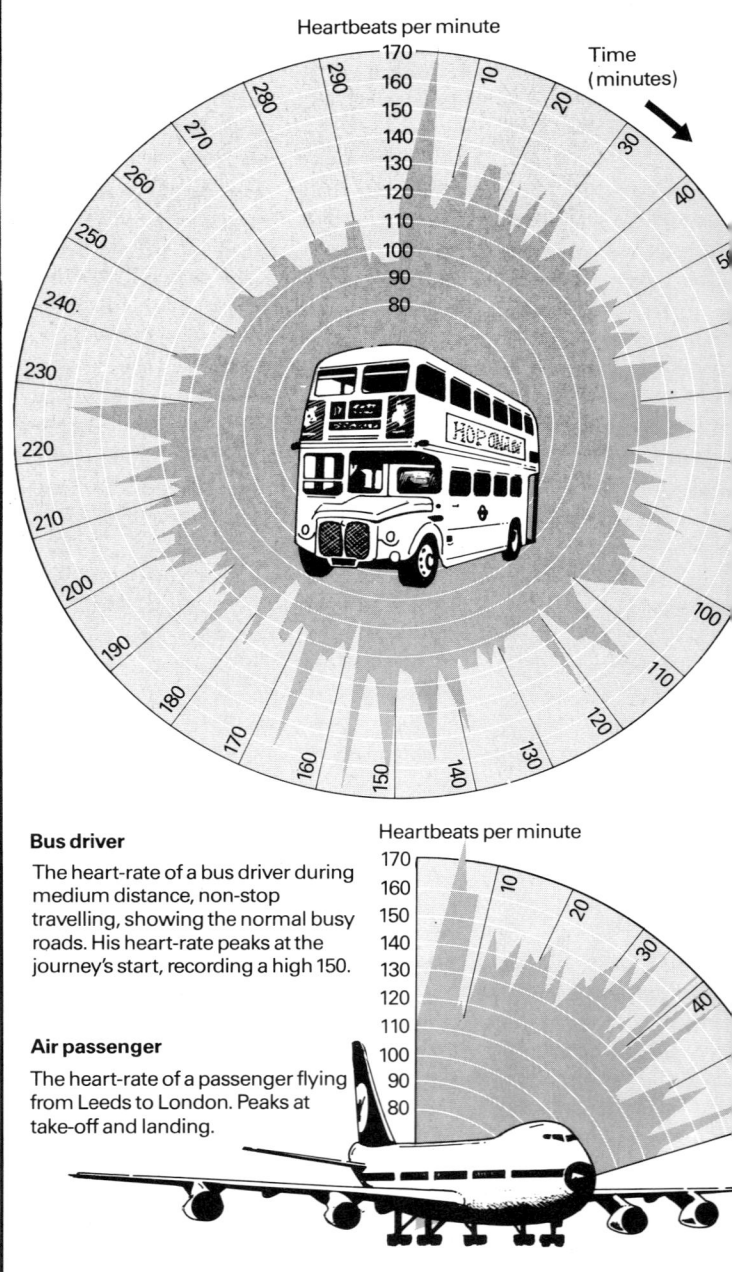

Bus driver
The heart-rate of a bus driver during medium distance, non-stop travelling, showing the normal busy roads. His heart-rate peaks at the journey's start, recording a high 150.

Air passenger
The heart-rate of a passenger flying from Leeds to London. Peaks at take-off and landing.

ill – possibly just minor illnesses like flu or colds, but nevertheless illnesses. In a way his findings echoed what folk wisdom has always said: if you are 'run down' or 'got down' by events, you catch whatever germs are around.

Dr Rahe then went further. He decided that it was too vague just to say that life events which required change made a human being more likely to develop some kind of illness. So he tried to draw up a scale of events, which gave a numerical value to each event so that the effect of an event on the average person could be measured. Four hundred Americans helped him work out the relative stressfulness of such events as divorce, the sack, mortgage difficulties and even Christmas (see Stress Quiz, page 68).

This way of measuring stress is extremely useful, but it cannot allow for individual differences. There is no doubt that personality, and the way we react to stress, makes a great deal of difference. It is interesting to note, for

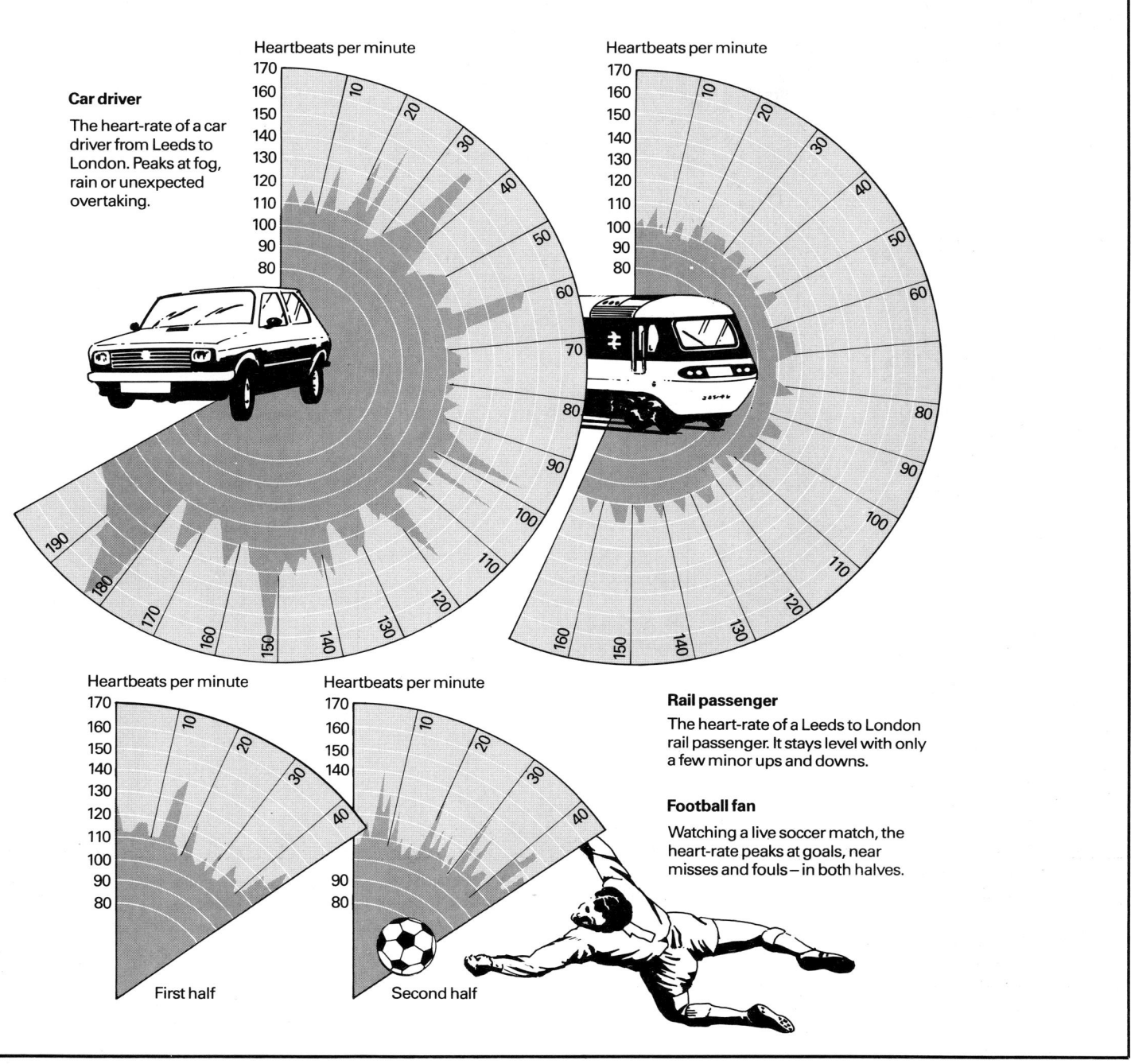

instance, that migraine sufferers tend to be people who are not only ambitious but perfectionists, intolerant of unpredictability, indecisiveness and uncertainty, and reluctant to sacrifice standards.

In the same way, heart disease has been associated with a particular – and not dissimilar – collection of personality traits. Two American heart experts, Dr Meyer Friedman and Dr Ray Rosenman, have dubbed the typical heart disease personality the 'Type A'. The Type A man suffers from 'hurry sickness'. He does things rapidly, he is always conscious of time, impatient, doing two or three things at once, guilty about relaxing, obsessed with 'numbers' and measurements, competitively ambitious, deadline-conscious, and an obsessive worker.

THE EFFECTS OF STRESS ON THE HEART

Dr Stanley Taylor, consultant in Cardiology and Senior Lecturer at the University of Leeds, has made a special study of the effects of stress and hypertension on the heart. He has spent over five years investigating the way everyday situations affect people with and without heart conditions. The graphs above are taken from his researches and they show the dramatic effects on the heart-rate of perfectly normal subjects when travelling by various means between Leeds and London. He also looks at the effects of a football match.

The graphs show the heart-rate, measured in beats per minute, of the normal healthy subjects who were monitored while driving their own cars between Leeds and London, a distance of about two hundred miles. The peaks of the heart-rate relate to normal motorway hazards such as bunching of cars in the fast lane, overtaking, rain, hazardous moves by other drivers, and driving at high speeds. There was a sustained increase in heart-rate while driving in

STRESS QUIZ

Are *you* under stress? You can measure the amount of stress in your life, using Dr Richard Rahe's stress scale. He has calculated the amount of stress that is caused by major life-events, and given each a numerical value. Have any of these events happened in your life in the last six months? If so, score for each that occurred, then check your total to see if your life is overstressful.

1.	Death of spouse	100
2.	Divorce	73
3.	Marital separation	65
4.	Jail term	63
5.	Death of close family	63
6.	Personal injury or illness	53
7.	Marriage	50
8.	Fired at work	47
9.	Marital reconciliation	45
10.	Retirement	45
11.	Change in health of family member	44
12.	Pregnancy	40
13.	Sex difficulties	39
14.	Gain of new family member	39
15.	Business readjustment	39
16.	Change in financial state	38
17.	Death of close friend	37
18.	Change to different line of work	36
19.	Change in number of arguments with spouse	35
20.	A large mortgage or loan	31
21.	Foreclosure of mortgage or loan	30
22.	Change in responsibilities at work	29
23.	Son or daughter leaving home	29
24.	Trouble with in-laws	29
25.	Outstanding personal achievement	28
26.	Spouse begins or stops work	26
27.	Begin or end school or college	26
28.	Change in living conditions	25
29.	A change in personal habits	24
30.	Trouble with the boss	23
31.	Change in work hours or conditions	20
32.	Change in residence	20
33.	Change in school or college	20
34.	Change in recreation	19
35.	Change in church activities	19
36.	Change in social activities	18
37.	A moderate mortgage or loan	17
38.	Change in sleeping habits	16
39.	Change in number of family get-togethers	15
40.	Change in eating habits	15
41.	Holiday	13
42.	Christmas	12
43.	Minor violations of the law	11

HOW TO SCORE
Below 60: your life has been unusually free from stress lately. **60 to 80:** you have had a normal amount of stress recently. This score is average for the ordinary wear and tear of life. **80 to 100:** the stress in your life is a little high, probably because of one recent event. **100 upwards**: pressures are piling up, either at home or work, or both. You are under serious stress, and the higher you score above 100 the worse the strain.

the cities and on the motorway, with frequent peaks of 110–140. Stress is indicated by heart-rates of over 100–120 beats per minute, depending on the age of the subject. Normal resting heart-rate is between 70 and 80. (The effects of the same test on those with heart disease were obviously more worrying, with up to 150 beats per minute.)

When the subjects were being driven in the front seat of a car doing the same journey, maximum heart-rates ranged from 90–110 with situations of sudden or potential danger.

When they were travelling from Leeds to London by plane their heart-rates were recorded at 100–150. The high rates were associated with events such as the closure of the aircraft's door before take-off, with landing procedures and sudden changes in altitude. Rail travel was by far the least disturbing with the heart-rate rarely going above 80 beats per minute.

Dr Taylor's subjects showed very little or no physical activity when the heart-rate was at its highest, and it is interesting that a subject was unaware of what was happening to his heart, even when the heart-rate was up to 150 beats per minute.

People were also monitored while watching live and televised football matches. The peaks here relate to goal-scoring, near misses, fouls on home-side players and misinterpreted decisions by the referee. The television viewing of live transmissions of the matches show a lower heart-rate than if you were actually seeing the match live.

But it is not just stress that is the enemy: it is how the individual responds to stress. The theory is that the key may lie in the body's automatic response to emotions like fear, anxiety, anger or even joy. 'In modern society, wrath, reinforced by sloth and gluttony, is the deadliest of the seven sins,' says Dr Malcolm Carruthers, another British heart specialist who has measured the body's response to various stressful activities such as driving and flying.

Primitive man, faced with an experience that aroused emotion, would either attack or run away. Modern man has also got this 'flight or fight' reaction. Strong emotion produces adrenaline and noradrenaline, hormones that pour into the system. The heart beats more strongly and the blood-vessels narrow to make more blood available for the muscles. Breathing becomes faster. The whole body is ready for action.

Unfortunately, physical action is not usually required. We cannot fight the boss or the income-tax demand – nor can we simply run away from a marital quarrel. So the body's emergency response turns inward on itself, taking a toll of the body, either immediately or sometimes later after the emotions have disappeared, resulting in nervous diarrhoea, indigestion, or even a rise in blood pressure.

Doctors who believe that many of the changes in illness statistics, like the increasing amount of migraine and heart disease, are due to stress, blame modern life for producing this reaction too often. Caught in a traffic jam on the way to work, worried by a boss's demand for better performance, made anxious by the news that the firm is going to make people redundant, the modern executive is permanently on the alert. His or her body is going into this emergency response over and over again, and never being able to react in a physical way with a good fight or a fast getaway.

Stress may also harm human beings by producing fatigue, which in turn makes the individual vulnerable to illness. Most people react to stress by something which is called the general adaptation syndrome. The first reaction is shock, followed by resistance, during which the body marshals its forces to deal with the stress. Finally, this energetic reaction will end in exhaustion and collapse, if the stress continues long enough. When stress overloads a person, fatigue and exhaustion result. 'At this point, there is a lowering of resistance to infection,' says Dr Carruthers. 'When people drive themselves on through tiredness to the point of exhaustion, that's when the harm is done.'

But the good news is that we can learn to cope with stress. For those who are in the grip of a serious illness like heart disease, it may mean avoiding stress – giving up shift work, cutting down on too much driving or overseas travelling, or even changing jobs to something less stressful. For the rest of us, coping with stress means taking more heed of the messages of the body – stopping when tired instead of forcing oneself on, getting enough rest and sleep, learning to switch off from anxieties and tension by proper relaxation. For those who are habitually tense and anxious, relaxation or meditation classes may be necessary.

Relaxation

For stresses that cannot be avoided, a different strategy is needed. A regular relaxation period every day is what Dr Friedman and Dr Rosenman recommend for their Type A potential heart-attack victims, and it does seem to work. Measurements on people practising meditation, which involves mental and physical relaxation, have shown that their oxygen consumption drops, their breathing slows down, their heart beats more slowly and (if they are people with high blood pressure) their blood pressure drops. However, other researchers have found that the same amount of time spent sleeping seems to have a similar effect.

Even more interesting was a trial carried out by Dr Chandra Patel, a British doctor. She treated twenty patients suffering from high blood pressure by persuading them to carry out twenty minutes of meditation and relaxation twice a day. She compared their progress with a group of similar hypertension sufferers, who were getting the same regular attention from her but not doing any meditative relaxation. The blood pressure of the regular meditators dropped over a yearly period, and their need for drugs was reduced. The patients who were not doing the meditation did not improve, and they needed just as many drugs at the end as they had at the beginning.

Deep relaxation, like the sort experienced by meditators, is therefore the key. Of course, it may be a skill that you already possess. Hot baths, a quiet drink with the feet up, a real rest after sport or gardening – these are ways many people relax. Others find that these are not enough and find difficulty in relaxing body and mind into real quietness.

So how can we learn to relax? Here are some of the ways people have been helped to relax. Everybody has different preferences, so choose the one you think might appeal. Relaxation should be enjoyed, otherwise it will not work.

MASSAGE
Try rubbing the back of your partner's neck and shoulders using the thumbs to roll up the muscles towards the head.

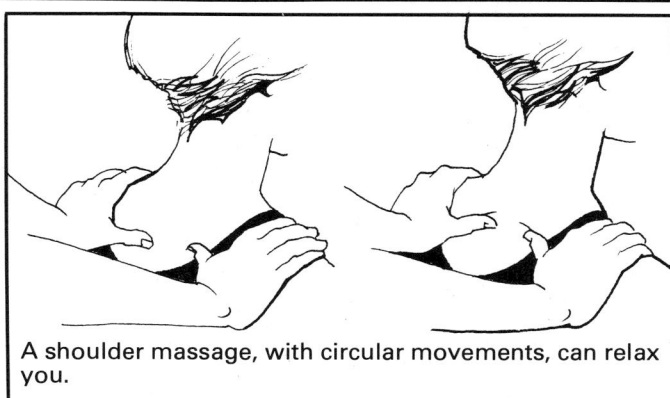
A shoulder massage, with circular movements, can relax you.

Or massage the back and buttocks with the flat of the palm in a regular firm rhythm. Feats such as walking up and down somebody's back are strictly for the professionals. If you do belong to a health or sports club where massage is available after exercise, indulge yourself.

MUSCLE CONTROL
Classes are sometimes available to teach muscle control. It is relatively easy to know when the muscles are tensed, but difficult to feel when they are relaxed. Relaxation classes can help teach this. In principle, if one can relax each major muscle group, one's mind will relax, too, and deep relaxation will follow. Classes can sometimes teach the 'trick' of relaxing, which can be turned on at will during stressful experiences. It is worth checking to see if any classes are held in your area.

The most common method of learning to identify a relaxed muscle is the 'tense-and-let-go' method. For instance, when shoulders are tensed, they tend to rise up towards the ears. By deliberately hunching them into a tense position then letting them go, it is possible to feel what a relaxed muscle should be like. Try sitting down hands on lap, and legs slightly apart. Then clench the jaw, and relax it; frown and screw up the face, and relax it; squeeze your thighs together, then let them relax outwards; clasp your hands and then relax them. A good system using these kinds of exercises and others has been worked out by British physiotherapist Mrs Jane Madders (see Appendix Three).

Some people find deep breathing useful. If you are emotionally upset, your breath comes in short sharp pants from the top of the rib-cage; so deep breathing from the diaphragm is the opposite. Place your hands at the bottom of the rib-cage so that the fingers lightly touch. Take a deep breath inwards, pulling the air into the diaphragm so that your fingers are drawn apart as the diaphragm swells. Do this three or four times.

Some people find three or four deep breaths useful before a potentially stressful experience. A variant of this kind of relaxation 'trick' is recommended for Type A potential heart-victims by Friedman and Rosenman. If

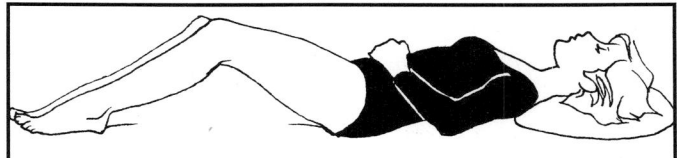
Try deep breathing when lying on the back with knees half bent

STRESS AND RELAXATION/RELAXATION

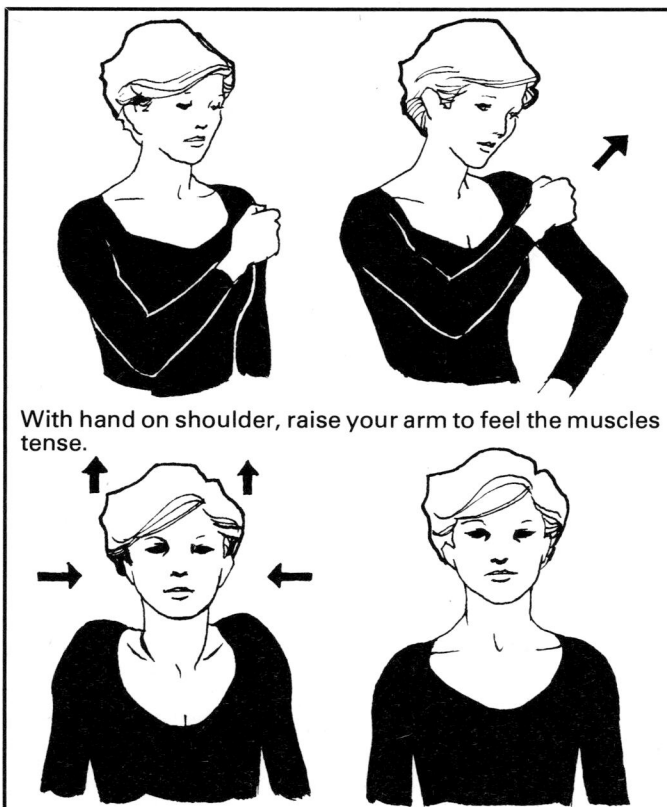

With hand on shoulder, raise your arm to feel the muscles tense.

Hunch shoulders towards the ears, tensing muscles, then relax. Stress exercises from *Relax*, by Mrs Jane Madders (BBC publications)

faced with a particularly long-drawn-out stressful experience – like writing a long report or having to do a series of complicated manual manoeuvres – take the occasional break from it, to stop the nervous tension building up. Stop doing it altogether, and read a newspaper for a while. Stroll out of the office or workroom for a chat with a friend. Take a proper tea or coffee break – *not* with the work still before you. Some people find that Biofeedback machines can help them learn to relax (see Appendix Three).

AUTOGENIC TRAINING

This could be described as a European version of the deep meditation practised by Eastern cults. It is a deep-relaxation technique invented by a German psychiatrist in 1932, where the emphasis is purely on the physical relaxation rather than the spiritual meanings of meditation. By attending classes for eight weeks, you can learn to put yourself into a kind of self-hypnosis. The aim is to counter-act stress and fatigue by this low-arousal state. Classes at the London centre are under medical supervision, and there are also a few practitioners outside London (see Appendix Three).

MEDITATION

Relaxation by meditation is becoming more common in Britain. It is practised in yoga and Zen Buddhism, and among various Eastern spiritual organizations. The best known is probably transcendental meditation, practised by the followers of the Maharishi, made famous by the Beatles. Siddha meditation is a slightly different variant practised by the followers of the Swami Muktananda.

The principle is to use a mental device – a mantra, a single word, or a visual symbol – to relax the mind, from which bodily relaxation will flow. In its simplest form it means giving the mind something fairly unexciting to think about to blot out distracting thoughts. When such a thought comes into the mind, it is replaced by the mantra, the word or the symbol. It is probably easiest to learn this technique in a class. Check if local education services have any yoga lessons or write to the transcendental meditation and siddha meditation centres (see Appendix Three).

SLEEP

Few things are more important than a good night's sleep. After a good sleep you are much more alert and capable of working or enjoying yourself to your full capacity. When you are short of sleep you are slower, duller and less fun to be with. However, different people need different amounts of sleep: most adults average just under eight hours' sleep per night but old people need less and young people need more.

During sleep, the body is busy repairing itself. Growth hormone pours into the blood and stimulates the various tissues and organs of the body to repair themselves and grow. This is one reason why growing children need more sleep than adults. Even the brain is growing and repairing itself during sleep, and while it is doing this the blood-supply to the brain increases and a person goes through a more wakeful period of dreaming sleep. Good sleep is essential for this process of bodily renewal, and if a person is deprived of sleep for a number of nights, then they will oversleep later in order to catch up. If a person does not catch up on lost sleep, then they lose their ability to concentrate and to deal with anything but the simplest problems.

When we are awake, the hemispheres of the brain are very active, enabling us to respond to what we feel, hear and see. The activity in the brain hemispheres is dependent upon stimulation coming from the brain-stem, which lies at the point where the brain is attached to the spinal cord. Thinking and consciousness occur in the hemispheres, but without the constant stimulation of the brain-stem activity in the hemispheres declines and we fall asleep.

The brain-stem itself works as if it were a clock with a twenty-four-hour cycle of activity. However, some people seem to have a twenty-five-hour cycle and tend always to stay up late, and others have a twenty-three-hour cycle and tend to go to bed early and wake early. The hemispheres also stimulate the brain-stem and may override it. This happens when we are worried or excited – the hemispheres then stimulate the brain-stem to keep up its activity so that it is very difficult for them to switch off. On the other hand, a monotonous, warm environment makes us sleepy because the hemispheres cease to stimulate the brain-stem, which in turn ceases to stimulate the hemispheres.

There are two kinds of sleep. We start the night with deep sleep, but after one and a half to two hours we experience lighter dreaming-sleep, when our eyes make rapid movements and our electric brain-waves are faster than in ordinary sleep. Psychologists call the period of dreaming-sleep paradoxical or 'rapid eye movement' sleep. When people are woken up during this period they say they have been dreaming; these periods of dreaming-sleep recur about every one and a half hours during the night. Both

RELAXATION/STRESS AND RELAXATION

types of sleep are needed, and if someone is deprived of dreaming by being constantly woken up whenever they dream, then the following night they will have more dreaming-sleep.

Inability to sleep properly may be a sign that a person is worried, depressed, drinking too much or taking insufficient exercise. The majority of people who complain about their inability to sleep properly are worriers. They are people who feel they carry a great burden of responsibility, have great ambitions or perhaps carry a burden of guilt. Relaxation may help people with these problems.

A little alcohol may help a person to sleep at night. It is effective as an occasional remedy for difficulty in getting to sleep. However, regular or heavy drinking in the evenings can cause sleeping problems. A person who has had plenty of drink is liable to wake up early in the morning, when the effects of the alcohol are wearing off.

One of the best ways of getting a good night's sleep is to get some exercise in the evening before going to bed: take a walk, go jogging or if you cannot get out of the house try running up and down stairs.

People who suffer from depression often find it extremely difficult to sleep. Depression sometimes follows a personal crisis such as a death or a feeling of failure, or continues after a physical illness such as flu or jaundice. A person who is depressed often feels at their worst in the morning and wakes up at 2 a.m. and again at 4 a.m. with their mind racing. During the daytime a person who is depressed does not have normal energy and is not able to do the normal tasks of life. When this has lasted for weeks and cannot be put right by a change in circumstances, then your doctor may be able to help (see page 73).

Other drugs can be prescribed to help a person to sleep, but turning to drugs for help over a long period is dangerous (see Drug Dependence, page 147). Barbiturate sleeping tablets should no longer be prescribed. They are addictive, and an overdose, particularly combined with alcohol, is extremely dangerous.

Nothing can better natural sleep, but, if your doctor thinks a sleeping tablet is a good idea – and it should never be the first choice – first try the commonsense measures listed below, and then nitrazepam (Mogadon). This drug depresses the activity of the brain-stem and also relieves anxieties by its effect on the hemispheres, and so it makes sleep easier. However, like other sleeping drugs it reduces the amount of time spent dreaming and reduces the intensity of dreams. When coming off sleeping tablets, dreams become more vivid and it may take up to two months before sleep returns fully to normal.

Sleeping tablets taken before going to bed continue to have an effect the next day. They may cause a person to feel dreamy and to lack concentration; they may cause simple errors to be made in driving or any kind of brain-work or mechanical work. This effect may last until lunch-time the next day. Old people particularly (see Chapter 10) may become confused if given sleeping tablets or tranquillizers.

Sleeping tablets should always be considered to be a short-term solution. There are many alternative ways of promoting sleep. For example:

1. More exercise. Take a walk or jog before sleeping.
2. Have a milky drink or a snack before turning in. Avoid tea, coffee, rich or spicy food late at night.
3. Wear ear-plugs or install double glazing to cut out noise.
4. Read a book until you drop off. If you wake worrying, read to take your mind off the problem.
5. Some people use a mental task, like counting sheep, mental arithmetic or reciting poetry, to help them drop off. Relaxation or meditation exercises can be used in bed.
6. Keep warm with bedsocks, hot-water bottles or electric blankets.
7. Do not smoke in the bedroom. Stuffy air can prevent sleep.
8. If the bed is uncomfortable, buy a new one or put the mattress on the floor.
9. If anxiety keeps you awake and a book doesn't help, it may be worth getting up for a hot drink, then starting afresh to try to sleep.

Time-lapse photography shows the way human beings change their position during sleep. Most people shift position every 90 minutes or less. Frequent movements probably prevent pressure damage to skin and nerves.

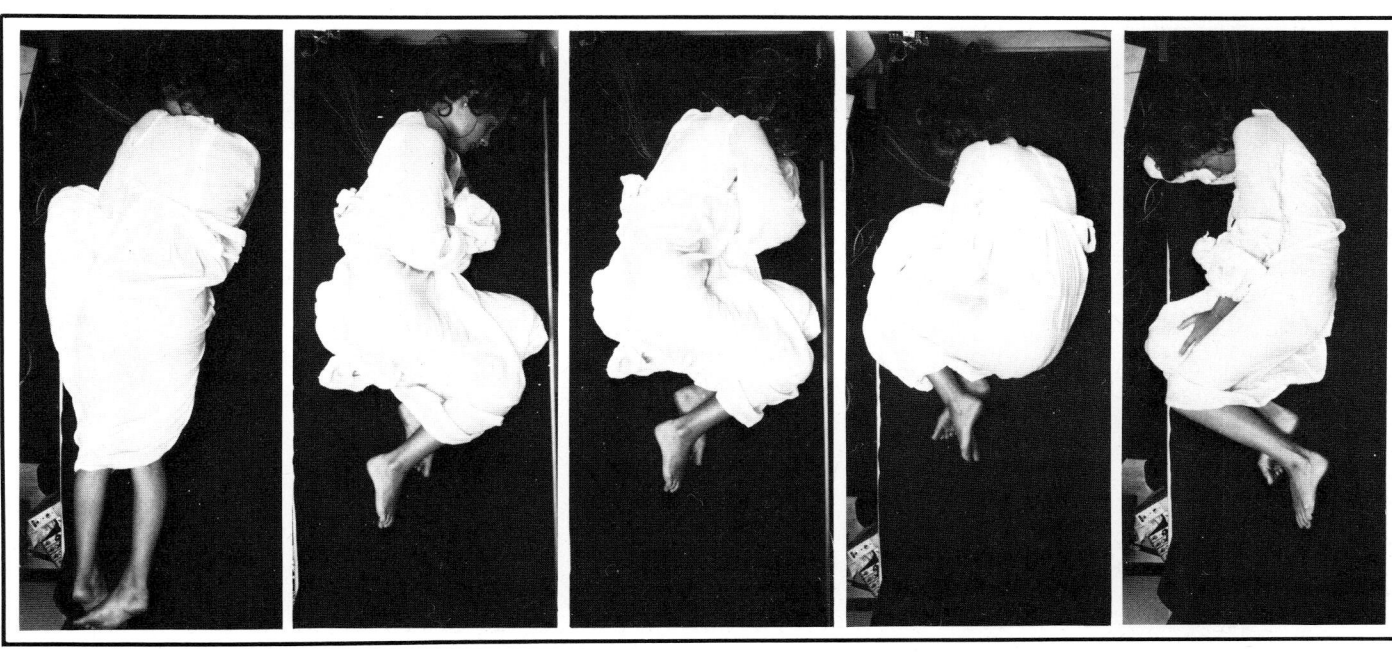

Headaches

Headache is one of the commonest of all complaints, and may be caused by anything from bad lighting to conflict between people creating psychological tension. Sometimes a headache is simply an excuse for a dignified retreat from the scene, but it can also be a sign of serious illness. Whatever the cause, the pain is a biological sign compelling the person to withdraw, a warning that something is wrong. The pain of headache usually arises in the structures around the brain, not the brain itself which is insensitive to pain. The blood-vessels that go to the brain, the membranes which cover it, and the muscles of the scalp are the usual sources of pain. Any stretching in these structures will cause a pain which may be localized in one spot or spread to the whole head. In the worst cases it is a blinding pain which prevents the victim from doing anything.

Vascular headaches arise in the blood-vessels which go to the brain and the muscles of the head. Arteries are sensitive to substances produced in the body which circulate in the blood-stream. These substances, metabolites, may cause excessive dilation of the blood-vessels in the brain in sensitive people; this stretches nerves in the blood-vessels, causing pain. Vascular headaches generally throb in time with the heartbeat. The pain may seem to come from deep inside the head but more often comes from the front or back.

Muscular headaches are caused by pains developing in the muscles of the scalp and neck. These may be the result of having to hold the head in an awkward way while working or a result of bad lighting. But more often they are the result of spasms in the muscles caused by tension, and so are often called tension headaches. Anxiety is the basic cause. The pain which results is sometimes described as a vice-like grip on the head, or like pressure from a tight band. The intense contraction of the muscles compresses the blood-vessels, so reducing the blood-supply and causing metabolites to accumulate locally which later dilate the blood-vessels, causing pain. Awareness of the source of the problem can enable a person to take simple measures to avoid tension (see Relaxation, pages 69–70).

Eye-strain is sometimes the cause of headaches. If you have any difficulty in seeing clearly, then you should get your eyes tested; if you already wear glasses, perhaps you need new lenses (see Eyes, pages 119–21).

Toxic headaches often occur when a person is ill with, for example, a cold or flu, but they can also be caused by food or alcohol. When too many toxic products are produced in the body, as in illness, and cannot be removed sufficiently quickly by the kidneys, then they may cause the blood-vessels in the brain to expand, giving a vascular type of headache. Alcohol taken in quite small quantities can trigger appalling headaches in sensitive people; more rarely, sensitivity or allergy to certain types of food such as cheese, red wine, eggs or fish is a cause (see Allergies, pages 164–8).

Migraine headaches are particularly severe but only a minority of people suffer from them. The migraine attack usually consists of two phases. In the first phase the blood-vessels in the brain constrict, and this may cause temporary disturbance of vision or, very occasionally, temporary weakness. Then the blood-vessels dilate and severe headache follows, together with a feeling of nausea, vomiting and sometimes diarrhoea. The person is quite unable to carry on normally while this is happening and must rest. Migraine headaches can be treated by a variety of drugs, so consult your doctor. You can also get help and advice from the Migraine Trust (see Appendix Three). They will provide a list of specialist clinics, to which your family doctor can refer you.

Self-help starts with the study of your migraine attacks. You should keep a diary, recording both the day and the time of the attack, as well as a daily record of your activities and food. By looking back over the twenty-four hours before the attack, you may be able to identify what brings on migraine. It is not always easy, since for many people it is a combination of factors which starts the migraine.

Trigger factors – the causes of an attack – include: worry; depression; shock; excitement: emotion; over-exertion; physical or mental tiredness; bending or stooping; lifting heavy weights or straining; change of routine; late rising; travel; weather change or a different climate; high winds; bright sunlight or lights; watching TV or films; hot baths; noise; intense smells; sleeping tablets; alcohol; lack of food or dieting; irregular meals; menstruation or the pre-menstrual period; menopause; high blood pressure; continued use of the pill; toothache or other pains in the head or neck. Certain foods, such as chocolate, citrus fruit, fried foods, pastry and cheese, also can trigger attacks.

Once the trigger factors are identified, try to avoid them. Do not get hungry and be careful what you eat. Women who suffer pre-menstrual headaches should be sure to eat something every three hours during the day (see also Pre-menstrual Tension, page 175). Avoid extreme temperatures and stressful events, if possible. Learn to relax and do not get overtired. Once an attack has come, take a pain-killer and lie down. Sleep is part of the natural recovery from migraine.

WHEN TO CONSULT YOUR DOCTOR

Headache may also be a symptom of some underlying illness, such as high blood pressure and occasionally more serious conditions. If you suffer from frequent headaches or if any unusual headache persists, or recurs or rapidly becomes worse, see your doctor for advice about treatment. Always consult a doctor about headaches which follow a blow to the head.

TREATING YOUR HEADACHE

If you have a severe headache, it may be best not to try and carry on bravely. People with headaches are hypersensitive to noise, more irritable and likely to be accident-prone. If you are able to rest, that is the best thing to do. Aspirin is an extremely effective treatment for headache, although it can cause stomach irritation and should not be taken day after day without consulting your doctor. Aspirin also should not be taken with alcohol since this can irritate the stomach. Paracetamol is an alternative to aspirin which seldom causes stomach irritation. A slightly stronger remedy available in Britain without prescription is Compound Codeine tablets, which contain a mixture of aspirin and codeine. Many proprietary preparations containing aspirin also contain caffeine, the active drug from coffee, which should be avoided if you wish to sleep your headache off.

Depression

Everybody gets depressed occasionally. Human life brings with it stresses and strains that are bound to make us unhappy. Loved ones die, jobs are lost, marriages or love affairs break up, and families quarrel among themselves. To be unmoved by these events is not to be fully human.

Confusion arises, however, because the word 'depression' is used in two different ways. Its most normal use is among ordinary people to cover ordinary feelings. People say they are depressed when they mean that they are feeling unhappy, down at the mouth, miserable or gloomy. They are talking about a normal unhappy mood which they expect will pass. Most of us feel mildly depressed after we have been ill, or when we are tired, and some people have mild feelings of depression that come along for no good reason. Women sometimes find that depression is part of pre-menstrual tension (see page 175).

The word 'depression' is also used to cover something much more severe. Severe depression makes the person ill with its mental suffering. Outsiders, who are used to the feelings of ordinary mild depression, sometimes do not understand just how acutely painful and prolonged are the mental sufferings of somebody with a depressive illness.

Severe depression can be triggered off by head injuries or concussion; some infections; operations on valued parts of the body – like having a leg amputated; hormonal changes; epilepsy; old age; and the aftermath of a non-fatal stroke or thrombosis. Some people may be psychologically more vulnerable than others to severe depression. Those who are cut off from human companionship – women kept at home with young children, widows and widowers, isolated single parents – are also more likely to get severe depression.

MILD DEPRESSION

Tragic life events like bereavements, marriage failure, or job loss can set off a mild depression. Society acknowledges that it is normal to feel unhappy after such events. We expect people to feel depressed when they have suffered loss, hardship or disappointment. Occasionally success can paradoxically set off mild depression too, probably because success is stressful as well as failure.

The normal first reaction to a tragic event like a death is shock, and a kind of numbness. Quite often a death in the family does not come entirely unexpectedly and so there has been a time during which the relatives were anticipating it. Even so, it is still usual for them to feel a great sense of loss followed by numbness.

The next stage is often anger. The bereaved person is angry that the loved one has been taken away and may experience feelings of unfairness or anger against people who have not suffered such a loss. Those trying to befriend somebody who has been bereaved may find this stage unexpected and even rather upsetting. Sometimes denial sets in too and the bereft person refuses to believe what has happened.

Finally, these painful feelings are superseded by feelings of acceptance and letting go. The anger burns itself out, and the person comes to terms with their loss. Then the stage is set for a return to normal living.

Friends and relatives are usually helpful and sympathetic to somebody whose depression has a fairly obvious cause like bereavement. They will rally round, show their affection and generally lend a shoulder to cry on. This kind of depression, which is the mourning for a loved person, can continue for quite some time. Many widows, for instance, feel that it takes up to two years before they are fully recovered. Friends will need patience, as well as affectionate concern. There are also organizations which can help, like Cruse, an organization for the widowed (see Appendix Three). On the whole, it is more difficult for friends and relatives to understand a severe depression, which comes on without any real cause, than one which is a natural reaction like mourning after bereavement.

SEVERE DEPRESSION

This kind of depression is marked by its persistence and its acute painfulness for the sufferer. Occasionally, a depressive illness grows out of a mild depression of the kind described above. Post-natal depression is usually a mild kind of maternal blues, which can occasionally persist and become a severe depression. At other times, severe depressive illness seems to be triggered off by relatively trivial events, or it may simply settle upon somebody without any apparent cause at all.

SYMPTOMS
These include guilt and a feeling of unworthiness, a loss of confidence, inability to concentrate, indecisiveness about even minor decisions like what to wear or eat; poor memory; agitation and anxiety; weeping; suicidal thoughts; irritability; fear of being alone; hopelessness; extreme weakness; tiredness and lethargy; delusions; fears about death; slowness of thought; loss of sexual desire; reduced appetite; insomnia and waking in the early hours of the morning; feeling worse in the morning and getting better in the day; loss of interest in life; self-neglect; a preoccupation with bodily symptoms and bodily functions.

People who feel like this urgently need professional help. Unfortunately, when depression sets in, the lethargy can be so overwhelming that even seeking help seems too much effort. Friends and relatives should encourage the sufferer to see the family doctor, offering to accompany him or her if necessary. It is probably best to ask the doctor to refer the depressed person to a hospital, since some studies have shown that family doctors sometimes do not treat depression very well. People who are severely depressed need anti-depressants, rather than tranquillizers or sleeping pills (see Suicide, pages 74–5). Hospital treatment is not only more effective, but it will also mean that a suicidal person is kept under proper supervision, so that he or she is less likely to do themselves harm. People are still frightened of hospitals, and there is still some stigma attached to being treated there. However, it is worth reminding the sufferer that most patients in mental wards are not there compulsorily, but are there of their own free will. If you are a voluntary patient, then you can discharge yourself at any time.

Self-help for depressives is usually more than they can manage, if their illness is severe. However, trying to keep eating the right sort of food and taking regular exercise will do some good. The most important thing of all is to seek help from a doctor, remembering to tell him just how terrible you feel, so that he knows you are severely affected. It is in the nature of a depression for the sufferer to feel that there is no hope. *This despair is part of the illness*, and the real circumstances are quite different. Depression does not last for ever. Remember that, though you may now feel as if there is nothing to live for, if you can simply keep living through one day after another, this despair will lift. The illness can be cured, and you will be happy once more.

There are self-help groups for those suffering depression (see Appendix Three). You may also find that relaxation groups are helpful too. The Samaritans will talk to anybody who is feeling depressed, whether mildly unhappy or acutely despairing. Sometimes it is impossible to seek help at the lowest point in a depression: the time to look for help may be either before or after the low point, when you have enough energy to do so. If you are feeling acutely depressed, make sure that you are getting in touch with a respectable self-help group. The wilder kinds of group therapy and encounter groups should be avoided by anybody whose mental suffering is acute. A good self-help group, like Depressives Anonymous, will bring you in touch with people who do understand; they have been in the depths of depression, just as you are. Their experience may help you live through the worst and return to happiness.

WHAT FRIENDS AND RELATIVES CAN DO
1. Remember that you are dealing with an illness. The sufferer may be behaving in a way which is entirely unreasonable and even very annoying. But it is pointless and unkind to be irritable or angry with a sick human being. You may have to keep reminding yourself of this.
2. Help the sick person to get proper professional help from a doctor. Offer to accompany them to the doctor's surgery. Help them keep any hospital appointments. Relatives who are worried about the treatment a patient is receiving can always confide their anxieties to the doctor or hospital. This may be worth doing if you suspect that the sick person has not managed to be entirely frank with the doctor.
3. Try to help them eat. It is discouraging to see somebody refusing a meal you have just cooked. Do not get angry. Cook the kind of food they might like and make sure the meal is always put before them even if they do not eat it.
4. Lend a listening ear. Depressed people cannot *change* their feelings, so it is useless to try to tell them to do so. Listening may help them a little. But do not let their troubles overwhelm you. Stay detached, though loving.
5. Help depressed people to avoid decisions, if they are tormented by indecisiveness. Do not ask them what they want to eat or wear – put the meal in front of them and put out their clothes. Do not try to plan family activities with them. Organize these yourself, and then ask if they will join in. Make it clear they are wanted and loved, but do not be upset if they refuse.

Suicide

Suicide accounts for about one in five deaths from unnatural causes. Britain has a very low suicide rate compared with other developed countries but nevertheless in recent years the figures have begun to climb upwards again.

In the 1960s and early 1970s, the number of suicides was steadily falling, particularly among the older age group. Nobody can be quite sure why. One theory was that the establishment of the Samaritans, a befriending service, had prevented deaths. Other researchers pointed to the change from poisonous coal gas to natural North Sea gas. A third possibility was that better hospital treatment meant that would-be suicides were being rescued from death.

Those who study suicides and suicide attempts agree that two rather different acts are concealed in the statistics. There are the people who definitely intend to kill themselves. They make proper plans to do so, and often succeed. Then there are the people whose suicide attempts are not intended to end in death. Of course, some people who truly intend to die are rescued, and so do not appear among the death statistics. Among the completed deaths are also those of people who did not intend to die, and whose suicide attempt succeeded 'by mistake'.

Some researchers, therefore, distinguish between suicide and para-suicide, which they call 'deliberate self-harm'. There are about twenty cases of deliberate self-harm for every completed suicide, and their number is growing. Sadly, those who take these not-quite-suicidal overdoses are often in more danger than they think. Drugs combined with alcohol are very dangerous indeed, and some drugs, like paracetamol, produce a slow painful death rather than a quick loss of consciousness. More women than men commit deliberate self-harm; more men than women succeed in killing themselves.

This distinction between seriously intended suicides and those attempts that are not meant to succeed is not much use to ordinary people who come into contact with suicidal individuals. Every mention of suicide *must* be taken seriously. From a purely human point of view any individual whose distress has reached this point urgently needs help.

Identifying those at risk of suicide has been the subject of much study. People who commit suicide include many who are suffering from psychological troubles. About three-quarters of those who go on to die from suicide have consulted a doctor in the three months before their death. Frequently the doctor has failed to recognize the danger, sometimes even prescribing the tablets that are later used in the suicide.

The most common disorder that leads some people to take their own lives is depression. Depression is a mental illness which can be treated. For the majority of sufferers, it is an illness which will be cured, and the person who was depressed will go on to lead a normal and healthy life.

Therefore, if a person can be prevented from committing suicide, there is a good chance that he or she will eventually recapture happiness and health. Sometimes, when people are severely depressed they are too lethargic to commit suicide. Paradoxically, the danger time for suicide can come when the depressed person is beginning to recover.

Loneliness and isolation also seem to affect people who commit suicide. Elderly people without children, young people in lodgings, or those living without any family, are all at more than average risk. Those who have moved house, or who have moved from one country to another, are also vulnerable to suicide. Bankruptcy, unemployment, redundancy, the death of a loved one, or even the anniversary of such a death, can all trigger a suicide attempt.

Alcoholism and drug abuse are also quite common among those who take their own lives. Indeed, drug addiction is sometimes called 'slow suicide'. In these cases the drink or drug problem must be tackled (see Alcoholism, pages 148–53, and Drug Dependence, page 147). People who are suffering from a serious illness, chronic pain, or an illness they believe to be fatal, sometimes kill themselves. If the illness can be treated, their depression will lift as well. Once again, if they can be seen through the crisis, happiness will return.

Identifying those at risk is not as difficult as it might be. A large proportion of those who kill themselves *tell somebody beforehand that they are going to do it*. It is entirely wrong to think that those who talk about it don't do it. The reverse is true. Any talk of suicide, or even a hint of it, should be taken *very seriously indeed*.

DANGER SIGNS OF SUICIDE
People at risk display some of the following features. If two or more of these are present in the same person, then he or she needs professional help at once.

1. Depression. The individual is withdrawn and cannot relate to others.
2. A family history of suicide.
3. An earlier suicide attempt.
4. The person has a definite idea of *how* the suicide will be committed. He or she may be tidying up their affairs in readiness, and giving away treasured possessions.
5. Anxiety, as well as depression, is present.
6. The person suffers from a painful physical illness, chronic pain or severe disablement.
7. He or she is dependent upon alcohol, illegal drugs or prescribed drugs.
8. There is a feeling of uselessness. In the elderly, there may be a lack of acceptance of retirement.
9. Social isolation, loneliness, or uprooting. There is the possibility of having to live with few human contacts.
10. Severe insomnia.
11. Financial worries.
12. No philosophy of life to help them cope, such as a comforting religion.
13. Recovery from depression. When a person appears to be getting better, he or she may at last have enough energy to commit suicide.

WHAT FRIENDS AND RELATIVES CAN DO
1. Talk about the person's suicidal feelings. People are often afraid to do this in case they 'put ideas' into the depressed person's head. But you cannot put the idea of suicide into someone's head, if it is not already there.
2. Take their feelings seriously. The ability to listen, no matter how distressing the outpourings, is perhaps the greatest kindness a friend can give. Do not condemn or get angry. Do not try to force solutions upon them or give too much advice. Severely depressed people cannot pull themselves together or change their mood by will-power. Encourage any positive thoughts that they themselves may have.
3. Encourage them to seek help. Severe depression needs treatment. Sometimes an offer to accompany them to the doctor may be helpful. Encourage them to keep any appointment made with a psychiatrist. Remind them that their unhappiness will eventually pass. Treatment for depression takes time to work.
4. Encourage them to contact the Samaritans. Not only do the Samaritans offer a friendly listening ear at all times, but they also offer befriending services. If a person is severely depressed, they will offer regular and frequent phone contact for as long as it is needed.
5. Seek help and advice yourself on how to cope from the Samaritans. Dealing with a suicidal or severely depressed person can be bewildering, tiring and upsetting. The Samaritans can advise you, give you support, or just help you come to terms with the other person's distress. They will also help relatives and friends of people who have committed suicide.
6. Seek help on behalf of the suicidal person. It may be worth telling the family doctor, for instance, so that he is alerted to the possibility of a drug overdose. In the case of young people at college or school, there may be a sympathetic school counsellor or a tutor who can keep an eye out for their distress.
7. Be reliable in whatever help you give. Do not make promises of help that you cannot fulfil. If the suicidal person has chosen you as a confidant, then you must do your best to fulfil that role.

THE AFTERMATH OF A SUICIDE ATTEMPT
It is now generally agreed that anybody who has tried and failed to commit suicide, however trivial the attempt, needs psychiatric help. Unfortunately, in some hospital wards suicide attempters are not always treated sensitively. Doctors and nurses may feel that the deliberately ill are less welcome patients than those who have ordinary illnesses.

Officially every suicide attempter should be seen by a psychiatrist. Good hospitals arrange this before the patient leaves. But, more often than not, patients are merely offered an out-patient appointment some days later. Only about half of these appointments are kept.

Friends and relatives may be able to encourage the person to keep such appointments by offering to accompany them. Indeed, all suicide attempters should be encouraged to seek help after, as well as before, such attempts. Contact with the Samaritans, student counselling services or the National Marriage Guidance counsellors, may help people come to terms with their problems. Those whose suicide attempts were associated with drink or drugs should be encouraged to seek help for these problems (see Appendix Three, under Alcoholism and Drug Dependence).

4: DIET

Nutrition

USING THE RIGHT FUEL

One in every three deaths among people over thirty-five could be postponed if dietary theories now widely accepted by the medical profession were put into practice. This might mean another ten years of life for those people who are at present picked off before their time by heart disease or cancer.

Man, it seems, is not adapted to eating the large quantities of fat and meat he now consumes. It has been known for some time that the accumulation of fats in the blood-vessels makes us prone to heart attacks and strokes. But it now appears that poor adaptation to large quantities of fat in the diet also makes us vulnerable to certain cancers.

A 'Prudent (low-fat) Diet' was first publicized in 1957 by a New York doctor when he launched the Anti-Coronary Club. It was later endorsed by the American Heart Association, and more recently in Britain by the Royal College of Physicians. Expert committees in some fourteen countries have now endorsed the low-fat diet for prevention of heart disease. And now the low-fat diet has won further approval from cancer experts as well.

In addition to eating too much fat, we also eat too much sugar and too little roughage – the indigestible fibre in vegetables and grains. Too much sugar rots the teeth (see pages 124–7) and may also have an adverse effect on the heart. Too little roughage causes slow bowel movements and constipation, which may eventually cause piles and diverticular disease, a common disease of the bowel in Western countries which is almost unknown in people living on unprocessed foods. Lack of roughage in the diet leads to these and other consequences, which Dr Denis Burkitt, British Medical Research Council scientist, has called diseases of civilization.

According to all these ideas, the majority of people in Western countries are eating an unhealthy diet which can only be put right by a diet revolution. This revolution has already begun: wholemeal bread and soft margarine made with 'polyunsaturated' vegetable oils are now available in most food shops. But most people need more information and ideas in order to cook the most nourishing and healthiest meals for themselves. In this chapter we summarize the evidence which shows that a diet revolution is needed. We also give practical advice on alternative healthier ways of eating; in Appendix One we give recipes which demonstrate that healthy eating need not be dull or unimaginative eating.

HEART DISEASE: THE EVIDENCE AGAINST SATURATED FATS

The first observation suggesting that the rich Western diet is the cause of heart and blood-vessel disease came in 1916 from a Dutch physician, C. D. De Langen, who found that the Javanese had much lower quantities of cholesterol in their blood and were much less prone to hardening of the arteries, blood clots, gallstones, and heart disease than were Westerners. These diseases were common among Dutch settlers in Java, the rich Javanese and those Chinese who ate Western food. Dr De Langen recommended a low cholesterol diet. This work was only suggestive, but since then many more detailed studies have been made which have come to essentially the same conclusion.

The Japanese also seldom suffer from heart disease, and this has led to the suggestion that the Eastern races of man may have an inherited resistance to these diseases. However, this has been disproved by the observation that Japanese living in California, who live and eat like other Americans, are more or less as equally susceptible to heart disease as other Americans. Japanese living in Japan normally eat little or no dairy produce and relatively little meat. They eat more fish, vegetables and carbohydrate than people do in the West.

Yemenite Jews coming to Israel had much lower quantities of cholesterol in their blood and were much less prone to heart disease than Jews from Europe. However, after a number of years the Yemenite Jews adopted the European diet with large quantities of fat. The cholesterol in their blood went up and they became more vulnerable to heart disease.

Heart disease is most prevalent in Western countries. Finland, Scotland, South Africa, the United States, Australia, New Zealand and Canada head the list, with England and Wales not far behind. Countries with least heart disease are Bulgaria, Greece, Italy, Poland, Portugal, Romania and Taiwan, with Japan at the bottom of the list. There are, of course, many differences between the diets of these countries. However, sifting the evidence suggests again that the most important difference which accounts for the prevalence of heart disease in Western countries is the amount of saturated animal fat eaten in these countries. Everything points to a Mediterranean or Oriental diet being far healthier than the customary diet of Northern Europe, America and the white Commonwealth.

In many countries, there is a positive correlation between heart disease, or the age at which people die, and

> **DIET GLOSSARY**
>
> **Carbohydrates** include sugars, starches and related substances which are chemical compounds of carbon, hydrogen and oxygen. Carbohydrates are made by plants from carbon dioxide and water, using the energy from the sun. Potatoes, pasta (spaghetti, etc.), bread, rice, and any grain are rich in carbohydrate. Starch from these foods is broken down into sugars in the body before being used as a source of energy for maintaining the body, for growth and for everyday activities. Cellulose, the main constituent of paper, is also a carbohydrate found in all plants, but it cannot be digested by people, although it can by certain animals such as cows. Nevertheless, cellulose and other undigestible carbohydrates are now thought to be an important part of the diet, as a source of fibre which aids the passage of material through the bowel.
>
> **Cholesterol** is a substance resembling fat, although strictly speaking it is not a fat from the chemical standpoint. It is common in most tissues of the body and is probably the starting point for the synthesis of certain hormones. Cholesterol is the main component in atheroma, which accumulates in the body and causes coronary artery disease. The only common food to contain high quantities of cholesterol is egg yolk.
>
> **Fats and oils** are chemically similar compounds of carbon, hydrogen and oxygen, which is combined in them in a characteristic way different to the carbohydrates. There are many different types of fats and oils. However, the only difference between fats and oils as a whole is that oils are liquid at room temperature. Most animal fats are hard at average room temperatures. Fats contain twice as much energy, weight for weight, as carbohydrates and so it is important to cut down on fats when dieting. However, fats and oils are important in cooking because they carry flavours, and so they should be mixed judiciously with carbohydrate foods.
>
> **Proteins** are the essential 'building blocks' of the living cell and comprise about 12 per cent of the weight of the human body (water 70 per cent, fat 15 per cent). Proteins are made up from some twenty-two different amino acids. Proteins can be made by the body into an enormous variety of shapes to do various different jobs. Enzymes, the biological catalysts of the body, are all proteins and there are many thousands of them in the body – each one different. Proteins in the food are broken down by digestion into amino acids, which are then rearranged into new proteins needed by the body. If unnecessarily large quantities of protein are eaten, then they are used as a source of energy and broken down into simple substances such as carbon dioxide, water and urea, which is excreted in the urine. Amino acids are composed of carbon, hydrogen, oxygen, nitrogen and sometimes sulphur. All necessary protein may be obtained from bread, grains and beans, although meat, fish and eggs are good sources.
>
> **Vitamins** are substances needed by the body which the body cannot make for itself from raw materials. Vitamins are only needed in small amounts, mostly as catalysts helping along vital chemical reactions. Shortage of vitamins causes deficiency such as scurvy (shortage of vitamin C), rickets (shortage of vitamin D), beri-beri (shortage of vitamin B_1) and others. A good mixed diet contains all the necessary vitamins. It is much more important to try to obtain a good mixed diet than to attempt to supplement the diet with vitamins. In fact, too much vitamin A or D can be harmful and excess of the others will serve no purpose. However, there are special circumstances when extra vitamins may be prescribed by a doctor.

their consumption of sugar. However, the amount of sugar people eat and the amount of fat they eat are closely linked. The amount of sugar people eat is also closely linked with the amount they smoke. For this reason it is difficult to know whether sugar has a bad effect on the heart. Heart disease is not particularly common in countries such as Venezuela, Mauritius or the Caribbean, where there is a high consumption of sugar, which suggests that there is no need to worry about the effect of sugar on the heart. The Royal College of Physicians says that there is no firm evidence linking sugar consumption to heart disease.

However, everyone agrees that excessive consumption of sugar, particularly between meals, has a bad effect on the teeth. Excessive consumption of sugar also leads to obesity, which in turn is associated with diabetes and high blood pressure. Therefore it is a good idea to cut down on the use of sugar in cooking, to restrict sweet snacks and drinks between meals and, if overweight, try to cut down on sweet things.

CANCER: THE EVIDENCE AGAINST FATS

The Japanese have one of the lowest rates of breast cancer in the world. Their chance of contracting it is only a quarter that of English women, and a sixth that of women in Oakland, an affluent town near San Francisco. Cancer of the prostate, testis and ovary are also relatively rare in Japan, where they cause about a tenth of the deaths that they do in Western countries. These cancers, together with breast cancers, are the 'hormone dependent' cancers: their growth is apparently controlled by the quantities of several different hormones produced by the sex organs and the pituitary gland in the brain.

Until a few years ago, many scientists thought that the Japanese must have an inherited racial resistance to these cancers. Then it was discovered that Japanese women living in the United States were four times more susceptible to breast cancer than Japanese women living in Japan. Japanese living in the United States also have an increased incidence over native Japanese of cancers of the prostate, testis, ovary and bowel.

Could it be that the change from a rice and fish diet to an American diet rich in meat and fat has made Japanese immigrants more vulnerable? Bowel cancer might obviously be caused by something we eat, but the suggestion that breast – or prostate, testis or ovary – cancer might also have a dietary cause at first seems incredible. However, this is the conclusion that cancer experts are now coming to.

Britain has one of the highest incidences of breast cancer in the world; some twelve thousand women die in Britain every year of the disease. Breast cancer is commonest in

DIET/NUTRITION

Europe, Australia, New Zealand, Britain, the USA and Canada – countries which consume most meat, fat and sugar – and is least common in the Far East and South America. Argentina is an exception: breast cancer is almost as common there as in the United States or Britain. Meat consumption is high in Argentina but sugar consumption is low, pointing to meat and perhaps even to beef as a major cause of breast cancer when eaten regularly in large quantities. In Europe, the poorer countries with large peasant populations such as Spain, Greece and Yugoslavia have least breast cancer.

Dr John Berg of the University of Iowa Cancer Research Center says:

One can go so far as to suggest, speculatively, that mankind generally evolved under conditions of prudent – low fat and protein – nutrition, and that the present affluent diet from childhood onward may overstimulate the endocrine (hormone-making) system, producing the same effect that one would obtain running a diesel engine on high-octane fuel.

Cancer of the bowel, which kills some sixteen thousand men and women in Britain a year, may also be caused by a high-fat diet. Countries which have a high incidence of breast cancer and heart disease also tend to have a high incidence of cancer of the colon (large bowel) and the rectum. Scotland, which has a high-fat diet relieved by relatively few fresh vegetables, holds the world record for colon cancer. Deaths from breast cancer in Scotland are also among the highest in the world, as too are deaths among women from heart disease.

An individual may become ill either with bowel cancer or heart disease, but usually not with both. This at first sight seems odd if both are caused by a high-fat diet. Dr Ernst Wynder of the Naylor Dana Institute for Disease Prevention in New York, one of the pioneers in the field, theorizes that people may fall into two types: those who take cholesterol from the food into the blood and deposit it in the heart and arteries, which leads to arteriosclerosis; and those who do not absorb so much cholesterol, or excrete larger quantities of cholesterol products into the intestine and bowel where it causes cancer.

Dr Michael Hill of the Central Public Health Laboratory, Colindale, London, suggests that a high-fat diet causes the production of large quantities of bile acids, which may be changed by bacteria in the bowel into substances which cause cancer. He has found that people who excrete large quantities of bile substances are at greater risk of developing bowel cancer. Dr Hill says that his results imply that cancer of the bowel and rectum is a preventable disease – even though the causal mechanism is not fully understood – and he endorses the low-fat diet.

Seventh Day Adventists have half to two-thirds the average incidence of cancer deaths, and almost half the incidence of heart disease, stroke and arteriosclerosis, compared with other Americans. Adventists do not smoke and do not drink alcohol, which accounts for their low frequency of cancer of the lung, mouth, oesophagus and bladder. (They also do not drink coffee, but coffee has no proven hazards in animals or man.) However, even if they are compared with non-smokers in the general population, they still have a much lower frequency of cancer of the breast, ovary, prostate and bowel. This is almost certainly the result of the Adventists' vegetarian diet.

All Adventists are strict in not drinking alcohol or eating pork, but a vegetarian diet is not obligatory for them and those who are vegetarian usually eat eggs and milk. On average, the amount of fat in their diet is cut by about a quarter. Dr Roland Phillips of Loma Linda University, California (an Adventist foundation) has discovered that Adventists with heart disease or bowel cancer eat more meat and dairy products than the average Adventist. Adventists who suffered breast or bowel cancer were found to have eaten more fried foods in the past, and to have eaten more refined foods such as white bread, cake and pie. The Adventists who did not get cancer ate more green leafy vegetables and beans.

These studies all point in the same direction. People who eat a low-meat, low saturated-fat diet tend to have a low incidence of cancer as well as heart disease, and it can be safely concluded that someone who eats this diet is likely to be healthier and to live longer than someone on the average Western diet.

FATS AND OILS

Oils are chemically similar to fats; the difference is simply that oils are liquid at room temperature whereas fats are solid. The fats and oils in our diet can be divided up into three categories important for health: saturated, mono-unsaturated and polyunsaturated. Animal fats, which are usually hard at room temperature, consist mostly of saturated fats (see table, page 79) whereas most vegetable and fish oils consist largely of mono-unsaturated and polyunsaturated oils. However, not all vegetable oils are mono- or polyunsaturated. Palm and coconut oil, which are widely used in making biscuits and artificial cream, are relatively highly saturated and hard at room temperature. Most authorities agree that the amount of saturated fat in the diet should be restricted, because excessive consumption of saturated fat is associated with heart disease and certain cancers. This can be done by eating less fatty meat and less butter, cream and top-of-the-milk, less hard margarines, fewer eggs and more vegetables – particularly peas and beans – and also by including more fish and poultry rather than beef or lamb in the diet.

Consumption of polyunsaturated fats reduces the amount of cholesterol in the blood and the tendency of the blood to clot. Therefore it is important to replace animal fat as much as possible, by using polyunsaturated fats such as

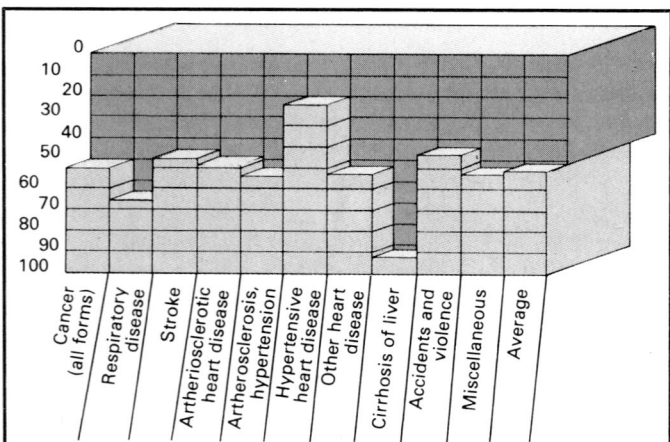

Outstanding health record of Seventh Day Adventists in the USA. Death rates of Adventists expressed in percentages below rates for the general population.

sunflower oil, safflower oil, corn oil, groundnut (peanut) oil *(arachide)* or soya-bean oil for cooking, and by using soft (polyunsaturated) margarine (see below) instead of butter.

Olive oil is mono-unsaturated and low in saturated fat and so is described as neutral from the health point of view. People who live in the Mediterranean region have a remarkably low incidence of heart disease and breast cancer, particularly in those parts of the Mediterranean where most olive oil is consumed. So it can be concluded that olive oil is good for health.

The polyunsaturated 'soft' margarines are made from oils such as corn oil or sunflower oil, which are rich in polyunsaturates. The oils are made harder by mixing with a small amount of hard oil, or by treating some of the oil with hydrogen to make it harder. They are then emulsified with some water or whey to give a creamy consistency. The brand leader, Flora, is made from sunflower oil, but is not so polyunsaturated as sunflower oil itself through being mixed with some harder oil. The makers of Flora guarantee that it consists of at least 50 per cent polyunsaturates. There are now many brands of soft margarine. Some are made from corn oil, which is also a good source of polyunsaturates. In choosing a soft margarine, look for a declaration on the label of the kind of oil being used and a specification that it contains 40 per cent or more polyunsaturates. Nevertheless, other soft margarines such as Blue Band or Stork SB, with lower quantities of polyunsaturates, are still better than butter (only 3 per cent polyunsaturated) for use as your everyday spread.

Egg yolks contain large amounts of cholesterol, so it is wise to restrict the number of egg yolks in the diet to a maximum of three a week. Vegetarians may safely eat more because they are likely to be eating less fat. However, a vegetarian who eats a lot of dairy produce including eggs may be on just as hazardous a diet as someone eating a lot of meat. Both meat-eaters and vegetarians should aim to get a substantial part of their protein from bread, grains, peas and beans, which are low in fat.

Offal such as liver and kidney contains a lot of cholesterol, but this is compensated for by the fact that these meats contain less fat, and the fat that is in them is more polyunsaturated. Brains contain a great deal of cholesterol but they are eaten too infrequently to worry about. Game such as rabbit, hare or venison is always very lean and contains little saturated fat, so it is highly recommended.

Cooking with oils

Corn Oil: This is the least satisfactory of the recommended vegetable oils for cooking purposes. For salads, the flavour is rather powerful. If you do not find the flavour attractive, try mixing in some olive oil for cooking or salads.

Olive Oil: Olive oil is delicious for everything, but is expensive. It has a lovely fruity flavour which varies tremendously from country to country. Some people like the heavy green Greek oil, others the delicate golden Provençal oil, while there are those who swear that the deep yellow Tuscan oil is the pearl. However, it is wasteful to use this oil for frying, since it loses its delicious flavour at high temperatures. Use it for rubbing onto meat or fish before grilling, for marinades, for lubricating freshly cooked pasta, and of course for all salads.

Salad Oil: An interesting salad oil can be made by mixing four tablespoons of sunflower oil with two dessertspoons of walnut oil, which has a delicious flavour.

Composition of fats and oils. Fats and oils high in polyunsaturated and mono-unsaturated constituents are the best for health.

	Saturated	Mono-unsaturated	Poly-unsaturated
Beef	48%	44%	3%
Chicken	32	37	26
Lamb	54	37	4
Pork	36	42	17
Liver	34	27	34
Herring	19	10	66
Milk, butter, cheddar	62	30	3
Eggs	33	45	17
Margarine			
Blueband	39	41	20
Flora	19	31	50
Kraft Golden Corn	20	39	41
Stork	41	54	5
Stork SB	26	59	15
Vegetable oils			
Coconut	91	7	2
Corn	17.5	29	56.5
Ground nut	13	61	24
Olive	11	74	10
Palm	53	38	9
Palm kernel	85	13	2
Safflower	11.5	13	75.5
Soya bean	17	25	58
Sunflower	12	20	68
Walnut	16	28	51

The total percentage is sometimes less than 100 because of the glycerol present. Chemically, the fat molecule consists of a chain of carbon atoms linked to each other, with each also linked to two hydrogen atoms. In *saturated fats* each carbon atom has the maximum number of hydrogen atoms attached to it. *Mono-unsaturated fats* have one pair of carbon atoms in the chain which each have only one hydrogen atom attached, all the other carbon atoms have two hydrogen atoms. *Polyunsaturated fats* have two or more pairs of hydrogen atoms missing from the chain.

Soya Oil: A good oil for frying, but it starts to taste and smell a bit strong at high temperatures. It has the right consistency for salads. This is the oil used in Japan, where they have so little heart disease. Highly recommended.

Sunflower Oil: The oil is excellent for frying as it is almost tasteless and does not smell. It gives a very crisp result. As it is so light and thin it makes a rather dull salad dressing. It is the most versatile of the recommended polyunsaturated oils but it is expensive.

Walnut Oil: It gives a sweet, nutty and entirely delicious flavour in salads. Try it on a lettuce-and-chicory salad with a few walnuts strewn in. This is a heavy oil which does not keep particularly well, so do not hoard it: keep it in the refrigerator. Too expensive to use in cooking except to add flavour.

BREAD AND FLOUR

Before 1870, most people in Europe and America ate bread made from stone-ground flour, which contained appreciable quantities of bran – the fibrous part of the grain.

(Sources: *Manual of Nutrition* (HMSO); Van den Berghs; Procter & Gamble)

DIET/NUTRITION

However, mass-production of white refined flour by mills in the 1870s, together with a decline in the amount of bread eaten, has meant that people on average eat about a fifth of the amount of cereal fibre in their diet now than they did a century ago. This change in our diet has been blamed for many of the diseases of civilization which are unknown in people living on an unrefined diet.

The importance of bran in our everyday diet has been pointed out by Dr Denis Burkitt, of the British Medical Research Council, and Surgeon Captain T. L. Cleave, formerly of the Royal Navy, who during the Second World War kept the sailors 'regular' aboard his battleship *George V* with the help of bran. Dr Burkitt's interest in fibre was aroused by his work in Africa, where he noticed that native Africans seldom suffered from many diseases common in Western countries.

Appendicitis was rare in Africans until they began to eat the refined Western diet deficient in cereal fibre. Appendicitis also used to be rare in Western countries before the advent of roller milling. When fibre is deficient in the diet, the content of the bowel becomes hard and it is difficult for the bowel to move the content along. The bowel may then become obstructed, causing appendicitis. Another disease called diverticular disease also occurs as a result of the bowel becoming obstructed. In straining to pass the content along the bowel, small 'blow outs' – diverticula – may occur in the bowel wall, just as a rubber tyre may blow out where there is a weakness. People who have diverticular disease usually improve dramatically when given a diet containing plenty of fibre. Fibre provides bulk in the diet which acts as a natural lubricant, making it easy for the bowel to move.

The first and most obvious effect of insufficient fibre in the diet is constipation. People who eat a diet containing plenty of fibre tend to pass large, soft and often unformed stools. If a person regularly needs to strain to move the bowels and the stool is hard, then they probably do not have enough fibre in the diet. Straining to move the bowels increases pressure in the abdomen, and this may damage valves in the veins in the legs, causing varicose veins and haemorrhoids (piles).

Excessive removal of fibre from food also encourages people to eat a diet too rich in highly refined starch and sugar. This leads to overweight, and often to other health problems such as diabetes. Fibre in the diet may also prevent absorption of cholesterol, and so may protect against heart disease. Proponents of the theory suggest that fibre in the diet may also protect against bowel cancer and gallstones. The importance of fibre in the diet is now generally accepted, although it is not yet agreed by experts whether lack of fibre is a cause of bowel cancer and heart disease.

It is not difficult to get sufficient fibre in the diet. The easiest way to get more fibre is to eat wholemeal bread and wholemeal breakfast cereals such as All-Bran, Shreddies, Weetabix, Shredded Wheat, porridge or muesli; vegetables are also a useful source of fibre. Bran itself can also be bought from health stores and, increasingly, from many supermarkets. This can be added to breakfast cereals or put in soups and stews. Wholemeal flour can also be used in a great many ways in cooking. Health-food enthusiasts may prefer stone-ground flour but there is no evidence that this is better than ordinary wholemeal flour made in metal-roller mills. It is not necessary to eat wholemeal foods all the time, but try to make them your staple.

Cooking with wholemeal flour

100 per cent wholemeal flour contains the entire wheat grain, including the bran. It is the heaviest and most strongly flavoured wheat flour. Wheatmeal or brown flour contains from 80 to 90 per cent of the whole wheat grain, but has some of the coarser particles, mainly the bran, extracted. White flour contains about 72 per cent of the whole grain, and has all the bran and most of the wheatgerm extracted. All the white flours are given extra vitamins to make up for those which have been extracted, including iron, thiamin and niacin; extra calcium is also added.

100 per cent wholemeal and wheatmeal flours have a warm, nutty and agreeable taste with more character and flavour than white flour, which means that for some dishes, where what is needed is a fairly anonymous pastry crust or delicate basic sauce, they can be a bit much. They are more solid than white flour, so when you want to use wholemeal flour for pastry or bechamel sauce, make sure that the food that it is to be eaten with it is robust enough to take it. An onion or leek or cheese quiche or an apple tart would be fine, but if you were using, for instance, smoked salmon or mushrooms, a white crust would perhaps be more suitable. A cheese sauce to go with cauliflower, or a parsley sauce to eat with poached haddock or turbot, would be excellent, but put in lots more cheese or parsley than usual.

Cakes, scones, biscuits, and so forth, can be made very well with wholemeal flour, but are best made with quite a lot of shortening, which should be one of the recommended soft margarines, or they do become very solid (see recipes in Appendix One). Noodles can be made with wholemeal flour and be very tasty, whereas pizzas, pancakes, soufflés, éclairs are among the things that do not lend themselves so well to the change. So the best thing to do is to experiment, and where you really like the results, then switch to wholemeal or wheatmeal flour.

VEGETABLES

Vegetables are useful sources of minerals, vitamins and fibre, and also provide some polyunsaturated fat. Vegetables in the diet may actually protect a person against cancer. A number of surveys have shown that people who eat plenty of fresh vegetables – such as lettuce or celery – are less likely to get stomach cancer. The importance of vegetables in the diet for prevention of cancer has now been demonstrated in animals, and has led to the discovery of a new class of substances which protect against cancer.

Dr Leo Wattenburg of the University of Minnesota School of Medicine discovered that rats which were fed a balanced, *highly purified* diet containing all known vitamins and nutrients, were not able to make certain enzymes (biological catalysts) in the liver which had the vital function of inactivating cancer-causing chemicals. However, when the rats were fed a crude diet containing alfalfa (an animal-fodder plant), they were able to produce the enzymes in their livers. Further experiments showed that rats which are induced to make this enzyme in their livers have increased protection against cancer when chemicals known to cause cancer are added to their diet.

Dr Wattenberg then tested other vegetables, and found that several members of the *Brassica* family, including cabbage, Brussels sprouts, turnips, broccoli and cauliflower, caused the protective enzyme to be made in rats'

TWELVE RULES FOR HEALTHY EATING

1. Eat less meat. Reduce the frequency and the serving-size of beef and lamb portions. Do not eat meat more than once a day and preferably less often.

2. When you do eat meat, select lean cuts and remove all visible fat before eating. Grill rather than fry.

3. Eat more poultry and fish. Avoid sausage, frankfurters, spam, bologna and other processed meats which are usually high in fat.

4. Reduce severely the amount of cream, butter, cream-cheese and ice-cream. Restrict the amount of cheese. Choose semi-skimmed (stripey-top) milk or pour off the cream.

5. Eat low-fat dairy products such as skimmed milk, cottage cheese, yoghurt. Use soft margarines high in polyunsaturates.

6. Restrict the number of eggs to no more than three per week.

7. Reduce consumption of commercial biscuits and cakes made with hard fats.

8. Use recommended oils – corn, soya, or olive – for cooking.

9. For the sake of your teeth, reduce intake of heavily sweetened foods such as sweets and biscuits.

10. Eat some fresh fruit every day and, if you can, eat fruit at every meal.

11. Eat more vegetables, particularly peas and beans – fresh or dried – which are a good low-fat source of protein.

12. Eat wholemeal bread as your staple. Eat wholemeal breakfast cereals. Take extra bran if the rest of your daily diet is rather refined.

---

livers. He found that spinach, dill and celery were effective, but that the vegetables varied in their effect according to their freshness, variety and the soil in which they were grown.

Finally, Dr Wattenberg was able to identify the actual chemicals in the vegetables which cause the protective enzymes to be formed. They turned out to belong to a well-known family of organic chemicals called indoles. Dr Wattenberg also found that citrus fruits (oranges and lemons) contain chemicals called flavones which, like indoles, cause the protective enzymes to be formed in the liver.

Other plant products may protect against cancer. Beans and seeds are rich in plant proteins called lectins which increase movements of the bowel. They have been found to protect animals against cancer in laboratory experiments. Beans also seem to have an important effect in lowering the amount of cholesterol in the blood. Professor Ancel Keys of the University of Minnesota found that Americans given a diet with the same amount of protein, carbohydrate and fat as eaten in Naples had higher amounts of cholesterol in their blood than Neapolitans until they were fed beans. So beans are not only important in being a low-fat substitute for meat; they also seem to have a positive effect in lowering cholesterol, and it does not seem to matter what type of beans are eaten. Beans are best introduced into the diet slowly for people not accustomed to them, because they do cause some people to suffer from a lot of wind – at least at first.

Several different experiments have shown that onions or garlic contain chemical substances which alter the ability of the blood to clot. This has led to the suggestion that onions and garlic are valuable in preventing the formation of blood clots, which are a cause of coronary heart attacks and strokes.

To get maximum benefit from the vitamins in vegetables, cook briefly so that they are still a little crisp to the taste. Overcooking destroys the vitamin C in vegetables and washes other nutrients into cooking water which may be discarded. The water used to cook vegetables may also be utilized as stock for stews so making sure that minerals and vitamins are not lost to the diet.

DIET/NUTRITION

A BALANCED DIET

It is essential for a healthy diet to eat a variety of food so that you get all the vitamins, minerals and nutrients you need. Therefore at each meal you should aim to eat as great a variety as you can.

Carbohydrate or starch, which is present in bread, pasta, potatoes, rice and other grains, is necessary for energy; these are also good sources of protein, which is necessary for body-building. Sugar is also a source of energy but it provides nothing but what have been called empty calories. So keep sugar to the minimum.

Proteins – available in most concentrated form in lean meat – are made up from chemical building-blocks called amino acids, and are broken down again into amino acids during digestion. Different proteins contain amino acids in different proportions, and plant proteins do not contain amino acids in the ideal proportion for direct use by man, but this does not matter, because the extra amino acids which cannot be used in body-building are burnt up as energy. However, protein is scarce in some parts of the world, and then it becomes more important to make the best possible use of the proteins in the diet by providing the different amino acids in the optimum proportions at the same time. This can be done by mixing beans (which are low in the amino acid methionine) and other vegetables, particularly grains (which are low in another amino acid, lysine), in the same dish. Beans served on wholemeal toast with a little polyunsaturated margarine provide better nutrition than steak and chips. The protein is just as good but there is no saturated fat. Beans served by themselves are also a good source of protein and energy.

Fats are also a source of energy; weight for weight, fats provide twice as many calories as protein or carbohydrate. Therefore, by cutting down on fat in the diet, you can eat a little more protein and carbohydrate and so continue to eat the same bulk. A certain quantity of fat in the diet is essential for health, but in practice no one is likely to eat too little fat except under famine conditions, because food without a minimum of fat tastes dry and unpleasant.

A balanced diet contains adequate amounts of protein, carbohydrate and fat as well as sufficient vitamins and minerals. To obtain a balanced diet, make sure that you eat each day: some foods giving concentrated protein (meat, milk, cheese, fish, beans); some vegetables, fruits, potatoes, to provide vitamin C and other vitamins, nutrients and fibre; some margarine and vegetable oil; and some wholemeal cereals or bread to provide more protein, energy, vitamins and fibre.

Old people sometimes eat such small quantities of food that they become deficient in essential nutrients. It is important for everyone, and particularly old people, to take plenty of exercise so that they have a good appetite and can eat enough food to get sufficient minerals and vitamins without putting on weight. Avoid highly processed foods such as biscuits, which are deficient in vitamins and minerals.

Vegans who eat no meat or dairy produce, as opposed to vegetarians who usually eat eggs and milk products, may become deficient in vitamin B_{12} if they do not take care. They need to eat yeast extract or some other source of essential B_{12}. In pregnancy, and before, special care should be taken to eat a good mixed diet (see Chapter 1).

LOW-FAT COOKING

The healthiest of people are often those peasants who cannot afford to eat meat every day and have learnt to make meat go far when they do have it. In Appendix One, we give some of those recipes which use meat as a flavouring rather than as the main ingredient of dishes: for example, moussaka; stuffed tomatoes or peppers; and risotto. In fact, meat is frequently much more delicious when used in this way, delicately flavoured with herbs and vegetables. Neapolitans eat their spaghetti with tomato sauce as a daily staple, and they are remarkably free of heart disease. It is no coincidence that the richer meat sauce known in Italy as *ragu* is generally attributed to Bologna, where the incidence of heart disease is much higher.

The way food is cooked can dramatically affect the fat and oil content of what we eat, as the three meals below show. The same ingredients (8 oz raw beefsteak, 6 oz peeled potatoes, 3 oz mushrooms, 2 oz onions and 3 oz tomatoes per person) are used in the first two meals. In the third, less meat is needed, and so two more vegetables have been added.

Frying

Lightly fried steak; potato chips; fried mushrooms; fried onions and fried tomatoes.

This is the fattiest meal possible with these ingredients. It is high both in calories and fats because the meat, even lean steak, contains a lot of 'invisible' fat and the vegetables simply soak up oil or fat. Just by frying the onions and mushrooms, over 21 g of fat is added to the meal. Chips have three times as many calories as boiled potatoes. If you must fry food, use sunflower oil, corn oil or soya oil, which are less harmful than animal fat. And even lean meat contains so much fat that, if fried in a non-stick pan, it is not necessary to add further fat.

Total: Fat 71 g (2.5 oz). Calories: 970.

nutrition/DIET

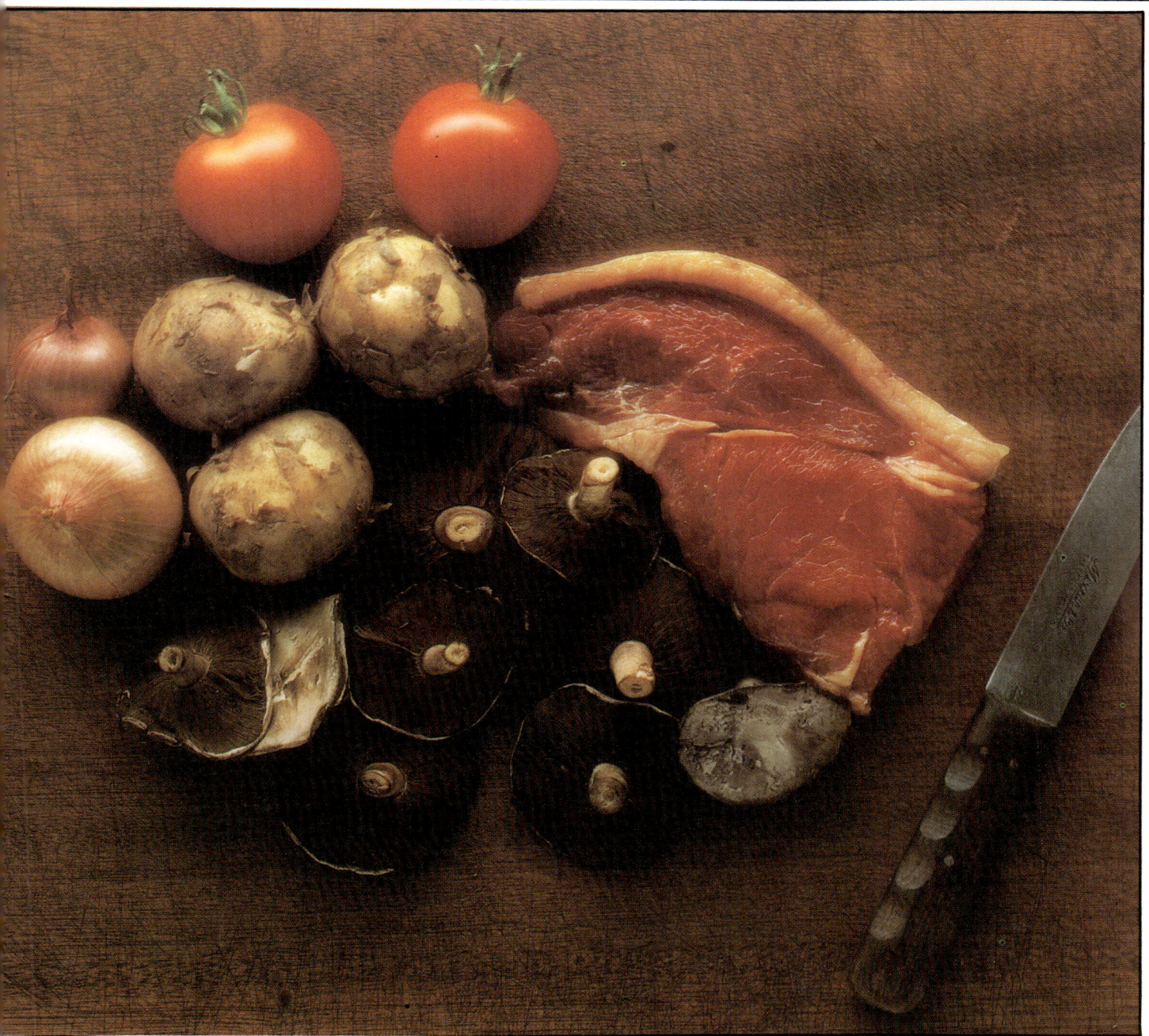

Grilling
Grilled steak; boiled potatoes; tomato, mushroom and onion salad. (Alternatively, grill the tomatoes and mushrooms and boil the onion.)
By grilling the steak, boiling the potatoes and eating the other vegetables raw in a salad, you can halve the fat content of the first meal, even using exactly the same ingredients. Because the vegetables contain only negligible amounts of fat, the only source of fat in the meal is the meat. This should be grilled on a raised wire-mesh rack to allow as much fat as possible to run out. ¼ oz of margarine on the boiled potatoes would add 6 g of fat (and 56 calories) to the total below. Similarly, french dressing made with ¼ oz olive oil on the salad would put the fat content up a further 7 g (adding an extra 66 calories).
Total: Fat 36 g (1.3 oz). Calories: 634.

Stewing
A casserole of steak, onion, mushrooms, tomatoes, potatoes, carrots and peas.
With this kind of meal, meat goes a lot further and so 4 oz, half the original amount, is ample for each person. In its place, other vegetables can be added – in this case, 2 oz carrots and 2 oz fresh or frozen peas, per portion – to make it a lot tastier. The steak is cut into pieces and arranged in layers with the vegetables. Some of the sliced potatoes should be kept aside for the top layer. Water and seasoning are added and the casserole baked in a slow oven for about 2½ hours. The lid of the casserole should be removed for the last half-hour to brown the potatoes. This meal has only one-sixth the fat content of the fried meal, and you could have almost three helpings of it before you would take in the same amount of calories.
Total: Fat 12 g (about ½ oz). Calories: 362.

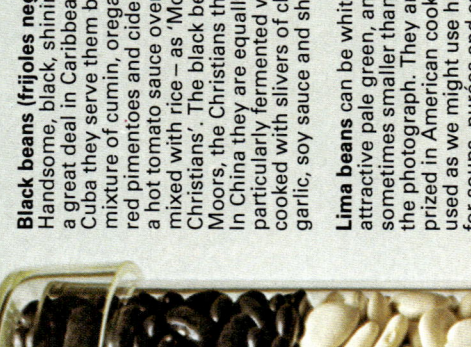
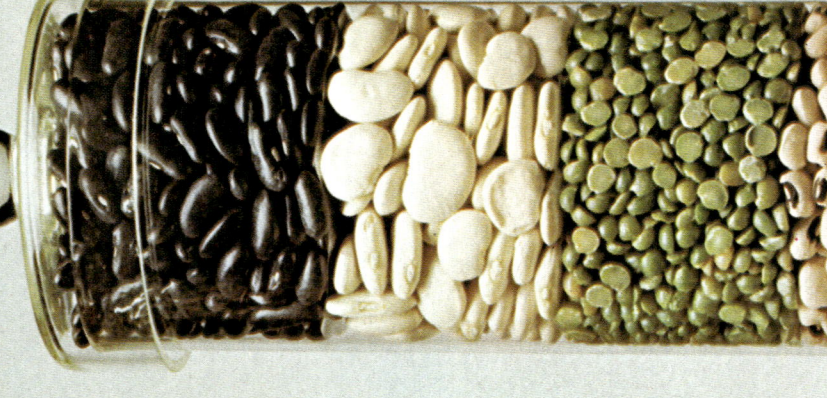

Black beans (frijoles negros). Handsome, black, shining beans used a great deal in Caribbean cooking. In Cuba they serve them bathed in a mixture of cumin, oregano, onions, red pimentoes and cider vinegar with a hot tomato sauce over the top, or,– mixed with rice – as 'Moors and Christians'. The black beans are the Moors, the Christians the white rice! In China they are equally popular, particularly fermented with salt then cooked with slivers of chicken, ginger, garlic, soy sauce and shallots.

Lima beans can be white or an attractive pale green, and are sometimes smaller than the ones in the photograph. They are greatly prized in American cookery and are used as we might use haricot beans – for soups, purées and salads – often with sour cream added.

Split green peas. These skinned and split peas are the ones for pease pudding; for dried green pea soup with mint; for purée of peas to serve with a piece of roast pork or glazed ham; or of course for thick Dutch Pea Soup, afloat with chunks of smoked sausage or frankfurter.

Black-eyed beans (closely related to black-eyed peas) have a delicious, homely, earthy flavour that blends particularly well with spinach, with ham and with garlic. In the Deep South of America, black-eyed peas are traditionally served with pork and candied sweet potatoes, or with fried ham and red-eyed gravy.

Aduki beans. Known as the Prince of Beans in the Orient, aduki beans are distinctly sweet-flavoured and are used in China to make a sweet soup, served in a long glass, like an ice-cream sundae, with grated ice and cream. They are also made into a cream that is something like a chestnut purée, which is used as a filling for wedding cakes.

Brown lentils. These large brown lentils are excellent, robust in flavour, a little floury in texture and a perfect accompaniment to lamb, pork or ham. They soak up oil or butter in large quantities, and are improved by a handful of parsley at the last moment.

Pearl beans or small haricots. These are the original 'baked beans', and traditionally cooked with salt pork,

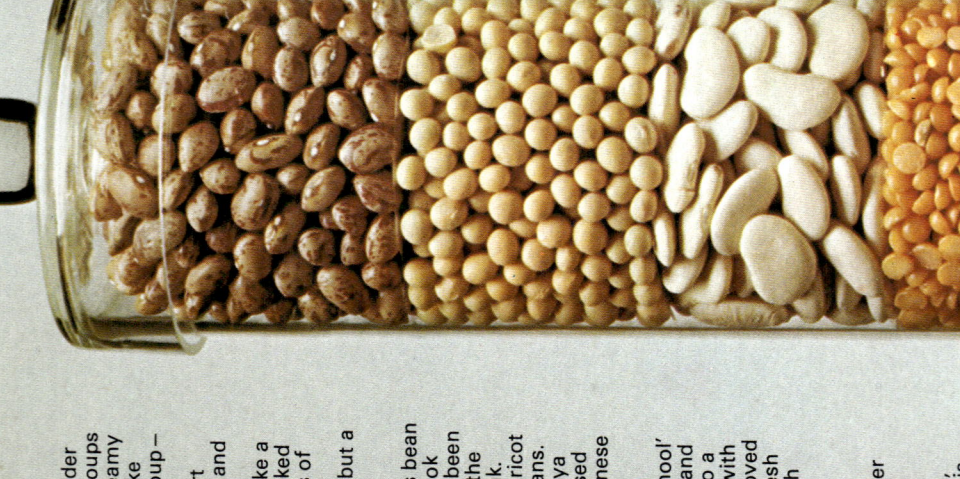

Brown Borlotti beans. Fairly tender beans, useful for making bean soups as they cook to a nice floury, creamy consistency. Can be used to make minestrone or Venetian Bean Soup – beans cooked with ham bones, onions and cinnamon, with short noodles added towards the end and served with plenty of grated Parmesan. In Piedmont they make a complete meal out of beans cooked all night in the oven, with pieces of bacon and, again, cinnamon. Saluggia beans are very similar but a little smaller.

Soya beans. The most nutritious bean of all, round dried soya beans look more like beans once they have been soaked. ½ cup of soya beans is the protein equivalent of 5 oz of steak. They can either be boiled like haricot beans or sprouted like Mung beans. Soya beans provide oil, flour, soya bean curd, soy sauce, and are used extensively in Chinese and Japanese cooking.

Butter beans. These familiar 'school' beans have a distinctive flavour and are traditionally served cooked to a soft consistency as a vegetable with roast pork. They are much improved if drained and given a bath of fresh tomato sauce, and flavoured with celery towards the end of the cooking.

Split yellow peas are used in Atter med Flask – Swedish yellow-pea soup, flavoured with thyme and marjoram, ginger, streaky bacon, onions and cloves. In Sweden it is eaten on Thursdays in memory of King Eric XIV who died on a Thursday in 1577 after his brother had slipped poison into his yellow-pea soup.

Chick peas or Garbanzas. Chick peas, which can be as hard as bullets after six hours' cooking, need plenty of soaking (at least 24 hours) and plenty of simmering (at least 3 hours). They are eaten whole as a snack, with beer; made into stews with chicken and saffron; or crushed and mixed with sesame seed paste (tahini), lemon and oil to make houmous.

Mung beans are mainly known as bean sprouts. Soak 6 oz of beans overnight in cold water. Drain, and place swollen beans on tray so that air can circulate. Cover beans with wet cloth and keep in a dark place. Rinse beans, tray and cloth with water every morning and evening. In

Wonderful world of beans

...and are traditionally used in place of white haricots in the making of baked beans. They can be grown and dried successfully in your own garden. Although a dreadful nuisance to shell, they can then be kept for months.

Small lentils. These are mauve, but there are also black, white, green, mottled, yellow, pink and orange lentils – over sixty varieties. Lentils are delicious boiled as a vegetable to serve with game, pork or rabbit. They make a lovely spiced soup with cream and cumin, and take kindly to being curried. They do need fat though.

Dried white haricot beans (fagioli). These large haricot beans are the sort to eat with a gigot on a Sunday – cook them with garlic and a sprig of rosemary, and crush a few spoonfuls at the end to make a creamy sauce (or add a few spoonfuls of tomato sauce). The juices from the meat provide the necessary lubrication.

Red kidney beans. These handsome shiny lacquer-red beans are the ones for chilli con carne and for a hefty Italian bean soup, cooked with garlic and sage. They are also served cooked with tomato sauce, garlic and shredded cos lettuce, as a vegetable. Mexicans are particularly fond of chillified beans, refried and smothered with grated cheese. In Spain, kidney beans and rice are served in tomato sauce as a filling main course.

Whole green peas. The type used for traditional, mushy green peas, dried peas are a very underestimated food – served with boiled bacon or salt pork they make a most comforting and supportive lunch on an autumn day.

...earthenware pot, sprinkled with brown sugar half an hour before the meal, and allowed to caramelize, uncovered, before serving.

Dried broad beans, either white or brown, are to be found in Greek shops and are probably best bought ready-skinned. They must be well soaked and boiled and can then be served whole, in the Turkish way, as a salad with oil and vinegar, or puréed, sieved and mixed with lemon juice and salt for an *hors d'oeuvre*.

Split lentils. Bright orange or yellowish in colour, these are excellent for making dahl to serve with curry, since they cook quickly to a nice, mushy consistency. They are rather dreary, however, without plenty of spice, tasting fairly strongly of sacking. Watch out for small stones, which tend to abound in these lentils to make them weigh more heavily.

Flageolets. Haricots Flageolets are a delicate, pale green bean with a more subtle flavour than the ordinary haricot. Cook them to eat with lamb, or make a multi-coloured bean salad using red kidney beans, flageolets and ordinary haricots. Flageolets also make a particularly fine, pale green purée which looks very attractive decorated with chopped parsley. Serve it with lamb chops.

Ful Medames (Egyptian brown beans). 'Since time immemorial they have faithfully been served in the same manner; seasoned with oil, lemon and garlic, sprinkled with chopped parsley and accompanied by ... hard-boiled eggs, and since time immemorial people have adored them.' (Claudia Roden)

In Southern India pulses, spiced and fragrant, are an integral part of an essentially meatless diet. In China fermented beans, succulent bean curd and fresh bean sprouts are put on the table at almost every meal. In Brazil, Mexico, Spain and parts of Italy, and all through the Middle East, beans and lentils are a loved and favoured food in winter and summer alike, with bean salads a regular feature, while chick peas are daily cooked in stews like meat.

Nowadays the pulses we buy, on the whole, are of better quality than they used to be – not so hard, not so dusty, not so full of stones or weevils – and the preparation is very simple. Wash the pulses and put them to soak overnight, then bring slowly to the boil in soft water if it is available, and simmer until tender. Crush one between finger and thumb, or between the teeth, to test for tenderness. But a quicker way of cooking pulses, saving time all round, is to bring them to the boil slowly, simmer for 10 minutes, then remove from the heat and allow to cool for an hour. Now put them back on the stove and cook.

The cooking time will vary greatly according to when the pulses were harvested and how long they have been in store. As a general rule, lentils take an hour, beans one-and-a-half hours or more and chick peas up to three hours or even longer. Red kidney beans must be boiled for at least 10 minutes or they will make you ill – actually they take over half an hour before they are tender. Pulses need some lubrication – a piece of salt pork or bacon in the pot, or a generous portion of oil, or a tomato sauce with herbs.

The long cooking needed by pulses tends to exhaust the flavourings added at the beginning, so add a little more of the chosen spices and herbs towards the end of the cooking. Most beans are interchangeable, so for any recipe which specifies dried white haricot beans, you can just as easily use red kidney beans, pearl beans or flageolets. The beans or pulses above are among the many now available in Britain.

apart from mushy peas, split pea soup and baked beans, Britons are generally unimaginative in their use of the dozens of different peas, beans, lentils and so forth available now. Yet with a little experimentation, we could add a new dimension to the national diet, since pulses provide cholesterol-free protein as well as cutting down on butcher's bills – a little bit of meat goes a long, long way when buried in a large pot of lentils.

DIET/NUTRITION

THE NEW DIET: MEAL BY MEAL

Breakfast

The traditional British breakfast of bacon, sausage and egg is extremely high in fat. If you want to have a quick, hot breakfast, try baked beans on toast, or a small amount of well-grilled bacon with tomatoes on toast or fish such as poached haddock, undyed kippers, fish fingers or fishcake. Try to limit eggs to three a week. If you must have one, poach, scramble or boil it. Alternatively why not try hot porridge or a hot wholewheat cereal.

A cold breakfast of wholemeal cereal such as Shreddies, Shredded Wheat, Weetabix, porridge, or muesli is simple and healthy. They all contain bran, which keeps the bowel working smoothly. If you prefer cornflakes (and white bread), make sure you take extra bran or All-Bran. Eat raisins, prunes (but avoid tinned prunes, which come in a heavy syrup) or chopped banana instead of sugar with the cereal to add interest. For milk choose semi-skimmed fresh milk (stripey top) which tastes like ordinary milk and has all the nutrients of ordinary milk but most of the cream removed.

Stoke up with wholemeal bread on toast, marmalade and polyunsaturated margarine (such as Flora). For jam, use a brand such as Whole Earth, which is made without added sugar – better for the teeth and less fattening. This type of jam must be kept in a refrigerator once it has been opened.

Fill up with fruit such as apples or oranges. You can have as many cups of tea and coffee as you like. Coffee was suspected of having a link with heart disease and cancer but has now been cleared.

The main meal – lunch or dinner

Generally it is wise to eat meat only once a day, for the main meal, or preferably less often. Alternatives are fish, poultry or pasta with a light cheese or meat sauce; if you are overweight and find slimming impossible it may be healthier to be fat the Italian way (by eating pasta) rather than the British way (by eating steak and chips, butter and cream). And try to have at least one vegetarian meal a day.

Grill rather than fry meat. If you must fry, use as little fat as possible – a non-stick pan helps – and pour off excess fat to prevent it being absorbed. Roasting is good because it allows fat to drip off, but do not baste the meat with grease. Use non-fat drippings or stock to baste meat. Cut off excess fat before eating. Alternatively, ask your butcher to prepare the roast without any attached fat and cook in foil; this will take longer to cook than traditional roast. Use a special sauce-boat – *graisse et maigre* – to separate the juices from the fat.

Boiling or pot-roasting meat, or cooking as the French do *en daube*, is a good low-fat method because the fat may be skimmed off. Stews are also good if excess fat is cut off first. If you want to fry the meat first, use polyunsaturated cooking oil. The way you cook meat makes an enormous difference to the fat and calorie content of the whole meal.

Sauces: It is possible to make sauces without using fat, by using cornflour or arrowroot as the thickening agent. Alternatively, use polyunsaturated oil, such as corn oil, instead of butter. A vegetable purée can be used to make a sauce which will carry the flavour and moisten the food. Tomato is very good for this.

Poultry: Most of the fat is in the skin, which should be removed before eating and can often be removed in the preparation, but *not* before roasting.

Salad: If you like olive oil, use it. Or you can dilute it with polyunsaturated oil such as corn or sunflower oil in dressings. Alternatively, use seasoned natural yoghurt, preferably made with skimmed milk, as a dressing: this is delicious with cucumber but also as a dressing for lettuce or cabbage – as in coleslaw.

Desserts

Restrict commercially made cakes, pastries, biscuits and ice-cream, which are rich in sugar and saturated fat. Serve egg-based desserts only after a vegetarian first course. Never serve cream or fat-based toppings; try natural yoghurt as an alternative. Traditional British milk puddings are quite harmless – try making them with skimmed milk – but best of all, serve fresh fruit. Cut the amount of sugar in most dessert recipes by at least half; it may actually improve the flavour, which can be masked in a heavy syrup.

Cheese: A small portion only, unless you had a vegetarian main course. Cottage cheese is low in fat and so preferable in, for example, salads.

Alcohol: Only in moderation. Excess increases the flow of fats to the heart and causes you to put on weight. Light wines and beers in moderation may aid digestion and help you relax; spirits are more addictive and so can be a serious threat to health.

Light meals

The biggest mistake most people make is to have two large meals a day. One meal (other than breakfast) should be simple, consisting of, for example: a savoury rice or macaroni dish (if these incorporate meat it should be in small quantity, used more as a flavouring); or bread and soup; or baked potato and grated cheese. Always add salad and fruit if you can.

Tea

Cakes and scones can be made from polyunsaturated margarines such as Flora. We give some sample recipes in Appendix One. More can be obtained by writing to Flora margarine. Remember to use less sugar (about half) than specified in most cake recipes. Flapjacks, made from oatmeal (watch the sugar again), are also a wholesome, wholegrain food. Try also recipes for cakes which use puréed fruit as the binding agent and contain reduced quantities of fat and sugar, or even none at all. Banana cake is the best known of these, but there are others.

Snacks/supper

Go easy on cakes and biscuits; it is better to have a slice of wholemeal bread with polyunsaturated margarine and jam or yeast extract. A milky drink is fine, if you have kept your intake of fats down during the rest of the day; or make it instead with semi-skimmed (stripey-top) milk. A banana might be the answer if you are still really hungry. Carrots, nuts, raisins make good snacks for children and adults.

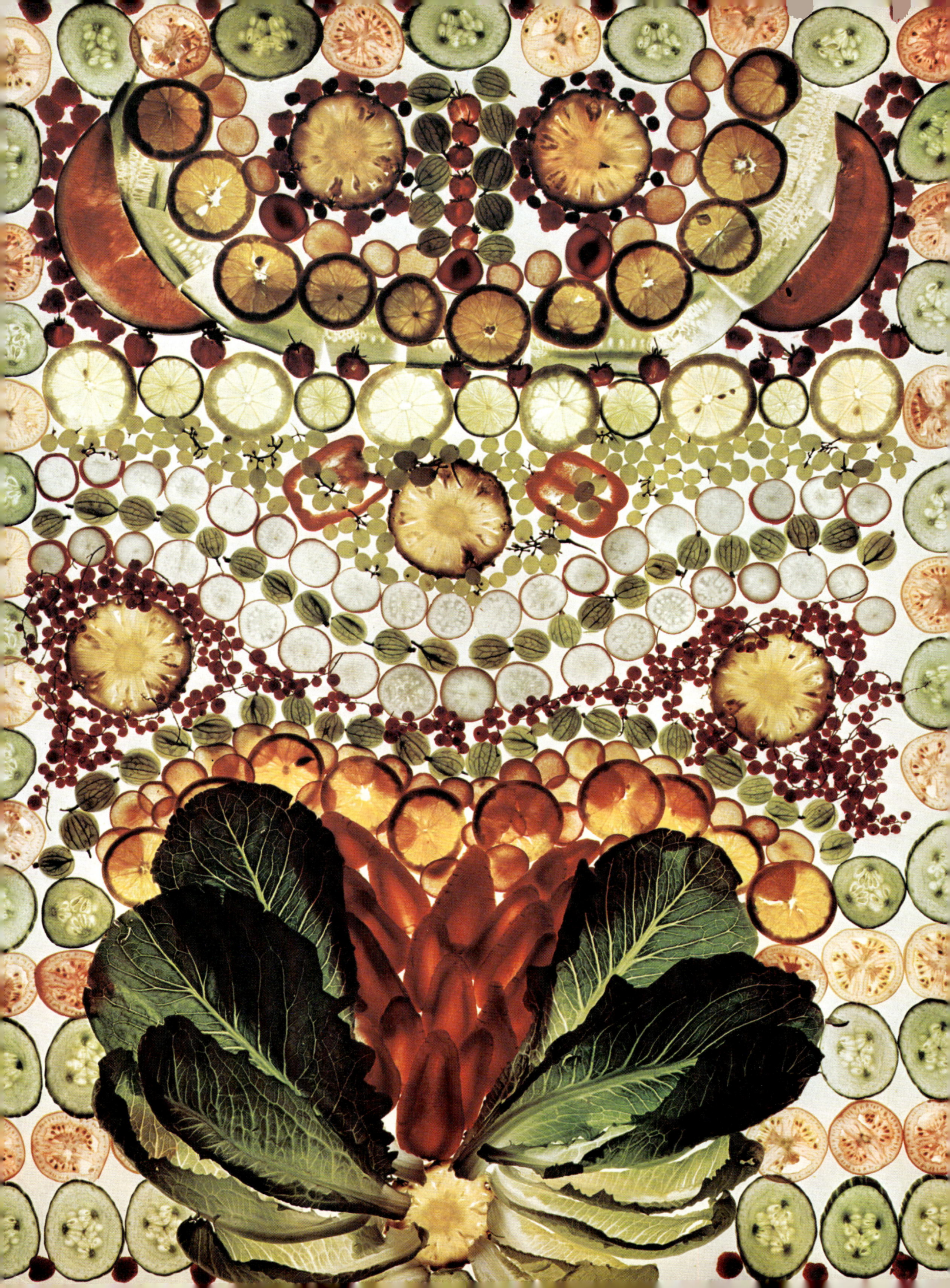

Slimming

The *Sunday Times* has pioneered and popularized a new type of healthy slimming. The aim of this type of slimming is not just to lose weight but to develop the right eating habits which are good for the body in the long run. It does not make sense to slim simply by cutting *out* bread and potatoes, which supply essential nutrients, vitamins and fibre. This advice has been given too often in the past and is now an unhealthy part of the folklore of slimming. Our diet works by cutting down first on excessive fat and sugar – the empty calories which are a threat to health. We have now extended this approach to give advice not just on how to choose and limit the food you eat but to suggest how you can change the way you eat.

Often, people fail to slim because their approach is simply to starve themselves – they lose weight but in the end they go back to their old eating habits which have not changed. To be successful you must first of all understand your own eating habits and decide that you want to change them. If you want to do it, we tell you how.

ARE YOU TOO FAT?

It is normal for an adult man to have about 10–20 per cent of his body-weight as fat and for an adult woman to have about 25 per cent fat. To carry a lot more fat than this is unnecessary and is associated with bad health. Unfortunately, it is impossible for you to measure the actual fat content of your body because this requires expensive equipment, but it is very easy to find out if you are too fat by some indirect methods:

1. Look at yourself naked in a full-length mirror. Can you see large folds of flesh? If so, you are too fat.
2. Use your thumb and first finger to pinch the back of your upper arm, halfway between your shoulder and your elbow. Can you pick up a fold with a total thickness of more than an inch? If so, you are too fat. (Men should also get someone to help them check the skinfold thickness a couple of inches beneath their shoulder blade. A fold thickness of more than an inch here also indicates they are too fat.)

These two methods rely on the fact that a large proportion of your total body-fat is found just below your skin. The other methods of deciding whether you are too fat depend on body-weight. It is unusual for any normal untrained man or woman to change their muscle or bone mass very much during adult life; the only fluctuating component of body-weight apart from water is body-fat. So, provided you have not recently started or stopped intensive sports training, you can assume that a permanent change in your body-weight reflects a change in your body-fat.

The graphs printed on page 89 show the best weights for men and women. These are based on the data collected by life assurance companies in America, and represent the weights for each height at which fewest people die. The white line shows the ideal weight for height and the shaded area on each side allows for differences in frame size (there is a 10 per cent allowance from ideal weight on each side). If you find that your weight for your height falls above this shaded area, then you are overweight and, indirectly, you are too fat. Your aim should be to reduce your weight so that it falls within the shaded area.

DOES FATNESS MATTER?

The answer to this question is 'yes', for the following reasons:

1. The data collected by life assurance companies has shown that a man or woman who is at least 20 per cent above ideal weight has a greater chance of dying earlier than a normal-weight person of the same age. The fatter you are, the likelier you are to die earlier. The same data also show that if you are fat now, however, you are not necessarily destined for a shorter life. If you reduce your weight to normal, your chances of living longer return to normal too.
2. Fat people more frequently get certain illnesses, particularly those connected with the heart and blood-vessels, and they are particularly prone to diabetes. Being fat probably does not cause these diseases directly but rather is a symptom that you are eating a diet which makes you prone to them. Eating less overall, and losing weight, generally means eating less of the fat and sugar which causes these diseases.
3. Also you might find that the doctor has more difficulty in diagnosing what exactly is wrong with you, because your increased fat hampers a normal examination. Similarly, the surgeons are not quite as keen to operate on fat people because even an ordinary operation carries a greater than normal risk.
4. Fat people put extra strain on their joints and ligaments, and this often results in them getting arthritis and back pain. They also tend to move more slowly than thin people because of their greater bulk and this means that they get involved in more accidents at home and at work.
5. Fat women, in particular, suffer because of their appearance. They feel less attractive and have difficulty in finding fashionable clothes.

STRATEGIES FOR SLIMMING

Most people who are overweight make a serious attempt once or twice a year to lose weight. Many do not succeed or, if they do, put the weight on again within a few weeks or months. Why is this? The reason is that most slimmers see the measures they are taking to lose weight as temporary. They are not actually attempting to change their basic lifestyle, so the weight loss does not become permanent. Slimmers cannot be blamed for this. In the past it has been assumed that it was only necessary for someone to be given the correct information about the calorie values of foods and what target to aim for, and then they could lose weight. Failure was considered to be due to lack of will-power.

Now we know that many factors influence a person's eating habits and that if a person is to lose weight successfully then he or she must first identify these factors and learn to control them. The reason most people fail to slim is that the factors which decide their weight have got beyond their control. It is essential to take steps to bring them back within control. For example, a man often does not choose the food or the quantity of it he is given – at lunch he eats a meal, or has to entertain, and in the evening his wife may expect him to eat a full meal with the rest of the family. A woman's weight may also be influenced by her husband. The husband may not be at home much and so the wife becomes depressed and uses food as an escape. A husband may bring a wife chocolates whenever she loses a few pounds. It may be more reassuring to a man to have a wife who is plump than one who is lean and attractive.

Research by Dr Stanley Schachter of Columbia University, New York, and others, has established that overeating is caused at least as much by the situation surrounding a person as by the person himself. For example, he has found that people who are overweight are much more likely to eat when food is in full view or already prepared than when it has to be cooked. People who overeat tend to eat certain problem foods, which appeal to them, such as ice-cream or biscuits. They eat more carefully when they know how much they are eating at, for example, a set meal – as opposed to a party where food is constantly being offered round. Husbands whose wives are overweight more often begin to talk about food and to offer it around. People who are overweight are more likely to eat than others when they are emotionally disturbed.

So, if the situation can be controlled, then overeating can be brought under control too. The first step to take is to analyse the situation and discover the factors which affect your eating. The way to do this is to keep a daily eating record. Every time you eat you should record:

1. what the time is
2. the food you ate
3. how much food you ate
4. where you were
5. what you were doing
6. who you were with
7. what feelings you had while you ate.

After keeping an eating record for a few days, you will begin to see patterns in your eating habits. For example, you may see that you ate a lot when you were by yourself and you felt lonely, or that you ate a lot of problem foods such as chocolates, biscuits or peanuts. Alternatively, it may be that you ate most in company and that you should seek ways of altering your social habits. For example, you might arrange to meet a friend in a park or sports club rather than in a café or pub.

HOW TO CONTROL YOUR EATING HABITS

You can begin to control your eating by developing a series of rules which you undertake to use for guidance. Occasionally you may break a rule. That does not mean that you have failed – start again. First you must learn to control all the circumstances that precede eating, then eating itself. Then the consequences of eating – your weight – will come under your control.

First stage
Choose a particular room in which to eat at home and only eat there.
If you choose to eat in the kitchen, then it means you must not eat in the living room even if you want to watch TV. If you want to watch, eat later. If you choose to eat in the

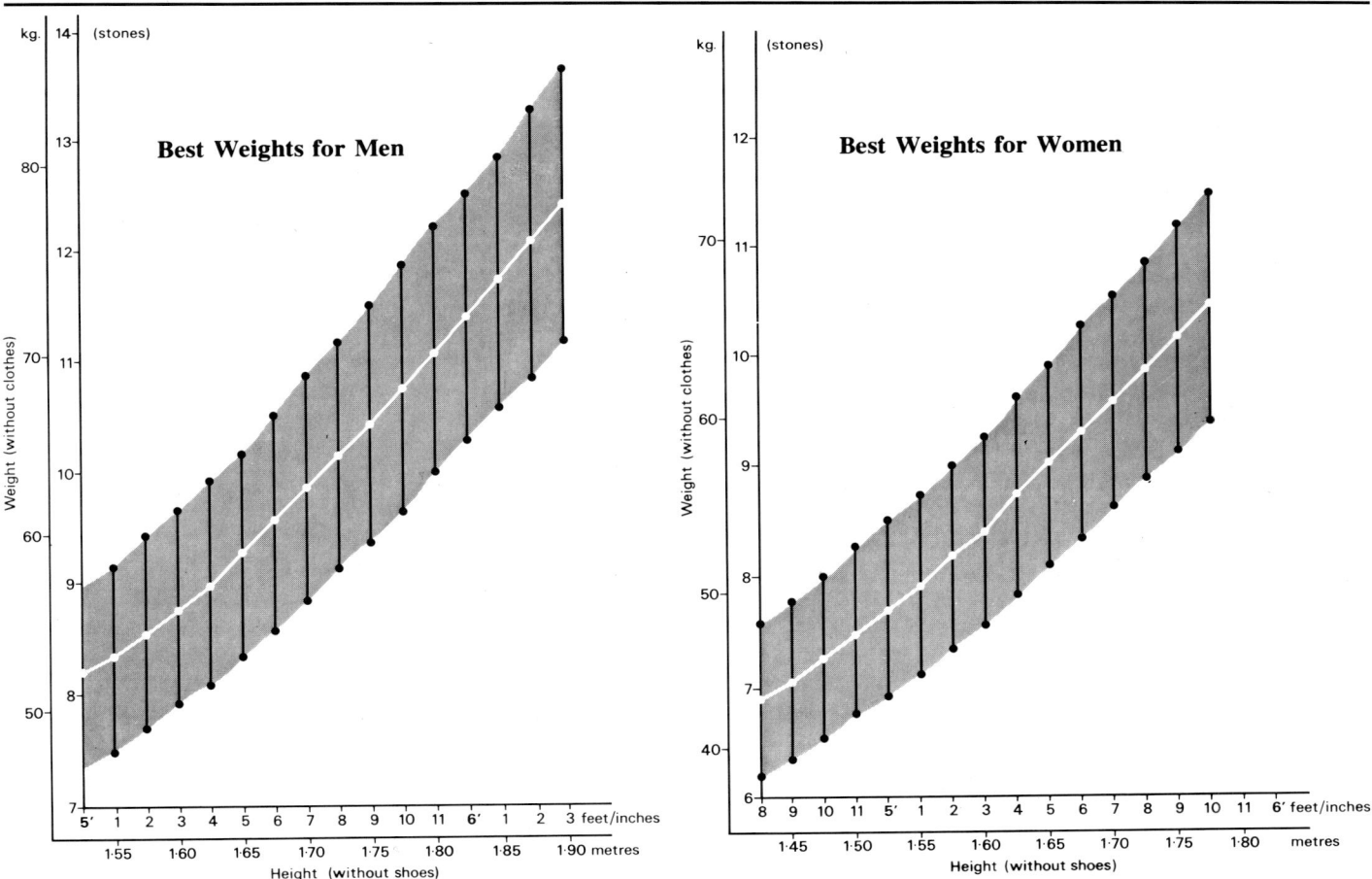

The shaded areas show the range of best or desirable weights, allowing for differences in sizes of body frames – large, average or small – for each height.

living room, then you must not nibble while you are in the kitchen.

Make up your mind to eat in only one place in the room, and when you eat avoid doing other things at the same time such as watching TV or listening to music. In this way, you will gradually reduce the number of situations which make you think of food. If you are in the habit of eating while watching TV, then switching on the set becomes a cue for the conditioned reaction of eating. In the same way, being in a particular room such as the kitchen may provide a stimulus which makes you want to eat.

Second stage
Buy non-fattening foods.
Sometimes you may find it impossible to resist buying fattening foods. Packaging and displays in shops make it very difficult to resist. If you do buy fattening foods, such as chocolates or biscuits, put them away out of sight and out of easy reach so that you have to make a very conscious decision to eat some. Don't, for example, keep sweets or biscuits in the living room or the glove pocket of the car. Shop from a list and only buy items which are on the list. You may find it easier to shop after you have eaten.

Third stage
Keep up the record of your eating and analyse your problems.
Some women, for example, eat a lot of their children's leftovers. Without thinking it through, they tell themselves that the food should not be wasted. Force yourself to throw the leftovers away and begin to give the children smaller portions. After work you may go for a drink with friends. Choose a small drink which contains fewer calories, drink halves of beer, and make up your mind to leave or have no more after the second drink. If that doesn't work, then you may have to change your habits more radically if you seriously want to slim.

Fourth stage
Enlist help from others – and train them.
Explain to your mate, your friends and the people who work with you what you are doing so that they can remind you if you forget. Tell them that you need praise not punishment and ask them to compliment you when you stick to your rules.

Fifth stage
Be sly but knowing.
Use a little deception to make small portions appear large. For example, use a small plate. But be sure to measure out what you eat so that you know how much you have eaten. Don't put serving dishes on the table, to make it more of a conscious effort to get a second helping. If you are a fast eater, you might try coming to the table late to avoid eating twice as much as everyone else.

Sixth stage
Know the six enemies: boredom, depression, loneliness, hunger, anger and fatigue.
Boredom, depression and loneliness are generally problems for people who are overweight because they tend to use food as a means of fighting these moods. But you can fight these moods off in other ways. For example, keep a list of friends to call, think of starting a new hobby or joining an evening class. Make a list of things to do when you are hungry. Hunger can be controlled by taking regular small meals. If you skip breakfast and have a small lunch, you are bound to feel very hungry in the evening. Then you may eat a large meal which more than compensates for all the food you have denied yourself. Eat three regular meals a day.

Some people who cannot express their anger find this inability makes them overeat. Exercise is a much better way of relieving tension and it uses up calories. If you do not have a particular sport, try walking – an excellent way of relieving tense feelings.

When people are very tired they often try to get more energy by eating. You may be tired because you are not getting enough sleep or because you need to relax more in the middle of the day. As a rule try to get eight to nine hours in bed a day even if you are not asleep all the time (see section on sleep, pages 70–1).

Seventh stage
Have safe snacks at hand
Keep safe snacks such as peeled carrots, shredded cabbage, celery, or cottage cheese ready in the refrigerator. You can make the snacks more interesting by, for example, carving the carrots into shapes, mixing cottage cheese with fresh herbs such as parsley and putting it into a mould. If you know you will want a snack at a certain time, you can try saving one item, such as a slice of toast, from a previous meal.

Eighth stage
Learn to eat more slowly.
Consider your eating habits. Do you tend to finish your meal while others are still only halfway through? If so, teach yourself to take smaller bites and to chew for longer. If this is too difficult at first, simply stop for two or three minutes, putting down fork and knife. After the pause, continue trying again to eat small mouthfuls slowly. Some people put more food into their mouth before they have finished chewing the first mouthful. Make sure you avoid this. Research has shown that it takes twenty minutes after eating for a person to begin to feel full and to lose the feelings of hunger. If you finish eating within twenty minutes you will still feel hungry at the end of a meal. Try to pause between courses.

Ninth stage
Increase the amount of exercise you get.
It is important to take more exercise so that you burn up fat and food. Studies have shown that many fat people do not eat more than slim people but they do take a lot less exercise. Try to build exercise into your life even if it only means walking home from work or going to a dancing class twice a week (for more information on exercise see pages 100–2 and Chapter 2).

Tenth stage
Choose your method of dieting.
We offer two different approaches to dieting:
1. The **Cut Down** diet. In this diet you are given lots of information on calorie contents of foods and drinks, and advice on the right calorie limit to set and the right things to choose, and you are then left to devise your own diet.
2. The **Cut Out** diet. In this diet you are given certain foods you can eat as much of as you like, other foods which are rationed and some foods which are forbidden.

Research has shown that both types of diet are popular; usually, but not always, the Cut Down diets appeal to women and the Cut Out diets appeal to men. You probably know which appeals to you already. We are going to give you instructions for both types of diet, starting with the Cut Down diet below and then the Cut Out diet on page 100 Even if you know that the Cut Out diet is for you, we advise you to read about the Cut Down diet because you should know the basic principles of calorie counting even if you prefer to follow a diet that does not involve any counting or weighing.

MONITOR YOUR PROGRESS AND REWARD YOURSELF

It is important to keep an exact record of your progress. This should show the calorie value of the food you have eaten, the calorie value of the exercise you are taking and your weight. You can display this as a graph. If you are lapsing in the amount of food you are eating or the exercise you are taking, the graph will tell you. When you see your weight falling on the graph, you will feel good and that in itself will be an encouragement for you. You can keep this graph for a week or so before you actually start dieting while you are trying to analyse some of your eating habits. This will give you a base line so that you will know how it varies from day to day and if you are making real progress.

It is important that you reward yourself for success. And success is not just losing weight. You must reward yourself for changing those small habits which are going to build up to success in the long run. For example, you should set yourself a goal which you know you can achieve such as putting into practice the first three stages of the above programme. When you have done that for a week, reward yourself with an evening out at a show, or by buying a record – or by finding time for something simple you really want to do. Then you can go on to the next three or four stages in the same way. And for each day or week of achievement try to treat yourself to something. Some people find it helps to award themselves tokens for each small achievement and so many tokens add up to a night out. Others find it helpful to award themselves a medal which can be worn proudly in front of the family. Enlist the help of family to make you feel good when you have earned your medal. You need all the praise you can get.

SLIMMING WITHOUT DIETING

It is the eternal hope of every fat person that someone, some day, will invent a method of slimming which does not involve a diet. Unfortunately, this has not happened yet although some clever ads would have you believe it! The term 'slimming' really means the breakdown of fat and this is only achieved physiologically by creating an energy gap between your calorie input and your calorie output. No amount of mechanical rubbing with massages and creams or vibrator belts will do any good whatsoever.

THE CUT DOWN METHOD OF SLIMMING

Average calorie requirements of men and women vary with their age and the amount of energy they expend in work and exercise (see diagram page 95). We must stress here that these figures are only averages and there can be quite a range of calorie requirements even when sex and age are the same. It is very difficult to measure total calorie expenditure directly on a daily basis, and our best estimates come from surveys measuring the energy intake needed to balance output and so maintain a constant weight. This is also your best method of estimating your own calorie output if you are not content to accept the average figure for your age and sex. But you will have to be very careful when you start to work out your calorie input. Everything you eat and drink must be counted, and do not forget that cooking can drastically alter the calorie values of raw foods.

Once you have some idea of your energy output, you must decide on a suitable 'energy gap' between your input and output. The size of this gap is your choice, but the chart opposite gives you some idea of the rate of weight-loss for different energy gaps. Suppose you consider yourself a fairly inactive forty-five-year-old woman, and you take the average value of 2,200 calories to be your energy output. If you set yourself an energy gap of 500 calories, this means that your energy input must be 1,700 calories; an energy gap of 700 calories reduces your allowed input to 1,500 calories, and an energy gap of 1,000 calories will limit you to 1,200 calories a day. (Don't ever be tempted to set your calorie limit lower than 800 calories.)

From the chart, you can see that, whatever energy gap you set yourself, you will lose more weight in the first week than in any other. This is probably because the first energy reserves that your body calls on when output exceeds input are its starch stores in the muscles. Since these starch stores have quite a lot of water associated with them, you will lose quite a few pounds of water in the first week, as well as a little fat. The amount of water you lose will depend on the size of your starch stores, and this in turn will depend on your previous diet; a diet rich in carbohydrates will fill up the stores. After the first week, it is much easier to predict the rate of weight-loss on a known energy gap because it is known that it takes a total energy gap of 3,500 calories to break down a pound of fat. So seven days on a 500-calorie energy gap will cause a fat-loss of one pound, on a 700-calorie energy gap the fat-loss will be nearly one-and-a-half pounds, and on a 1,000-calorie energy gap two pounds of fat will be lost.

The lines of weight-loss on the chart are straight because

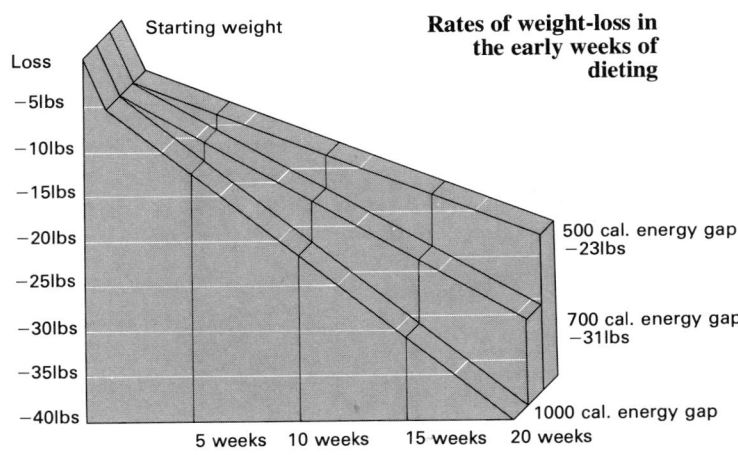

Weight-loss varies according to the 'energy gap' most suitable for you – see text above.

DIET/SLIMMING

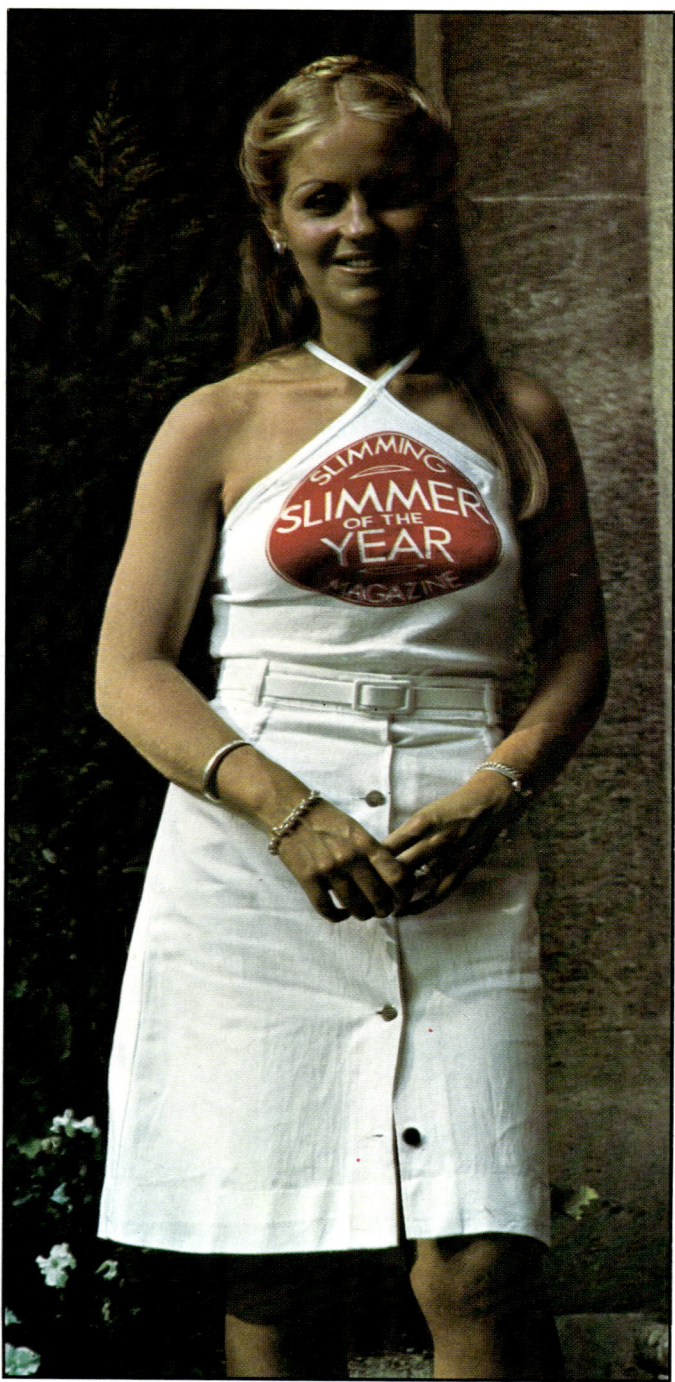

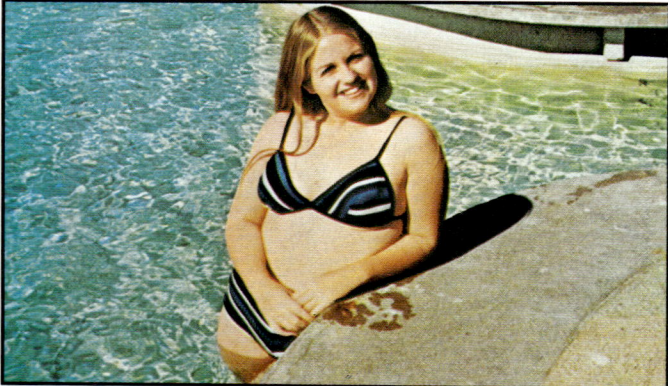

Gail Ingham, a British Slimmer of the Year, after dieting down to 8½ stone from the 15-stone teenager in the swimming pool.

they are based on theoretical calculations and assume that you stick rigidly to your energy gap. Of course, this will certainly not always be the case, but if you try to stick roughly to your energy gap over a matter of weeks you should find that your line of weight-loss will more or less follow the chart line. Gains and losses of water are another thing that will make your actual weight-loss line deviate from the one on the chart. In particular, women might notice a tendency for their weight to 'stick' in the week before a period even if they are maintaining their strict energy gap. This is almost certainly due to fluid retention and they will probably get a greater loss than they were expecting in the week after their period.

We have shown the lines on the chart continuing at the same rate of weight-loss for twenty weeks. If you need to diet for longer than this, you will probably find that your weight-loss tends to slow up and that your line begins to straighten out. This could be due to the fact that you are being less strict with yourself and that you are now setting a smaller energy gap. If you know that this is the reason, then the remedy is in your own hands. However, there is another reason why your weight-loss rate might slow up, and this is because your body might adapt to the reduced input and automatically reduce its energy output. So the energy gap that you set will get smaller through no fault of your own. By the time this happens (and it won't necessarily happen to you), you should be at least a couple of stone lighter and, hopefully, you will feel fitter and more active, so that it should be easy to increase your energy output.

If you have a large amount of weight to lose (over four stone, say), it is sometimes a good idea to use the 'staircase slimming' method. What you do is to make a definite effort to lose your first stone in a month (by setting a 1,000-calorie energy gap), then aim to maintain this new weight for a month (by eating the number of calories approximately equal to your output), then lose another stone in the next month and so on. This will not only be easier on your nerves (and possibly those around you) but will also allow your skin, which has been stretched by your excess fat, time to shrink back gradually to its original size.

Use the graphs on page 89 to help you to decide how much weight you ought to lose. Although it is advisable to get your weight within the shaded portion, it is more important that you should maintain whatever weight-loss you achieve. So if you are four stone above your ideal weight, it is far better that you should reduce your weight by two stone and keep it there, than lose the complete four stone but not be able to keep it off permanently.

When you have successfully reduced your weight, you will be able to drink and eat more because you will not need to create an energy gap any more. But do not be surprised if you cannot have as much as you could when you were fat: remember that your body needed that much extra fuel in those days when you were expending more energy carrying the extra weight around.

CHOOSING THE RIGHT CALORIES

As far as calculating fat-losses and gains goes, all calories are equal and calories from any food or drink which is surplus to your requirements are stored as fat. It follows, then, that a 1,000-calorie diet of anything will cause a weight-loss because this is bound to create a reasonable energy gap. However, it is particularly important that you should follow the general principles of a healthy diet when

SLIMMING/DIET

you are eating less overall, and this is why you should try to follow a few rules about the amount of fat, protein and carbohydrate that make up your calorie limit.

The Royal College of Physicians' report recommends that no more than 35 per cent of your total daily calories should come from fat and it is a good idea to apply this principle to your weight-reducing diet. Thus for every 1,000 calories that you allow yourself on your diet, no more than 350 of these calories should come from fat. Since 1 gramme of pure fat contains 9 calories, this restricts the fat in your 1,000-calorie diet to just under 40 grammes. To calculate the fat limit in a diet where the calorie limit differs from 1,000 calories, divide your calorie limit by 1,000 and multiply by 40 (e.g. a 1,200-calorie limit will have a fat limit of 48 grammes).

In this Cut Down diet we are only going to suggest that you stick to two limits, a calorie limit and a fat limit, because otherwise the counting would get far too complicated. However, do also bear in mind that calories from sugar are 'empty calories'; they supply energy and nothing else, and so you should keep your sugar-intake low if you want to stay healthy and ward off heart and dental disease.

THE LOW-DOWN ON HIGH-CALORIE FOOD

On pages 97–9 we give the all-important percentages of fat in various foods, as well as protein, calories and carbohydrate; the remaining percentage is usually water. You can calculate the *type* of fat you are eating by referring to the table on page 79. Check your daily calorie intake against the totals given on pages 97–9 and measure the precise proportions of fat, protein and carbohydrate in your diet.

DO BE SENSIBLE

It is possible to become obsessive about slimming. The condition known as anorexia nervosa is becoming increasingly common in teenage girls and young women. Sufferers from this condition go to all lengths to avoid eating and endanger their health in so doing. Do make certain that you know not only when to start but also when to stop! If you have a child who is seriously underweight and does not eat normally, take the child to your doctor.

THE CUT DOWN PLAN – day by day

To show you how the Cut Down plan works out in practice, we have set out plans for seven days which have a 1,000-calorie and a 40-gramme fat limit. They have been calculated so that all the breakfasts are about 200 calories, all the snack meals are about 300 calories and all the main meals are about 500 calories. This has been done to allow you to juggle the meals around to suit your fancy: e.g. you can have Day 1 breakfast, followed by Day 4 snack meal, followed by Day 7 main meal.

If you are planning your own calorie-counted meals using the chart, then there is no need for you to arrange your calories in this strict fashion. You can have ten small snack meals of 100 calories if you want to: it is up to you to cut down in the way it suits you.

The calorie and fat contents are calculated according to the metric measures and are 'rounded' to the nearest 5 calories and to the nearest 0.1 gramme, respectively. All weights are uncooked weights.

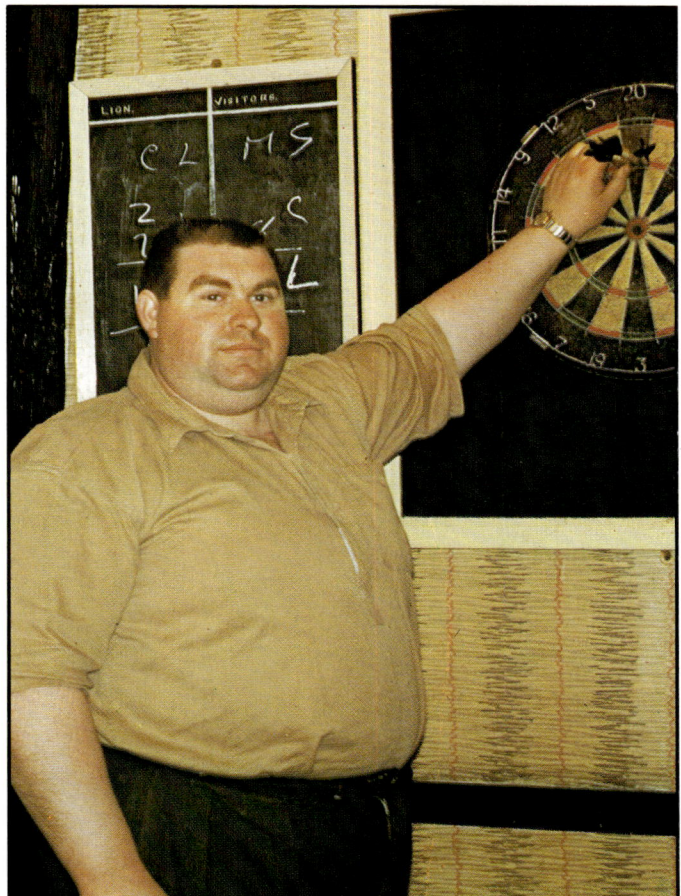

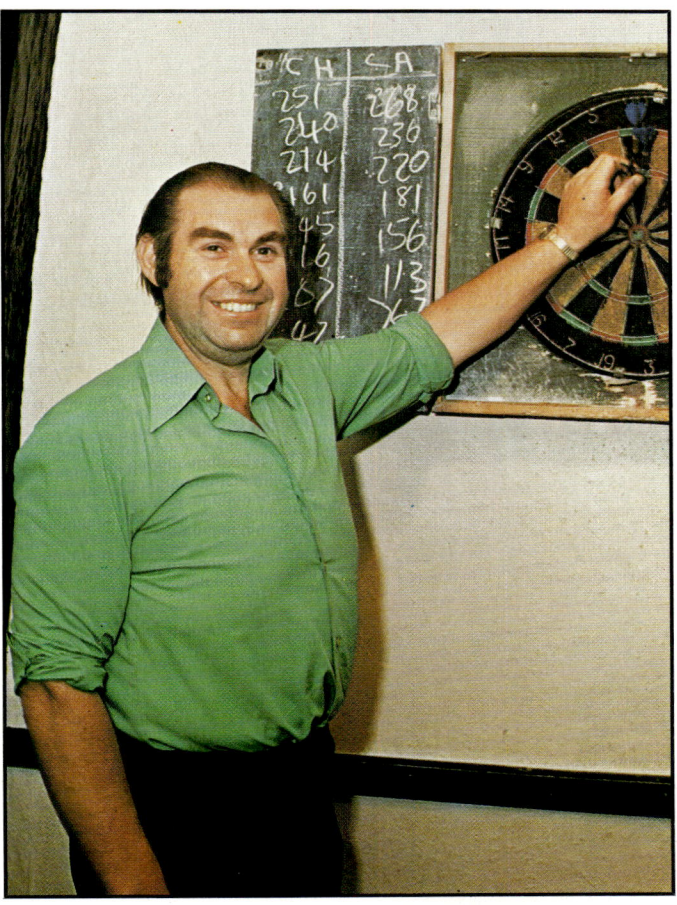

Handyman Claude Halls at play: from 33 stone to 12st. 12lb in just 14 months

DIET/SLIMMING

Day 1

Breakfast	Calories	Fat (g)
25 g (1 oz) cereal (wholemeal, if possible)	80	1.1
150 ml (¼ pt) milk	100	5.5
5 ml (1 teaspoonful) sweetener (granular)	10	—
	190	6.6

Snack meal		
50 g (2 oz) wholemeal bread, toasted	115	1.0
10 g (½ oz) soft margarine	80	8.5
100 g (4 oz) baked beans	95	0.4
	290	9.9

Main meal		
50 ml (1 glass) of dry sherry	60	—
1 portion lamb pie (see recipe)	360	23.7
100 g (4 oz) cabbage	10	—
100 g (4 oz) boiled potatoes	75	—
	505	23.7

Totals	985	40.2

Day 2

Breakfast	Calories	Fat (g)
1 egg (boiled)	90	6.6
25 g (1 oz) wholemeal bread	55	0.5
5 g (¼ oz) soft margarine	40	4.3
	185	11.4

Snack meal		
50 g (2 oz) Edam cheese	160	11.5
2 apples (200 g)	90	—
	250	11.5

Main meal		
100 ml (1 glass) of dry white wine	70	—
100 g (4 oz) chicken piece, grilled	205	10.3
150 g (6 oz) boiled rice (brown, if possible)	185	0.5
100 g (4 oz) peas	50	—
125 g (5 oz) yoghurt, low fat	70	2.3
	580	13.1

Totals	1015	36.0

Day 3

Breakfast	Calories	Fat (g)
1 kipper, grilled (100 g, 4 oz)	200	11.4

Snack meal		
75 g (3 oz) cold lean pork	245	17.8
50 g (2 oz) boiled potatoes	40	—
	285	17.8

Day 3 — Contd.

Main meal		
300 ml (½ pt) beer or cider	95	—
1 portion tomato casserole	165	5.3
100 g (4 oz) boiled pasta	115	0.6
150 g (6 oz) stewed apples, sweetened artificially	70	—
125 g (5 oz) natural yoghurt	70	2.3
	515	8.2

Totals	1000	37.4

Day 4

Breakfast	Calories	Fat (g)
1 egg, poached	90	6.6
25 g (1 oz) wholemeal bread	55	0.5
5 g (¼ oz) soft margarine	40	4.3
	185	11.4

Snack meal		
50 g (2 oz) prawns or shrimps	50	0.9
100 g (4 oz) cottage cheese	120	0.5
100 g (4 oz) lettuce	10	—
1 orange (100 g, 4 oz)	40	—
1 banana (100 g, 4 oz)	60	—
	280	1.4

Main meal		
100 ml (1 glass) dry wine	70	—
100 g (4 oz) steak, grilled	305	21.6
100 g (4 oz) sprouts	15	—
1 portion strawberry jelly	95	—
150 ml (¼ pt) slimmers' custard	80	0.3
	565	21.9

Totals	1030	34.7

Day 5

Breakfast	Calories	Fat (g)
1 grapefruit	30	—
150 g (6 oz) smoked haddock	145	1.2
	175	1.2

Snack meal		
300 ml (½ pt) beer or cider	95	—
150 g (6 oz) liver, grilled	215	12.2
100 g (4 oz) tomatoes, grilled	15	—
100 g (4 oz) baked potato	105	—
	430	12.2

Main meal		
300 ml (½ pt) soup, e.g. tomato	210	9.3
1 portion cauliflower cheese	205	8.9
	415	18.2

Totals	1020	31.6

SLIMMING/**DIET**

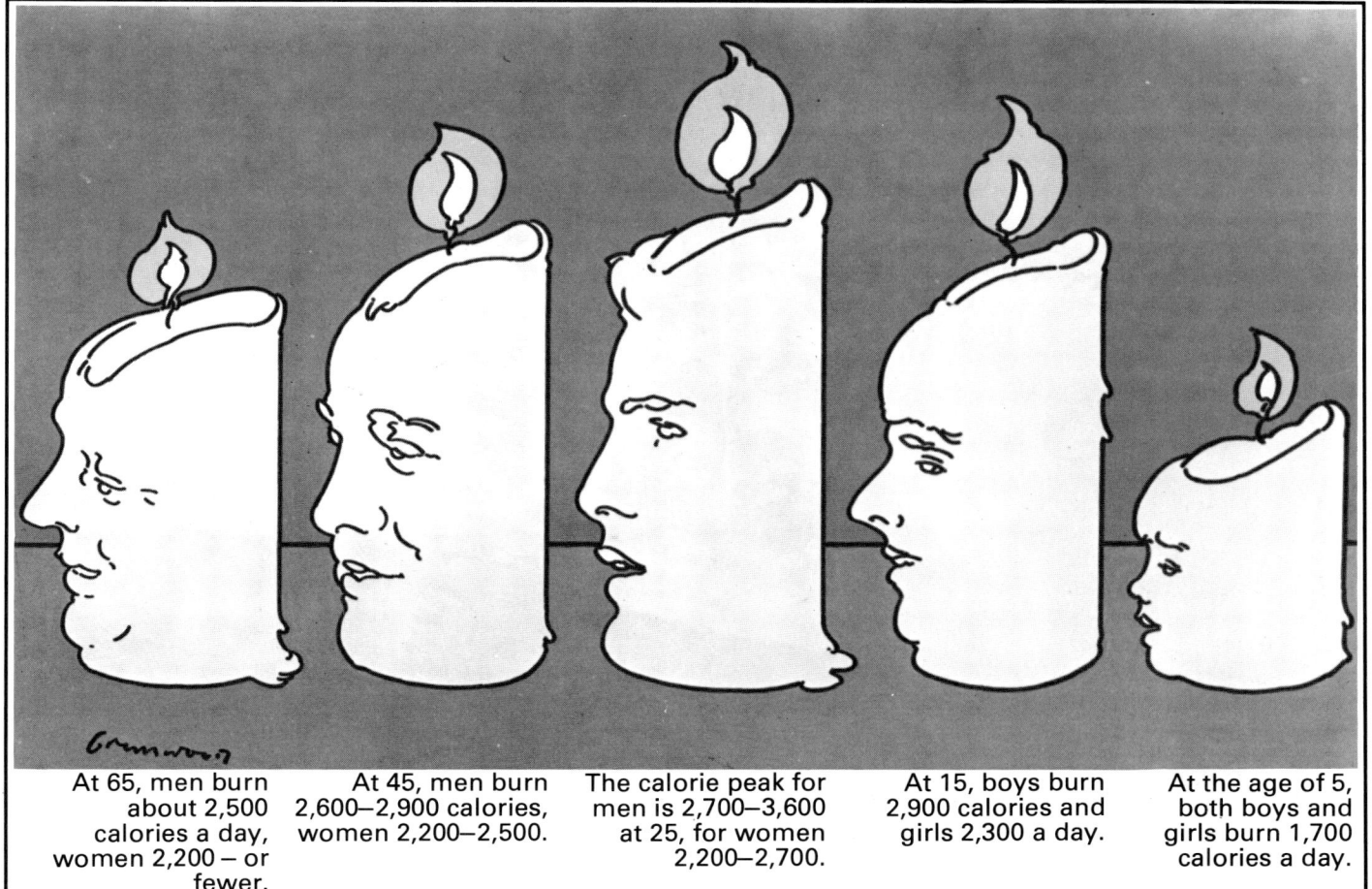

At 65, men burn about 2,500 calories a day, women 2,200 – or fewer.

At 45, men burn 2,600–2,900 calories, women 2,200–2,500.

The calorie peak for men is 2,700–3,600 at 25, for women 2,200–2,700.

At 15, boys burn 2,900 calories and girls 2,300 a day.

At the age of 5, both boys and girls burn 1,700 calories a day.

(These are average values. Calorie consumption varies in individuals with body build, body chemistry and the amount of exercise taken.)

Day 6

Breakfast	Calories	Fat (g)
1 portion plain omelette (1 egg)	90	9.3
50 g (2 oz) wholemeal bread	110	1.0
	200	10.3

Snack meal		
300 ml (½ pt) soup, e.g. tomato	210	9.3
25 g (1 oz) wholemeal bread	55	0.5
1 apple (100 g, 4 oz)	45	—
	310	9.8

Main meal		
1 portion stuffed haddock (see recipe)	370	5.8
100 g (4 oz) peas	50	—
100 g (4 oz) boiled potatoes	75	—
	495	5.8
Totals	1005	25.9

Day 7

Breakfast	Calories	Fat (g)
50 g (2 oz) wholemeal bread	115	1.0
10 g (½ oz) soft margarine	80	8.5
10 g (½ oz) jam or marmalade	25	—
	220	9.5

Snack meal		
50 g (2 oz) sardines, drained	150	11.3
25 g (1 oz) wholemeal bread, toasted	55	0.5
	205	11.8

Main meal		
50 ml (1 glass) dry sherry	60	—
1 portion kidney casserole (see recipe)	215	10.6
100 g (4 oz) cooked rice	120	0.3
1 banana	60	—
1 portion slimmers' custard	80	—
	535	10.9
Totals	960	32.2

DIET/SLIMMING

SLIMMING RECIPES

There is no shortage of detailed recipes for slimmers, and we list some of the best books in our bibliography. But often it is just a question of using common sense in adapting well-known dishes to the slimmer's particular needs. For instance, we kept the calorie count down to 205 per portion in the cauliflower cheese (Day 4) by using slimmers' milk or milk made from low-fat milk powder. The slimmers' custard (Day 3) not only uses the same kind of milk but also artificial sweetener instead of sugar along with the custard powder.

The calorie counts of some other dishes – notably tomato casserole, kidney casserole and lamb pie – could have been reduced further by using a low-calorie soft margarine such as Outline rather than a soft low-fat margarine like Flora which reduces saturated fat, not calories. We print below detailed recipes for three of the dishes. Do not think that these are the only ways to cook slimming versions of these meals. Build upon the principles of slimming cookery and use the food fact-finder on pages 97–9 to develop your own favourites.

Lamb pie for four

	Calories	Fat (g)
1 large onion	25	—
1 large carrot	20	—
10g (½oz) soft margarine	80	8.5
400g (1lb) minced cooked lean lamb	1085	70.0
2 egg yolks	150	13.1
150ml (¼pt) stock	15	—
2 egg whites	30	—
pinch of mixed herbs	—	—
seasoning	—	—
10g (½oz) Parmesan cheese	40	3.0
	1445	94.6

1. Chop onion and carrot finely.
2. Melt the fat and fry meat, onion and carrot in it.
3. Separate the eggs and add the yolks plus stock and herbs to the meat and vegetables.
4. Mix well and cook for a few minutes. Transfer to ovenproof dish.
5. Whisk up egg whites until they are stiff. Add seasoning and spread meringue over meat mixture.
6. Sprinkle Parmesan cheese over top of meringue.
7. Cook in a fairly hot oven (Reg. 5, 375°F) for about 15 minutes or put under a hot grill until the meringue is golden brown.

Calories per portion 360
Fat per portion 23.7g

Kidney casserole for four

	Calories	Fat (g)
25g (1oz) soft margarine	200	21.3
400g (1lb) of kidney	475	21.2
4 large onions	100	—
300ml (½pt) tomato soup	80	—
seasoning	—	—
chopped parsley	—	—
	855	42.5

1. Melt the fat in a frying pan or large saucepan.
2. Cut the kidneys into bie-sized pieces. Chop onions finely.
3. Toss kidneys very quickly in the melted fat. Add onions.
4. Add soup to pan, bring to boil stirring. Add seasoning to taste.
5. Reduce heat to a simmer, cover pan and continue cooking for a further 15 minutes.
6. Add the chopped parsley just before serving.

Calories per portion 215
Fat per portion 10.6g

Baked Stuffed Haddock for four

	Calories	Fat (g)
2 large haddocks (about 1200g or 3lb total)	1165	9.6
200g (½lb) chopped mushrooms	15	—
2 tomatoes, skinned and sliced	20	—
4 small onions, chopped	40	—
25g (1oz) breadcrumbs	60	0.5
1 clove of garlic, crushed	—	—
2 eggs	180	13.1
	1480	23.2

1. Prepare the fish: remove scales, fin, tail and internal organs if this has not been done already. Wash in cold water and dry on a towel or kitchen paper.
2. Prepare the stuffing. Mix mushrooms, tomatoes, onions, breadcrumbs and garlic and bind with the beaten eggs.
3. Fill the cavity of the fish with stuffing and secure with skewers or with needle and thread.
4. Put the fish in an ovenproof dish or wrap in foil, and bake for 30 minutes. (Reg. 4, 350°F).
5. Garnish with lemon slices and parsley.

Calories per portion 370
Fat per portion 5.8g

SLIMMING/DIET

Description of food and method of cooking	Protein percentage	Fat percentage	Carbohydrate percentage	Calories per 100g (3.5oz approx.)
Cakes and pastries				
Doughnuts	6.0	15.8	48.8	355
Ginger biscuits	5.9	16.7	71.2	447
Jam tarts	3.8	15.4	62.7	394
Pastry, flaky, baked	6.7	42.0	45.6	589
Pastry, short, baked	7.7	33.4	54.9	548
Plain fruit cake	5.8	16.3	53.9	378
Scones	7.7	13.2	57.3	369
Shortbread	6.1	27.2	64.9	521
Sponge cake	8.9	7.0	55.1	308
Puddings				
Apple pie	1.9	7.5	30.0	190
Jelly	1.9	0	19.1	82
Rice pudding	3.6	7.6	15.7	144
Trifle	3.3	5.6	22.4	150
Yorkshire pudding	7.1	9.4	27.0	218
Cereal and cereal foods				
All-Bran, Kellogg's	12.6	4.5	58.0	311
Biscuits, cream crackers	9.6	16.3	68.3	447
Biscuits, digestive	9.6	20.5	66.0	481
Biscuits, plain mixed	7.4	13.2	75.3	435
Biscuits, rusks	6.0	8.4	81.6	409
Biscuits, sweet mixed	5.5	30.7	66.5	556
Bread, wholemeal	8.2	2.0	47.1	228
Bread, brown	8.7	2.1	49.9	242
Bread, Hovis	9.0	2.3	47.6	237
Bread, Procea	10.7	2.4	50.3	255
Bread, white, large loaves	7.8	1.4	52.7	243
Bread, white, toasted	9.6	1.7	64.9	299
Cornflakes, Kellogg's	6.6	0.8	88.2	367
Cornflour	0.5	0.7	92.0	354
Custard powder	3.4	3.9	17.5	116
Flour, English wholemeal	8.9	2.2	73.4	333
Flour, white, household	11.2	1.5	77.5	350
Macaroni, boiled	3.4	0.6	25.2	114
Oatmeal, raw	12.1	8.7	72.8	404
Oatmeal porridge	1.4	0.9	8.2	45
Rice Krispies	5.7	1.1	85.1	351
Rice, polished, boiled	2.1	0.3	29.6	122
Ryvita	9.1	2.1	76.8	345
Semolina	10.7	1.8	77.5	352
Shredded Wheat	9.7	2.8	79.0	362
Soya. Full fat flour	40.3	23.5	13.3	433
Spaghetti	9.9	1.0	84.0	365
Weetabix	10.9	1.9	77.0	351
Milk products and eggs				
Milk and milk products				
Butter, slightly salted	0.4	85.1	Tr.	793
Cheese, Camembert	22.8	23.2	Tr.	309
Cheese, Cheddar	25.4	34.5	Tr.	425
Cheese, Cheshire	25.8	30.6	Tr.	389
Cheese, cream	3.3	86.0	Tr.	813
Cheese, Danish Blue	23.0	29.2	Tr.	366
Cheese, Edam	24.4	22.9	Tr.	313
Cheese, Gorgonzola	25.4	31.1	Tr.	393
Cheese, Gouda	22.6	26.6	Tr.	340
Cheese, Gruyère	37.6	33.4	T.	465
Cheese, Parmesan	35.1	29.7	Tr.	420
Cheese, processed	23.0	30.1	Tr.	374
Cheese, Stilton	25.6	40.0	Tr.	477
Cheese, Wensleydale	29.3	30.7	Tr.	406
Cream, double	1.5	48.2	2.0	462
Cream, single	2.4	21.2	3.2	219
Milk, fresh, whole	3.4	3.7	4.8	66
Milk, fresh, skimmed	3.5	0.2	5.1	35
Milk, condensed, whole, sweetened	8.2	12.0	56.0	354
Milk, dried, skimmed	34.5	0.3	49.1	326
Yoghurt, low fat	4.7	1.8	4.9	54
Eggs, fresh, whole	11.9	12.3	Tr.	163
Egg white	9.0	Tr.	Tr.	37
Egg yolk	16.2	30.5	Tr.	350
Eggs, fried	14.1	19.5	Tr.	239
Eggs, poached	12.4	11.7	Tr.	160
Fats and oils				
Lard	Tr.	99.0	0.0	920
Margarine	0.2	85.3	0.0	795
Olive oil	Tr.	99.9	0.0	930
Meat, poultry and game				
Bacon, raw, average	14.0	37.4	0.0	405
Bacon, raw, gammon	15.3	28.2	0.0	325
Bacon, back, fried	24.6	53.4	0.0	597
Bacon, collar, fried	27.4	35.0	0.0	438
Bacon, gammon, fried	31.3	33.9	0.0	444
Bacon, streaky, fried	24.0	46.0	0.0	526
Beef, corned	22.3	15.0	0.0	231
Beef, silverside, boiled	28.0	20.0	0.0	301
Beef, sirloin, roast, lean only	26.8	12.3	0.0	224
Beef, sirloin, roast, lean and fat	21.3	32.1	0.0	385
Beef steak, fried	20.4	20.4	0.0	273
Beef steak, grilled *	25.2	21.6	0.0	304
Beef steak, stewed	30.8	8.6	0.0	206
Beef, topside, roast, lean only	26.7	15.0	0.0	249
Brain, calf, boiled	12.0	5.8	0.0	103
Chicken, boiled	26.2	10.3	0.0	203
Chicken, roast	29.6	7.3	0.0	189
Duck, roast	22.8	23.6	0.0	313
Goose, roast	28.0	22.4	0.0	323
Grouse, roast	30.1	5.3	0.0	173
Guinea-fowl, roast	32.5	8.2	0.0	210
Ham, boiled, lean only	23.1	13.4	0.0	219
Ham, boiled, lean and fat	16.3	39.6	0.0	435
Ham or Pork, chopped	15.2	29.9	Tr.	340
Hare, roast	31.2	7.0	0.0	193
Hare, stewed	29.2	8.0	0.0	194
Heart, sheep, roast	25.0	14.7	0.0	239
Kidney, ox, raw	17.0	5.3	0.0	119
Kidney, sheep, fried	28.0	9.1	0.0	199
Liver, raw, mixed	16.5	8.1	0.0	143
Liver, calf, fried	29.0	14.5	2.4	262
Liver, ox, fried	29.5	15.9	4.0	284
Lamb chop, grilled, lean only	26.5	17.5	0.0	271

* Weights of food are measured after cooking. For this reason grilled meat comes out with more calories per 100g than fried meat. This is because in grilling, more moisture is lost than in frying and therefore more of the weight after cooking is accounted for by protein and fat.

DIET/SLIMMING

Description of food and method of cooking	Protein percentage	Fat percentage	Carbohydrate percentage	Calories per 100g (3.5oz approx.)
Lamb chop, grilled, lean and fat	19.9	45.0	0.0	500
Lamb chop, fried, lean only	22.8	25.2	5.7	341
Lamb chop, fried, lean and fat	15.4	60.1	2.6	629
Lamb leg, roast	25.0	20.4	0.0	292
Partridge, roast	35.2	7.2	0.0	211
Pheasant, roast	30.8	9.3	0.0	213
Pork, leg, roast	24.6	23.2	0.0	317
Pork chops, grilled, lean only	25.3	23.7	0.0	325
Pork chops, grilled, lean and fat	18.6	50.3	0.0	544
Rabbit, stewed	26.6	7.7	0.0	180
Sausage, beef, fried	13.8	18.4	15.7	287
Sausage, pork, fried	11.5	24.8	12.7	326
Sausage, black	5.3	22.5	14.7	286
Sweetbreads, stewed	22.7	9.1	0.0	178
Tongue, sheep's, stewed	18.0	24.0	0.0	297
Tripe, stewed	18.0	3.0	0.0	102
Turkey, roast	30.2	7.7	0.0	196
Veal, cutlet, fried	30.4	8.1	4.4	216
Veal, fillet, roast	30.5	11.5	0.0	232
Venison, roast	33.5	6.4	0.0	197

Fish

Description of food and method of cooking	Protein percentage	Fat percentage	Carbohydrate percentage	Calories per 100g (3.5oz approx.)
Bass, steamed	19.5	5.1	0.0	127
Bream, red, steamed	19.7	4.0	0.0	118
Cockles	11.0	0.3	Tr.	48
Cod, steamed	18.0	0.9	0.0	82
Cod, fried	20.7	4.7	2.9	140
Cod, grilled	27.0	5.3	0.0	160
Cod roe, fried	20.6	11.9	3.0	206
Crab, boiled	19.2	5.2	0.0	127
Fish paste	14.9	9.5	6.5	174
Haddock, fresh, steamed	22.0	0.8	0.0	97
Haddock, fresh, fried	20.4	8.3	3.6	175
Haddock, smoked, steamed	22.3	0.9	0.0	100
Halibut, steamed	22.7	4.0	0.0	130
Herring, fried	21.8	15.1	1.5	235
Kippers, baked	23.2	11.4	0.0	201
Lemon sole, steamed	19.9	0.9	0.0	90
Lemon sole, fried	15.4	13.0	9.3	219
Lobster, boiled	21.5	3.4	0.0	119
Mackerel, fried	20.0	11.3	0.0	187
Mullet, red, steamed	21.4	4.3	0.0	128
Mussels, boiled	16.8	2.0	Tr.	87
Oysters, raw	10.2	0.9	Tr.	50
Pilchards, canned (fish only)	21.9	10.8	0.0	191
Plaice, steamed	18.1	1.9	0.0	92
Plaice, fried	18.0	14.4	7.0	234
Prawns	21.2	1.8	0.0	104
Salmon, fresh, steamed	19.1	13.0	0.0	199
Salmon, canned	19.7	6.0	0.0	137
Sardines, canned	20.4	22.6	0.0	294
Scallops, steamed	22.4	1.4	Tr.	105
Shrimps	22.3	2.4	0.0	114
Skate, fried	15.0	16.4	7.5	242
Sole, steamed	17.6	1.3	0.0	84
Sole, fried	20.1	18.4	5.4	274
Sprats, fresh, fried	22.3	37.9	0.0	444
Sprats, smoked, grilled	25.1	23.2	0.0	319
Trout, steamed	22.3	4.5	0.0	133
Turbot, steamed	20.7	1.6	0.0	100
Whitebait, fried	18.3	47.5	5.3	537

Fruit

Description of food and method of cooking	Protein percentage	Fat percentage	Carbohydrate percentage	Calories per 100g (3.5oz approx.)
Apples, imported eating	0.3	Tr.	12.2	47
Apples, English eating	0.3	Tr.	11.7	45
Apples, cooking, baked	0.3	Tr.	10.0	39
Apricots, fresh	0.6	Tr.	6.7	28
Apricots, dried, raw	4.8	Tr.	43.4	183
Apricots, canned in syrup	0.5	Tr.	27.7	106
Avocado pears	1.1	8.0	2.5	88
Bananas	1.1	Tr.	19.2	77
Blackberries, raw	1.3	Tr.	6.4	30
Cherries, eating	0.6	Tr.	11.9	47
Cranberries	0.4	Tr.	3.5	15
Currants, red, stewed without sugar	0.8	Tr.	3.4	16
Damsons, raw	0.5	Tr.	9.6	38
Dates	2.0	Tr.	63.9	248
Figs, green	1.3	Tr.	9.5	41
Figs, dried, raw	3.6	Tr.	52.9	214
Fruit salad, canned in syrup	0.3	Tr.	25.0	94
Gooseberries, ripe	0.6	Tr.	9.2	37
Grapes, black	0.6	Tr.	15.5	60
Grapes, white	0.6	Tr.	16.1	63
Grapefruit	0.6	Tr.	5.3	22
Greengages	0.8	Tr.	11.8	48
Lemons, whole	0.8	Tr.	3.2	15
Loganberries	1.1	Tr.	3.4	17
Loganberries, canned	0.6	Tr.	26.2	101
Mandarins, canned	0.5	Tr.	16.6	64
Melons, Cantaloupe	1.0	Tr.	5.3	24
Melons, yellow	0.6	Tr.	5.0	21
Olives (in brine)	0.9	11.0	Tr.	106
Oranges	0.8	Tr.	8.5	35
Orange juice	0.6	Tr.	9.4	38
Peaches, fresh	0.6	Tr.	9.1	37
Peaches, canned in syrup	0.4	Tr.	22.9	87
Pears, English eating	0.2	Tr.	10.4	40
Pears, canned in syrup	0.4	Tr.	20.0	77
Pineapple, fresh	0.5	Tr.	11.6	46
Pineapple, canned in syrup	0.3	Tr.	20.2	77
Plums, Victoria dessert	0.6	Tr.	9.6	38
Plums, stewed without sugar (weighed with stones)	0.4	Tr.	4.8	20
Prunes, stewed without sugar (weighed with stones)	1.2	Tr.	20.2	81
Raisins, dried	1.1	Tr.	64.4	247
Raspberries, raw	0.9	Tr.	5.6	25
Rhubarb, stewed without sugar	0.4	Tr.	0.8	5
Strawberries	0.6	Tr.	6.2	26
Sultanas, dried	1.7	Tr.	64.7	249
Tangerines	0.9	Tr.	8.0	34

Source: *The Composition of Foods*, by R. A. McCance and E. M. Widdowson, (Medical Research Council/HMSO), reprinted by permission of the Controller of Her Majesty's Stationery Office.

Tr = only traces present.

SLIMMING/DIET

Description of food and method of cooking	Protein percentage	Fat percentage	Carbohydrate percentage	Calories per 100g (3.5oz approx.)
Nuts				
Almonds	20.5	53.5	4.3	598
Brazil nuts	13.8	61.5	4.1	644
Chestnuts	2.3	2.7	36.6	172
Cob nuts	9.0	36.0	6.8	398
Coconut, fresh	3.8	36.0	3.7	365
Peanuts	28.1	49.0	8.6	603
Walnuts	12.5	51.5	5.0	549
Vegetables				
Artichokes, globe, boiled	1.1	Tr.	2.7	15
Asparagus, boiled	3.4	Tr.	1.1	18
Beans, baked	6.0	0.4	17.3	93
Beans, broad, boiled	4.1	Tr.	7.1	43
Beans, French, boiled	0.8	Tr.	1.1	7
Beans, haricot, boiled	6.6	Tr.	16.6	89
Beans, runner, boiled	0.8	Tr.	0.9	7
Beetroot, boiled	1.8	Tr.	9.9	44
Broccoli tops, boiled	3.1	Tr.	0.4	14
Brussels sprouts, boiled	2.4	Tr.	1.7	16
Cabbage, red, raw	1.7	Tr.	3.5	20
Cabbage, spring, boiled	1.1	Tr.	0.8	8
Cabbage, winter, raw	2.2	Tr.	3.8	25
Carrots, old, raw	0.7	Tr.	5.4	23
Carrots, young, boiled	0.9	Tr.	4.5	21
Carrots, canned	0.7	Tr.	4.4	19
Cauliflower, boiled	1.5	Tr.	1.2	11
Celery, raw	0.9	Tr.	1.3	9
Chicory, raw	0.8	Tr.	1.5	9
Cucumber, raw	0.6	Tr.	1.8	9
Endive, raw	1.8	Tr.	1.0	11
Leeks, boiled	1.8	Tr.	4.6	25
Lentils, boiled	6.8	Tr.	18.3	96
Lettuce, raw	1.1	Tr.	1.8	11
Marrow, boiled	0.4	Tr.	1.4	7
Mushrooms, raw	1.8	Tr.	0.0	7
Mushrooms, fried	2.2	22.3	0.0	217
Onions, raw	0.9	Tr.	5.2	23
Onions, boiled	0.6	Tr.	2.7	13
Onions, fried	1.8	33.3	10.1	355
Parsley, raw	5.2	Tr.	Tr.	21
Parsnips, boiled	1.3	Tr.	13.5	56
Peas, fresh boiled	5.0	Tr.	7.7	49
Peas, canned	5.9	Tr.	16.5	86
Potatoes, old, boiled	1.4	Tr.	19.7	80
Potatoes, old, mashed	1.5	5.0	18.0	120
Potatoes, old, baked in skins	2.5	Tr.	25.0	104
Potatoes, old, roast	2.8	1.0	27.3	123
Potatoes, old, chip	3.8	9.0	37.3	239
Potatoes, new, boiled	1.6	Tr.	18.3	75
Potato Crisps	5.9	37.6	49.3	559
Spinach, boiled	5.1	Tr.	1.4	26
Spring greens, boiled	1.7	Tr.	0.9	10
Swedes, boiled	0.9	Tr.	3.8	18
Tomatoes, raw	0.9	Tr.	2.8	14
Tomatoes, fried	1.0	5.9	3.3	71
Turnips, boiled	0.7	Tr.	2.3	11
Watercress, raw	2.9	Tr.	0.7	15
Sugar, preserves and sweetmeats				
Boiled sweets	Tr.	Tr.	87.3	327
Chocolate, milk	8.7	37.6	54.5	588
Chocolate, plain	5.6	35.2	52.5	544
Honey, in jars	0.4	Tr.	76.4	288
Ice cream	4.1	11.3	19.8	196
Jam, fruit with edible seeds	0.6	0.0	69.0	261
Jelly, packet	6.1	0.0	62.5	259
Marmalade	0.1	0.0	69.5	261
Mincemeat	0.6	3.3	25.5	129
Peppermints	0.5	0.7	102.2	391
Sugar, Demerara	0.5	0.0	99.5	394
Sugar, white	Tr.	0.0	99.5	394
Syrup, golden	0.3	0.0	79.0	297
Toffees, mixed	2.1	17.2	71.1	435
Beverages				
Cocoa powder	20.4	25.6	35.0	452
Coffee, ground, roasted	12.5	15.4	28.5	301
Horlick's malted milk	14.4	8.0	70.8	399
Lemonade	Tr.	0.0	5.6	21
Lemon squash	0.1	Tr.	33.7	126
Lime juice cordial	0.1	0.0	29.8	112
Lucozade	0.0	0.0	17.9	67
Marmite	1.4	Tr.	0.0	6
Nescafé	11.9	0.0	11.0	90
Orange squash	0.3	Tr.	35.8	136
Ovaltine	13.2	6.3	72.3	384
Pineapple juice	0.4	0.1	13.4	53
Ribena	0.2	0.0	60.9	229
Tea, Indian	14.1	0.0	0.0	58
Alcoholic beverages				
Beers				
Brown ale, bottled	0.25	Tr.	2.95	28
Draught ale, bitter	0.25	Tr.	2.25	31
Pale ale, bottled	0.31	Tr.	1.99	32
Stout, bottled	0.31	Tr.	4.20	37
Ciders				
Cider, dry	Tr.	0.0	2.64	37
Cider, sweet	Tr.	0.0	4.28	42
Wines, Heavy				
Port, ruby	0.13	0.0	11.40	152
Sherry, dry	0.19	0.0	1.36	114
Sherry, sweet	0.31	0.0	6.88	135
Table Wines – white				
Champagne	0.25	0.0	1.40	74
Graves	0.13	0.0	3.37	73
Sauternes	0.19	0.0	5.89	93
Table Wines – red				
Australian Burgundy	0.25	0.0	0.42	72
Beaujolais	0.19	0.0	0.25	68
Chianti	0.13	0.0	0.19	65
Medoc	0.19	0.0	0.27	63
Spirits				
70% Proof	Tr.	0.0	Tr.	222

DIET/SLIMMING

THE CUT OUT METHOD OF SLIMMING

Not everybody likes to count calories when they are slimming because it involves quite a lot of accurate weighing and measuring, at least at the beginning. Some slimmers would rather sacrifice the flexibility that calorie-counting allows for the simplicity of a system where they divide various foods and drinks into certain categories, and have specific rules which tell them how to treat the items in these categories.

Most people who use this method of slimming cut out carbohydrates such as bread and potatoes. That is an effective method of slimming but is an unhealthy way to eat. Bread and potatoes are good sources of protein, nutrients and fibre as well as being a source of calories in the form of carbohydrate. The aim of a Cut Down diet should be to do without the empty calories in sugar and fats and high-calorie foods such as cakes and biscuits.

There are three categories in our Cut Out plan, and we have placed items of food and drink into these following the general principles for a healthy diet that we have already outlined in this chapter, i.e. a diet which is low in fat and cholesterol and sugar but which provides sufficient proteins, vitamins, minerals and roughage.

The first category is the one containing the unrestricted foods and drinks. All of them have a low fat and sugar content and contain relatively few calories.

The second category is called 'go carefully', because you must limit your overall intake of these foods as suggested. These foods and drinks are not alarmingly high in fat or sugar when eaten in reasonable quantities and they will ensure that you do not go without any important vitamins, minerals or roughage. If you eat high-fibre wholemeal bread and cereals you take in more bulk for the same number of calories and so should find your food more satisfying.

The foods and drinks in the third category are the ones you must *cut out* completely. They are the foods which are either very high in fat, or very high in sugar content, or sometimes high in both. Cutting out these items from your diet will do no harm whatsoever, in fact it should improve your health considerably.

It would be very surprising if this diet did not involve a considerable reduction in your calorie intake if you follow it carefully. You should lose weight at roughly one or two pounds a week (more in the first week), and your health will certainly benefit in many ways.

CUT OUT GUIDE

Unrestricted
Liver, kidney, heart, brain
Poultry (not duck), game
White fish and seafood
All green vegetables, such as lettuce, cabbage, celery
Root vegetables, such as carrots (but see below for potatoes)
All fresh fruit, except bananas and avocado pears
Cottage or curd cheese
Consommé, and low-calorie soups
Water, black tea and coffee, low-calorie drinks

Go carefully (No more than the indicated helping each day, and no more than four items from this category)

Milk	300 ml (½ pt)
Eggs	1
Soft margarine	25 g (1 oz)
Meat	100 g (4 oz)
Oily fish (e.g. herring, mackerel, sardines, tuna, salmon)	100 g (4 oz)
Cheese	100 g (4 oz)
Breakfast cereals (wholemeal)	100 g (4 oz)
Bread (wholemeal, if possible, if not brown)	2 slices (50 g, 2 oz)
Alcohol	1 normal measure of beer or wine
Soups	300 ml (½ pt)
Rice (brown if possible)	100 g (4 oz)
Spaghetti or pasta	100 g (4 oz)
Potatoes	100 g (4 oz)
Bananas	1 large
Avocado pear	half

Cut out completely
Cream
Butter, hard margarine, fats and oils
Cream-cheese
Patés and fatty meats, like salami
Sugar, sweets, chocolate
White bread (but not wholemeal or brown)
Corn Flakes, Rice Crispies and non-wholemeal cereals
Cakes, pies, pastry, biscuits, heavy puddings
Honey, syrup, treacle, jam, marmalade
Fruit tinned in syrup
Dried fruit
Crisps, savouries, nuts
Salad cream, mayonnaise
Rich creamy soups

EXERCISE AND SLIMMING

In the past, exercise has often been said to be rather a slow way of losing weight. This is because it has to be quite strenuous to burn up a lot of extra calories. As our illustration shows, it takes over two hours' walking to consume the amount of energy obtained from a 4 oz bar of milk chocolate. However, regular exercise causes an increase in the 'metabolic rate' of the body which continues after the exercise is completed. Taking an analogy with the steam engine: it is as if the furnace continues to burn fiercely for hours after a fast run.

In the past, the metabolic rate used to be thought constant over a period of time, if a constant amount of exercise were taken. Now, as noted in Chapter 2, there is some evidence that metabolic rate – like the thermostat on a furnace – can vary. It seems that when some people reduce their intake of food their metabolic rate also goes down, so that they rapidly reach a plateau where they no longer lose more weight – unless they exercise more and put up their metabolic rate. Weight-loss can stop at a particular point if there is a reduction in metabolic rate because the energy gap created by dieting may no longer exist.

Exercise is an important part of any weight-control programme because it can increase the metabolic rate – not

SLIMMING/DIET

Burning Up Calories

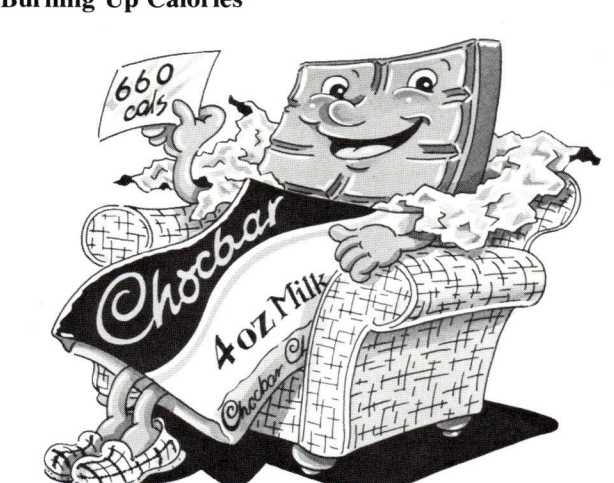

By eating a 4 oz (approx. 100 g) bar of milk chocolate about 660 calories are added to your daily total. If these are in excess of daily requirements, the length of time it takes to burn them off may make you think twice before indulging. If you don't burn off the calories they become body fat – 3 oz per chocolate bar. Exercise will burn off calories – but it takes longer than you think. To indulge in an extra bar of chocolate without gaining extra weight, one of the following activities should be performed for the time shown.

Activity	Duration
Walking at 4mph	2 hours 10 minutes
Cycling at 13mph	1 hour
Driving a car	4 hours
Digging the garden	1 hour 20 minutes
Swimming 20 yards a minute	50 minutes
Ironing clothes	2 hours 40 minutes

just during exercise but afterwards. Exercise thus counteracts the tendency of the body to reduce metabolic rate when food intake is reduced.

After strenuous exercise, such as football, the metabolic rate may be raised by 25 per cent for fifteen hours afterwards. During a half-hour game of squash, you may expend 450 calories. However, during the following two days you may burn up an extra 550 calories in addition as a result of the game – that is 1,000 calories from one game of squash. If you can undertake regular exercise every day or every other day, you can permanently increase your metabolic rate.

Exercise also builds up muscle and it is muscle which burns up energy, even at rest. So, apart from an immediate increase in metabolic rate – perhaps due to increased blood supply to muscles – exercise also causes a long-term increase in muscle mass, leading in turn to a further increase in metabolic rate. So build up the amount of exercise you take and you will have the satisfaction of knowing that you are also burning up more calories during rest and sleep.

When you lose weight from dieting, you may lose muscle tissue as well as fat if you do not exercise at the same time. If you do lose muscle tissue, then your metabolic rate will go down, and when you stop dieting – as most people do in the end – you will put on more weight than before because your muscles have wasted.

Furthermore, if you try to lose weight by dieting alone and take very little exercise it can be quite difficult to eat a proper balanced diet which gives you sufficient vitamins and nutrients. This may be all right in the short run, but it is always better to increase the amount of exercise you take and eat a more normal diet. If you can keep up the exercise, you should lose weight even if you do not reduce your food intake a great deal.

In the past, it was thought that exercise causes an increase in hunger. In fact, the opposite seems to be true. Signals from the body telling us when we are really hungry and when we are not seem to work better in active people. Farmers make use of this principle: when they want to fatten animals for market they keep them penned up. People are the same: when they are penned up, they eat more. Exercise also helps to get rid of the tension and anger which cause some people to overeat.

Whatever method of exercise you decide to use, remember that to be effective in weight reduction it must be:

1. *Reasonably vigorous*, so that it uses up more energy than just resting.
2. *Sensible for your age and ability*, so that you don't overdo things and injure yourself.
3. *Enjoyable*, so you don't resent doing it.
4. *Regular*, so that it makes a worthwhile contribution to your energy gap.

There are two main ways in which you can increase your energy output:
A. You can arrange to get more natural exercise, e.g. walking rather than driving, or climbing stairs rather than using the lift. Just half an hour a day of walking or climbing stairs will increase your energy output by about 900 calories in a week and this could get rid of 9 lb of fat in a year.
B. You can increase the amount of specific exercise that you do. This does not have to involve other people and organized sports. You can see from the chart that an hour's standard walking by yourself will do you as much good as an hour spent playing hockey or tennis. The chart gives you a rough idea of the energy values associated with different types of exercise. They cannot be more accurate because people vary in the amount of energy they use for the same task according to their sex, their size, their physical fitness and the effort they use. The values given are for an hour's activity in each case to make comparison easy, but this does not mean that you must do an hour of the activity – as little as half an hour's exercise is helpful if you do it regularly.

If you are healthy, you should aim to build up to an extra 500 or so calories of exercise per day. First work out how many calories of exercise you are getting already. You can do this by keeping a diary and working out the number of calories equivalent to your exercise from the table. Build up the amount of extra exercise you get slowly like this:

First week: 50 to 150 extra calories
Second week: 100 to 250 extra calories
Third week: 150 to 350 extra calories
Fourth week: 200 to 500 extra calories
Fifth week: 250 to 500 extra calories

Make sure you feel comfortable about the increase in exercise and that you enjoy it. You can get the extra exercise in various ways. For example half an hour of slow, easy walking would use up an extra 135 calories and in the first week that could be spread over several days. Within five weeks you should have built up to a minimum of at least one extra hour of slow walking per week. As you get more fit, you will probably find that you want to take up a sport of some kind, or perhaps dancing to use up more energy.

DIET/SLIMMING

HOW TO KEEP UP YOUR INTEREST IN EXERCISE

Chapter 2 details a number of different types of exercise that will make you fitter and leaner. The danger is that whichever type you choose, after a few days you will lose interest. To avoid this, make some careful plans.

Find a friend to do it with
It is more fun if you exercise with a friend. If your friend becomes inspired, his or her enthusiasm will carry you along when your interest may be declining temporarily.

Exercise naturally
Incorporate exercise into your life as a natural part of it. You may find it is just as quick to bicycle or jog to work as it is to wait for a bus or crawl in a car through traffic. Use stairs instead of waiting for lifts in the office. If your journey to work is a long one, try walking part of the way if possible.

Choose a convenient and enjoyable sport
Choose a sport which is easy to fit into your life because there are good facilities nearby and you enjoy it. For one person it might be ice skating, for another swimming, for another dancing.

Reward yourself
Try to make sure that your efforts to exercise are rewarded. Perhaps by going off with your sports club on an outing or to see an away game. Or, if you are walking to work, use the money you save to treat yourself to something that makes you feel good. Buy a miniature tape-recorder and headphones so that you can listen to your favourite music while walking.

NB: See Chapter 2 for more on exercise and why weight loss is only one of the joys of fitness.

NOTES ON SLIMMING

YOUR FIGURE

Women who lose weight successfully may still be dissatisfied because they do not lose it from the places that they want to lose it from. The bust becomes smaller but the hips seem to remain almost the same. This pear shape is perfectly normal, although unfashionable. Many methods of spot reduction are advertised which claim to remove fat from the hips – but there seems to be no real evidence that any of them work.

The various methods include: vibrator belts, massagers, slimming garments, and 'artificial exercisers' which use an electric current to cause muscles to contract. These various devices have been tested by *Which?* the Consumers' Association magazine; it found that none of them proved to be of the slightest use in reducing weight in particular places. Sweat garments may cause a small loss of weight. This is entirely due to loss of water which is rapidly replaced. Getting slim takes time and effort. There is no gadget which will do it for you.

Rather than waste money on gadgets, buy yourself a new brassière and a well-cut dress. This is more likely to achieve what you want. There are also some practical measures which can be taken to improve your figure. Look at Chapter 2 on exercise and undertake regular exercises which make use of the muscles of the lower abdomen.

SLIMMING CLUBS

There are a lot of different slimming clubs (see Appendix Three) which you can join. They charge a membership fee and a weekly sum. At the first meeting a new member is generally weighed and measured and given a target weight

HOW EXERCISE CAN HELP

Level*	Walking	Running	Sports & Games
Level A (about 175 cals per hr)	Ambling, strolling (1½–2½ mph)	—	archery, billiards, bowls (green), boule, cricket, croquet, golf, rifle-shooting, sailing, table tennis
Level B (about 270 cals per hr)	Slow, easy walking (2½–3½ mph)	—	badminton, bowling (ten-pin), canoeing, dancing, diving, gardening, rowing, softball/baseball, surfing
Level C (about 355 cals per hr)	Standard walking (3½–4 mph)	gentle jogging (3–5 mph)	basketball, bowling (cricket), cycling, digging, fencing, gymnastics, hockey, judo, karate, lacrosse, orienteering, rambling, skating, tennis, trampolining
Level D (about 435 cals per hr)	Brisk striding walk (4–5 mph)	Slow running (5–6 mph)	climbing, football, rugby, skiing
Level E (about 740 cals per hr)	Sprint walking (6–7 mph)	Standard running (7–8 mph)	competitive running, handball, squash, swimming, water polo

*NB: Remember that you would use up approximately 60 calories if you rest for an hour. All these figures include this value for resting metabolism. See also sports chart, page 63.

The human hump

It is not only the weight of the body that changes as we accumulate or lose fat. The shape of our body changes too — as the diagrams on the right illustrate. The numbers indicate the danger points where excess fat first reveals itself.

Accumulation of fat is the result of eating more food than the body needs for its daily expenditure of energy. Thus fat represents the body's main reserve of available energy. The body of a healthy 20-year-old man is about 20 per cent fat. This rises to 25 per cent by the time he is 50. The softer bodies of women contain a correspondingly greater proportion of fat. A 20-year-old girl's body is 25 per cent fat. This rises to 45 per cent by the time she is 50. Not only do women have a thicker layer of fat under the skin than men, it tends to be concentrated around certain areas, notably the breasts, buttocks and legs.

The body's fat pads are numbered on the pair of figures on the left. The 'middle-age spread' on the pair on the right results from an increase in the thickness of the fat layers in these pads.

This table gives, in millimetres, the desirable average thickness of fat for each pad.

Fat pad	Man	Woman
1 Shoulder	18	18
2 Outside arm	4	6
3 Inside arm	4	7
4 Hip	19	19
5 Top of thigh	16	28
6 Outside leg	5	7
7 Inside leg	6	11
8 Front of leg	3	4
9 Back of leg	7	13

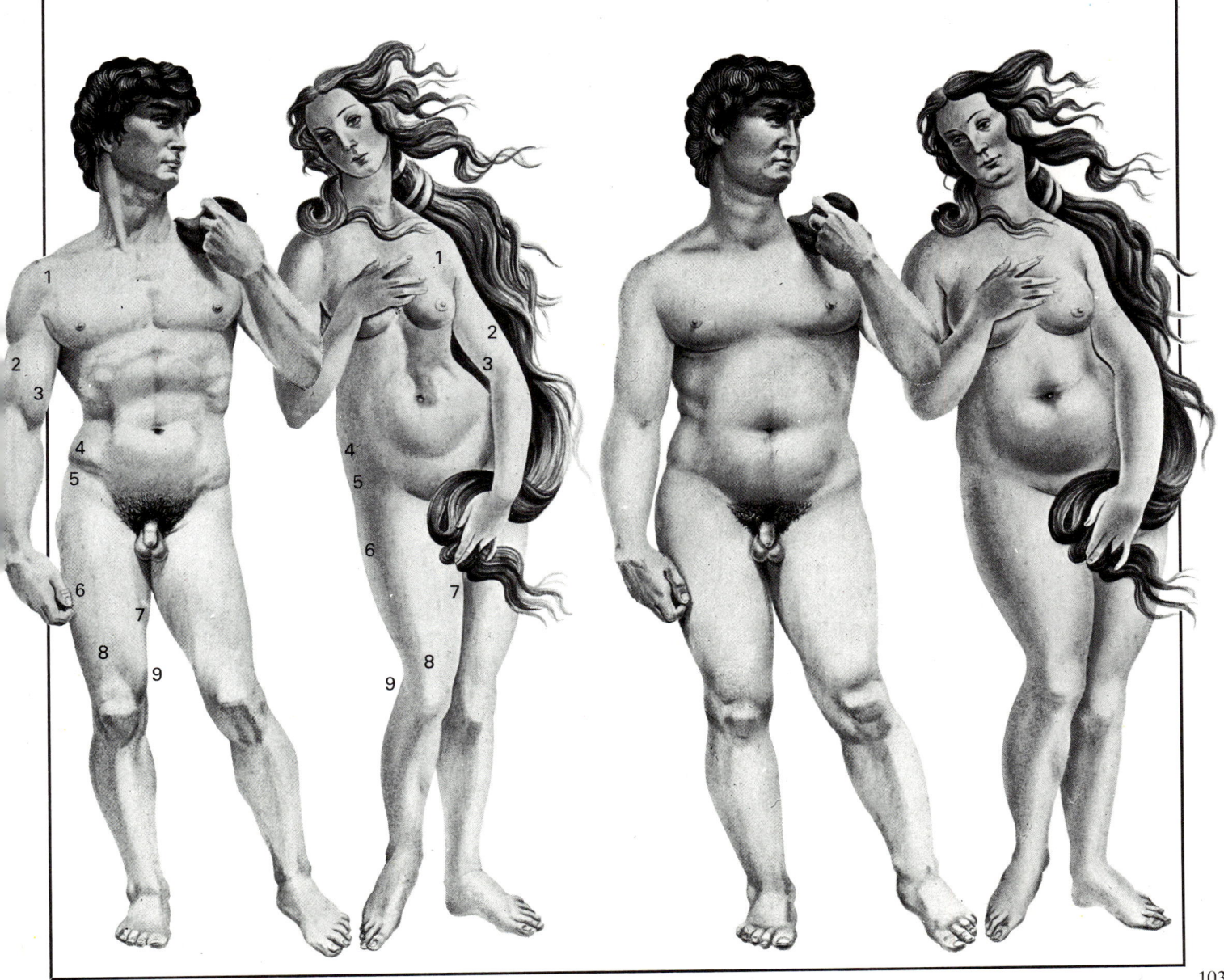

DIET/SLIMMING

to get down to. The next week your weight-loss will be read out with all the others. They do not however read out your actual weight. Then there is usually a discussion about some aspect of slimming led by a supervisor. Some clubs also have exercise sessions.

When you reach your target weight, you will be rewarded with a badge or coloured scarf. You are then encouraged to remain part of the group so that you can continue with controlled eating and do not immediately put on weight again. Joining a group is very helpful for some people because of the encouragement which may not be available at home. There is also the opportunity to discuss your problem with other people and get ideas about slimming meals. However, some people do not like them because they feel they are treated like children.

Why not start a group of your own with some friends? All you need is a weighing machine, a tape measure and a lot of enthusiasm. You can get everyone to contribute a little and have a low-calorie night out once a month.

AIDS TO HELP YOU DIET

Appetite-reducing drugs. Those you can buy without a prescription from a chemist are useless; those you get on prescription – fenfluramine (Ponderax), phentermine (Duromine and Ionamin), diethyl propion (Tenuate, Dospan, Apisate), and mazindol (Teronac) – can be quite helpful to some people in the short term, but others find that their side-effects reduce their use. The side-effects vary from sleepiness to tenseness. It depends on the drug and it depends on the individual; but the side-effects are quite minor compared to those of the now-banned amphetamines. Doctors vary in their readiness to prescribe appetite-reducing drugs. Drugs will only work if you diet at the same time. So you might just as well get on with the diet.

Substitute meals: You can buy these in biscuit form (e.g. Bisks, Limmitts), drink form (e.g. Slender) or complete meal form (e.g. Contour, Kousa, Heinz). The principle of them all is that they tell you exactly how many calories are in the product, and you count this in your calorie-controlled diet. They can be quite useful to some people, especially those who want a quick snack which does not involve too much cooking. However, there are plenty of other snacks that can be made or bought for the average 300 calories in these products, and you will find that you pay quite a lot extra for the convenience of having a calorie-counted product. Remember that they are meal *substitutes* and not meal *supplements*.

Sweeteners and low-calorie alternatives: The general principle behind these products is that a low-calorie substance is substituted for a high-calorie one. In general, saccharin substitutes for sugar, water substitutes for fat, and air substitutes for starch.

There is now a wide range of drinks (mixers, squashes, colas) sweetened with saccharin instead of sugar and reducing the calorie content to virtually zero. If you like your tea or coffee sweetened, you can get sweeteners in pellet, powder or granular form. The pellets are calorie-free but the powder and granular sweeteners contain sugar and saccharin so that they are not completely calorie-free (usually one-quarter of the normal value). Eating sweet things is an acquired habit, and it is possible to change your tastes slowly and learn to take your food and drink less sweet. This is a better strategy than using sweeteners because saccharin is under suspicion of being a cause of cancer, albeit a weak one, and cyclamates have other unwanted side-effects.

In low-fat spread (e.g. Outline), low-calorie sauces (Waistline, Heinz low-calorie salad-dressing) and low-calorie soups (Heinz, Boots), some of the fat-content of the parent product has been replaced by water, thus reducing the total calorie content of the product by about half.

Slimmers' breads and rolls (e.g. Procea, Slimcea, Nimble) contain the same number of calories on a weight basis as ordinary bread. However, they are lighter (i.e. contain more air) and so an average slice of slimmers' bread contains about half the calories.

The products in the last two categories will appeal to you if you eat bread, butter, etc. by volume. They enable you to eat your normal volume of food for half the calories. Of course, these special low-calorie alternatives might cost you more and you might not like them as much as the real thing. But if you do not have the will-power to cut your volume by half, then you will find them useful. We do not recommend them because you will find if you use them that you eat the same amount of butter or margarine but less bread. This simply increases the amount of unhealthy fat in the diet and does not save a lot of calories.

DIET MYTHS

The information and instructions we give you in this chapter should be all you need to lose weight successfully and keep it off. But you are bound to come across other diets in newspapers and magazines or be told about them by your well-meaning friends. Beware of these myths.

Diets which restrict low-calorie fluids: There are no calories in water and virtually none in artificially sweetened drinks, black tea and coffee. Provided you have normally functioning kidneys, your body will get rid of all the surplus fluid, so you can drink as much of these as you like. Severe fluid restriction could lead to chronic dehydration with some serious consequences.

Diets which tell you to overdrink: It is true that one of the reasons for an adequate water intake is to help remove waste products from the body. But it is *not* true that drinking a lot of water will actively cause breakdown of fat and speed its removal from the body. And drinking water before or after meals will make no difference to the calories you absorb from the meal.

Grapefruit and lemon diets: Grapefruit and lemon are low-calorie fruits and are therefore useful for slimmers. But there is no scientific evidence to suggest that they can speed up the conversion of fat to energy.

Diets where you can eat as much as you like: Some low-carbohydrate diets are worded very badly and give the impression that any food containing carbohydrate can be eaten *ad lib* without making you fat. See page 100 for the Cut Out plan, which is a low-fat, low-carbohydrate plan that *will* work.

Diets which claim that eating fat burns up fat: The only way in which fat is burnt up is when your diet creates a calorie deficit and body-fat is needed as a fuel. Dietary fat has no magical, direct effect on body-fat. If you eat more fat, you will get fatter unless you eat a lot less of other things.

THE COMMON EXCUSES FOR FATNESS: HOW MUCH WEIGHT DO THEY CARRY?

Glands, metabolism and inheritance

Some of the common excuses made by a fat person run along the lines of 'it's my glands', 'it's my metabolism' or 'it runs in my family'. These excuses can all be considered together because they might all contribute partly to the fatness in some people (but not necessarily those who use them as an excuse).

Obesity due solely to the malfunctioning of one particular endocrine gland is very rare, probably accounting for only one in ten thousand cases. It has been said that the only glands which are not working properly in a fat person are the salivary glands, which work too well! This is probably a little unfair because some studies of overall eating patterns have shown that fat people eat no more than thin people.

'Metabolism' is a very general term to describe the way in which food is turned into energy by the body, and studies of metabolic rate have indeed revealed vast differences between individuals, so that the amount of food they can eat without getting fat will also vary greatly. It has also been shown that individuals vary in their response to overeating. Some (the 'easy-gainers') will gain the theoretically calculated amount of weight when they are overfed while others (the 'hard-gainers') will gain less than predicted. Exactly why this happens is not known yet.

The fact that obesity runs in families is a well-documented one. However, it is so difficult to separate nature from nurture that it is difficult to say how valid an excuse it is. The studies of twins and adopted children which are usually undertaken to resolve this nature–nurture conflict give confusing results, although there is a definite indication that some genetic factor plays a part.

In summary, it seems that some people do have a genetically inherited tendency to fatness which manifests itself in metabolic changes. However, there is nothing to stop those with a tendency to fatness overcoming it, even though the task for them might be harder than it is for others.

Childhood obesity

Recently, scientists have been particularly interested in classifying fat people according to the age of onset of their obesity. This followed some reports in the early 1970s that the child-onset obese had more fat-cells than the adult-onset obese, and it was inferred by others that the child-onset obese would have greater problems with slimming as adults. The publicity given to this theory, while being useful in the prevention of infantile and childhood obesity, has been harmful in another way: being fat as a child has become quite a common excuse for adults who cannot lose weight easily. There is no truth in this excuse because (a) it has never been shown that the child-onset obese cannot lose weight and (b) further research has cast doubts on the original fat-cell theory.

Puppy fat

The term 'puppy fat' is used by some teenagers and their parents to describe increased fatness during adolescent years. It is true that the changes in sex hormones during these years will lead to an increase in body-fat in girls in particular, but any overeating during this time will lead to surplus body-fat and this cannot be blamed on the hormones.

Getting fat on the pill

Some women complain that they managed to maintain a reasonable weight until they went on the pill. Unfortunately, there is no large-scale survey which can validate this claim: usually, average weight-changes on different pills are given as zero because an equal number of women lose weight on the pill as those that gain it. However, it is known that certain pills cause some fluid retention in some women and this could cause a weight-gain of up to 7 lb (3 kg). If a weight-gain on the pill is due to fluid retention it will be fairly obvious as soon as the pill is withdrawn because the weight will drop very quickly. A change to a pill with a different hormonal composition will often be the solution to the problem.

Getting fat during pregnancy

A lot of women will say that having children was their downfall as far as their weight was concerned. Here again, it is impossible to separate the physiological factors associated with pregnancy with the changes in lifestyle that usually accompany pregnancy and the subsequent caring for children. A sensible weight-gain during pregnancy is between 22 and 28 lb (9.5 and 12.5 kg). A weight-gain above the maximum limit will almost certainly mean that the mother has added too much to her own fat-stores. Although it has never been shown that extra fat gained during pregnancy is different from normal fat, or that the mother's metabolism alters appreciably, some women find that they never lose this extra fat. Mothers who have a second child soon after the first might find it particularly difficult to lose the fat without a positive effort, because they lose track of what it was like to have a normal figure (see Chapter 1 for advice on diet during pregnancy).

Giving up smoking

It is true that a lot of people do put on weight when they stop smoking. A recent American survey showed that men who had given up smoking during a certain five-year period had gained much more weight on average than men who continued to smoke. However, this only shows an average trend and does not indicate that a weight-gain is a biological certainty. There is no evidence that smoking alters your metabolism by an appreciable amount, and those who do gain weight are often very willing to admit that they do eat more when they stop smoking, probably because they feel the need to have something in their mouth all the time. If this is your problem, try chewing low-calorie gum. It is generally agreed that smoking is a greater health risk than obesity, so it is worth making the effort to give up smoking.

Middle-aged spread

The average weight of both men and women increases with age although there is no physiological reason why it should do so. More often than not, surplus fat accumulates gradually with age because of a gradual decline in physical activity coupled perhaps with an increase in food and drink consumption. Small changes in your lifestyle, such as taking the lift instead of walking up the stairs each time, can make quite a difference in the long term.

5: MAINTAINING THE BODYWORK

The Back

The twenty-four separate vertebrae of the spine are probably the most troublesome bones in the body. In Britain alone, over a million and a half people go to their doctors with back pain every year. One result is that Britain loses thirteen million working days a year; by comparison, in 1981 industrial disputes cost four million days. Yet much back pain is avoidable.

It used to be believed that back pain was a consequence of our upright posture. Apart from being unhelpful – we cannot really spend our lives on all-fours – this belief is probably also untrue. We and our ancestors have been shuffling around on two feet for some millions of years, which should be long enough to have got used to the position.

The truth is that nobody knows for certain why backache is increasingly common. It could, like some headaches, be a sign of a more stressful world. It could be that, as part of the harder lives our parents and grandparents lived, backaches were accepted almost unnoticed.

But, if we do not know why complaints about back pain are more common, we do know a lot about the causes of back pain, and this can help us to avoid much of it.

BACK STRAINS

These are the most common source of back pain. Fortunately, they are also the least serious, because if reasonable care is taken they usually cure themselves.

We frequently risk these temporary injuries, since whenever we lift a heavy weight or move awkwardly – let alone when we do both together – we subject the muscles of our back to enormous stresses. Some of the bundles of fibres that make up muscles may become fatigued: ligaments and tendons may become torn. (Ligaments join bones or cartilages; tendons join muscles to bones or other muscles.)

Disabling muscle pain can be caused by lifting weights awkwardly or by twisting or bending the joints of the spine beyond their normal range. In general, the pain is felt immediately and is sufficient to stop the activity that is causing the damage. Usually, too, the damage will repair itself, given time. But complete rest is not the answer. Muscles benefit by movement, and they need a circulation of blood. The process of self-repair will therefore be helped by gentle exercise such as walking or swimming, and by mild bending and stretching. The pain itself can be relieved by keeping the muscles warm. This is why infra-red lamps are recommended for muscle strains, although hot baths and hot-water bottles are cheaper alternatives.

If the pain does not start to get better after a few days, it is usually sensible to see your doctor, in case the cause is something other than a simple strain.

DISC TROUBLE

Disc trouble is much rarer than muscular pains, and it is slower to mend. The discs are the shock-absorbers of the spinal system. The 'back' itself, including the neck, is basically twenty-four moveable vertebrae that together form the spine. They link to form an S-shaped curve. Each vertebra is linked to its neighbours by bony projections above and below. The rounded part of each vertebra is separated from its neighbour by a tough shock-absorber generally known as a disc, and more properly called an intervertebral disc.

The disc is a fairly rigid ring surrounding a pulpy centre. These discs operate healthily if the vertebrae they cushion remain in the proper alignment. If they are continually misaligned, and especially if they are heavily loaded while misaligned, the disc may slide, slip, or even burst. If the disc slips or bursts backwards it may cause pain, because it can then press on one of the nerves leading to the spinal cord. The spinal cord is the column of nerves that is an extension of the lower part of the brain, and it runs in a protective sheath down the spinal canal, passing through an approximately circular hole in the vertebrae and behind the discs. The roots of the nerves of the spinal column pass in and out of it, and carry nerve messages. As they pass between the bones of the spine, they are at risk of pressure from a displaced or burst disc, and the pressure may be sufficient to produce pain. Usually, the pain is felt in the part of the back where the disc has been disturbed; very occasionally, our idiosyncratic nervous system reports the pain as coming from an area of the skin to which the nerves of the spinal cord go.

POSTURE

The human body is self-repairing and to a certain extent muscles become stronger if they are frequently loaded. In the case of an arm or a leg, repeated movement against a resistance develops strength – and also the muscles sought by the 'body-builder'. But the muscles of the back show this strengthening less markedly. Repeated abuse or the cumulative effect of relatively small stresses may cause painful muscle strain.

Posture is generally important, as explained on page 110, but it is particularly important for the back. If we habitually sit in motor cars so as to put our back into a stressed position, or ride where there is a series of unpredictable

THE BACK/MAINTAINING THE BODYWORK

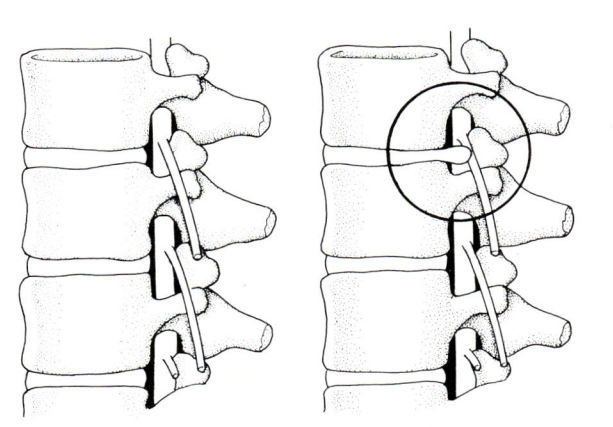

Between the bones of the spine are the cartilage discs. If a disc's outside cartilage ring weakens, its fluid centre bulges out, pressing against one of the spinal nerves.

shocks – over rough ground, for example – the stressed part of the spine may yield to the repeated onslaught, and the disc may move.

An activity as simple as washing up or typing can produce incapacitating back pain if it involves prolonged stooping: it need not involve 'heavy' work. Even walking, especially when carrying an awkwardly balanced load such as a suitcase, can strain the back. And because carrying an 'internal load' can be as harmful as carrying an external one, overweight people are much more vulnerable to back problems than those of normal weight.

BACK PAIN AND AGE

As we get older, our joints are increasingly likely to become inflamed and painful. About half the people over sixty suffer from this problem, known as osteo-arthrosis or osteo-arthritis, from time to time. It hits the joints of the neck and the small of the back as well as such joints as the hip and knee, which are discussed in more detail elsewhere.

Arthritis is not the only medical term associated with back pain in the later years. The word *rheumatism* is sometimes used by doctors as a label for virtually any kind of pain that involves muscles, ligaments, bones or joints. Rheumatism is not the name of a disease, only shorthand for a number of afflictions that can often be more precisely described. Lumbago, again, is not the name of a disease: it means simply 'pain in the lower part of the back – the lumbar region'.

As rheumatism and lumbago are not the precise names of diseases – the terms are clinically vague, in fact – there are no 'cures' for rheumatism or lumbago as such; the remedies depend on the precise nature of the problem. It is worth while consulting your doctor before spending money on drugs, lotions or equipment advertised as rheumatism or lumbago treatments.

Sciatica is the name given to pain felt in areas of the buttock, back of the thigh, and in the leg, ankle and toes, all of which are supplied by the sciatic nerve, which runs down the back of the leg. Like lumbago and rheumatism, sciatica is the name of a symptom. The pain may be caused by disc trouble in the lower back – the sciatic nerve is formed by the joining of a number of nerves from the spine – or by joint disease affecting the lower spine.

BACK PAIN IN WOMEN

The muscle strain that produces backaches makes no distinction between the sexes: men and women are equally vulnerable. However, there are a few causes of backache that are peculiar to women. The slackening of the joints of the pelvis that is associated with pregnancy can lead to pain in the back. Furthermore, the nerves from the lower end of the spinal cord feed into the womb, so period pain often includes backache. Some specifically female disorders, such as a prolapse of the womb or an infection in the tubes, may also produce pain in the back. Consult a doctor if you have any acute sudden pain in the back. But as a general rule, if it is back *movement* that elicits the pain in that region, then it is specifically the muscles or joints of the back that are the cause, rather than problems affecting other internal organs.

AVOIDANCE AND TREATMENT OF BACK PAIN

Back pain is debilitating, it can keep you from work and spoil your pleasure, but it is not normally serious, in the sense that people do not, in general, die from it. Usually it goes away on its own; sometimes, recovery can be helped by medical treatment. But it is always unpleasant: that is the natural function of pain, as otherwise you would ignore it. And there is always the risk that the damage may not cure itself completely, and that there will be a weakness in the back that is particularly vulnerable to a repetition of the damage.

There is, too, always a risk of injuring the back by subjecting it to unexpected stresses. A sudden awkward and energetic movement can present a hazard. Swinging a suitcase onto a luggage rack, or pulling one from the boot of a car, for instance, can strain muscles or suddenly load particular vertebrae so that the disc between them is damaged. Unfortunately, we cannot always avoid the risks. There are, though, ways of reducing the general vulnerability of the back.

The experimental evidence is slight – it is a difficult experiment to set up – but most people agree that, if you have a back that gives you trouble, it will give you more trouble if you are overweight. Carrying a couple of extra stone around is a steady minor abuse of the back which can eventually lead to disabling back pain.

Secondly, gentle exercise is as good for back problems as it is for many other afflictions. A supple, mobile back is less likely to give trouble than one that is stiff and unused to movement, and if you exercise your back there is a good chance that you won't damage it by the way you type or wash up or drive. Walking, swimming, cycling and yoga are all good exercises. If you are taking up exercises as prevention, you should start gently, of course, otherwise your attempts at prevention could themselves cause trouble. Take your exercise daily rather than in bursts on a Saturday.

In any case, you should aim towards a good posture, whether you are standing or sitting, walking or working. The ways to develop a good posture are explained below.

You should also learn techniques for everyday activities that will reduce the risk of back damage. Some backs are

MAINTAINING THE BODYWORK/THE BACK

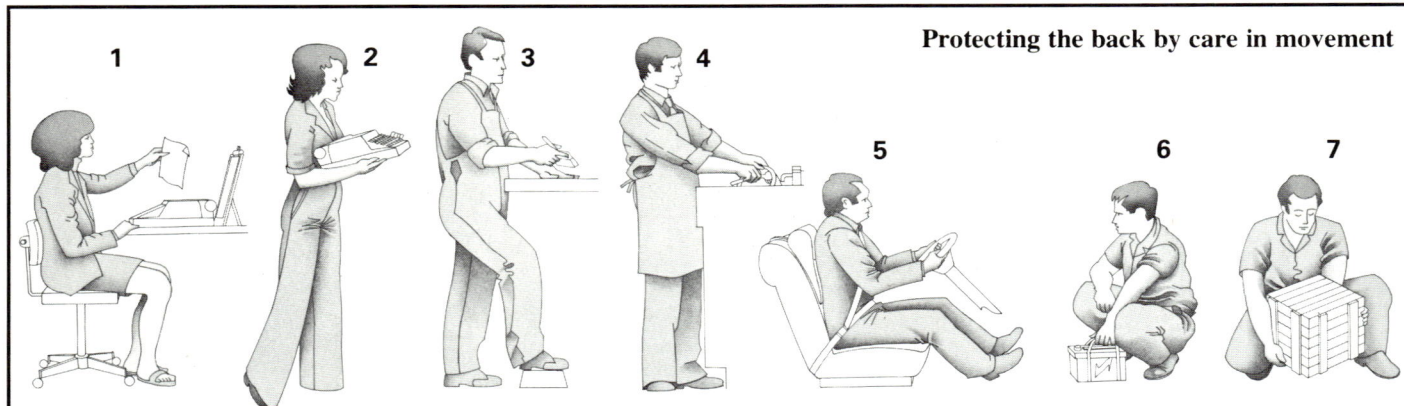

Protecting the back by care in movement

Everyday activities, at work, at home, or when driving a car, for example, can put stresses on the back that may lead to strains. Moving properly keeps the risk to a minimum.

weaker than others, and therefore more vulnerable. But everyone can lessen the likelihood of back pain by following the few simple rules illustrated by the drawings above. From left to right:

1. Many workers sit down at their work. They, or their bosses, should choose the chairs they sit in so as to reduce the risk of back pain. The chair shown here supports the lumbar – lower – spine well. This is important, because this is where pain is most common. Ideally, the back of the chair should be adjustable for people of different height. The seat of the chair illustrated is less satisfactory. It should be deep enough, front to back, to support the thighs, and the front should not dig into the thighs. The seat should, as shown, have a slight slope backwards, and the height should be such that the feet can rest comfortably on the ground, with the user's knees bent to no more than ninety degrees. The height of the seat, therefore, must be adjustable. Furthermore, the design of the seat must suit the line of vision and the actual activities of the person who uses it.

The chair shown is fairly typical of those provided for typists. Office workers who have to use uncomfortable chairs should try to improve them – with a cushion, for instance – to support the lumbar spine. Another worthwhile, though less easy, modification is for shorthand- or copy-typists to clip their notebooks or copy directly in front of them. The traditional method, which involves continuously looking at copy fixed to the side, keeps the spine twisted. If you can avoid this, even if only by changing the work from one side to the other, the stress on the back and neck is reduced.

2. *Lifting weights:* If you think of the spine as a curved, flexible rod that must be kept in shape by its muscles, you can understand the rules for weight-handling. When carrying even a rather commonplace weight, such as a typewriter, keep the weight in front of you, so that you do not bend the spine sideways. Moreover, you should keep the weight as near to you as possible. In this particular example, it is worth remembering that the keyboard is the lighter part of the machine: carry a typewriter keyboard-forwards.

3 and 4. When working at benches or sinks, as in these two drawings, the danger is one of frequent small abuses. You should not stoop over a sink; if you can, make sure that the sink is high enough and that you can get your feet underneath it. Most of us, unfortunately, cannot rebuild either

our sinks or our work-benches. We must therefore compensate for bad design by extra care. There are a few simple modifications that can help. We can, of course, reduce the stress on our backs simply by leaning on the sink with thighs or stomach, wearing some protection against the wet. Quite often, the working height of a sink can be raised by standing a plastic washing-up bowl on a block of wood inside the sink. Equally, a block of wood (figure 3) at the side of a work-bench will help to reduce back pain. It enables you to take the weight off one foot at a time and so vary your posture, rather than having to bend over your work.

5. Many people get backache while driving a car. This is not surprising; we are ill-designed for the positions that car-driving puts us into. There are a few people whose back is so sensitive to stress that they shouldn't really drive a car at all. Most people cannot avoid driving at some time or another, but they *can* minimize the risks to their back. The aim is to keep the back upright and supported, and the legs extended with support along the thighs. Ideally, the seat should be as high as it can be without getting riskily near to the roof; low seats mean that the hips and the lumbar spine must be unduly bent. The seat can often be raised on wooden blocks; an easy modification – a firm cushion on the seat – can give the same effect. You cannot usually do much about changing the amount of leg support your car seat gives, but carefully arranged cushions can improve the backs of most car seats. The seat backs should come up to the top of your head, but many car seats still do not. Head support can be added, but add one that reaches only to the base of your head, and which therefore supports the spine but not the head itself.

6 and 7. When heavier weights have to be moved, use your head to save your spine. Older people, and those who are unfit, should try to avoid lifting heavy weights if at all possible. If you are unused to the task, it is quite easy to damage the back by awkwardly lifting a weight of as little as twenty pounds. People who are travelling, for example, should think about the weight of their baggage when they are packing, rather than travelling in the hope that there will always be some strong-backed assistant at every stopping-place.

8. Babies and small toddlers can often produce back pain in their parents. Many women go through pregnancy being careful not to strain their backs, only to forget these

THE BACK/MAINTAINING THE BODYWORK

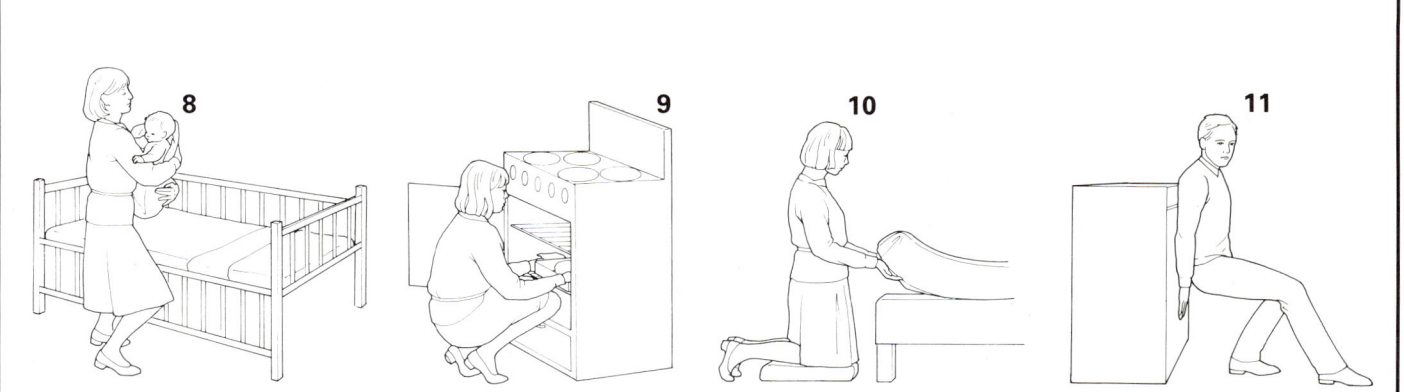

People tend to think that back pain comes from heavy work or unusual loads. But even the ordinary movements of housework can produce back pain.

precautions when they take the new baby home. Lift the baby from its cot as you would lift any heavy weight. Bend your knees, rather than stoop. Hold the child's weight close to the body. A cot with a side that drops down will make lifting up the child easier.

Baby carriers like rucksacks are usually safe, since they hold the weight close to the body either in the front or at the back. But you may need help in lifting the child up originally. Try to avoid rough-and-tumble games with toddlers, or games which involve swinging the child off the ground. Trying to lift up a rebellious toddler is also dangerous for the back.

9 and 10. Housework presents problems for the back sufferer. In general, it is best to change jobs frequently, spending less than half an hour on each job. If possible, fit your kitchen with a high oven so that you do not have to stoop to take out the Sunday roast. If the oven is low, then remember to bend your knees. Bedmaking is another trap for the unwary. Do not stoop over the bed. Kneel on the floor to tuck in the sheets. Duvets, instead of sheets and blankets, cut out bedmaking. Make sure your partner helps when you turn the mattress. Kneel to clean the bath rather than stoop to it. When vacuuming, brushing, mopping or sweeping, put your whole body into the movement. Standing still and just using your arms risks back strain.

The garden is the other place where back pain often strikes. It always pays back-pain sufferers to think out a job, before starting work. The gardener who walks round and stoops suddenly to pull a weed, may pull his back instead. Weeding is best done kneeling upon a rubber pad. 'When digging, concentrate on keeping the back straight. Plan a system of digging that avoids heavy wet sods being lifted and placed to one side so that you have to bend and turn your back,' advises Anthony Reed, training officer for the Back Pain Association. 'Do not take off that jacket or sweater, as cooling the body quickly when moving the spine multiplies the stress on it.' In general, vary work in the garden, rather than doing just one job all the time. Take regular breaks to rest. The temptation is always to do too much at once, in order to catch up with gardening jobs. Those with vulnerable backs cannot afford to make this mistake. Be careful about overloading the wheelbarrow. Make two journeys with small loads, rather than one overloaded. Be careful mowing the lawn. Wear strong shoes with a good grip and push the machine with the whole body, rather than just the arms. A smaller machine may mean more mowing, but a heavy machine is more likely to put a strain on the back.

11. Moving furniture can be difficult for back-pain sufferers. Rather than pushing with the arms, it may be best literally to put your back into it, leaning against the object with the back and using your body-weight to shift it.

When moving furniture such as wardrobes or cupboards, try to avoid lifting. See if they can be rocked and turned and inched around. If you do have to lift, keep the load on the spine in the direction it is 'built for': vertical, or as near so as possible. Don't stoop, but bend the knees, keep the spine straight. Lift, if you can, between the bent knees, so that the load is as near the body as possible, and lift by straightening the legs, where you have powerful and resilient muscles. In lifting, as with other tasks, the damage can come from one heavy load or a succession of small ones. In lifting a case from the boot of a car, you can use one hand to lift and the other to press against the car's body to relieve the strain on the back.

Pushing a car puts a heavy stress on the back, but two researchers at the University of Surrey have found that pulling involves very much less. The stress on the back can be derived from a measurement of the pressure inside the stomach, because it turns out that the stomach muscles, in men at least, play an important part in straightening the back. They compress the fluid contents of the stomach and thus assist the back muscles. You can measure the effort of the stomach muscles by using a radio pill that is swallowed, and the results make it quite clear how preferable pulling is. It is, of course, difficult to arrange to pull a car, but the muscles of the back are, fortunately, concerned only with the direction of the effort, not in the actual way the effort is exerted. Leaning with your back against a car and pushing it counts as pulling to the muscles, and minimizes the risk to the back.

BACK PAIN AND BEDS

We spend a third of our lives in bed, generally asleep, so it is important to make sure that the bed is beneficial to the back. So-called 'orthopaedic' beds are available, but these are not essential.

If you wish to buy an 'orthopaedic' mattress, be wary of advertisements, and high-pressure salesmen. Most well-known bedding manufacturers sell firm mattresses. All you need to do is go to a reputable store, ask about these and try them out there and then. Very highly priced, specially made mattresses are not usually necessary and may well be a waste of money.

All you need is a bed that supports the body. The base must be firm, since a sagging bed allows the spine to curve to an undesirable extent, but it should not be hard. *Any* bed can be prevented from sagging by placing two or three nine-inch planks across it under that part of the mattress which supports the trunk. The boards should be about a foot shorter than the width of the bed. Other ways to achieve the same desirable effect are to use a thick foam-rubber mattress on a hard base or a thinner one on a stiff-spring base. Any bed, in fact, which has a firm base and a mattress resilient enough to follow the contours of the body without letting it sag will help avoid back pain. In emergencies you can always put your mattress on the floor and sleep there: this gives all the firm unsagging support you need. Pillows are less important than the bed itself, but they are worth some thought. If there are too many pillows, they tend to get into odd places under the shoulders. They should also be soft rather than hard for comfort, while small pillows can be used to support the knees and the lower back when you lie down.

WHEN BACK PAIN STRIKES

Despite precautions, you may still be laid low with back pain. Always see your doctor before contemplating any of the many 'cures' which, considering the affliction is so widespread, have not surprisingly been proposed for back troubles. And, as the human system varies widely, so most of them have worked on someone. Acupuncture, which involves the use of needles on 'sensitive' points of the body, has worked; plaster supports have worked; osteopaths, who manipulate joints, have succeeded; and some sufferers have been helped by changes in diet. If we accept that back pain can also result from psychological tension, then some people will cure their pain by learning to cope more successfully with stress.

But none of these should be the first remedy you try. Sufferers should always first see their doctor. He or she should know you and the kind of life you lead, and can at least tell you how to avoid making the problem worse. In fact, if the pain is severe, get your doctor to come to see you. Keep warm, stay in bed on a firm mattress – get someone to slide some boards underneath if it is soft – and wait for the visit. The doctor may recommend drugs: analgesics or pain-killers help some people to sleep or exercise when they have a strained back; or the doctor's advice may be massage, manipulation, some form of physical support, or a mixture of all these different approaches.

Muscle or ligament strain is the most common diagnosis, usually because nothing else can be found wrong. There are then several possible approaches to treatment, all of which are worth trying although there is no agreed order of priority. The general rule is that rest is the first treatment to be tried. Young people are generally advised to strengthen muscles and restore the full range of movement, though some preliminary treatment including rest will almost certainly be needed. Physiotherapy, heat treatment and massage may also help. If the pain still persists after several weeks, perhaps a surgical corset may be recommended – especially for older people. If there is local tenderness, then injections of hydrocortisone and local anaesthetic may be advised. In other cases manipulation by an osteopath may bring relief, but always ask your doctor about this first. Time cures most backaches but sometimes nothing seems to work and the sufferer has to live with it. An operation is not advisable unless a doctor has found something positive in their investigations. Once you are 'cured', always remember that you are probably more vulnerable than before. You are also likely to know at least one activity which is risky – the one that set off the attack – and therefore to be avoided if at all possible.

POSTURE FOR HEALTH

Good posture is an important part of good health. It is something that we can all improve for ourselves without any special equipment or drugs. Improving your posture is more than a step to improving your health; it will also improve your personal appearance. Some people think of posture as simply the body's position when standing to attention. Posture is not just this. It is the attitude of the body, whether it is lying down, walking, sitting or moving in any way. A good posture is one that gives the highest efficiency for each individual with the lowest amount of muscular effort. As individuals vary, so will posture. One can therefore describe a good posture only in general terms.

A good posture is one which gives the body easy balance and poise; is aesthetically pleasing; enables the muscles to work to the best advantage and in harmony with each other; and provides the internal organs with room in which to work.

A bad posture is one where the balance of the body is maintained by muscles ill prepared for the task. The result not only looks unpleasant: the muscles have to work more than necessary; and the internal organs are cramped.

You can feel the difference between a good and a bad posture by trying to stand in the right way. The body's weight should be distributed so that the line of gravity falls just behind the ear, through the cervical vertebrae, through the shoulder and in front of the thoracic vertebrae, through the lumbar vertebrae and the hip-joint, and just in front of the knee to about 1½ inches (4 cm) in front of the ankle-joint. To get this ideal posture, every part of the body has to be placed gently in the right position. The head should be centrally placed, neither leaning on one side nor jutting forward. The shoulder must be relaxed and low but neither hunched nor pressed back. The pelvis should be tilted so that the stomach is gently (but not fiercely) held in. The feet should face forward. Try standing like this in front of a mirror.

In order not only to see but also to *feel* what a good posture is like, try some bad attitudes. It is often assumed that standing to attention is a good posture. Thrust the chin up, the shoulders back and the chest out. You will feel that the shoulder muscles are rigid rather than relaxed – an unnecessary muscle-effort. They will probably also have crept upwards. Though the thrust-out chest gives plenty of room for the lungs, it also hollows the back unnecessarily, putting a strain on the spine. It is significant that armies, recognizing that standing to attention is a strain, make use of the 'At ease' position.

At the other extreme is the slouching attitude. Round and hunch your shoulders forward, sinking the chest downwards and backwards. Usually your head will automatically jut forward, and your pelvis tilt too. If you try to take a deep breath, you will find there is not enough room to inflate the

THE BACK/MAINTAINING THE BODYWORK

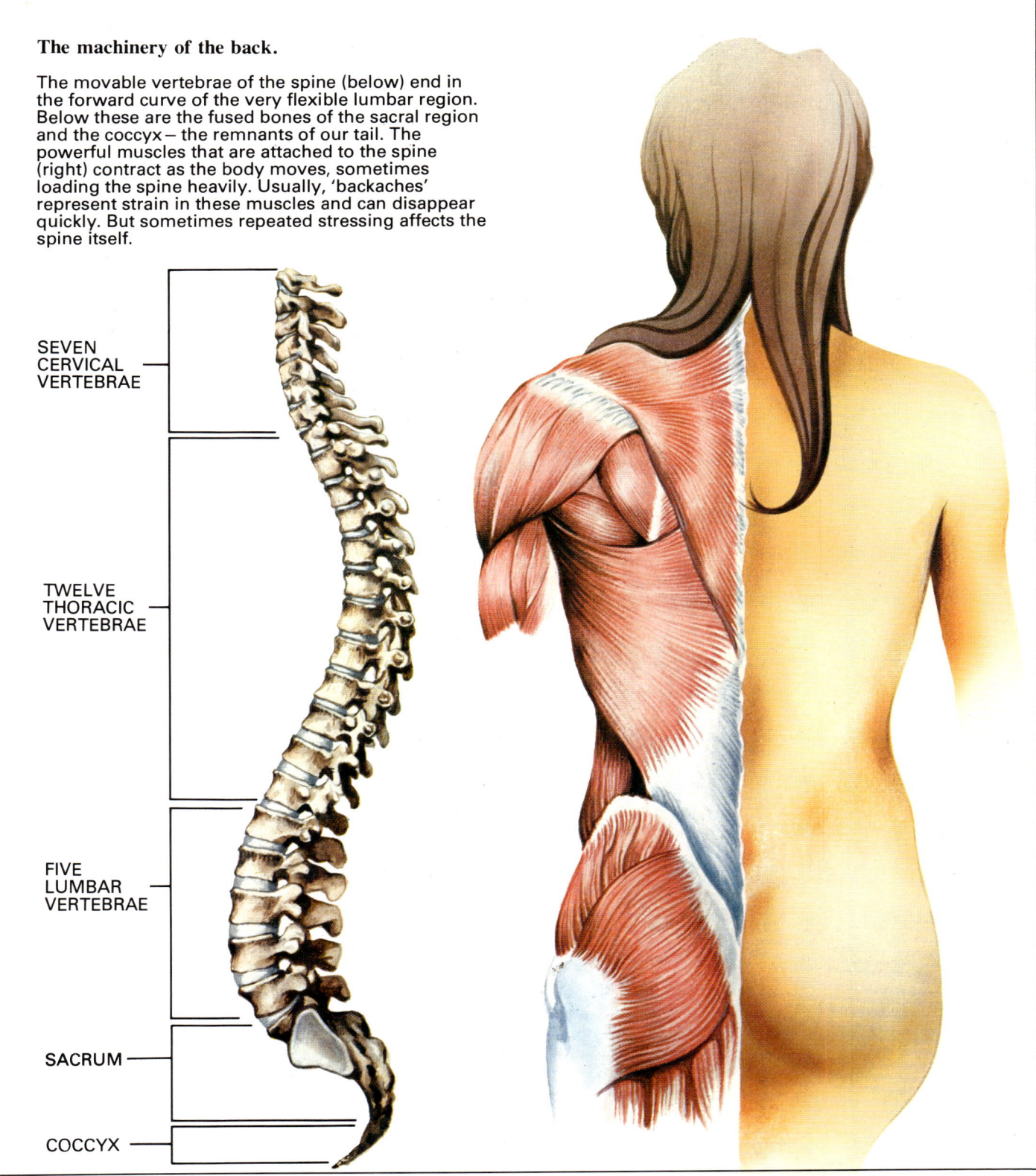

The machinery of the back.

The movable vertebrae of the spine (below) end in the forward curve of the very flexible lumbar region. Below these are the fused bones of the sacral region and the coccyx – the remnants of our tail. The powerful muscles that are attached to the spine (right) contract as the body moves, sometimes loading the spine heavily. Usually, 'backaches' represent strain in these muscles and can disappear quickly. But sometimes repeated stressing affects the spine itself.

SEVEN CERVICAL VERTEBRAE

TWELVE THORACIC VERTEBRAE

FIVE LUMBAR VERTEBRAE

SACRUM

COCCYX

lungs fully. The weight of the head is a strain on the upper spine, and the pelvic tilt means that the lower spine is under unnecessary strain.

Obviously a good posture applies to moving or sitting as well as standing. In all activities the same principles apply: balance, minimal muscle-work, room for internal organs and proper weight distribution.

Sitting: Sit with legs firmly planted on the floor, slightly apart, the body positioned evenly on the buttocks, which are set well back into the chair. Try to make sure this is the way you watch television or read, although you will obviously change position from time to time. Rest the head on the back of the chair if possible.

Walking: An erect posture gives room for the lungs to work. Keep a rhythmical stride, stepping out freely and letting the arms swing naturally. If you have to carry

MAINTAINING THE BODYWORK/THE FEET

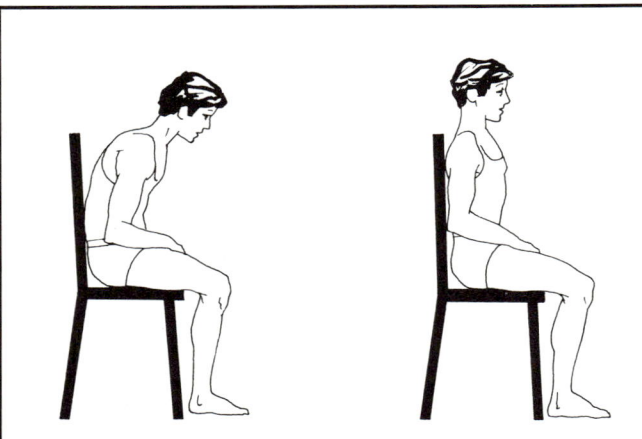

For sitting, the body should be positioned evenly on the buttocks, which are set well back into the chair (*right*).

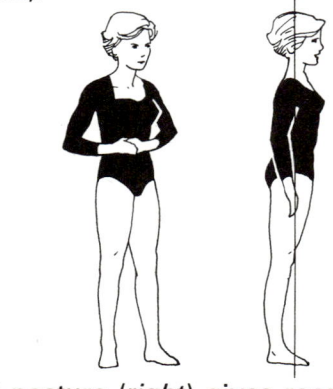

An erect posture (*right*) gives room for the lungs to work.

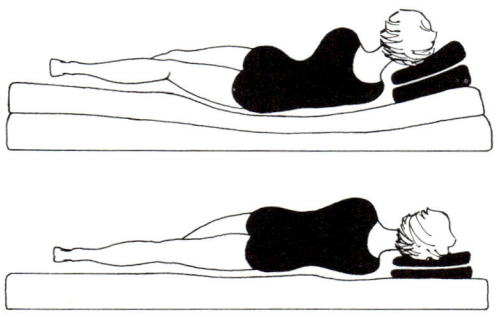

For sleeping, the mattress should be extra-firm and not sag. The neck should be supported, and in line with the rest of the spine.

anything heavy, try to split a load into two bags or suitcases, so that you can balance one on either side rather than have to walk with the weight all on one side.

Sleeping: Invest in an extra-firm mattress. Do not assume it will last a lifetime. Buy a new one if it begins to sag or go lumpy. The base of the mattress should be hard: put in enough planks to support the whole mattress, not just one under where you think your back will be. Make sure the neck is supported, if you sleep on your side. The shoulder should be on the mattress with enough pillow or pillows to hold up the neck in line with the rest of the spine. Some people find special neck-pillows helpful. You can make one by taking a loosely filled pillow and tying it in the middle into a butterfly shape.

Some people re-learn 'body attitudes' by special teaching in what is called the Alexander Technique (see Appendix Three). But this can be expensive. It is certainly possible for most people to improve their posture by following these simple rules:

1. Practise a good posture, when standing, sitting or kneeling, whenever you remember.

2. Check any habitually bad body-movements and attitudes, and try to convert them into properly balanced ones.

3. Give the muscles a fair chance of rest by having adequate sleep.

4. Dress sensibly. Working clothes should permit free movement and be such that if necessary you can hold 'dirty' weights closely.

5. Take up some sport, exercise or dancing. Anything which teaches bodily co-ordination and rhythm helps towards good posture.

6. Cultivate a healthy and optimistic mental attitude. It is not for nothing that we describe a negative and angry person as having 'the hump'.

7. Lose any extra weight you carry. This will relieve one burden on the spine. Pregnancy, by adding an extra weight load, can give temporary posture problems (see Chapter 1). Walking is perhaps the best exercise. Don't worry unnecessarily. But make sure that when the baby is born, you go back to your old upright posture without too much hollow in the back.

The Feet

A healthy body owes a great debt to the feet. Your feet propel you through the day, down streets, up stairs, over sportsfields – but all too often the only 'care' they receive is a fortnightly assault on stubbornly tough toenails.

Feet, then, are a down-trodden part of the body. They are squeezed into badly fitting shoes, constricted by sweaty, tight stockings or socks, and made to function for days at a time in fashionable footwear that would make an infantry regiment mutiny. No wonder they wreak their revenge with corns and bunions in old age.

Foot lib should begin with babies. Give a child badly fitting shoes and too-tight socks, and you have doomed him or her to foot deformity for life. Add fashionable shoes for the next twenty years and you have probably doubled the size of the developing bunions. Yet all feet need is a little bit of freedom.

CHOOSING THE RIGHT SHOES

The first step in towards healthy feet is to take proper time and care in choosing shoes. Since more and more shoe shops are self-service, you will often have to rely on your own judgement, rather than an assistant's advice. The Consumers' Association magazine *Which?* compiled an eight-point checklist for shoe buyers.

1. Wear the same sort of socks or stockings as you are

THE FEET/MAINTAINING THE BODYWORK

normally going to wear with the shoes.

2. Try on both shoes of the pair and, if they have laces, do them up properly – facings should not touch.

3. Standing up (or at least putting your weight on to your feet), check where your longest toe comes to. There should be *at least* half an inch inside the shoe at the end of your toe. If not, the shoe is too short.

4. Stand on tiptoe. As you do so, there should be no, or very little, movement between your foot and the heel of the shoe. If there is, the shoe is too big over the instep.

5. As you stand on tiptoe, look at the front part of the shoe. If a big deep fold develops, the shoe is too deep.

6. Feel the widest part of your foot through the shoe. If there is spare space on either side, the shoe is too wide. If your foot makes the shoe bulge, the shoe is too narrow.

7. Can you move all your toes freely inside the shoe? If not, the shoe is too narrow, or too shallow at the toes – try a different style.

8. See if you can push your toes up against the front of the shoe leaving a gap behind the heel. If you can, the shoe is too big over the instep – try another style.

Even if you do have well-fitting shoes, you can still hurt your feet if you wear the wrong shoe for the wrong job. 'It's a question of wearing football boots for football, trainers or plimsoles for physical education – not running around all day in trainers,' says Arthur Swallow, a chiropodist and lecturer at the London Foot Hospital. 'If you can only afford one pair of shoes, then it must be lace-ups. They are best for the feet. Lacing holds the heel of the foot back into the heel of the shoe and gives the toes room to function.' Changing your shoes at least once a day will also relieve the foot. High heels worn all day and evening might do damage; but high heels worn just for an evening will do little harm.

FOOT CARE

1. **Wash feet daily with warm water, and dry between the toes:** Dust with talcum powder. It is relaxing, apart from being good for the feet. If you get blisters, don't break them. Stop wearing the shoes that caused them. If the blisters break, cover them with a sterile dressing.

2. **Change stockings and socks daily:** Men are particularly bad about this. Not only do socks that are worn too long make your feet smell, they also go stiff and rub against the skin.

3. **Go barefoot as much as possible, within reason:** Tramping around the woodlands and fields will simply leave you with scratches, thorns and possibly worse. But a good way to give your feet a rest is to go barefoot in the house, or on the lawn whenever it is warm enough. Babies, indeed, should never wear shoes till they start to walk: check then that their bootees or socks are not tight.

4. **Cut toenails in a relatively straight line:** Do not cut too far down into the nail grooves.

5. **Refresh sweaty feet with an astringent lotion, such as surgical spirit:** Moisten dry feet with hand or face cream.

FEET AND EXERCISE

Aching or blistered feet will ruin jogging, walking or any other kind of exercise. Take care of the feet, first of all by making sure that your sports shoes fit correctly. On the whole, it is worth paying more for shoes designed for a particular sport.

Start your exercise gradually to give your feet a chance to adapt. Jogging five miles on the road or taking a twenty-mile hike will tire feet that are not used to it. Start with just a gentle jog or walk. You can toughen your feet in advance by gently rubbing them with surgical spirit and letting it dry on. Walkers should wear two pairs of socks – either two medium-weight or a thin under-pair and a thick over-pair. Make sure the outer socks are larger by half a size. Wool and cotton absorb sweat better than nylon.

FEET AT RISK

Elderly people and those who are suffering from impaired circulation, diabetes or rheumatoid arthritis need to take special care of their feet. Diabetics and those who do not have much sensation in their feet may not notice minor injuries. If these are left untreated, serious health risks can ensue.

Diabetics and the elderly should also be wary of using slippers around the house. Because slippers are loose-fitting, the toes can be thrust forward against the front of the shoe. Abrasions or bruising may result. Always wear a proper shoe about the house. Blind or poor-sighted people should also be especially careful to check for minor foot injuries.

Diabetics should look out for these danger signs: any colour change whether paler or darker in the leg or foot; any discharge from a break or crack in the skin or from a corn, or from beneath a toenail; any swelling or throbbing in any part of the foot.

All foot trouble *must* be taken seriously by diabetics. If in any doubt at all, they should go to a state-registered chiropodist or their family doctor. Those who have a history of foot troubles would do well to have a regular routine check-up.

OTHER FOOT TROUBLES

Athlete's foot: A fungus infection, athlete's foot is usually cured by proprietary liquids or medicines. Hot sweaty feet are more vulnerable to it. Keep bath towels separate, as athlete's foot is contagious. Use a piece of kitchen towel over the bathmat.

Callouses: These can be treated at home. They appear where there has been pressure on the foot. The thickened skin can be gently rubbed away with a pumice stone, but both pumice and foot should be wet.

Corns: These should usually be treated by an expert. Proprietary corn paints and plasters are sometimes dangerous, especially to the elderly and diabetic. **Bunions, warts** (or verrucae) and **ingrowing toenails** will all benefit from treatment by a state-registered chiropodist.

Chiropodists can also help with pads, slings, and shoe-fillers. Those with very deformed feet may need special surgical boots. People who have difficult feet to fit with shoes may find help from the Disabled Living Foundation's list of footwear suppliers (see Appendix Three).

The Hair

Hair matters to us all more than we probably realize. Too much of it or too little, or hair in the wrong places, can cause considerable emotional distress. What can we do to keep our hair and our feelings about it healthy?

Hair itself cannot be 'hurt' or diseased, though it can show signs of disease elsewhere in the body. Many problems about hair are really problems about our attitude to it. Left to itself, hair manages quite well. It is shed regularly, and new hair starts forming in the base of the hair follicle and eventually pushes out the old. Its colour, waviness, length and texture are part of a general body-programme which makes hair on the arms, for instance, shorter than hair on the head.

Hair can be washed twice a week without upsetting the natural balance of body oils. It can be waved, permed and generally cut without much trouble. The worst that might happen is that it might break off a few inches from the scalp, if it is over-permed. Even so, it will grow again. Any sudden loss of hair should be reported to the doctor. There are a variety of possible causes, including pregnancy, drug side-effects, illnesses or glandular abnormalities. Usually when the cause has been removed, the hair just grows again. But it is important to go to a doctor, not to a so-called hair clinic or trichologist. They are not qualified to diagnose illnesses.

BALDNESS

Baldness is part of the body's genetic programme that is fixed at birth. Many men suffer from what is known as 'male pattern baldness' as they grow older, and some women also go thin on top. Although baldness can be alarming, it quite often stops at a certain point. So if the hair at your temples is receding, it does not mean you will end up as bald as an egg. There is no cure for baldness. Yet a variety of 'hair clinics', 'treatment centres' and 'hair specialists' still offer baldness cures. When the Consumers' Association magazine *Which?* sent two ordinary balding men round some of these establishments, an extraordinary series of diagnoses ranging from 'blocked follicles' to psoriasis were made. Yet a dermatologist had examined both men and pronounced nothing more than the usual male pattern baldness. Shampoos, creams, massage, lotions, electro-therapy, ultra-violet and infra-red radiation were among the expensive remedies these clinics were pushing.

Sometimes it may seem as if clinics *do* work. This is because some people suffer a 'transient moult'. Their hair is shed then grows back again. If in the meantime they have been to a clinic, they think it is the result of the treatment, not knowing that the hair would have re-grown anyway.

If you must cover up your baldness, a hairpiece is probably the easiest answer. Hair transplants also work, but they are expensive and do not always look much better. Besides, you have got to use the hair from the side and back of your head, and when this is transplanted it might fall out too. 'The disease lies not in the baldness,' says Dr Ian Caldwell, a British dermatologist, 'but in the lack of ability to accept it.'

UNSIGHTLY HAIR

Hair in the wrong places is the main female worry. Very occasionally this is caused by a glandular abnormality, so if hair suddenly sprouts it is worth checking with your doctor. Normally, like male baldness, it is just part of the genetic make-up of the individual. The only permanent way to remove hair is by electrolysis. In Britain this is rarely available on the National Health Service, so you will have to pay for treatment at a commercial clinic. Make sure that the electrolysist is a member of a reputable trade organization. Do not try to do it yourself with a home kit. Bad electrolysis can leave scars.

Electrolysis works by inserting a needle into the root of the hair, then killing the root with an electrical impulse. It is a slow process and can be expensive, so make sure you get a realistic estimate of the time and cost of treatment before committing yourself. There are commercial sharks that prey on women's worry about superfluous hair, just as some do on men's fears of baldness.

There are many old wives' tales about removing hair. Shaving it off does not make it grow stronger: it makes it feel stronger or more bristly because of the blunt ends of hair. Likewise if you take out a hair with a tweezer, you will not find two growing in its place. Tweezing, however, does distort the follicle and may make subsequent electrolysis more difficult.

HAIR DYES

These have become controversial ever since some American research suggested certain dye chemicals might cause cancer after being absorbed through the skin. So far there is no firm evidence that they do, and no firm evidence that

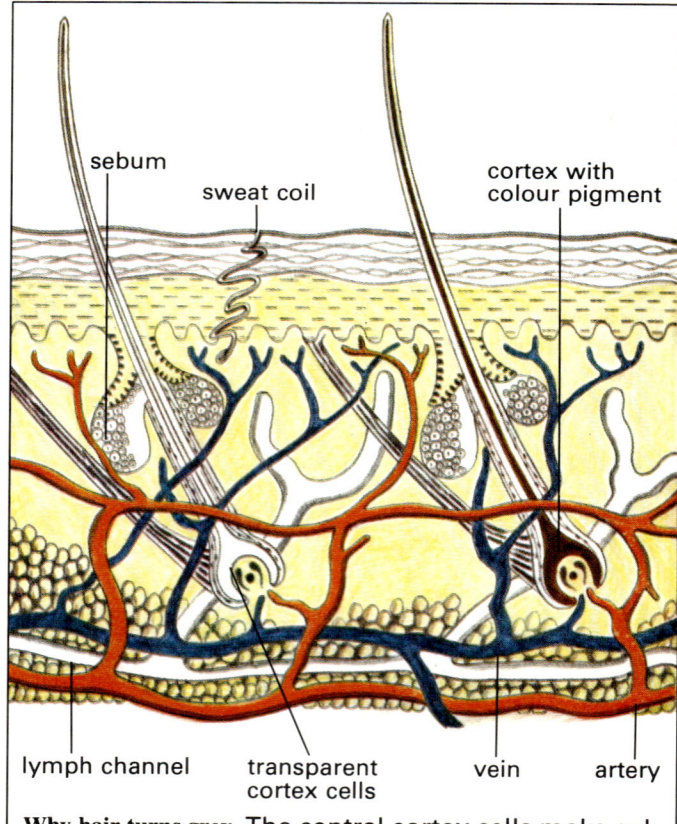

Why hair turns grey. The central cortex cells make colour pigments. With age, these become transparent.

THE HAIR/**MAINTAINING THE BODYWORK**

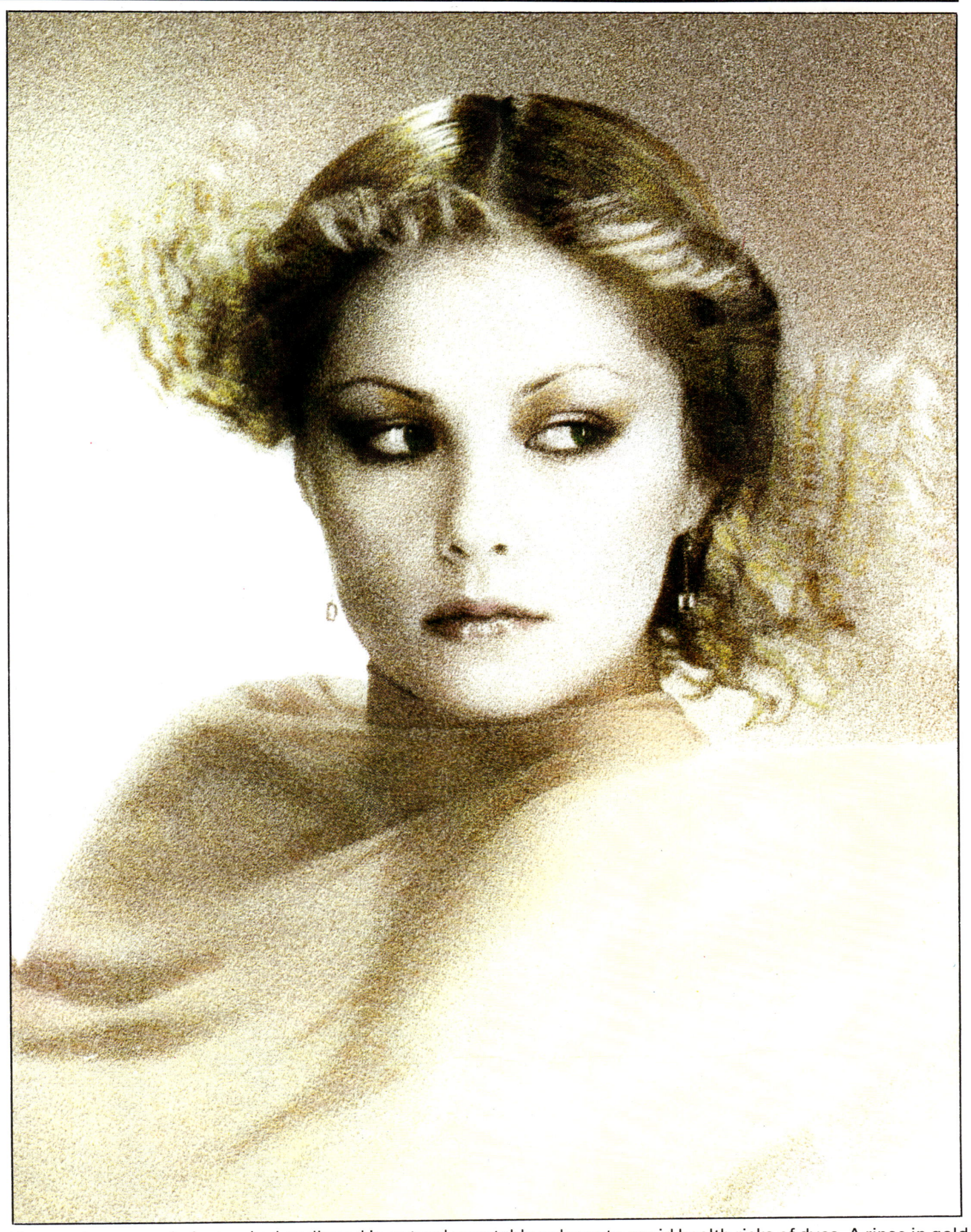

You can have your hair streaked or dipped in natural vegetable colours to avoid health risks of dyes. A rinse in gold and green (or even pink and purple) can be reversed with a shampoo. Or buy a switch of coloured hair to pin in an exotic streak.

they do not. Indeed, the problem of proving that anything causes cancer in human beings is particularly difficult, since it may take several decades before the disease emerges. The main scare centres round a series of chemicals that have been found to cause mutation in bacteria. Substances that cause cancer in humans also cause mutation in bacteria; but there are also some substances that do *not* cause cancer in humans which nevertheless have this effect on bacteria. So the bacteria test only works as a rough initial screen. Only one of the dye chemicals, 2,4-diaminotoluene (or meta-toluylenediamine), has been shown to cause cancer in animals so far.

The simplest way to play safe is just not to dye your hair. Vegetable dyes, hair darkeners (to make grey hair darker), or that old stand-by henna are probably all right. So, too, is plain bleaching peroxide, but quite often this comes packaged with a colouring dye as well. Indeed at the hairdressers, you may not know (and neither may the hairdresser) exactly what you are getting. So avoiding dyes is the easiest way to be sure.

If you feel you must dye your hair, do so as little and as infrequently as possible. Have it done with a streaking technique which means the dye does not get on the skin of the scalp: as long as the dye does not touch the skin, it cannot enter the body, and can therefore do no harm. Use rubber gloves to put the dye on. British manufacturers claim to have stopped using 2,4-diaminotoluene, but make sure by avoiding any dye that has 'toluylenediamines' mentioned on the pack.

Unfortunately, not all dyes have their chemical contents mentioned. Write to the manufacturers to ask if they contain any of the following, or avoid any which mention these chemicals on the pack: 4-nitro-ortho-phenylenediamine, 2-nitro-para-phenylenediamine, 2,4-diaminotoluene (meta-toluylenediamine), 2,4-diamino-anisole, 2,5-diaminotoluene (para-toluylenediamine), 2,5-diaminoanisole, para-phenylenediamine, ortho-phenylenediamine, meta-phenylenediamine, 2-amino-5-nitrophenol, 2-amino-4-nitrophenol.

Quite apart from any possible cancer risk, some dyes can set up an allergy. So before you use any hair dye, make sure you have a patch-test on your skin.

Some hairdressers think it is enough to patch-test only on the first occasion of using a dye. They are wrong. A test should be made *every single time* that a dye is used. Sometimes allergies develop after many, many times of use.
Anybody who works with hair dyes should be very careful indeed. Gloves should be worn at any time that a dye is being handled.

DANDRUFF
Dandruff is not a disease. The white flakes are simply dead skin-scales off the scalp. It is more likely to be noticeable when the hair is greasy, so wash your hair more often. If you have severe dandruff look for a shampoo that contains either zinc pyrithione or selenium sulphide. These seem to be the only ingredients that really make any difference. However, medicated shampoos can cause scalp irritation, and frequent washing with a mild shampoo may be more effective.

LICE
Most of us think of lice or nits as something that cannot happen to our children. Yet the head-louse is on the increase and no respecter of persons. Perfectly clean, nice and well-brought-up children can, and do, catch lice. Indeed the head-louse is having a population boom in almost every developed country. The head-louse, or nit – *Pediculus humanus capitis* – is an ingenious and determined insect. A full-grown louse is about the size of a matchstick head, with six legs. Each leg has a claw with which it clings onto the hair near the scalp. On the louse's head is a needle-like apparatus, with which it probes into the skin till it finds a blood-vessel. It sucks up the blood, meanwhile pumping an anti-coagulant into the wound to make sure the blood keeps flowing. By the time the small bite begins to itch, the louse has moved on to another drinking hole.

The eggs are laid on hairs close to the scalp and fixed there with an insoluble glue. After eight to ten days they hatch out into larvae of a lighter colour. Nine days later these mate, the males mating several times, since there are more females in the population. Each female then lays about five to eight eggs daily and can produce a total of up to three hundred. These are light-coloured balls the size of pinheads, known as nits. The louse has evolved different strains, suitable for different hair. European lice have claws adapted for clinging to European hair, while African lice have claws that are better for oval African hair. These two strains can mate and produce hybrids.

The spread of the new super-louse, resistant to DDT, has been enormously helped by people's reluctance to admit to lice. The main reason why people are so ashamed of them is because they believe lice are only found on dirty people. In fact the reverse is true: the head-louse actually prefers clean, non-scurfy hair, so that it can get at the scalp more easily. Nor can lice be caught from seats in public transport, cinemas or other public places. Since the insect moves by clinging onto hairs, it cannot travel far. Lice are spread by head-to-head contact. Even long hair, sometimes blamed for lice, is not the cause. Short hair spreads lice just as well, if not better, since the louse always lives close to the skin rather than at the end of the hair.

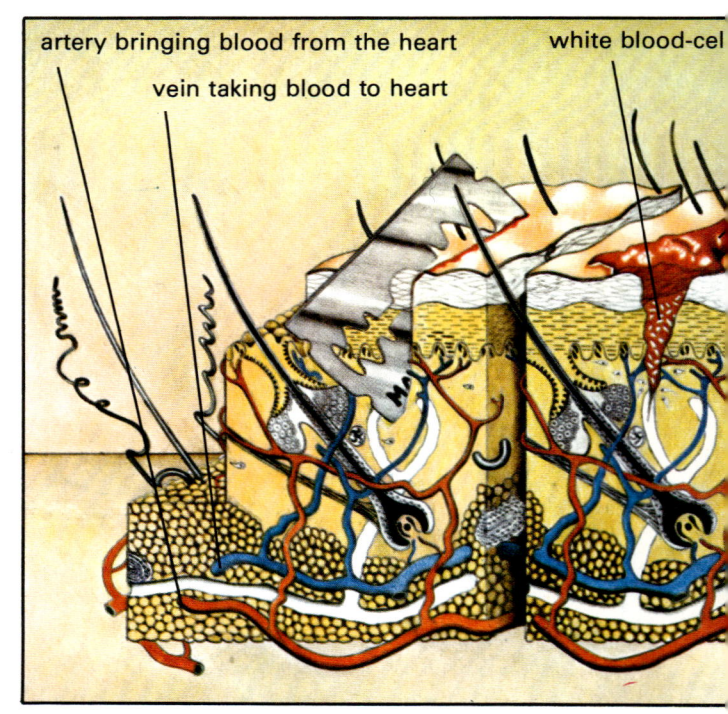

Symptoms: The first sign is itching. If you look carefully you will see the dead lice which fall out of the hair after scratching, and may see the live insects which move quickly amongst the hair. White nits, the eggs of the lice, can also be seen. These first appear at the hair roots, but in severe cases may occur in clusters along the length of the hair.

Leave malathion lotion on for at least twenty minutes and preferably for twenty-four hours. The longer you leave it, the less likely is re-infestation. The malathion kills not only the adult lice and the larvae, but also the eggs. To comb out these, after you have treated them with malathion, you need a metal-tooth comb. Comb out the hair while it is still wet, pulling the comb through the hair after starting right at the scalp. Merely combing, without using malathion, will not do the trick. Malathion is a potent insecticide which may be absorbed through the scalp, so it is not advisable to use it as a preventive in the absence of infestation.

The Skin

The body's first line of defence against disease is the skin. Its protective layer has to fend off germs, withstand temperature changes, cope with injuries, yet at the same time report back to the brain, via the nerves, what goes on in the tactile world outside.

The skin is made up of a barrier of cells, with a support system of nerves, glands and blood-vessels below it. The top layer is called the epidermis and is made up of living cells that, in turn, rise to the surface and die. So the surface layer of the epidermis is continually being shed. This layer is kept soft, flexible and to a certain extent free from infection by a kind of natural cosmetic emulsion. The sweat-glands feed liquid into the hair follicles, secreting more or less according to the body's mental and physical activity. The sebaceous glands secrete a kind of grease called sebum into the same follicles and out onto the surface. This mixture of grease and liquid lubricates the skin.

Some people, especially adolescents, suffer from too much sebum and have greasy skins. Others, especially the elderly, suffer from too little of it and have dry skins. Greasy areas look greasy and may produce acne; dry skins look flaky and may be sore. Most of the time the body, if left to itself, will get the mixture of grease and moisture right. But we do not leave the body to itself. We have been brainwashed into washing too often. Most dermatologists reckon they see far more skin-problems from clean people who wash too much, than from dirty people. So how often should we wash?

Face-washing once a day with soap and water is enough. If your face is greasy, wash more often: teenagers often need to wash three or four times a day. If your face is dry, use a cleansing lotion. Simple liquid paraffin obtainable from chemists is the cheapest, but do not mistake this for the paraffin-oil used in heaters. A moisturizing cream may help too, but a cheap one is just as good as an expensive one. All that a moisturizing cream does is to put back water and grease onto the skin.

Daily baths are all right, but older people may need to take them less often. As their body-oil decreases, a daily bath can produce dry skin which itches and cracks. If this happens to you, cut down on baths. Use a bath oil (any oil, even cooking oil, will do, though the smell may not be pleasant). Do not use bath salts or powders since these increase the dehydrating effect on the skin.

Diet probably does not make a great deal of difference to the skin in Western countries, although old people quite often suffer from mild scurvy, causing irritation of the skin and gums. This is easily treated by eating more fruit and vegetables, or drinking orange juice or vitamin C drinks.

Sunshine is another thing that many people think is good for skin. It is not. A sun-tan is merely the skin's way of

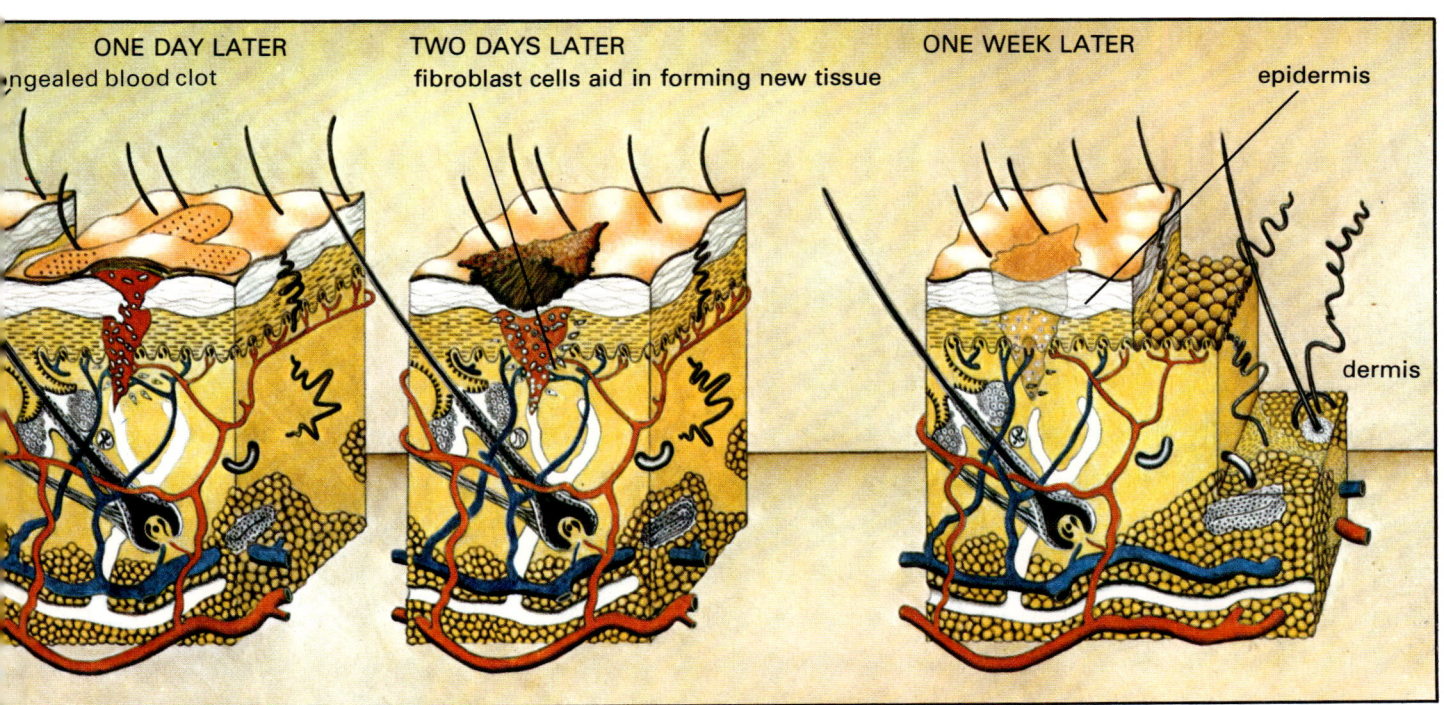

protecting itself against harmful rays. Be sensible about tanning. Anything which makes the skin blister and burn is too much. If you are going to be out in brilliant sunshine, use a sunscreen lotion or cream to protect you against harmful rays. One of the most effective sunscreens is Piz-Buin No. 6 lotion or cream. Wear a hat, light shirt with long sleeves and trousers if you have no sunscreen. In Britain there is rarely enough sun to make us worry about more than the occasional burn. In hotter climates, cancer of the skin may be a danger for people whose skins are continuously exposed by working out-of-doors. The remedy is simple: do not let your bare skin be exposed continually for long periods.

The magical claims for cosmetics are mostly illusory. What you pay for is the perfume, the packaging and the *je ne sais quoi*. So some rules are worth remembering.

1. Skin cannot be 'fed' from the outside, only lubricated.
2. Soaps with 'added fat' are not likely to do anything. The fat is in small quantities, and anyway we rinse ourselves after washing, thus rinsing off the fat.
3. 'Natural' ingredients such as avocado, strawberries and peaches will not do any harm. But neither are they likely to do much good.

Skins can suffer from diseases, and if you get one go to the doctor just as you would with any other disease. People have the false impression that skin diseases do not matter. Children with an unexplained rash should be taken to the doctor: any rash on an adult's skin that lasts more than a week should also be seen by a doctor. Here are some of the most common problems:

Acne: Usually suffered by teenagers, who are told that age will clear it up. Age does, but it can leave scars behind. So, if your acne is severe, go to a doctor for help. He can prescribe antibiotics, lotions and, occasionally for spotty girls, the birth-control pill. If acne is not that severe, do not spend a lot of money on specially medicated soaps and lotions. Ordinary soap will dry up the greasy skin that produces acne.

Contact dermatitis or contact eczema: A rash, with patches of red, itching and sometimes sores. The cause may be an allergy, which you can develop even to substances you have been safely and happily using for years. A dermatologist will help you track down the offending substance. The skin will never forget the allergy, so you will have to avoid touching that substance in the future (see Chapter 7).

Eczema: Atopic eczema is the term given to a similar rash when its cause is constitutional. Some people seem to have an inherited tendency to eczema, and it is often associated with asthma and hay fever. Babies are particularly prone to it, but the condition often clears up in later life. Eczema is not infectious or contagious. Go to a doctor for help and keep in regular contact with him. The steroid creams that are often prescribed can be strong, so use them sparingly and according to his instructions. Never lend or borrow such creams.

Psoriasis: This is the other major skin disease. Again it is neither infectious nor contagious. Red patches covered with silvery scales appear on the skin, often on the knees, elbows and scalp. Psoriasis comes and goes for no apparent reason and a doctor's prescription for ointments will be necessary. Careful sun-tanning helps some people.

The Joints

There are no fewer than 187 joints in the body – all of them working to make the rigid skeleton flexible. Keeping your joints working efficiently is something that the body does automatically. But you *can* help its maintenance-work.

The name usually given to any disease or trouble with the joints is arthritis. It is a loose term that covers many different types of trouble, but it can roughly be divided into two main groups of diseases: rheumatoid arthritis and osteo-arthritis (properly known as osteo-arthrosis).

Rheumatoid arthritis is a generalized disease, which usually leads to ill health and affects many joints at the same time. Osteo-arthritis, on the other hand, just affects the joints without any general ill-health. It can be a 'wear-and-tear' disease, affecting just one joint at a time, or affect many joints – perhaps on a hereditary basis. The cause of neither is fully understood, but both diseases become increasingly common as people grow older.

Treatment can help control the diseases but since arthritis is not fully understood there are no certain 'cures' and no certain ways to avoid getting it. Arthritis can also be part of many other diseases. There is, for instance, a transient form of arthritis that occasionally accompanies German measles.

Some general rules, however, are of interest. Diet does not usually make much difference, though you will find a host of old wives' tales about raw onions, orange juice, and the like. A balanced diet with plenty of vegetables and not too many fattening foods is all that is needed. Don't get overweight. Although the extra pounds do not *cause* arthritis, they make it more severe in the joints that have to carry the extra pounds, particularly the hips and knees.

Gout is an exception to the general rule. People who have an inherited tendency to gout will probably find that it may worsen, if they eat and drink too much. Even so, there are some unlucky people who, although teetotal vegetarians, still get gout.

For many years it was thought that exercise was likely to produce arthritis. Since some forms of osteo-arthritis were 'wear-and-tear' diseases, doctors concluded that exercise would just add to the 'wear'. Yet a recent study in Finland showed the opposite. Seventy-four former athletes were X-rayed for signs of osteo-arthritis. The athletes were, on average, about fifty-five years old and had competed for twenty-one years. They were compared with non-athletes of a similar age – in fact, hospital patients but excluding those who had complained of problems with their hips.

Only three athletes – or 4 per cent of the total – had true osteo-arthritis, compared with 8.7 per cent of the hospital patients. Among the three unlucky athletes was one who had competed for only eight years, giving up after he had collected an Olympic gold medal.

The sample was admittedly small and only applied to osteo-arthritis, not rheumatoid arthritis. However, a study of English footballers seemed to bear out some of its conclusions. Some fifty professional footballers, fifteen ex-pros and 1,490 former players were involved in the study, which found that only 3.2 per cent had arthritis.

Even more interesting was the fact that it was the standing leg, not the kicking leg, which was more likely to suffer.

THE EYES/**MAINTAINING THE BODYWORK**

The Eyes

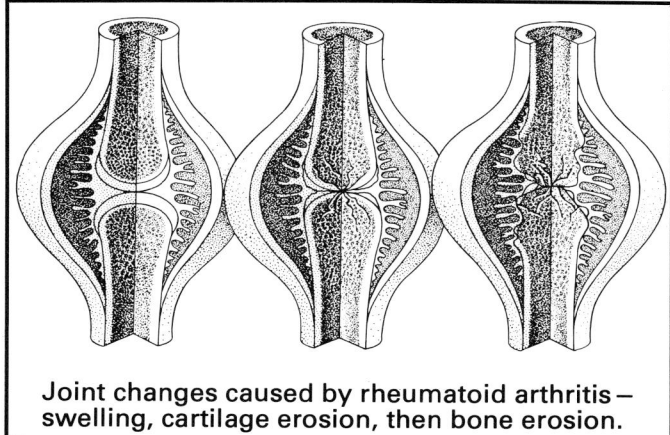

Joint changes caused by rheumatoid arthritis – swelling, cartilage erosion, then bone erosion.

This implied that it was *being* kicked rather than kicking that did the damage. As it was already known that injury to a joint can result in subsequent arthritis, athletes' arthritis may be due to injuries, not sport itself.

Indeed, the Finland survey suggests that exercise can be positively good for joints – perhaps because the joint cartilage is nourished by a joint fluid. This nourishment is facilitated by movement.

Eldery people are particularly vulnerable to such problems since tendons and ligaments become weaker in old age and more vulnerable to injury. Sometimes problems begin suddenly, but more often pain begins insidiously, particularly in the joints which do most of the weight-bearing – the knees and the hips.

Stiffness in the joints can in many cases be eased by simple remedies such as flexing the muscles before getting up in the morning, sleeping in a warm bedroom, hot baths and regular but not violent exercise. Walking is often sufficient to loosen stiff joints in the legs, while other joints can be kept mobile by generally flexing appropriate parts of the body.

Finally, if you do get problems apparently arising from the joints – pain, perhaps accompanied by swelling, heat or redness – go and see your doctor. Much can be done, if arthritis is treated early, to limit the problem. If you are merely being treated with pain-killers, do not be afraid to ask your doctor for a second opinion. The British Arthritis and Rheumatism Council, a body which raises funds for research, has pointed out that there is a shortage of rheumatism and arthritis experts, particularly in some areas of Britain. But it is worth insisting to see a consultant doctor if you feel your arthritis is getting severe.

POOR EYESIGHT

The eye works like an automatic camera. Light reflected from an object in front of the eye enters the eye through the lens. The lens is flexible and can be moved by a tiny muscle so that an image of the object is accurately focused on the back of the eye. The iris just in front of the lens acts like the diaphragm in a camera, and prevents too much light from entering. The back of the eye, the retina, contains light-sensitive nerve endings which pass messages back to the brain, informing the brain of the quantity and colour of the light falling upon them. So the retina is comparable with the film in a camera. The most sensitive part of the retina, the fovea, is near its centre. When a person looks directly at an object, the image of the object is focused on the fovea, where it can be seen most clearly.

Just like a camera, the eye must be 'made' to precise proportions. If the eye is a fraction of a millimetre too short or too long, then the image will not be precisely focused on the retina. This incredible accuracy has to be maintained from birth, when the eye is 14 mm long, until adulthood when the eye has grown to 24 mm long.

If the eyeball is too long, so that the image is focused in front of the retina, then a person is short-sighted. Short sight may develop at any time but particularly while a person is growing. It is readily corrected with glasses, which give clear distance vision that is essential for driving. If the eyeball is too short, so that the image again cannot easily be focused upon it, then the person has long sight. A small degree of long sight can frequently be compensated for by the eye itself while a person is still young and the lens of their eye flexible. But when such a person gets older, he or she finds it increasingly difficult to see things near-to, and may require glasses for reading or close work.

Poor eyesight can also be caused by a third condition called astigmatism. When someone suffers from astigmatism, they see an object as blurred and distorted, although they do not realize this until their eyesight is corrected with glasses.

There is no way of preventing the development of long sight, short sight or astigmatism. To some extent these conditions may run in families, but more often they are probably simply the result of chance effects on growth and development of the eyes. It is important that any defect in vision is corrected as early as possible so that children do

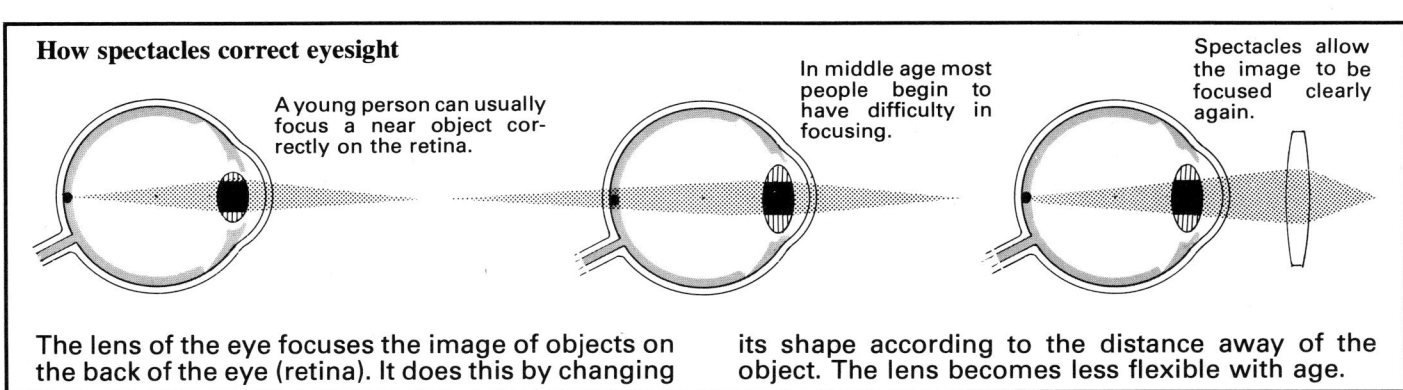

How spectacles correct eyesight

A young person can usually focus a near object correctly on the retina.

In middle age most people begin to have difficulty in focusing.

Spectacles allow the image to be focused clearly again.

The lens of the eye focuses the image of objects on the back of the eye (retina). It does this by changing its shape according to the distance away of the object. The lens becomes less flexible with age.

MAINTAINING THE BODYWORK/THE EYES

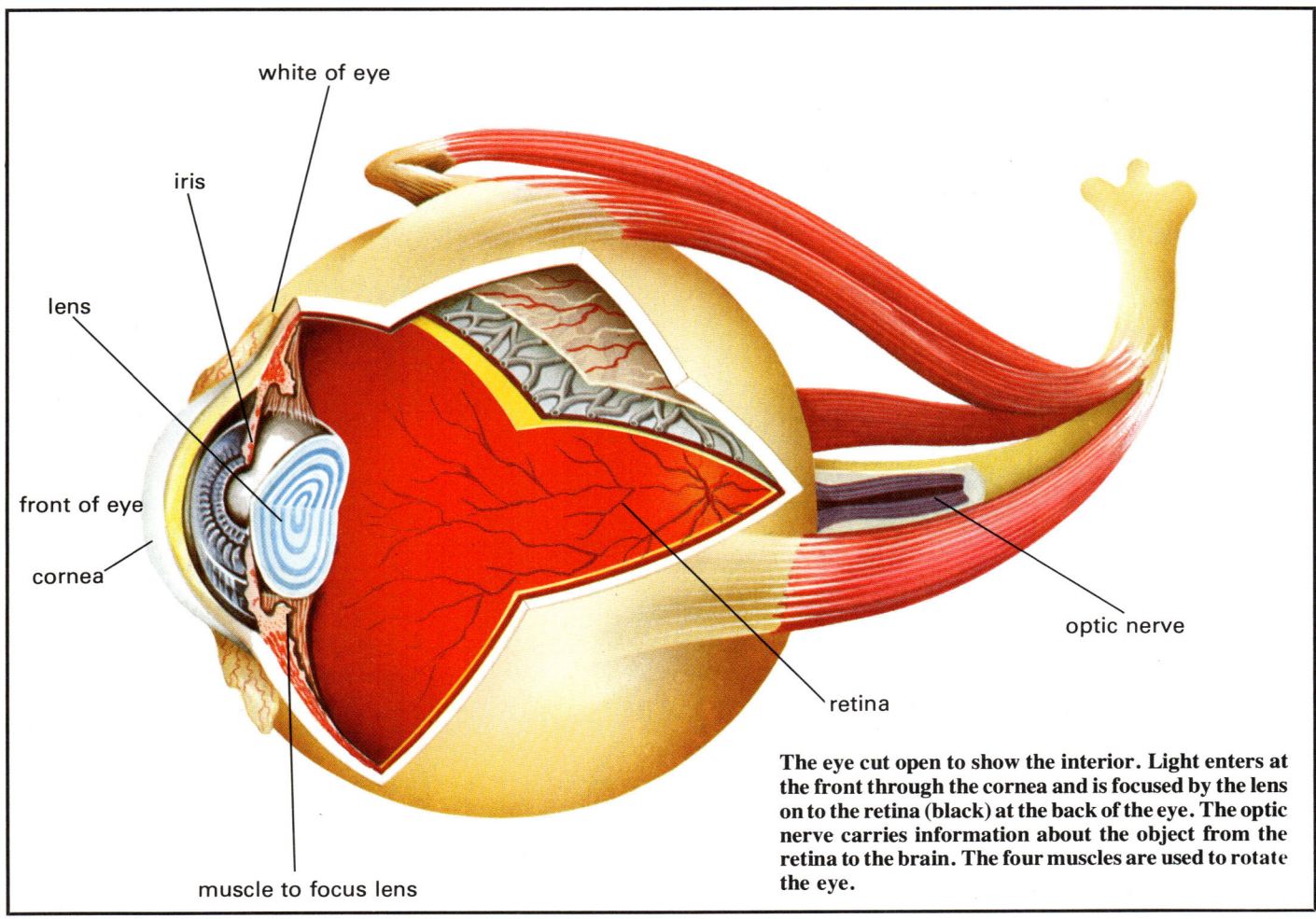

The eye cut open to show the interior. Light enters at the front through the cornea and is focused by the lens on to the retina (black) at the back of the eye. The optic nerve carries information about the object from the retina to the brain. The four muscles are used to rotate the eye.

not have any unnecessary difficulties in learning to understand their surroundings or to read. Children should have their eyes checked at any age if a defect is suspected. Ideally, all children should have their eyes checked before starting school. A rough test is often done at the school itself, but this is sometimes left until most children can recognize letters, at six or seven; by that time a short-sighted child may already have suffered difficulty in learning because of poor sight. If parents, brothers or sisters have poor sight, then a child should have a full check-up before going to school. If a child has any difficulty in learning to read, a full eye check-up is advisable.

The lens in the eye starts out in children with the consistency of a liquid such as treacle, but as a person gets older the lens becomes less flexible and ends up in old people almost as dense as the nails of the fingers. This means that as a person gets older they find it increasingly difficult to see close objects. Most people who have normal eyesight up to the age of forty begin to need glasses by their middle forties, especially for reading in artificial light. Check-ups every two to three years are advisable after the age of forty-five.

People are not usually aware of poor eyesight until it is corrected, and so some simple tests are useful. Anyone who cannot read a telephone directory at nineteen inches using *each eye separately*, has difficulty reading newspaper print with *each eye separately*, or cannot read a car number-plate at twenty-five yards with *each eye separately*, may need glasses and should get their eyes checked, (see Appendix Two for details of ophthalmic services available under the National Health Service).

Good lighting from behind is essential for easy reading. Eye exercises may help a person to interpret blurred images better and so may improve eyesight in that sense, but the most important way of correcting blurred vision will always be with glasses. Contrary to popular belief, it is not possible for an adult to strain his or her eyes, either by using them excessively or by using them in poorly lit conditions.

INFECTION
A bloodshot eye is often caused by a small blood-vessel bursting; this should not be a cause of worry and will heal without treatment. When the eye is red, or sticky, or watery, and also painful, you should consult a doctor. The irritation may be caused by a foreign body in the eye or by an infection, often a virus. Any mild inflammation of the eye or soreness which does not clear up in two days should also lead you to consult your doctor. Most eye infections are contagious, and so it is important that a person with infected eyes uses separate towels and face flannels.

ACCIDENTS
In many jobs it is important to wear protective glasses to prevent damage to the eyes. Strong infra-red light, such as

that given off by molten metal, can burn the lens or the retina, causing cataract or other forms of blindness. Ultra-violet light generated during welding may cause flash-burns to the cornea, which may cause temporary blindness: always use protective goggles or shields. Intense ultra-violet light reflected from snow can cause the same condition, when it is known as snow blindness; this can be prevented by special sunglasses (cheap sunglasses may not absorb harmful rays). Intense light reflected from water or sand may also cause discomfort, but is unlikely to do any permanent harm. Polaroid or reflecting sunglasses or a broad-brimmed hat provide the best protection.

Protection of the eyes against injury from foreign bodies is particularly important for people employed in workshops and factories. Special spectacles with side-cups may be sufficient but more elaborate protection in the form of face- and head-shields is available (see Chapter 7 for information on how to obtain advice about industrial safety). Do-it-yourself enthusiasts should take special care and invest in protective glasses. The greatest danger comes when hitting metal with metal, as when using a hammer and cold-chisel, because small chips of metal may fly into the eye at high speed.

A person who wears glasses and is also exposed to the possible hazard of flying objects hitting the eye should invest in plastic or toughened glasses with special side-cups for extra protection. It is vital that whatever eye protection is used is comfortable to wear, otherwise it will tend not to be used. If a chemical enters the eye, wash the eye out immediately with water by immersing the head in a basin and opening the eyelids with the fingers so that all the chemical is removed. Alternatively, the person may sit down with their head back, and while they hold the eye open a helper may gently pour about two pints of water over the eye; a teapot is ideal for this. Seek hospital attention at once unless the chemical is known to be mild.

PREVENTION OF BLINDNESS

Two of the most common causes of blindness in Western countries are glaucoma and the retinal changes associated with diabetes. These can usually be treated if discovered early. The common type of glaucoma usually gives no warning signs, and is only picked up during a routine eye examination. People who have a close relative with glaucoma should have their eyes examined regularly after the age of forty, as this disease tends to run in families. The less common acute glaucoma may be indicated by pain in the eye, headache, transient blurring of vision, especially in dim light, and the presence of coloured haloes around lights. The occurrence of any of these symptoms should lead a person to consult a doctor. Diabetics should have regular eye examinations, and close relatives of diabetics should have regular checks for diabetes, because this disease also tends to run in families.

Even more common than glaucoma and diabetes as causes of blindness are macular degeneration and cataract. Patients with macular degeneration are usually elderly and notice a slow deterioration in their ability to read and to recognize people's faces. They can often be helped by glasses or by other aids for low vision. Cataract, a condition in which the lens of the eye becomes opaque, produces a gradually increasing mistiness of vision which, if necessary, can be treated by an operation.

The Ears

Deafness is a terrible handicap, affecting to some extent one in every ten adults, and anything that can be done to prevent it is worthwhile. Most communication is based on speech, and inability to follow conversation means social isolation and often difficulty in finding work. Our ears are very delicate and easily damaged in a number of ways – many of which can be avoided. Simple hearing tests can in most cases quickly indicate which sort of hearing loss a person has.

PERCEPTIVE DEAFNESS

Sound-waves entering the ear are transmitted to the inner ear, known as the cochlea. The cochlea is connected with the brain via the auditory nerve. Damage to the cochlea produces a perceptive deafness (also called sensori-neural or sometimes nerve deafness). This is the commonest type of deafness. It cannot be cured by surgery, but can be helped by a hearing aid.

CONDUCTIVE DEAFNESS

This occurs when sound is blocked in its passage to the cochlea. The cause may be something simple, like wax blocking the outer-ear canal, or there may be disease of the eardrum or the middle ear. Many forms of conductive deafness may be corrected by surgery, and for this reason a specialist's opinion should always be sought. A hearing aid is often very useful for those suffering from this type of deafness.

CONGENITAL DEAFNESS

Being born deaf is a special handicap. Although many children who are born severely deaf learn to lip-read and to use what residual hearing they have, without the ability to hear their own voice their speech is often very strange and sometimes unintelligible to strangers. Thus, provision of a hearing aid can often help in speech production. The deafness may be due to a genetic abnormality that is inherited. If early deafness occurs in your family, or that of your partner, it may be advisable to seek genetic counsel before planning a family. One form of inherited deafness called otosclerosis, which causes severe conductive deafness in adult life, can now be cured by surgery.

German measles caught by mothers during pregnancy, particularly in the first three months, produces a high incidence of nerve deafness in children.

During childbirth it is not uncommon for the baby to become temporarily deprived of oxygen. The ear is very sensitive to the lack of oxygen, and deafness may result. It is now possible to detect hearing ability very early in childhood, using a computer to make special electrical measurements. Eventually, these methods will be available as a screening test for all young babies. When there is any doubt about a child's hearing ability these tests should be used, and if necessary a programme can be begun to make use of what hearing there is.

MAINTAINING THE BODYWORK/THE EARS

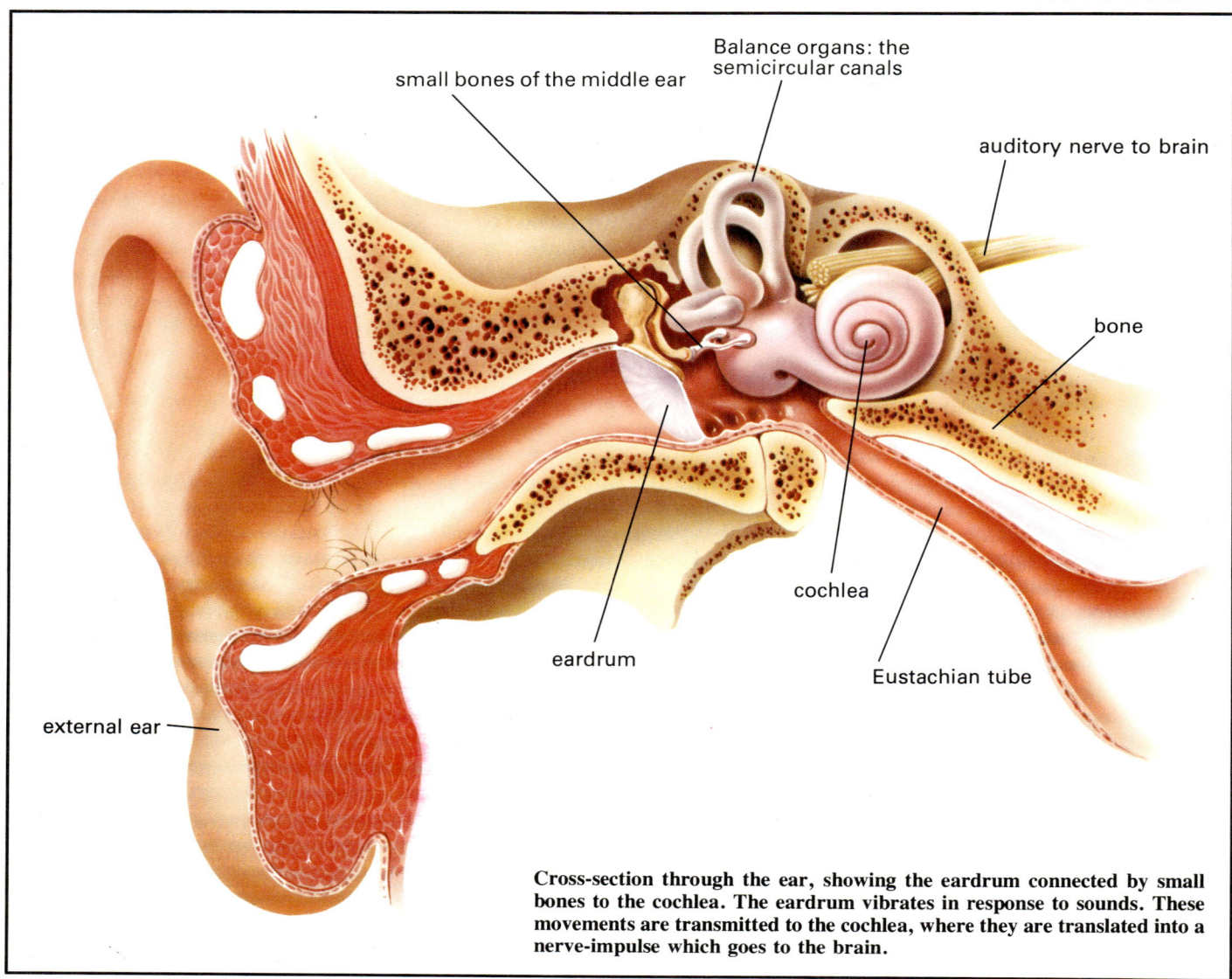

Cross-section through the ear, showing the eardrum connected by small bones to the cochlea. The eardrum vibrates in response to sounds. These movements are transmitted to the cochlea, where they are translated into a nerve-impulse which goes to the brain.

PROBLEMS WITH EARS

EARACHE IN CHILDHOOD
This can be alarming, but infection rarely nowadays results in permanent hearing impairment. This is largely due to the use of antibiotics. Any earache in a child which is not relieved by a pain-killer such as aspirin, or is associated with general illness or temperature, should be referred to the doctor. If there is a profuse and smelly discharge from the ear, this too is serious and needs immediate attention to avoid damage to the middle ear.

Mumps and measles very occasionally result in profound deafness. Measles can be avoided by vaccination (see page 32).

INJURY
Small children tend to push things into their ears and into those of their friends. More damage may be done in removing these than by pushing them in. Never make an attempt to remove them yourself but seek expert advice. The best way to remove foreign bodies from the ear is either by gentle syringeing or the use of a small suction apparatus. Poking and probing usually causes pain and bleeding, and pushes the object further down the ear.

A blow over the ear from a ball or from the flat of the hand may rupture the drum and occasionally disrupt the small bones of the middle ear. A conductive deafness results and there may also be pain and bleeding. For this reason never hit anyone over the ear. In fact, many perforations of the eardrum caused by a blow heal without treatment, but expert advice is always needed. More serious blows to the head which cause head injury may also result in deafness. Sometimes this is due to damage to the middle ear which may be correctable, but more commonly there is concussion of the inner ear, and the cochlea receives permanent damage. If there is a skull fracture this may involve the inner ear, and bleeding from the fracture may damage it permanently. Always wear proper head-protection when working in heavy industry, when riding a motor cycle or in any other potentially dangerous situation.

WAX
Wax can also cause conductive deafness but usually only if it is pushed down the ear canal. It is a popular misconception that the outer ear should be cleaned out with cotton buds, corners of towels and fingers. This pushes the wax, which is normally produced in the outer-ear canal, further down against the eardrum. In this position it causes uncomfortable blockage of the ear and mild deafness. If this

THE EARS/MAINTAINING THE BODYWORK

happens, medical advice should be sought and the wax removed by expert syringeing.

Irritation in the ear is also common and this may provoke more finger- and towel-poking. In addition to causing blockage by wax, infection may be introduced into the outer part of the ear. The majority of these cases can be avoided by leaving the ear canal entirely alone. If you do develop an irritation in the outer ear, seek medical advice.

NOISE EXPOSURE

It has been known since the first century AD that loud noise can damage the ear, but still many people exposed to this risk fail to wear simple ear-protection. The louder the noise, the shorter the length of exposure that is necessary to produce hearing loss. To begin with, this loss is temporary but eventually it becomes permanent. Noise arising from many leisure activities, from shooting to pop music at concerts or discos, can be sufficiently loud to cause hearing problems and even deafness. Seek expert advice (see Appendix Three).

Noise exposure in industry can produce permanent deafness, although the full effects may not be felt for many years. Where noise levels in a factory exceed 90 decibels – equivalent to the sound of a road-drill at five yards – ear protection should be worn at all times. A rough guide is that no one should be exposed to noise for any length of time which is so loud that normal conversation is impossible – although workers in such conditions often learn to lip-read and cease to be aware of the intensity of noise. A great deal can frequently be done to reduce noise in factories by surrounding noisy machines with baffles, or introducing noise-absorbing materials – but this is a job for experts. A wide variety of ear-plugs and ear-muffs are available which, while they do not exclude all sounds, do reduce them to safe levels.

In addition to deafness, excessive noise may produce

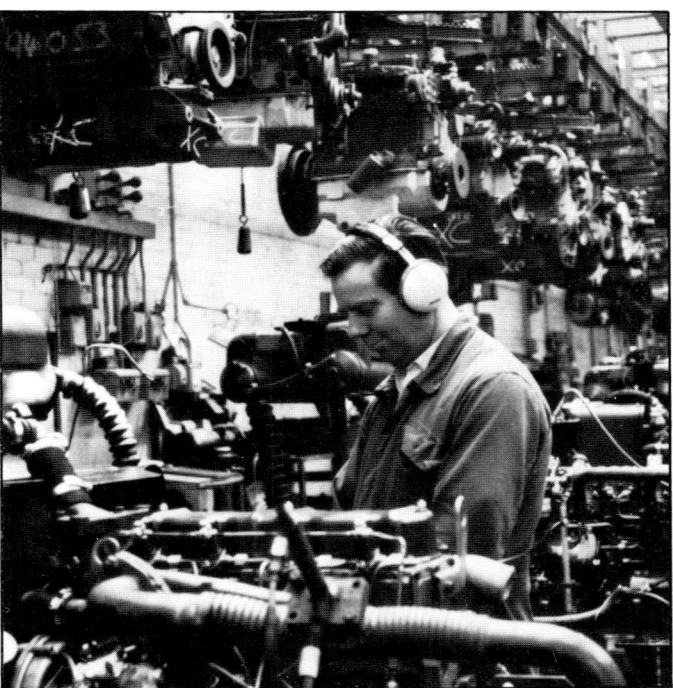

Loud noise is a major industrial hazard that can cause serious damage to hearing: always wear ear muffs, as this factory worker is doing, when noise exceeds 90 decibels (see page 156).

severe tinnitus. This takes the form of ringing, buzzing, or machinery-like noises generated in the damaged ear. It continues incessantly and can be extremely disturbing. In the initial stages the tinnitus will only occur after a noise exposure, and serves as a warning that you may be working in a hazardous environment. Tinnitus can occur as a consequence of almost any form of deafness. Tinnitus 'maskers' may be of benefit – these can be obtained through the National Health Service.

SUDDEN DEAFNESS

Sometimes, profound deafness occurs quite suddenly. It usually affects only one ear, and it is often difficult to find an exact cause. Sometimes the blood-supply to the cochlea is interrupted, owing to a spasm or a small clot in a blood-vessel. Prompt treatment aimed at increasing the blood-supply to the sensitive cochlea can sometimes restore hearing. It is always very important to seek specialist advice following sudden deafness.

AGE

Many people suffer increasing hearing loss for high-tone sounds as they get older. Although this is part of the natural ageing process, a hearing aid can be of assistance, but to gain the greatest benefit you should seek help as soon as you notice a deterioration in your hearing.

BALANCE

Dizziness often accompanies a hearing loss. The organs of balance and hearing are linked, as shown on the diagram. You should consult your GP if you have any unexplained dizziness; this may respond to treatment.

TRAVEL

Avoid flying with a cold if you possibly can. If you must, use a decongestant spray – available from chemists – for an hour or two before and during the flight to avoid pain in ears and possible complications. Consult a specialist if any pain, deafness or giddiness lasts longer than twenty-four hours.

HOW TO MANAGE A HEARING LOSS

The first thing is to get expert advice. If the hearing loss is conductive, it may be amenable to treatment or surgery; a hearing aid may help and should always be tried. Everyone makes use of visual clues during conversation, especially if there is a lot of background noise. People with a hearing loss should make greater efforts to watch the face of the person speaking to them.

The speaker should make every effort to speak clearly and not to shout. Make sure you are in a good light and that your face is not covered by a hand or pipe. All these things make lip-reading much more difficult. Above all, it is important to be patient. Deaf people find their difficulty in communicating extremely frustrating. Try not to treat them as if they were weak-minded.

The Royal National Institute for the Deaf can be a great source of assistance, offering advice on a wide variety of environmental aids, such as doorbell lights or vibration alarm clocks (see Appendix Three).

MAINTAINING THE BODYWORK/THE TEETH

The Teeth

Cleaning your teeth is a bore. That is partly why so many people have such rotten teeth. But we also make our teeth worse every day by eating the wrong things and, if we clean our teeth at all, often looking after them in the wrong way. The result: three in ten people in Britain over the age of sixteen have no natural teeth whatsoever. And many of those who still have their own teeth, regularly suffer from pain, bad breath and infected gums. Yet neither pain nor a toothless middle age are inevitable.

DIET: THE POSITIVE WAY TO PROTECT YOUR TEETH

You may never flash a film star's smile, but you will be saved a lot of pain and embarrassment if you think about what you eat. The basic rule is this: cut down on sugar. And cut out sweet things between meals. There is ample evidence to prove the link between sugar and tooth decay. Tooth decay became worse as the sugary content of our diet increased over the last hundred years. Eskimos, for instance, rarely suffered from tooth decay until they adopted the sweeter 'Western-style' diet. And there was less tooth decay during the Second World War when sugar was scarce and sweets rarer still.

If you must eat sugary things, do so at mealtimes. In 1954 the inmates of a Swedish institution were subjected to an experiment which showed that sweet things taken at mealtimes caused less decay than sweet things taken between meals. Drenching the teeth in sugar liquid makes the plaque produce more acid, which dissolves the protective enamel of the teeth. Many people believe that the unhealthy effects of a sweet diet can be avoided by eating honey instead. No such luck or, at least, no such evidence.

A sweet tooth is a habit which can be gradually altered by cutting down on sugar in cooking; the amount of sugar in cakes, for instance, can usually be halved without making much difference. But it is better never to allow children to develop a sweet tooth. Cut out all sweet snacks between meals and avoid sweetened drinks, especially the syrupy ones of the blackcurrant or rose-hip type. Beware, too, of babies' rusks, which may consist of almost 50 per cent sugar described – so that you would not know – as 'soluble carbohydrate'. Offer children (and adults) fruit or nuts as alternative snacks. An apple a day will not by itself keep the dentist at bay but it is certainly better for teeth than sweets.

If cutting out sugar is the most negative way towards better teeth, adding fluoride to our diet is the most positive way to reduce decay. Figures from the Netherlands, for example, show that fluoridation of the water-supply has reduced the amount of dental decay by some 50 per cent and the number of extractions by 85 per cent. Fluoride is a chemical compound which, in essence, hardens teeth to increase their resistance to decay. It can do this in two ways:
1. **Added to the diet:** This is especially effective for children since their teeth are still growing. The fluoride is absorbed into the bloodstream and incorporated in the tooth enamel.
2. **Brushed onto the teeth:** This makes the surface enamel of the teeth more resistant to decay.

Adding fluoride to the water-supply is the simplest and best way for a community to add fluoride to the diet, but it is also the most controversial. An alternative open to individuals is to buy it in tablet form from chemists. These can be swallowed one a day or, a better idea for children, crushed and added to food. And use fluoride toothpaste.

PLAQUE

Plaque is your enemy. It is a sticky white substance, consisting of millions of bacteria, which grows on the surface of everyone's teeth, feeding on the debris and food in the mouth. Plaque commonly accumulates between the teeth and at the edge of the gums where the attack begins. It attacks on two fronts. First, bacteria in the plaque produce an acid which attacks the enamel surface of the teeth causing them to decay. Second, it produces poisons which cause the gums to recede leading to pyorrhea (see below).

Acid from plaque bacteria gradually dissolves a hole in the enamel where other bacteria take over, causing caries, the familiar tooth decay. This is the major dental problem for people under thirty. If the caries is not removed by the dentist, then the decay will continue until it reaches the living pulp deep within the base of the tooth. Up to this point, the tooth will be painful only if it is stimulated by hot, cold or sweet food. But when the softer dentine beneath the enamel becomes infected, real toothache begins. When the pulp at the centre becomes infected, the tooth will become extremely painful. But this pain will suddenly cease as pressure builds up, cutting off the blood-supply and killing the nerves in the pulp. The relief is only short-lived. The infection passes through the minute nerve channel to create an abscess which causes more swelling of the gum and jaw.

SAVE YOUR GUMS

'I had to have all my teeth out although the dentist said they were perfect.' This unlikely tale is only too often true. Gum disease is the major problem for people over thirty, and again plaque is the cause. It collects at the base of the teeth, continually attacking the gums, and forms tartar, a hard white, brown or black deposit which irritates the gums, causing further soreness and swelling. The first symptoms are bleeding gums and a pink toothbrush; the gums themselves may be painless. These warning signs should be taken seriously and an urgent visit made to the dentist.

You can treat mild gum infection between just a few teeth yourself by removing offending plaque with a toothpick or floss and by thorough cleaning. Gum disease that is allowed to become really advanced through neglect is called pyorrhea, and it may have to be treated surgically by scraping and cutting away the unhealthy tissue. If gum disease is not treated it spreads to the root of the tooth which loosens in its socket and finally falls out. Regular careful toothbrushing is the only way to save your gums, although dentists can help through scaling and polishing.

CLEANING YOUR TEETH

Most of us skimp the tooth cleaning chore and many do it incorrectly, often doing more harm than good. To clean teeth effectively you must remove plaque from the crevices, gaps between the teeth and from around the edge of the gums. Plaque takes a long time to build up so it is probably sufficient to clean once a day, *if* you do a thorough job. Too many people push the brush in and out of the mouth, backwards and forwards. This wears a trough in the teeth and can damage the gums. To brush correctly, manipulate the bristles between the teeth into areas where the plaque accumulates. Give the crevices and the edges of the

THE TEETH/**MAINTAINING THE BODYWORK**

What a mouth

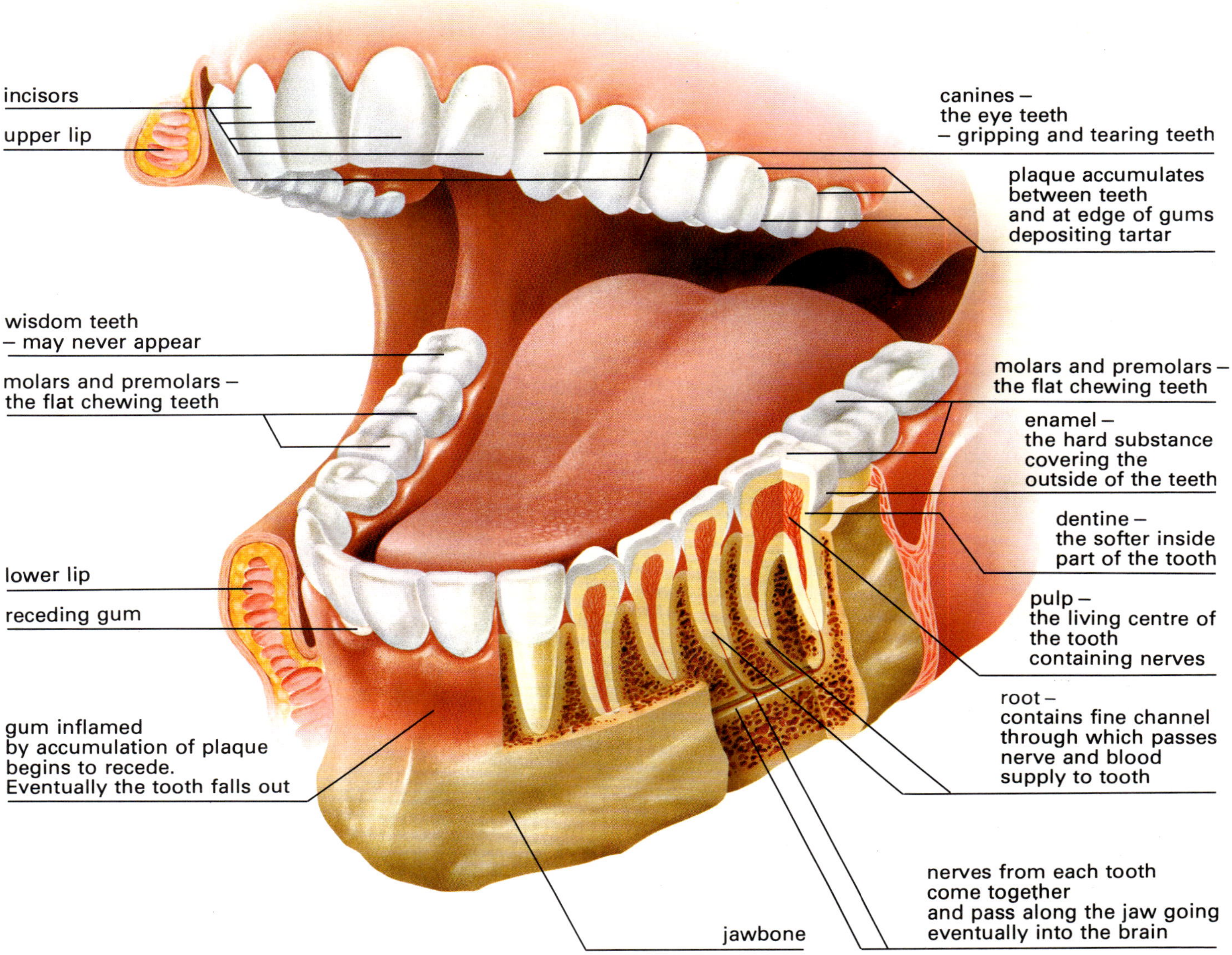

- incisors
- upper lip
- canines – the eye teeth – gripping and tearing teeth
- plaque accumulates between teeth and at edge of gums depositing tartar
- wisdom teeth – may never appear
- molars and premolars – the flat chewing teeth
- molars and premolars – the flat chewing teeth
- enamel – the hard substance covering the outside of the teeth
- dentine – the softer inside part of the tooth
- lower lip
- receding gum
- pulp – the living centre of the tooth containing nerves
- gum inflamed by accumulation of plaque begins to recede. Eventually the tooth falls out
- root – contains fine channel through which passes nerve and blood supply to tooth
- jawbone
- nerves from each tooth come together and pass along the jaw going eventually into the brain

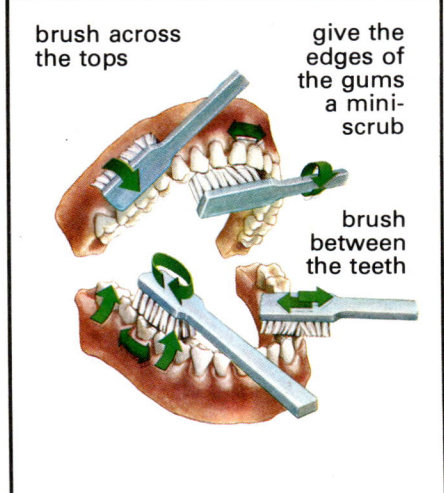

- brush across the tops
- give the edges of the gums a mini-scrub
- brush between the teeth

Brush with small circular movements first, then up and down, but not backwards and forwards.

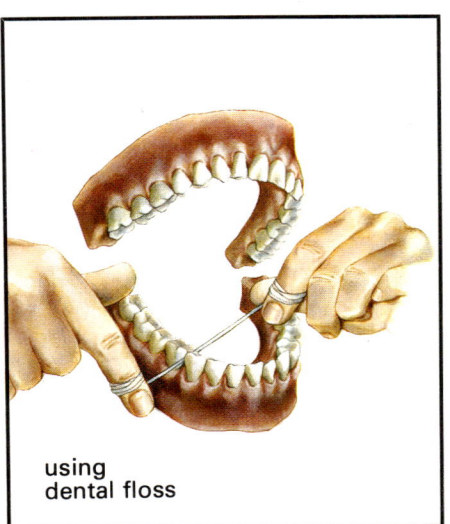

using dental floss

Dental floss is useful for removing stubborn pieces of food from *between* the teeth.

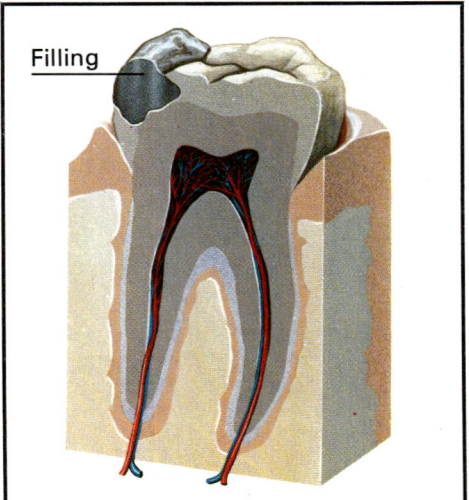

Filling

Cross-section of a molar tooth showing a filling – the most common of all dental repairs.

MAINTAINING THE BODYWORK/THE TEETH

gums a mini-scrub in a small circular motion, and then brush upwards and downwards to remove plaque from between the teeth.

There are sixteen surfaces of the teeth which should be cleaned: the insides, outsides and tops of the big chewing teeth in the upper and lower jaws, and the inside and outside of the cutting teeth at the front. It is no good just cleaning the outside as many people do. It should take you at least three minutes!

Is an electric toothbrush a con? Yes and no. They don't do anything that an ordinary toothbrush cannot do. But they do have the right scrubbing action and they are useful for disabled people who find it difficult to make the necessary arm movements.

Which brush is best? Use a soft or medium, nylon or bristle brush, not a hard one, since this can damage your gums. Choose a brush with a small head (one inch or less), because it is easier to ensure that each tooth is getting individual attention.

Are fluoride toothpastes best? Yes. Fluoride in toothpaste hardens the exposed surface-enamel of the teeth and this enables them to resist decay.

Dare you pick your teeth? Once only Hollywood tycoons (*circa* 1933) picked their teeth. Now nearly everyone does it, either discreetly in public or privately. A toothpick does two things: it removes awkward debris, and massages the gums where they meet the tooth. Choosing a toothpick is largely a matter for personal preference, but it must be the right size. If your gums have receded some way, you may need a thick pick; if the gaps are small, a slimmer one.

Is dental floss worth the fuss? Yes. Some stubborn pieces of food cannot be shifted with toothpicks and then you must use dental floss – a strong thread which can be passed between the teeth. You must do it in front of a mirror and take care not to damage the gums. Removing the stubborn plaque helps to prevent bad breath.

WHAT ABOUT THE KIDS?

Most important is to discourage children from eating sweets and taking sweet drinks between meals. Encourage them to drink water. This is more important than brushing, which is not really practicable until children are four or five – it should then begin as a game. Tooth-brushing should become routine, if possible, by the age of six, when the first adult teeth appear at the back of the mouth, before any of the milk teeth have been lost.

DOS AND DON'TS

Do visit your dentist twice a year for a check-up.

Do eat fruit or nuts if you must eat between meals.

Do brush your teeth properly at least once a day.

Do cut down on sweet things to eat and drink.

Don't put sugar in babies' bottles or drinks.

Don't give sweets as presents to children (or adults).

Don't give a baby a sweetened dummy to suck.

Don't be embarrassed about using toothpicks.

Don't take a sweet drink last thing at night.

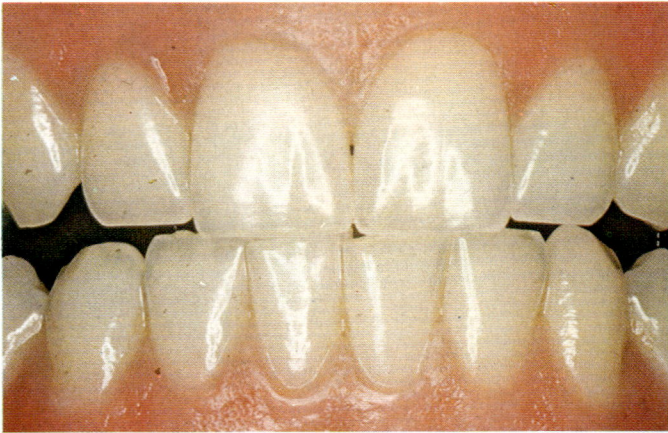
Perfect teeth: white and gleaming, all present (32 in all) with no gaps, and tight healthy gums.

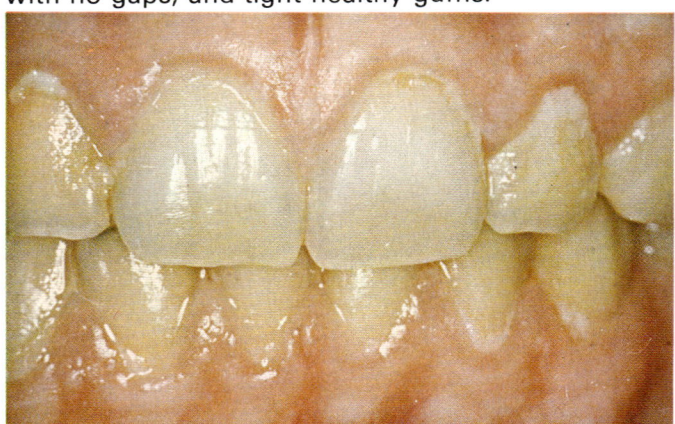
These teeth have not been cleaned for three days, and the result can be seen more clearly below.

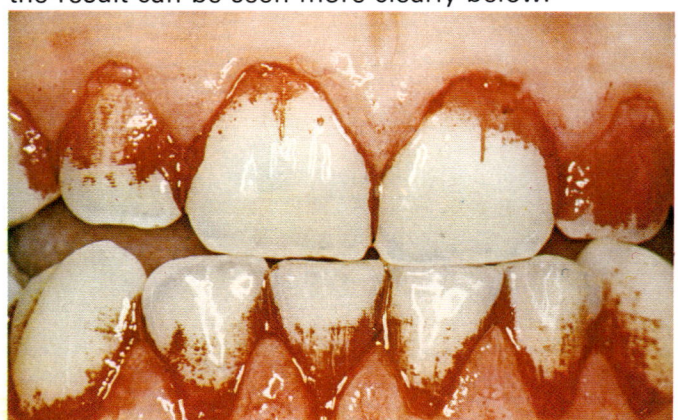
The same teeth washed with a pink 'disclosing' solution to reveal the full horror of plaque.

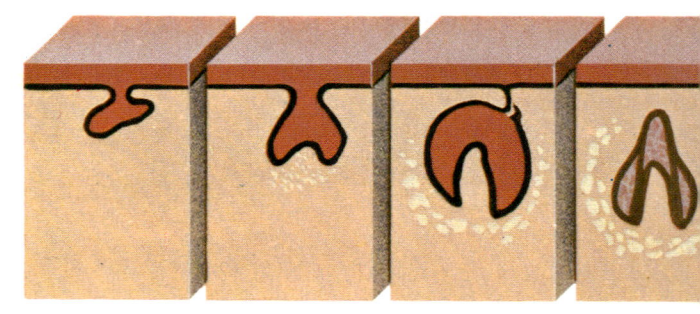
Stages in the growth of a tooth, originating (*left*) in the sk and above the skin.

*Photographs used by permission of the Royal Dental Hospital, London, and R. M. Callender of Gibbs Dental Research, London.

THE TEETH/MAINTAINING THE BODYWORK

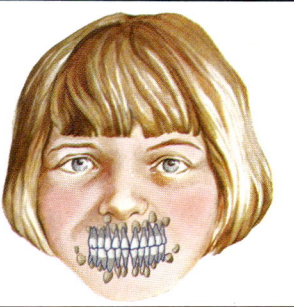

'Adult' teeth are present beneath the skin long before they begin to push out the baby teeth when a child is around six years old.

TOOTHACHE

So you have eaten the right things, brushed away zealously night and morning, picked away assiduously after meals, devotedly used fluoride toothpaste, regularly seen your dentist – and your teeth are hurting like hell. Don't despair and give up all your good habits; remember, you have probably had bad habits for longer. But do see a dentist urgently.

If you are really unlucky, of course, the toothache will strike at the weekend. You may be able to get emergency treatment at a large hospital with a dental casualty department. Most people will not be so lucky and will have to bear it until Monday. This is what you can do to help relieve the pain:

1. Take aspirin, compound codeine tablet or any proprietary pain-killer. *Swallow* it – never hold it in the cheek against the aching tooth since this will cause a painful ulcer or aspirin burn on the gums.
2. Try not to lie down, since this increases the blood-pressure in the head, and the pain.
3. Hot mouthwashes of salt and water may relieve the pain a little if gums are the problem (but not if the tooth is sensitive to heat) and continue to brush.
4. Finally, if things look really bleak, you could try a little whisky or other spirits. But if you have already taken some aspirin, spit out the whisky and use it simply as a mouthwash. Otherwise the combination of alcohol and aspirin may cause serious stomach irritation, which since the toothache will also still be there may not make drowning your sorrows seem quite such a good idea.

AT THE DENTIST'S

Not even the prettiest nurse, the softest music, the most comfortable bed-type 'chair' or the most riveting television programme is ever going to make the dental surgery particularly popular. Dentists are trying all these ideas to woo their patients, but none have had remotely the impact of the high-speed drills developed over the last twenty years. These mean the nastiest part of the dentist's work is over more quickly and less painfully. Anaesthetics are better, too, but be wary of the total anaesthetics favoured by some dentists. The British Dental Association says these should not be used unless another dentist or doctor is present to help in cases of difficulty. Local injections in the gum are certainly safer and normally just as effective. The three most common running repairs undertaken by dentists are:

1. **Scale and polish:** This removes the tartar and thus gives the gums a new lease of life and prevents decay. If you are lucky, scaling and polishing will be all the dentist prescribes on your six-monthly visit. If you're not so lucky, don't despair: remember those high-speed drills.

2. **Fillings:** The dentist begins by removing the decayed matter from the cavity with the drill. He then dries the cavity before filling it, usually with a mixture of mercury, silver, tin, zinc and copper known as mercury amalgam. It sets hard within about three minutes and continues to harden for several hours afterwards. The cavity must be shaped so that the filling cannot fall out after it sets, and so that the teeth can actually bite; the filling must be shaped so that food doesn't collect between the teeth. Mercury amalgam is grey in colour, so some people prefer white fillings, especially for the front teeth. These use a silica, plastic or composite material and are more expensive. Gold fillings are dearest of all and are usually used, if at all, in the back teeth for their toughness.

3. **Crowns:** When a tooth is badly damaged, the only way to repair it may be to make an entirely new 'crown'. The existing tooth is ground down to a peg and then an artificial crown is glued onto the peg. The new crown is made from plastic or silicone and can be matched with the existing teeth; or, if you're that way inclined, it can be made of gold. Whatever the colour, it takes several sessions with a dentist, and the more complicated the job, the higher the cost.

Remember that you should in any case see your dentist twice a year. Remember, too, that postponing a visit to the dentist doesn't make your teeth any better. The odds are that it will be still more painful next time.

WARNING SIGNS

If you notice any of the following symptoms, you should consult your dentist immediately:

1. Bleeding of your gums when brushing and flossing.

2. Persistent bad breath.

3. Soft, swollen, or tender gums.

4. Pus between the gums and the teeth.

5. Loose teeth.

6. Gums shrinking away from the teeth.

7. Any changes in the fit of your partial or complete dentures.

8. Any change in the spaces between your teeth or in the way your teeth come together.

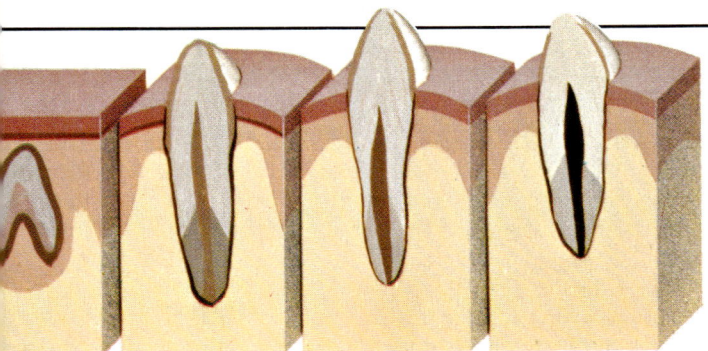

itself before its later development beneath

6: THE MAJOR HAZARDS

Smoking

If you are a smoker trying to give it up, you are a member of a large club. Four out of ten adults in the UK smoke, and half of them want to give it up. Unfortunately, about one half of male smokers and one third of female smokers continue to their last breath, even though they know how painful that last breath is likely to be.

The high failure-rate in attempts to give up smoking is because, for most smokers, it is more an addiction than a simple pleasure. Many smokers might deny this. But smoking is obviously not a pleasure in the sense that eating fish and chips or listening to Mozart or riding on roundabouts can be pleasures. People are not normally bad-tempered because they have not had their first Mozart record or roundabout ride of the day. And there cannot be many people so driven by a passion for fish and chips that they scour a deserted town late at night looking for a source of supply.

Breaking an addiction is different from giving up a pleasure. The reasons for breaking this particular addiction are numerous. For, whatever the disagreement about the extent of smoking's contribution to various illnesses, there is no medical expert in the world who claims that it does you good.

Why give it up? Everyone knows about the link between smoking and lung cancer, but not everyone appreciates what this means. Young people, in particular, can be vague about this hazard. This is a pity since they will have smoked, if at all, for only a short time and will not be strongly addicted.

Cancer is a disease in which the cells that make up some part of the body, in this particular case the lungs or larynx (voice box), multiply wildly, without any control. The sufferer, in the early stages, will be unaware of this, but in the case of cancer of the larynx will soon notice a persistent cough or a change in the quality of the voice. In the case of lung cancer, the sufferer may spit up blood when coughing, or develop a severe pain in the chest.

Operations for lung cancer are only possible in one in five cases, and less than one in twenty are cured. In Britain, almost a hundred people die every day from lung cancer: over thirty-eight thousand people a year. This is nearly six times the number who die on the roads, and should be reason enough to give up smoking, especially as half the victims are under sixty-five. But lung cancer is only one penalty of smoking.

Another is chronic bronchitis. It may sound more like a complaint than a disease but it, too, kills twenty-four thousand people a year. Bronchitis begins as a smoker's cough, clearing from the air-passages of the throat and lungs a slimy mucus produced by the irritating smoke that eventually starts to clog the lungs themselves. The smoke also damages the small air-tubes and the air-sacs, so that the victim cannot get enough air into the lungs and the blood cannot get the oxygen the body needs without desperate efforts to breathe. The shortness of breath may be so severe that the victim of chronic bronchitis cannot walk far without severe discomfort. In extreme cases, a victim may

The effect of one cigarette in patients with coronary artery disease.

One cigarette increases the heartbeat from about 77 beats per minute to 88 beats per minute, blood-pressure increases slightly and fats in the blood increase in concentration. These factors acting together cause the accumulation of fatty deposits (atheroma) in the arteries, leading to atherosclerosis and heart disease.*

*Source: Paper presented by Dr S. H. Taylor, University Department of Cardiovascular Studies and Department of Medical Cardiology, Leeds General Infirmary, to International Symposium, St Moritz, January 1976.

be confined to bed and only be able to move around the house on his hands and knees.

Other complaints caused by smoking are severe heart and blood-vessel diseases which kill many thousands of people every year. Smoking also causes cancer of the mouth and bladder, which together with cancer of the larynx account for several thousand deaths a year. If these do not kill, they can cripple. Some people suffer from these illnesses without ever having smoked in their lives, of course.

But *without exception* the risk increases dramatically if you do smoke. You are twice as likely to suffer from heart disease, for instance, and four or five times as likely in the thirty-five to forty-four age group, if you smoke. Pregnant women have a particular incentive to give up smoking: it can harm the unborn child, as explained in Chapter 1.

The list of afflictions is so grim that many people need read no further, but avoiding diseases is not the only reason for not smoking. Very soon after you stop, you will discover that you feel better, suffer less of the clogged-up feeling common among smokers, and are better able to taste and enjoy food. And at whatever stage you stop smoking, it will lessen your chances of falling victim to the smoking-related diseases described above.

It really is worth giving up. The first benefit you will notice is that cough and phlegm will gradually decrease and you become less liable to chest infections. If you suffer from breathlessness, that may also decrease on giving up. In some people permanent damage has been done and their breathlessness does not improve much; even for them, however, it stops getting worse, and a real benefit is still gained from being less liable to infection.

The long-term risks of premature death through lung cancer or bronchitis also begin to improve on giving up. A classic study of British doctors who gave up smoking shows that their health steadily improved. After five years the risk fell to about one half of the risk for men who continued to smoke, and after fifteen years the risk had nearly returned to normal. The heavy smoker has a two out of five chance of dying before retirement, while for the non-smoker the risk is one in five.

The 1976 follow-up study of the smoking habits of thirty-four thousand British doctors, started over twenty years ago, confirms the risk of smoking cigarettes. Between a third and a half of those who continued to smoke died prematurely of it. The earlier they stopped, the less likely was a premature death, although they never reached the survival rates of life-long non-smokers. Not starting is best, but giving up is always worthwhile.

The latest report of the Royal College of Physicians, *Smoking or Health*, says that smoking is continuing to decline among professional men and managers – only one in three now smoke, whereas almost two out of three manual workers smoke. However, the number of working women who smoke is continuing to increase. The report states that a smoker loses on average five and a half minutes of his life for every cigarette smoked. The report warns that tobacco smoking is a form of drug dependence different from, but no less strong than, dependence on other drugs of addiction. It says that the majority of adolescents who try smoking become dependent on it, and so special efforts must be made to protect children against acquiring the habit in their formative years.

If you feel any responsibility for others, you will also want to stop smoking. If you smoke, anyone who shares space with you will effectively smoke the equivalent of perhaps five cigarettes a day by inhaling the smoke-laden air. The nearer and dearer people are to you, the more likely it is that they will share the afflictions your cigarettes produce. Husbands, wives, lovers and children may thus suffer the irritations and ill-effects of smoke. A Scandinavian survey of families found that if neither parent smoked, and both were vocally opposed to smoking, only 10 per cent of the children took up the habit; if both parents smoked and were permissive about smoking, 70 per cent of the children followed their parents.

REDUCING THE RISKS

The simple answer is 'Just stop'. It is not that simple, of course, otherwise more people would succeed. You may be one of the lucky ones who can stop quite easily once they have really decided to. About one in three smokers are like this. You will have to *want* to stop smoking. Nobody can succeed against their will. Most anti-smoking experts say the only long-term guarantee of success is to stop altogether: compulsive gamblers and alcoholics face the same recommendation. But some half-measures are better than nothing. For instance, the most dangerous constituent of a cigarette is tar, which is known to contain the cancer-producing substances. And the most dangerous part of a cigarette is the final third, where the tar and nicotine tend to condense. These two facts alone suggest the following simple and sensible 'half-measures':

1. Leave long stubs.
2. Smoke filter cigarettes with a low tar-rating.
3. Avoid inhaling.
4. Smoke fewer cigarettes.
5. Take fewer puffs from each cigarette.
6. Never leave the cigarette dangling in your mouth.

If you can cut down the volume of smoking to, say, five a day, then the effect of your action will obviously help. But few people in practice can keep themselves for very long to the 'one or two a day after meals' that they claim, and few are successful at leaving long stubs or avoiding inhaling. Moving down the tar table seems like a good idea but most smokers compensate by inhaling more and so end up with just as much tar in their lungs. Except with the very low tar cigarettes, little or nothing may be gained. It is much better to aim for a complete break, and there are some ways of making the going a little easier. Begin by trying to recognize the kind of smoker you are.

WHAT KIND OF SMOKER ARE YOU?

Here are some statements made by people to describe what they get out of smoking cigarettes. How often do you feel this way when smoking? Answer every question, and score as follows: Always – 5; Frequently – 4; Occasionally – 3; Seldom – 2; Never – 1.

A. I smoke cigarettes in order to keep myself from slowing down.
B. Handling a cigarette is part of the enjoyment of smoking.
C. Smoking cigarettes is pleasant and relaxing.
D. I light up a cigarette when I feel angry about something.

THE MAJOR HAZARDS/SMOKING

E. When I have run out of cigarettes I find it almost unbearable until I can get them.
F. I smoke cigarettes automatically without even being aware of it.
G. I smoke cigarettes to stimulate me, to perk myself up.
H. Part of the enjoyment of smoking a cigarette comes from the steps I take to light up.
I. I find cigarettes pleasurable.
J. When I feel uncomfortable or upset about something, I light up a cigarette.
K. I am very much aware of the fact when I am not smoking a cigarette.
L. I light up a cigarette without realizing I still have one burning in the ashtray.
M. I smoke cigarettes to give me a 'lift'.
N. When I smoke a cigarette, part of the enjoyment is watching the smoke as I exhale it.
O. I want a cigarette most when I am comfortable and relaxed.
P. When I feel 'blue' or want to take my mind off cares and worries, I smoke cigarettes.
Q. I get a real gnawing hunger for a cigarette when I haven't smoked for a while.
R. I've found a cigarette in my mouth and didn't remember putting it there.

Scoring: Enter the points scored on each question below and then add up each of the six totals:

$$\overline{A} + \overline{G} + \overline{M} = \overline{\text{Stimulation}}$$

$$\overline{B} + \overline{H} + \overline{N} = \overline{\text{Handling}}$$

$$\overline{C} + \overline{I} + \overline{O} = \overline{\text{Pleasure}}$$

$$\overline{D} + \overline{J} + \overline{P} = \overline{\text{Support}}$$

$$\overline{E} + \overline{K} + \overline{Q} = \overline{\text{Craving}}$$

$$\overline{F} + \overline{L} + \overline{R} = \overline{\text{Habit}}$$

WHAT THE SCORES MEAN

Any higher than 11 indicates you smoke for that reason. Scores of 7 or less are low, scores in between are marginal. The higher your score (15 is the highest), the more important a particular factor is in the reasons or motivation for your smoking.

Stimulation: If you score high or fairly high on this factor, it means that you are one of those smokers who is stimulated by the cigarette; you feel that it helps you wake up, organize your energies, and keep you going. If you try to give up smoking, you may want a safe substitute such as a brisk walk, moderate exercise or a cup of coffee whenever you feel the urge to smoke.

Handling: Handling things can be satisfying, but there are ways to keep your hands busy without lighting up or playing with a cigarette. Why not toy with a pen or pencil, or try doodling, or playing with a coin, a piece of jewellery or some other harmless object.

Pleasure: It is not always easy to find out whether you use the cigarette to feel good, to get real, honest pleasure out of smoking. About two-thirds of smokers score high or fairly high on the 'pleasure' factor and about half of those also score as high or higher on the 'support' factor. Those who do get real pleasure out of smoking often find that sufficient consideration of the harmful effects of their habit will help them to stop. They substitute eating, drinking and social activities – within reasonable bounds – and find they do not seriously miss their cigarettes.

Support: Many smokers use cigarettes as a kind of support in moments of stress or discomfort, and on occasions it may work; the cigarette is sometimes used as a tranquillizer. But heavy smokers, those who try to handle severe personal problems by smoking many times a day, are apt to discover that cigarettes do not help them deal with their problems effectively. When it comes to stopping, this kind of smoker may find it easy to give up when everything is going well, but may be tempted to start again in a time of crisis. Again, physical exertion, eating, drinking, or social activity – in moderation – may serve as useful substitutes for cigarettes, even in times of tension. The choice of a substitute depends on what will achieve the same effect without having the same appreciable risk.

Craving: Giving up smoking is difficult for people who score high on this factor, that of psychological addiction. For them, the craving for the next cigarette begins to build up the moment they put one out, so tapering off is not likely to work. They must stop dead. It may be helpful for them to smoke more than usual for a day or two so that the taste for cigarettes is spoiled, and then isolate themselves completely from cigarettes until the craving is gone; this may take several months. Giving up cigarettes may be so difficult and cause so much discomfort that once they do stop, they will find it easy to resist the temptation to go back to smoking.

Habit: This kind of smoker is no longer getting much satisfaction from cigarettes, but just lights them, frequently without even realizing he is doing so. He may find it easy to stop permanently if he can break the habit patterns he has built up. Cutting down gradually may be quite effective if there is a change in the way the cigarettes are smoked. The key to success is becoming aware of each cigarette you smoke.

Conclusion: If you do not score high on any of the six factors, the chances are that you do not smoke very much or have not been smoking for very many years. If so, giving up smoking – and staying off – should be relatively easy. If you score high on several categories you apparently get several kinds of satisfaction from smoking, and will have to find several solutions. Those who score high on both the Support and Craving factors may have a particularly hard time in giving up smoking and in staying off. They can try the half-measures suggested above, and after several months of this temporary solution they may find it easier to stop.

Many people smoke 'automatically'. As they pick up a telephone, or finish a meal or settle in a car, or start to drink coffee, or even as they wake up, they suddenly find they have a cigarette in their hands. If you have noticed these habits you will not be surprised to find 'something missing' when you stop. People who smoke out of 'habit' should therefore try to change their routine. Don't smoke first thing in the morning. Try to delay your first cigarette by an extra fifteen minutes each day. Go for a short walk after dinner. Simply leaving a gap where once you smoked is a bit

SMOKING/**THE MAJOR HAZARDS**

unnerving: establishing a new routine will help break the addiction.

Changing to pipes and cigars, which can be less harmful, is not really the best way to avoid the risks. First, it is not available to everyone. Our society may be permissive, but it still looks at a pipe-smoking woman with a bit of surprise. What is more, most of the statistics about the relative safety of pipe- and cigar- smoking are based on people who have always smoked them and have never inhaled deeply. Former cigarette smokers continue to inhale when they smoke a pipe or cigars and so there is little or no benefit in such a change for them.

There is no substitute for actually stopping smoking, and if you are to stop, there is no substitute for clearly wanting to. Some people go to smoking withdrawal clinics, for example, with a vague hope that somehow or other the clinic will make the decision for them. If you do sincerely want to become a non-smoker, there is a wide range of aids. There is no miracle cure, and the idea that there is one is harmful: people can try something, fail, and decide that their case is hopeless. Virtually every method of giving up has at best a low success-rate: it works for roughly 30 per cent of those who try it. But the 70 per cent are not the same people for every method. Somewhere or other, there is a method for almost everyone, and if you have not succeeded with one, try another. If you have not been able to make the decision to give up before, that does not mean you will not be able to this time. A lot of people have to try a few times before they give up smoking for good.

There is a range of what may be called pharmaceutical aids available from chemists. If you want to try them, you will have to pay for the tablets or solutions yourself; on the other hand, they are much cheaper than the cigarettes you would smoke during the cure, let alone during the rest of your life. 'Aversion compounds' form one group of chemical aids. These usually contain a silver salt that makes cigarette-smoke taste foul: no one will continue smoking while using the tablets, mouthwash or gum, but of course a lot of people abandon the treatment. There are also tablets containing lobeline, a chemical that the manufacturers claim gives the satisfaction of nicotine without the harmful or addictive effects. They obviously do so for some people, and while it is difficult to be sure what fraction of users this represents, it could turn out to be the method that works for you.

Some smokers find nicotine chewing gum (brand name Nicorette) helps them to give up. This gum, which can be obtained from your doctor on a private prescription, contains a small amount of nicotine, the most addictive substance in cigarette smoke. The nicotine from the gum is absorbed through the mouth into the blood and so helps to satisfy the body's craving for it. However, the gum does not give the same satisfaction as cigarettes, and after a few weeks or months most people find it easy to stop chewing. A lot of people have found the gum very helpful, but again it is not infallible. It will not help you to give up unless you have made the decision yourself. Also, the gum does not taste very pleasant; it is quite expensive (though cheaper than cigarettes); and you have to chew it in a special way – very slowly.

Many people find that their resolve weakens without support, and smoking withdrawal clinics may help them. The clinics are free, or virtually so, and will often supplement their psychological approach with some of the pharmaceutical aids (see Appendix Three).

People, it is sad to report, will offer you cigarettes when they know you have given them up. Be firm, or abusive, or full of suspicious insight: why are they doing this? Or if they insist, accept the cigarette and tear it up. People who still smoke owe it to others not to offer cigarettes to anyone who is trying to stop. In fact, it is not a bad general rule never to offer cigarettes, as it leads to over-smoking in the same way as dutifully buying your round of drinks leads to overdrinking. And as some people's smoking is limited by the cost, don't give cigarettes as presents, and don't bring people cheap cigarettes from foreign trips. Don't, finally, smoke when children are about: your example, as well as your smoke, is harmful. Anyone who smokes owes a lot of consideration to those who do not. And a smoker who thinks enough about this obligation may even decide to give the habit up.

LOW-TAR CIGARETTES

Until recently everyone hoped that the risks of smoking might be reduced by persuading smokers to change to low-tar cigarettes. Low-tar cigarettes produce less tar and nicotine than high-tar cigarettes when smoked by a machine which smokes each cigarette in exactly the same way. However, smokers are not machines, and it is not difficult for a determined smoker to get as much nicotine and hence tar from a low-tar cigarette as from a high-tar cigarette. To do this, the smoker only has to puff harder, inhale deeper and hold the puff down longer. So changing to low-tar cigarettes can be self-defeating unless you make a determined effort at the same time to avoid inhaling more deeply – but most smokers find this even harder than giving up. Without thinking a smoker alters his smoking habit until he gets the 'satisfaction' – the relief of nicotine addiction – which he seeks. For this reason we have not reproduced the government tar tables in this book. The risks of smoking can be more reliably reduced by smoking fewer cigarettes or leaving longer butts, and best of all by giving up altogether.

YOU CAN GIVE UP SMOKING

On the following three pages we give advice on how to give up smoking published by the Health Education Council (78 New Oxford Street, London WC1A 1AH) and available from them as a free booklet.

Stopping smoking takes time. There are four stages:

1. You think about your reasons for stopping.
2. You prepare to stop.
3. You do it. Just stop.
4. You work on staying stopped.

Stage 1 can take anything from a few days to a few years. Stages 2 and 3 can be over in hours or may take weeks. Stage 4 is vital – it may be some months before you can be confident that you will never want another cigarette.

If you get to Stage 4 and then slip back, just start again from the beginning. Many people have to try a few times before they stop smoking for good.

If you've tried before and failed, still have another go. If you're not sure you can make it, think of this: there are eight million people in this country who have stopped smoking. So you can do it too.

How to Give Up Smoking

1. THINK ABOUT STOPPING

The big question is: do you *really* want to stop? Because this is the key to success. Make up your mind you are going to stop, and you will. Lots of people have been surprised how easy it was to stop once they had really made up their minds.

To help you make your decision, think about what you gain by stopping.

RIGHT AWAY
● You will be free from an expensive and damaging habit.
● You'll have another £5–£10 a week to spend.
● You'll smell fresher. No more bad breath, stained fingers or teeth.
● You'll be healthier and breathe more easily – for example, when you climb stairs or run for a bus.
● And you'll be free of worry that you may be killing yourself.

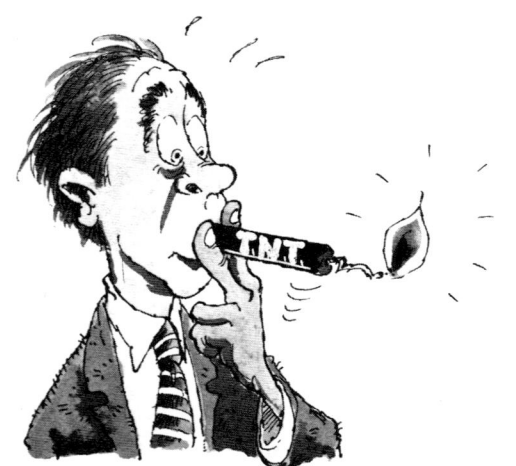

You'll be free of the worry that you may be killing yourself.

FOR THE FUTURE
● You will lose your smoker's cough.
● You will suffer fewer colds and other infections.
● And you will avoid the dangers that smokers have to face.

Many people killed by smoking could have lived 10, 20, even 30 or more years longer. On average, people killed by smoking lose 10 to 15 years of their lives.

Among 1,000 young men who smoke, about 6 will be killed on the roads but about 250 will be killed before their time by tobacco.

Women who smoke when they are pregnant run a greater risk of miscarriage or of their baby being born premature or underweight.

If you stop smoking before you have got cancer or serious heart or lung disease from smoking, then you will avoid nearly all the risks of death or disability from smoking.

FAMILY AND FRIENDS
Once you stop smoking, your family and friends gain too.
● They can enjoy fresher air.
● You'll be nicer to be with. Remember the slogan 'Kiss a non-smoker and taste the difference.'
● Children who live in smoke-free homes are much less likely to get colds and even pneumonia.
● If you don't smoke, your children are less likely to start.
● And although the main risk of smoking is to the smoker, non-smokers who live with a smoker have a higher chance of getting chest diseases.

For you, your family and friends, the benefits of stopping start on the day you stop smoking, and go on for good.

SO WHAT'S STOPPING YOU?

'I've tried before but the craving was too strong.'
However strong the craving may be at first, it will eventually go away so long as you don't give in to it. It goes away much more quickly if you don't sneak the odd cigarette.

'Right now is a bad time to try.'
It's true that there are some bad times for stopping – for example, when you're under a lot of stress. So try to choose a good time. But take care. Make it soon. It's easy to go on finding excuses for not stopping.

'I might fail.'
You won't know till you've tried. Anyway, even if you don't make it the first time, you will if you keep at it. Quite a lot of people try several times before they succeed.

'Yes. I'll give up. Some time.'
Give up now. The longer you go on smoking, the more damage you'll do to yourself. And you'll make it more difficult to stop.

SMOKING/THE MAJOR HAZARDS

'I'll lose my only pleasure in life.'
Just wait to see how much better it is to be a non-smoker. After you've beaten the habit, life will be much more worth living. For example, you'll taste and enjoy your food more.

'I can't inflict it on my family. I'd be impossible to live with.'
Think of what you're inflicting on your family now with all that pollution. A few weeks' bad temper is worth it for a longer, healthier life.

'I wouldn't be able to cope without cigarettes.'
Try it and see. You coped well enough before you smoked and you will again once you have stopped.

'I'll put on weight if I stop.'
Yes, you might put on weight, but you'll probably lose it again within a few months, especially if you take a little extra care about what you eat. Smoking is much more harmful to you than putting on weight, so it's vital to solve that problem first.

'I know someone who smoked like a chimney and lived to 84.'
But people don't talk about all the smokers who never even reach retirement.

'But I'm only a moderate smoker.'
Unfortunately, even a few cigarettes a day are dangerous.

'I smoke low tar cigarettes.'
Don't let anyone fool you. Low tar cigarettes are still very dangerous. The only safe cigarette is an unlit one.

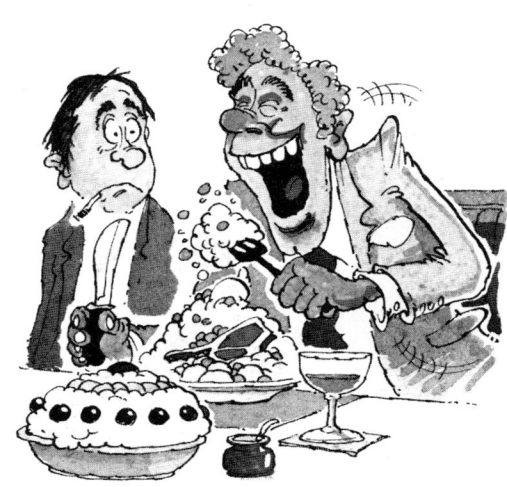

You'll taste and enjoy your food more.

2. PREPARE TO STOP

BREAK THE HABIT
Smoking is a habit that's closely linked to certain times and places. If you break these links, you can break the habit. The best way of doing this is to avoid the situations where you want a cigarette. If you can't avoid them, then you will have to fight off the temptation.

Sit down and think about when and where you usually have a cigarette. For example, do you always have one after breakfast? After other meals? In breaks at work? When you're watching television? With friends in the pub? Once you stop smoking, these times and places are going to be the danger spots, so work out now how you are going to cope with them.

It will also help if you can make new habits to break the old one of smoking. So plan some new activities to replace smoking – things to distract yourself, things to do with your hands, and different ways to cope with tension.

Some people find it helps if they cut down on cigarettes before they actually give up. It's one way of preparing for the day you stop for good. But don't look on cutting down as an alternative to giving up, and don't do it for more than a couple of weeks at the very most. The danger is that you go back to smoking as many as you did before.

GET SOME HELP
Try to get some help from your friends and family.
● Get them to sponsor you to stop.
● Make a bet with someone that you will stop for so long – say, three months.
● Make an agreement to stop with someone else.
● Talk to your family. Tell them what you are going to do and why. Ask them to help by being patient.

PICK A DAY
Decide when you are going to stop. Make it a day when you will not be under much stress. The day before, get rid of all your cigarettes, ashtrays and lighters.

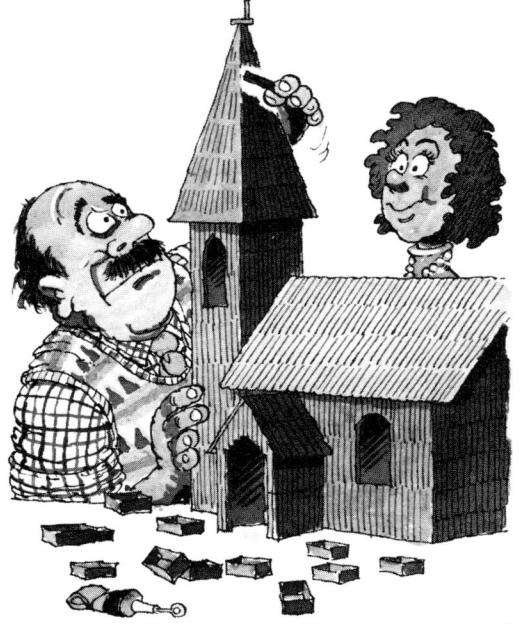

Plan some new activities to replace smoking.

THE MAJOR HAZARDS/SMOKING

3. STOPPING

A BIG DAY
Stopping smoking for ever seems like a big step. So just take it one day at a time.

Make the first day a big day.

Maybe stay in bed extra late – or get up specially early.

Have a long bath.

Have fruit juice for breakfast – the taste is fresh and the acidity will help get rid of the nicotine.

Plan a treat for the end of the day as a reward for not smoking.

CHANGE YOUR ROUTINE
Put your planning and preparation into practice. Try hard to change your routine so you avoid the situations in which you know you'll get a strong urge to smoke. The more you change your routine, the easier it will be to stop. You won't have to avoid the danger situations for ever but just for a few weeks until you have learnt to cope better with the urge to smoke.

DO SOMETHING ELSE
If you do feel a strong urge to smoke, then the important thing is to do something else instead.

If you just sit there wanting a cigarette, and worrying about it, you'll probably end up smoking. But if you get up and do something else, you'll find it easier to resist the temptation. For example, if you usually smoke after a meal, get up straightaway – even if it's only to do the washing up. If you can't do something, try and *think* about other things. Distract yourself from the idea of smoking and it will go away.

Find your own little dodges to help you get over the first few weeks. Some people find it helps to have something to do with their hands, like knitting, or playing with a bunch of keys. Some people find something to chew or suck. Some drink a glass of water every time they want a cigarette.

SIDE EFFECTS WILL PASS
Remember that up until now you have probably taken 100 to 400 puffs of tobacco every day and your body has got used to a constant supply of nicotine. At first you may be irritable and unable to concentrate. You may get wide swings of mood, happy one minute, depressed the next. You may get stomach upsets, and even a bad cough as the cleaning action in your lungs gets started. If you do get any of these side effects, don't worry. It may take some time to establish the habit of not smoking. Any side effects are all part of the process of getting better and should pass in a few weeks. If they do go on longer, then check with your doctor.

You may get no bad effects at all! Many people find they get all the benefits of stopping with very few or none of the problems.

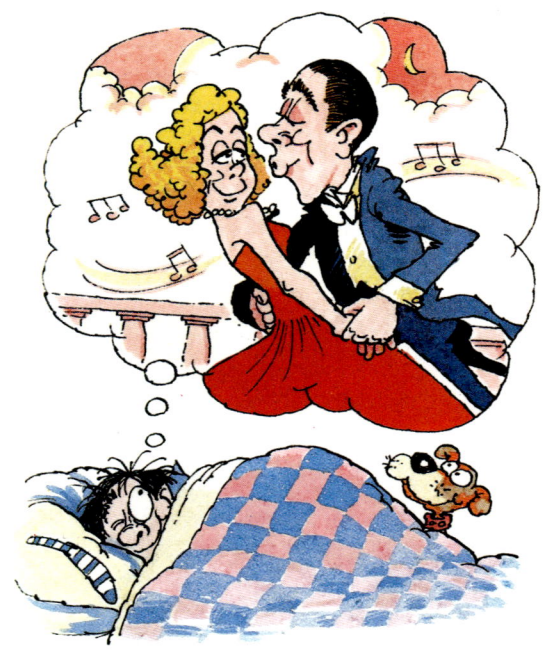

Maybe stay in bed extra late . . . plan a treat for the end of the day as a reward.

NOW YOU'VE STOPPED

KEEP AT IT
After your first enthusiasm has worn off, *keep at it*. Don't let yourself slip back. Don't smoke any cigarettes at all.

Practise looking in the mirror and saying 'No thanks, I don't smoke.' That way you'll be able to cope with smokers who want you to smoke so that *they* will feel less guilty.

Put aside the money you would have spent on cigarettes and watch it grow.

Give yourself lots to do. Clean the house, do some decorating, get out more. Go to places where you wouldn't think of smoking.

Do something active. Play some sport. Go for walks or for a run. Get others to join you so you can share the pleasure.

Keep reminding yourself of the benefits you've gained by stopping: you smell fresher, you breathe clean air, you have more money, and most important of all, you are much less likely to die young.

SMOKING/THE MAJOR HAZARDS

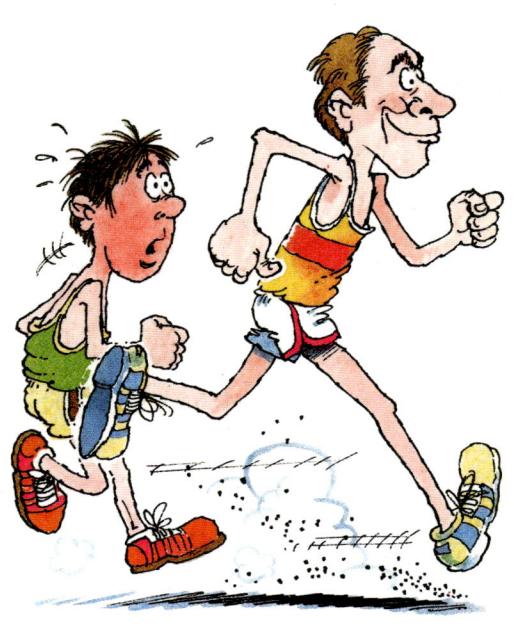

LEARN TO RELAX
You can help yourself to relax. Lie down and check every muscle in your body one by one. Start with your feet, your calves and so on. If you find a muscle that is tense, tighten it up hard, hold it for a few seconds, then let it relax.

Work over your whole body, finishing with your face and scalp. You'll be surprised how much tension you find in your body. Or try this: Sit in an upright chair in a quiet room. Shut your eyes and listen to your breathing. Count your breaths. If you find your mind wandering off to think of other things, just go back to counting your breaths again.

Go for a run. Get others to join you so you can share the pleasure.

4. STAYING STOPPED

Now people are no longer making a fuss over how well you've done. They think it's all over. But for you, this is the time that really counts.

DON'T BE TAKEN IN
If you found it easy to stop, you may think you could have the odd cigarette and stop again any time you want to. Don't kid yourself. For one thing, next time might not be as easy. Also, there's a part of you that wants to start smoking again and will find all sorts of excuses to smoke – 'One cigarette won't hurt,' 'This wasn't a good time to stop,' 'Maybe I'll wait until I find a painless cure,' and so on.

Don't be taken in by these excuses. There is no magic cure. It's up to you. You just have to work at breaking the habit for good.

TREAT YOURSELF
Every time you feel like smoking, remind yourself how much healthier you are now you've stopped. And wealthier too. Treat yourself or the family with the money you've saved. If you've stopped smoking with someone else, keep on helping each other.

KEEP AN EYE ON YOUR WEIGHT
Now's the time to keep an eye on your weight. If this is a problem for you, cut down on sweet and fatty foods as

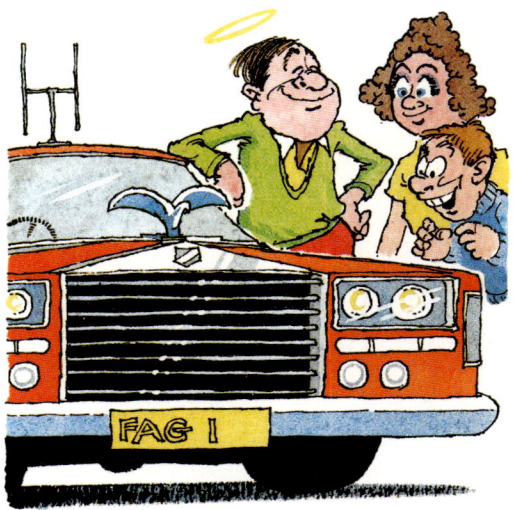

Treat yourself or the family with the money you've saved.

much as you can. If you want to eat more, concentrate on salads and fresh fruit and vegetables. Be careful. Don't use putting on weight as an excuse for going back to smoking. If you've beaten smoking, you can certainly tackle your weight.

Text reproduced by permission of the Health Education Council and the Scottish Health Education Group

Heart Disease

WHAT IS HEART DISEASE?
One half of all deaths in most Western countries are caused by atherosclerosis, the underlying condition responsible for coronary heart disease, strokes and other blood-vessel diseases. Atherosclerosis is also the cause of much crippling illness and senile decay; it may also cause chest pain and leg pain on walking. But now the means of preventing, delaying or perhaps even reversing the disease are beginning to be understood.

Atherosclerosis is caused by the accumulation of a sludgy deposit called atheroma in the lining of arteries all over the body, including those arteries which supply blood to the heart – the coronary arteries. The build-up of atheroma (which contains a lot of cholesterol) causes the walls of the arteries to thicken and narrow. This accretion of fatty material may begin in childhood but the ill-effects are not usually found until the forties when men, apparently in the prime of life, begin to be struck down by coronary thromboses.

The reason for atheroma clogging up arteries is usually a diet that has been too rich in saturated animal or saturated vegetable fats. The condition is accelerated and aggravated by smoking, high blood pressure and stress. (The precautions that everyone can take to reduce the chances of heart disease in middle age are outlined below, along with the details of medical measures designed to produce marked improvements in health for angina sufferers and those coronary victims who get a second chance.)

Atheroma restricts the supply of blood flowing through the coronary blood-vessels to the heart muscle, so that any physical or emotional stress which puts an additional burden on the heart may precipitate a crisis. This occurs when a rapidly beating heart needs more blood than is available to provide the heart muscle with sufficient oxygen. The narrowed vessels cannot supply it and so the heart is deprived of oxygen, causing patches of tissue to die which are replaced by inelastic scar tissue. One in every four people dies suddenly of heart trouble without any previous warning. Even when a person is aware of possible heart trouble, two out of three of those who die do so too quickly for medical help to reach them.

The immediate cause of a heart attack may be a blood clot – otherwise known as a thrombosis. This cuts off the blood-supply to the heart muscle. Blood clots form easily in people who have a lot of atheroma because the normal 'duck's back' lining of the blood-vessels, which prevents clotting, is lost. However, many people survive a 'warning attack', because the area of heart muscle which dies following the interruption of the blood-supply is small.

ANGINA
Some people learn that their heart is not working properly when they first suffer an attack of angina. This is a pain in the centre of the chest which may spread to the neck, midriff and arms. It is brought on by exertion, emotion or cold weather and goes away with rest, and can generally be distinguished from heartburn, which is caused by indigestion.

In angina the supply of blood to the heart is unable to keep up with demand. When a person who suffers from angina takes exercise, the heart muscle works harder and requires more oxygen. If blood-vessels, narrowed by atheroma, restrict the blood-supply, then the heart muscle will be deprived of oxygen and will begin to burn up fats and sugars inefficiently, so that waste products accumulate. These stimulate nerves in the heart, causing a violent pain.

Angina may be caused by anything which makes the heart beat faster: sport, sexual intercourse or any other kind of excitement. A heavy meal, particularly if it is fatty, may bring on an attack. Smoking and exhaust fumes may cause angina, since carbon monoxide from the smoke replaces some of the oxygen in the blood. Smoking also increases heart-rate and blood pressure, in the same way as emotional or physical stress, so that the heart may require more oxygen than can be supplied.

Angina can be relieved by medical treatment with drugs such as nitro-glycerine which expand the blood-vessels of the heart. Other drugs, the beta blockers, prevent the heart responding to adrenaline and impose a type of speed-limit on the heart so it cannot respond in the normal way to exercise or emotion. Operations have also been devised to relieve angina. It is sometimes possible to take a piece of vein from the leg and graft it onto the heart, by-passing a local blockage in one of the coronary arteries. However, if the harmful lifestyle is not changed, the graft itself may silt up and the problem return. So it is important for angina sufferers to keep strictly to a diet, to abandon smoking, to avoid stress, to reduce weight and to take as much exercise as they can without pain in order to improve circulation.

STROKES
Atheroma may cause trouble elsewhere in the body. A blood clot cuts off the blood-supply to part of the brain, causing a stroke. Only half of the people who have a stroke are alive a month later. The survivors may be partially paralysed, and their speech or other functions controlled by the brain may be badly affected. The factors which lead to a high risk of stroke are the same as those for heart disease: particularly smoking and high-fat diet.

OTHER SYMPTOMS OF HEART DISEASE
Arteries narrowed by atheroma can reduce the blood-supply to leg muscles and cause cramping pains during mild exercise – a condition known medically as intermittent claudication (limping).

Arteries generally become narrower and harder as atheroma accumulates. They are unable to respond flexibly to the demands of the heart during exercise, and so a person with narrowed arteries tires very quickly. Eventually, arteries become so narrow that the blood-supply is inadequate even without exercise. When this happens to blood-vessels in the brain, a person gradually loses normal mental functions and control of the body. This is the tragic waste of life we see as senile decay.

ARE YOU AT RISK?
Your chance of suffering from heart disease can be calculated from the chart overleaf based on a chart devised by the Michigan Heart Association.* As no single predominant cause of heart disease has yet been identified, the degree of risk depends on the combined total of several separate factors. So study the eight columns, mark the appropriate box in each and then add up your score.

*Risk. © Michigan Heart Association.

HEART DISEASE/THE MAJOR HAZARDS

SEX	BLOOD PRESSURE	FAT % IN DIET	EXERCISE	TOBACCO SMOKING	WEIGHT	HEREDITY	AGE
Female under 40 1	100 (upper reading) 1	Diet contains no animal or solid fats 1	Intensive work and recreational exertion 2	Non-user 0	More than 5lb. below standard weight 0	No known history of heart disease 1	10 to 20 1
Female 40–50 2	120 (upper reading) 2	Diet contains soft margarine, no fried food 2	Moderate work and recreational exertion 2	Cigar and/or pipe 1	−5 to +5lb. standard weight 1	1 relative over 60 with cardiovascular disease 2	21 to 30 2
Female over 50 3	140 (upper reading) 3	Diet contains some butter or hard margarine, some fried food 3	Sedentary work and intense recreational exertion 3	10 cigarettes or less a day 2	6–20lb. overweight 2	2 relatives over 60 with cardiovascular disease 3	31 to 40 3
Male 5	160 (upper reading) 4	Diet contains a lot of butter, or hard margarine, or fried food 4	Sedentary work and moderate recreational exertion 5	20 cigarettes a day 4	21–35lb. overweight 3	1 relative under 60 with cardiovascular disease 4	41 to 50 4
Stocky male 6	180 (upper reading) 6	Daily diet contains butter, or hard margarine or fried food 5	Sedentary work and light recreational exertion 6	30 cigarettes a day 6	36–50lb. overweight 5	2 relatives under 60 with cardiovascular disease 6	51 to 60 5
Bald stocky male 7	200 or over (upper reading) 8	Daily diet contains butter, or hard margarine, and fried food 7	Complete lack of all exercise 8	40 cigarettes a day or more 10	51–65lb. overweight 7	3 relatives under 60 with cardiovascular disease 7	61 to 70 and over 8

1. If you are a smoker who inhales deeply and smokes to a short butt, add 1 to your total.
2. If you have passed an insurance company medical recently, your blood pressure will probably be below 140.
3. Don't forget that cream, butter and eggs are high in animal fat.
4. To calculate the hereditary factor, only count parents, grandparents, brothers and sisters as relatives.

If you are an aggressive person, live under a lot of stress or suffer from gout or diabetes, then these factors will increase the risk of heart disease. But they are too complicated to calculate on a points system.

Scores:
6 to 11 – well below average risk
12 to 17 – below average risk
18 to 24 – average risk
25 to 31 – moderate risk
32 to 40 – dangerous risk
41 to 63 – imminent danger: see your doctor

HOW TO PREVENT HEART DISEASE

All forms of heart and blood-vessel disease are difficult to treat medically. The best hopes of preventing or alleviating them derive from a change of lifestyle. Apart from controlling diet and giving up smoking, it is particularly important to reduce the stress of daily living. Apart from causing a build-up of atheroma, stress can cause sudden death by interfering with the heart rhythm. Some people are addicted to a stressful life. They are ambitious, aggressive or uptight; they are not satisfied until they have drained themselves of all energy. Some doctors call this the coronary personality and this type of person faces a growing risk unless and until he or she learns to alter their lifestyle (see Relaxation, Chapter 3).

What this means, according to authorities such as Britain's Royal College of Physicians and the American Heart Association, is summarized below; fuller details of each category will be found elsewhere in this book. People who scored highly in the coronary risk quiz at the start of this chapter are strongly advised to take immediate steps to alter their way of life. But do not try to do it all at once; you are likely to find it too great a change, and give up. Try to change your lifestyle slowly, over a period of weeks, months or even years. Even a small change may make a large difference.

DIET
Whatever your age or state of health, reduce the saturated fat in your diet.

1. Eat less meat and then choose lean meat, although even that contains 30 per cent invisible fat. Remove visible fat. Grill rather than fry.
2. Eat fewer eggs – one per day maximum. Eat more poultry, fish.
3. Use butter sparingly, prefer soft margarine high in polyunsaturates. Cut down generally on dairy products such as top-of-the-milk and cream.
4. Use polyunsaturated oils for cooking, e.g. corn, soya

THE MAJOR HAZARDS/HEART DISEASE

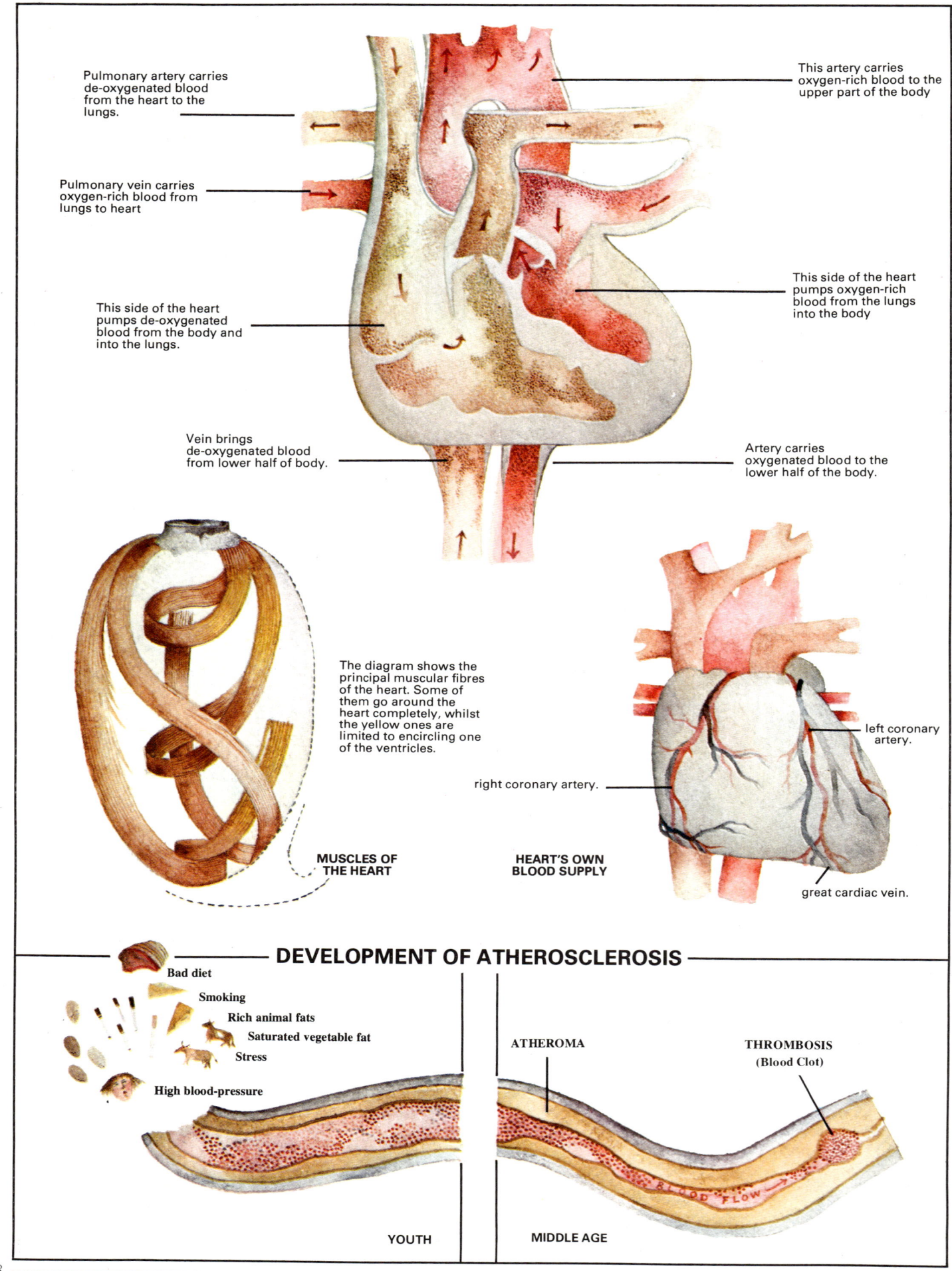

bean, sunflower or safflower oils. Olive oil is also acceptable. Avoid hard margarines, lard. Oils simply labelled vegetable oil may contain a lot of saturated oil.
5. Eat more vegetables, fruit.

WEIGHT
The reason overweight people run a greater risk of coronary heart disease is because they are less likely to take physical exercise and more likely to have a badly balanced diet. It is more important to balance your diet correctly by cutting down on fats than to worry about weight itself.

It makes sense to lose weight, but make sure you do not cut down mostly on starchy (carbohydrate) foods: cut down on saturated fats or by calorie counting. Fats are a highly concentrated source of calories so if you cut down on fatty foods you can still maintain the bulk of your normal diet while being less likely to feel hungry. Cut down, too, on sugar and alcohol.

SMOKING
The risk of coronary heart disease among smokers is twice that of non-smokers, and four or five times higher in middle age (thirty-five to fifty-four). But if you cannot give up smoking:

1. Smoke filters with progressively less tar.
2. Smoke less than five cigarettes a day.
3. Do not inhale; this is particularly important if you switch to cigars or a pipe.

STRESS
Acute emotion may precipitate angina or a heart attack. In extreme circumstances, a person may lose the will to live; their heart beats irregularly, then stops.

1. Guard against stress. Try to manage your life differently to avoid unnecessary, unproductive stress.
2. Try to cultivate methods of relaxation. Yoga or meditation may help.
3. Make sure of a good night's sleep. Make time to relax before going to bed. Sleep in once a week and catch up on lost rest. If necessary use an occasional sedative.
4. Discipline yourself to avoid exhaustion and fatigue. Be strict in refusing to take on more than you can do.

EXERCISE
Everyone should exercise regularly. Middle-aged people, who may not have exercised for years, can begin gradually. A medical is not essential except for older people, those who are seriously overweight or heart sufferers. If you develop unexpected symptoms during exercise, however, consult your doctor.

1. Get breathless some time every day. Climbing stairs instead of using lifts or escalators is a good way.
2. A minimum of fifteen to twenty minutes' vigorous exercise twice weekly (not normally on consecutive days) is necessary for your health. A daily walk is also excellent exercise. Gradually increase the distance, pace and slope.
3. Simple keep-fit exercises once or twice a day will work the main muscle groups in turn (see Chapter 2).

CONTRACEPTION
Women over forty, those who have relatives with coronary artery disease, and women who smoke more than ten cigarettes a day should avoid the pill and use another form of contraception if possible (see Chapter 8).

HOW TO RECOVER FROM HEART DISEASE

Some people are lucky. They survive a heart attack to win a second chance to live. The clinical possibilities of improvement have been demonstrated in research involving monkeys at the Universities of Iowa and Chicago in the United States. The monkeys were first given a diet high in saturated fat and cholesterol, and their arteries became narrower. When the monkeys were returned to what the researchers called a 'prudent' low-fat diet, their arteries widened again and their health improved. It is more difficult to establish that the same reversal of heart disease occurs in people. But there is evidence that the arteries of patients with high blood-fats can get wider again after many months of dietary treatment. As the coronary arteries get wider it is possible that the danger of heart disease gradually decreases.

During the Second World War, when there was a general shortage of meat, eggs and animal fats, there was a marked decrease in fatalities from heart disease in every European country involved except Denmark. The Danes had stopped exporting dairy produce and so maintained something like their usual diet.

The Royal College of Physicians recommends a diet for people who already suffer from heart disease which is stricter than that recommended simply for prevention of the disease. The hope is that this diet may actually reverse heart disease, although this is not yet proven.

These dietary measures for treatment of heart disease should be taken in addition to those for prevention.

1. Restrict meat meals to eight a week.
2. Always use soft margarines high in polyunsaturates.
3. Use skimmed milk.
4. Eat no more than three eggs a week.
5. Keep down cheese intake; use cottage cheese.
6. Restrict cakes, pastries and biscuits unless they are home-made with suitable fats.

A vegetarian diet seems to be particularly effective in reducing the chances of heart disease. The Seventh Day Adventists, who mostly eat a vegetarian diet with eggs and milk and occasionally meat, have a much-reduced incidence of heart disease and many other diseases. They also tend not to smoke or drink, which explains much of their good health and lower cancer rates but not all.

Other, more extreme, diets are sometimes recommended and may be beneficial, although they have not yet been proven scientifically. A diet consisting almost entirely of unprocessed vegetables and grains is recommended by the Longevity Research Institute in California. Their star patient, eighty-seven-year-old Mrs Eula Weaver, was chronically ill until she went on the diet. Mrs Weaver could not walk more than a hundred feet without getting severe pains in her chest, and her legs were swollen to twice their normal size. She was found to be suffering from high blood pressure and arthritis. After following the diet for several years, Mrs Weaver won six gold medals in the veterans' Olympics at Irvine, California. At eighty-seven years old she was running two miles a day, riding ten to fifteen miles on a stationary bicycle and working out twice a week in a gym. Mrs Weaver attributed her rejuvenation to the diet and exercise regime recommended

THE MAJOR HAZARDS/HEART DISEASE

by the Institute. It consists of peas, beans, other vegetables and unprocessed grains such as rice, wheat, oats, buckwheat and corn. The patients also eat some cottage cheese made from skimmed milk and eat up to three pieces of fruit a day. They eat one ounce of fish *or* fowl every five days but no meat, eggs, milk, full-cream cheese or any extra fats and oils. This limits the fats and cholesterol in the diet to a fraction of that eaten in conventional diets.

The amount of exercise taken is gradually increased in the Longevity regime. Patients go for short walks three times a day and later every hour, until finally they are able to jog gently. Mr Nathan Pritikin, director of the Institute, says that this regime has been remarkably successful in rehabilitating heart patients who were waiting for by-pass surgery and has also been successful for treating patients who have had by-pass surgery and have since relapsed. People who are suffering from claudication (limping caused by artery disease) have also made spectacular recoveries.

Doctors will be sceptical of these results until they are repeated in other research establishments. In the meantime anyone can try this type of extreme diet for themselves. The Vegan Society has pioneered a diet which contains no meat or animal produce. If you follow it rigorously there is no danger to health, but a little meat – particularly liver – once or twice a week will help to give you the B vitamins which must otherwise be supplied in the form of yeast extract.

HIGH BLOOD PRESSURE

At least one person in a hundred has severe high blood pressure and many more – perhaps one in ten people over forty-five – suffer from mildly increased blood pressure which is a threat to health. However, a person with high blood pressure often complains of no symptoms until the high blood pressure causes a stroke or heart failure. High blood pressure is aggravated by a stressful lifestyle, and an individual can do a great deal to avoid it by cultivating a relaxed approach to life and a healthy diet.

The pressure of blood in the body depends upon the force of the heartbeat and upon the tension in the thirty thousand miles of arteries which spread throughout the body. Blood pressure is measured by putting a cuff around the arm and inflating it to a pressure which stops the flow of blood. Two readings are taken: one for the blood pressure at its highest when the heart is actually contracting, and one at its lowest when the heart is resting between one contraction and the next.

Blood pressure varies a great deal according to physical and mental activity. If the person has been running, working hard, or worrying, then their blood pressure will be higher: this is quite normal. However, this variation makes it difficult to measure a person's resting blood pressure accurately; all the doctor can do is measure the blood pressure on several different occasions. If it is always raised, then this indicates that a person has high blood pressure which may be confirmed by other tests. Blood pressure is raised if it exceeds about 160 millimetres of mercury for the high reading and 95 for the low reading. This would usually be written by the doctor in the form 160/95.

The first signs of high blood pressure may be dizziness, headaches, or impairment of memory or concentration.

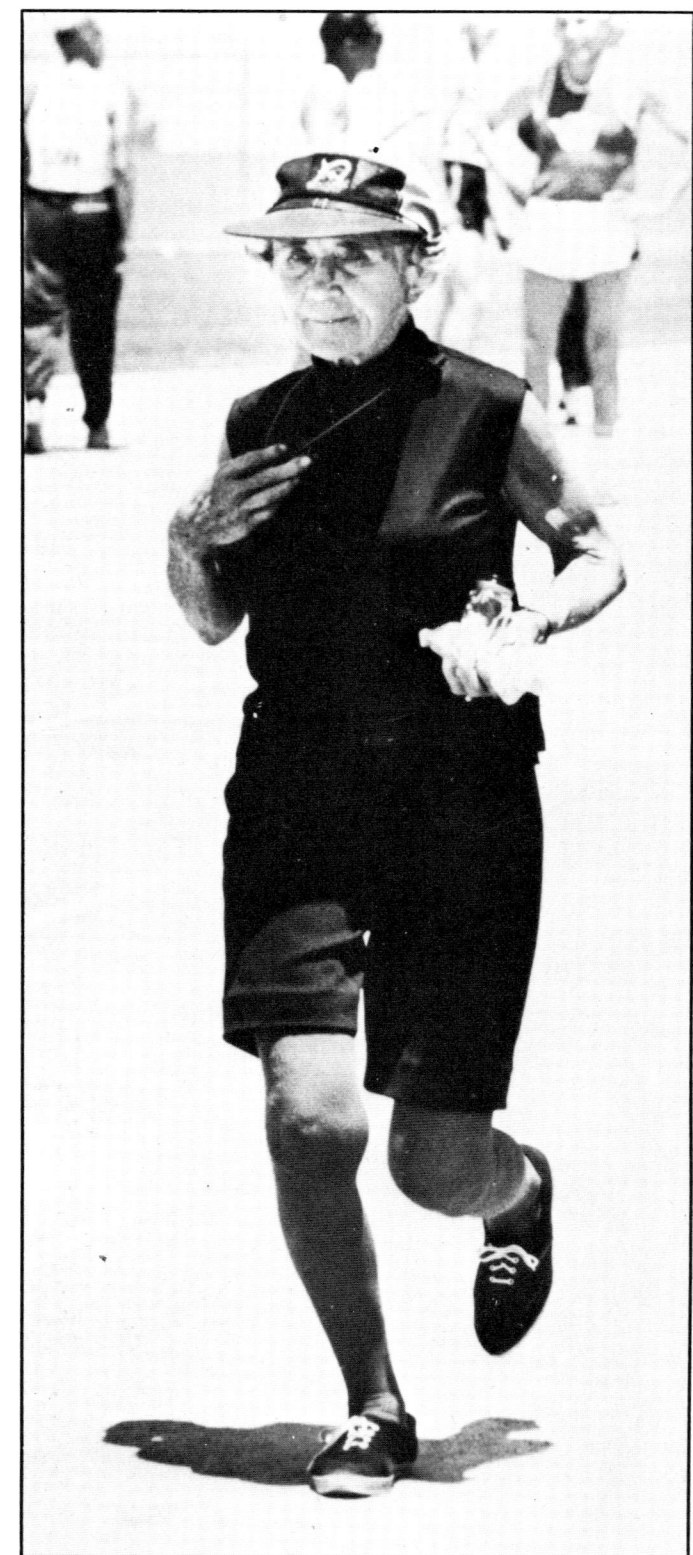

Star patient Eula Weaver, 87, was crippled. Now she wins medals in the senior Olympics. Exercise benefits the heart and circulation.

However, many people with high blood pressure feel perfectly well and only come to notice through routine examinations for insurance or eyesight, or other health checks. When high blood pressure builds up in the blood vessels in the brain, one may burst, causing a stroke. Alternatively, heart failure or damage to the eyes or kidneys may eventually result. These dangers are not

HEART DISEASE/THE MAJOR HAZARDS

immediate but steps must be taken to reduce them in the long term.

A full examination by a specialist is usually advisable when high blood pressure is found, in order to try and identify a cause. In the majority of people no cause can be found. In some cases kidney disease is found to be responsible; more rarely, there may be disease of one of the endocrine glands which secrete hormones into the blood. Women at menopause sometimes suffer from high blood pressure – this generally requires hospital investigation.

Salt in the diet is an important cause of high blood pressure. Investigations of several different kinds have now persuaded doctors after years of doubt that this is so. The Japanese have a diet high in salt. However, Japanese living in the North Island eat much more salt than those in the South and their blood pressure is on average higher. Solomon Islanders living beside the sea cook their food in sea water and eat about 11 g of salt a day. They tend to have a much higher blood pressure than closely related people who live inland and cook their food in fresh water.

The average person consumes 12 g of salt a day – much of it in consumer foods prepared already salted. However, doctors at Stanford University, California, have shown in their Heart Disease Prevention Program that moderate salt restriction by people living in two northern California communities resulted in lower blood pressures. Our sense of taste adapts to different quantities of salt in the diet. But people who are accustomed to having large quantities of salt in the diet are unable to distinguish large additions of salt to the food. If salt in the diet is gradually reduced, people who were accustomed to very salty food will become sensitive again to small additions of salt to the diet and be able to detect once more when food is oversalted.

To reduce salt in your diet, first avoid all salted foods such as nuts, chips, salted popcorn, pretzels and cocktail snacks. Then stop using table salt and pickles. Finally, try to reduce the quantity of convenience foods such as tinned vegetables, sauerkraut, tinned soups, certain breakfast cereals, and salted meats such as ham, corned beef and sausages. Drinking alcoholic beverages is another cause of high blood pressure.

One of the commonest identifiable factors contributing to high blood pressure is the stress caused by emotional problems. Apprehension, fear, anger and prolonged resentment can all cause stress or raise blood pressure. The effect on blood pressure may be temporary and it may return to normal when the period of stress is over. However, the cause of stress often seems to be difficult or impossible to find. Sometimes people develop a style of life which is impossibly stressful, and then they must learn a new way of living.

It is important for a person who suffers from high blood pressure to learn to relax (see pages 69–70), but it is also important for them to review their life and look for ways in which they can avoid stress. To begin with, it is important to aim at having nine hours in bed at night, and to wind down by reading something relaxing. Do not exercise immediately after a heavy meal. Delegate as many of your responsibilities as you can. Avoid working in the evenings or at weekends. Take leisurely holidays which involve a minimum of travelling, and especially try to avoid driving, which can be particularly stressful. Compulsive drivers should try to minimize driving at weekends in order to have a thorough rest.

It is important for someone who suffers from high blood pressure and is also overweight to try to reach a normal weight. If a person has more or less normal weight it is still a good idea to adopt the low-fat diet and avoid overeating, by cutting down a little all round, and to avoid drinking excessive amounts of alcohol. It is best to give up smoking completely. Normal sexual activity can usually be continued, although it is best to discuss this with the doctor. It is best to avoid sex when unduly tired or suffering from any shortness of breath or pain, which may be signs of stress.

Regular walking is good for people with high blood pressure because it lowers blood pressure by dilating the blood-vessels in the lower limbs. Swimming, running and cycling are also good exercises for people with high blood pressure, but care must be taken not to begin exercising suddenly after high blood pressure has been diagnosed. An exercise programme should be introduced gradually (see Chapter 2). Isometric exercises such as weight-lifting, wrestling and water skiing clamp down on the muscles and so put up blood pressure – they should be avoided.

Many drugs are available for treating high blood pressure although a lot of them cause one side-effect or another. Most effective drugs for treating moderate high blood pressure are diuretics, which increase urine flow and so remove more salt from the body. If side-effects do occur, it is usually possible to change the drugs so that they are avoided. Sometimes a person with high blood pressure may find that one day a week in bed resting, drinking fruit juice and taking very little solid food is a great help. Whatever treatment your doctor suggests, it is important to cultivate methods of relaxation.

How to deal with a heart attack

During a heart attack a severe pain is felt in the chest. This is often mistaken for indigestion. If the heart stops beating, the person collapses and turns pale or blue. Prompt action may save life.

Some doctors claim that it is possible for someone who is suffering a heart attack to restart their own heart and keep it going by coughing sharply and repeating as necessary. If there is no one else to help, cough sharply. If possible, phone for help.

If you are near someone who collapses with chest pains, put the patient on their back and lift the legs so that blood goes to the heart and thump the chest. Call an ambulance quickly. Loosen clothing around the person's neck, check the mouth for foreign bodies, remove false teeth. If breathing does not restart after thumping the chest, give mouth-to-mouth respiration: hold the nose and breathe into the mouth until the chest has risen; watch the chest fall, then repeat the operation.

If the victim does not begin to recover spontaneously, someone with experience of first-aid can look for signs that the heart has stopped: dilated pupils and no pulse in the neck. An experienced person may then attempt to restart the heart with cardiac massage. Cardiac massage squeezes the heart rhythmically to keep it going until expert help can be obtained. But inexperienced people are not advised to try this. (For more information see Emergency, Chapter 11.)

Cancer

Cancer is not one disease but many, perhaps as many as a hundred or more, each affecting different parts of the body and each one caused in a different way. Now that infectious diseases have been largely conquered by better housing, vaccinations and modern drugs, cancer remains one of the major killers of our time. About one hundred thousand people in Britain die from various cancers every year. Yet most cancers can be cured successfully if caught in their early stages. Everyone knows their own body best and should pay close attention to any changes which could be a sign of cancer. This does not mean becoming a hypochondriac but simply taking your own health seriously and watching for things which do not go away. Most cancers give early signs that they are developing, although the smallest lump which can be felt already contains a thousand million cells. These are too often missed because they are confused with the common symptoms of less serious complaints.

Warning signs: The International Union Against Cancer has identified eight warning signs of cancer. They may be caused by other less serious conditions but they may also be caused by cancer.

1. Chronic, persistent cough or hoarseness.
2. Any sore or ulcer which does not heal.
3. Unusual bleeding or discharge.
4. Any unexplained change in bowel or bladder habit.
5. Chronic indigestion or difficulty in swallowing.
6. A lump in the breast, neck, armpit or anywhere else in the body.
7. A change in a mole or wart.
8. Any unexplained loss of weight.

If you have any of these signs, do not panic. The explanation may be quite simple, but consult your doctor for advice without delay. Specific warning signs for different cancers and the chances of successful treatment are given below.

CANCER OF THE SKIN

Warning signs: Any change in the skin which grows larger; a sore which does not heal; moles or birthmarks which begin to grow, to bleed, to change colour, or become painful.

There is no need to be alarmed if you have a small skin cancer, as most of them are easily dealt with and cause no trouble. Skin tumours occur most frequently on exposed areas of the body, particularly in fair-skinned people who are exposed to sunshine. These people should take care to wear a hat or to keep in the shade where possible.

Rodent ulcer is the commonest type of skin tumour. It starts as a small raised lump which flattens out and grows at the edges while the centre ulcerates. It is easily cured but should not be neglected. A similar type which has more irregular edges *(squamous cell carcinoma)* is more serious because it can spread to the lymph glands. But it can be dealt with easily if medical attention is sought promptly.

The most dangerous type of skin tumour is black in colour and called *melanoma*. If it is caught early and a lot of apparently normal tissue around it removed with it, then the prospects of cure are nevertheless good. There are many other completely harmless skin blemishes, particularly in old people, but if in doubt consult your doctor.

CANCER OF THE BREAST

Warning signs: Any unusual lump or thickening in the breast, or any alteration in the shape of the breast; swelling in the armpit; retraction of the nipple. A bloodstained discharge from the nipple may have a variety of causes, but consult your doctor.

Many women delay seeking advice for breast lumps because they fear that treatment will make no difference. In fact early treatment of breast cancer can effect a complete cure, and a breast lump should always be treated as an emergency. However, the majority of lumps are not even malignant.

All women should examine their own breasts once a month (see below). Women who are particularly at risk should also try to get their breasts examined professionally in a screening clinic (see Appendix Three for details). Those most at risk are women who have a relative who has had the disease; women with no children or with only one child; women who had their first child after thirty-five; those who have had benign breast lumps; women whose breasts have a knotty fibrous texture; and women with a late menopause whose periods continue after fifty-one years of age. New methods of treating breast cancer are being developed, and even late breast cancer can be given treatment which will extend life for years.

Self-examination of breasts

Every woman over twenty should examine her breasts at least once a month, and more frequently if possible, so that she will notice any change as soon as it is detectable. Some lumps can be detected in this way which do not show up on an X-ray. Lumps may be best detected by a woman who examines her own breasts regularly, because she will notice any change. The consistency of the breasts changes during the menstrual cycle: some fluid-filled cysts get larger before a period and then go down or disappear altogether a week later. There is no need to worry about these. If a *persistent* lump appears, consult your doctor without delay; if you are unsure, wait for one cycle and go to the doctor if it does not go away. A few days after menstruation when the breasts are smallest is a good time to look for lumps.

How to examine yourself

Undress to the waist and stand or sit in front of a mirror. Look at your breasts first with your hands at your side, and then look again with your hands raised above your head, turning from side to side. Then put your hands on your hips and look again. Good lighting is important. Look for any differences between the breasts. Size is not important: breasts are frequently not exactly the same size. Look for a flattening or bulging in the surface or a puckering in the skin. Gently explore any part which looks different by feeling with the fingers. Any discharge from the nipple when it is gently squeezed, or any sore or scaly part, should lead you to consult your doctor. Lastly, lift each breast up in turn and examine the under-part in the mirror.

Now lie down on a bed – or you can do the next bit in the bath – and lift up one arm, putting your hand behind your head and keeping the elbow flat. Examine the breast on that side, gently feeling each quarter of the breast in turn.

CANCER/**THE MAJOR HAZARDS**

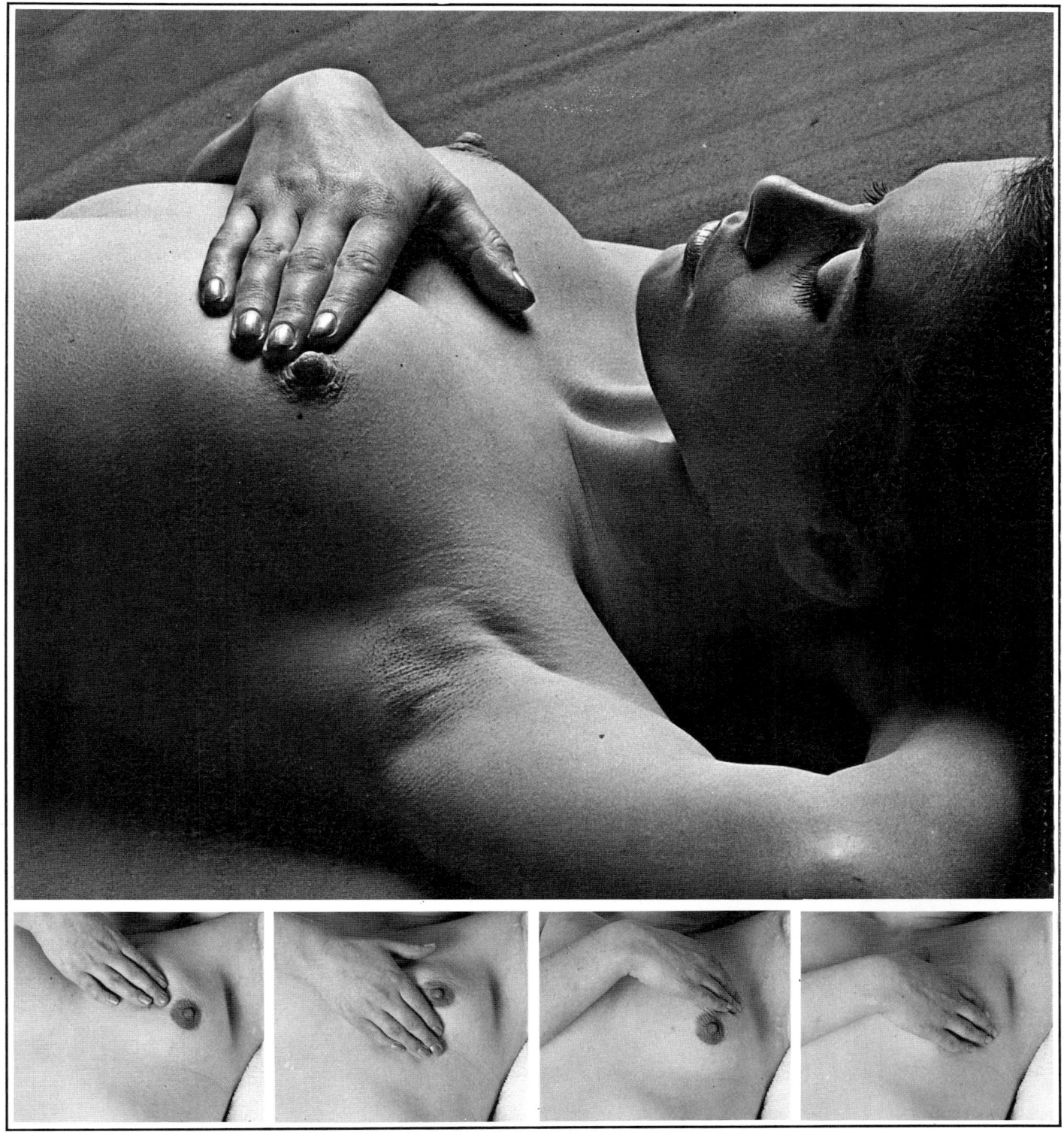

Repeat with the arm at the side. Then repeat the whole procedure for the other side, using the opposite hand. Tumours are most commonly found between the nipples and the armpit, so give that area special attention. Any slight thickening or lump which is different from normal and does not go away, however tiny, should be reported to your doctor for an expert opinion. If you do find a lump, your doctor will probably refer you to a specialist who may take an X-ray or ask you to have an operation for removal of the lump for tests. *Remember: the majority of lumps are not cancer, but also remember that by leaving the problem it will not go away*. Self-examination of breasts is most important because most lumps are discovered by women themselves.

If the lump is a cancer, the surgeon may need to remove the breast. Such an operation is often profoundly disturbing for a woman and support from the husband and family at this time is most important for a woman's well-being. At the time of the operation it may be possible to insert a breast replacement under the skin, thus preserving the breast shape. If this is not possible, a variety of attractive breast replacements, many of the same silicone type, are available and will return a woman's figure to an entirely natural line. For some early breast cancers, it may be

THE MAJOR HAZARDS/CANCER

possible to perform a simple operation with removal of only the lump and nearby lymph nodes followed by radio-therapy.

CANCER OF THE LUNG

Warning signs: Lasting cough; blood in spit; pain in chest; loss of weight. Rare in non-smokers. Recurrent chest infections. Loss of appetite; loss of weight.

There is as yet no good way of detecting lung cancer at an early stage and chances of recovery, except for a very few, are poor. Prevention is the only answer. It has been calculated that life expectancy may increase by a year for every three cigarettes fewer a person smokes per day. After a person gives up, their health slowly improves and the chances of getting lung cancer and other diseases caused by smoking slowly decline.

CANCER OF THE MOUTH, THROAT, NECK AND LARYNX

Warning signs: Any lump or swelling in the mouth or neck, a mouth ulcer or hard lump which refuses to go away; lasting hoarseness of the voice; persistent discharge of blood from the nose.

All these tumours can be treated successfully if caught early but if ignored may spread to the glands in the neck and become more difficult to treat. Pipe-smoking, cigarette-smoking, or even badly fitting dentures, may all cause irritation of the mouth, leading to cancer. Cancer of the larynx (voicebox) is commonest in people who both smoke and drink heavily. The larynx may have to be removed but it is possible to learn to speak again by a special method involving the swallowing of air, or with the help of an electronic gadget. Swellings in the neck are most commonly caused by infections. However, sometimes a swelling persists in the thyroid gland and it may occasionally be caused by a tumour. Surgical treatment is usually very effective.

Feel the glands of the neck with the finger-tips. These glands often swell during a throat infection and should not then be a cause of worry. If swelling persists indefinitely, consult your doctor.

CANCER OF THE OESOPHAGUS AND STOMACH

Warning signs: Persistent indigestion; difficulty in swallowing, particularly of dry foods; loss of weight and anaemia; poor appetite; vomiting and pain in the stomach; bleeding in the stomach may cause the stools to become black and tarry-looking.

These cancers are treated by surgery which can be successful if the warning signs lead to early treatment. People can live very well and eat almost normally even after large parts of their stomach have been removed. The cause of stomach cancer is not known but something in food or drink is suspected; the poor preservation of food is one possibility. Investigations include X-rays of the digestive tract and often its examination through a fibre optic tube.

CANCER OF THE COLON AND RECTUM

Warning signs: Constipation or diarrhoea or both, or other unexplained change in bowel habit; blood or pus in the stool; pain in the bowel; anaemia; loss of weight and general ill-health.

Early diagnosis of cancers of the bowel and rectum is important because the chances of dealing with it effectively by surgery are good. Any bleeding from the rectum should be investigated by a rectal examination, even though in the vast majority of cases – at least ninety-nine out of one hundred – it is caused by piles. A good doctor will do this but unfortunately many still do not. If the cause of bleeding cannot be established by the family doctor, a specialist examination should be requested. The cause of cancers of the bowel is probably a diet too rich in fat and low in fibre.

CANCER OF THE WOMB, CERVIX OR OVARY

Warning signs: Unexpected bleeding from the vagina; irregular bleeding between periods; prolonged bleeding during or after period; bleeding after intercourse. Swelling of abdomen, frequent calls to toilet.

Cancer may occur in the womb itself or in the neck of the womb (the cervix), the part where the womb is attached to the vagina. Women who have had children, and women who have had more than the average number of sex-partners, are most at risk from cancer of the cervix.

Cancer of the cervix can now be diagnosed by the cervical smear test. Women are now automatically tested as part of their pre-natal examination, or during gynaecological examinations or sometimes by their family doctors. When cervical cancer is found in its early stages it can be prevented from spreading by a simple operation. Cancer of the womb is also dealt with simply by surgery. Women most at risk of getting cervical cancer seem to be the most reluctant to come forward for screening.

The cause of cervical cancer is not known for certain, but all evidence suggests that it is connected with intercourse and with personal hygiene; the cause may be a virus or other infection spread by intercourse. Regular washing in the normal way may help prevent it, but measures such as douching are not recommended because they may cause other problems.

Ovarian cancer can grow quietly without causing symptoms. The abdomen may become persistently swollen without any notable weight gain, or due to pressure on the rectum and bladder it may feel as though there is a need to open the bowels or pass water frequently. This is another tumour which if detected early on has extremely good chances of cure.

CANCER OF THE BLADDER OR KIDNEY

Warning signs: Blood in the urine but no pain; a small amount of blood in the urine may make it a pink or smoky colour.

The chances of curing bladder tumours are good if it is caught in the early stages, because many such tumours are not malignant. Careful investigation is required to establish the type of tumour and to rule out other conditions such as bladder stones; the inside of the bladder can now be visually examined through a small tube. One cause of bladder tumours is chemicals which were once used in the rubber and dye industries. Smoking increases the vulnerability to bladder tumours. Blood in the urine accompanied by pain in the abdomen could be a sign of a kidney tumour. These are rare but with modern treatment the chances of cure are extremely good, especially in children.

PROSTATE ENLARGEMENT
Warning signs: Difficulty or discomfort in urination and increased frequency of urination; getting up in the night to pass only a small quantity of water. Difficulty in starting and stopping urine flow.

The prostate gland, found only in men, secretes part of the seminal fluid. It is situated at the base of the bladder around the tube which brings the urine to the outside. It often becomes enlarged in old age and occasionally a tumour develops, but these are slow-growing and can usually be treated easily and discomfort relieved.

LEUKAEMIA
Warning signs: Anaemia, tendency to bleed, severe tiredness, fever and sore throat are the commonest initial signs; these may be accompanied by ulcers in the mouth, pains in joints and muscles, and swollen glands.

There are several different types of leukaemia but all are the result of an increase in the number of white cells in the blood. Some develop very quickly over a short period but others may develop slowly over the years. Treatment of leukaemia has improved enormously in the last ten years, and there is now good prospect of a cure of certain types. The cause of leukaemia is not known but it is thought that some type of virus or radiation may be responsible.

CANCER OF THE BONE OR SOFT TISSUES
Warning sign: Lasting swelling or pain in the bone.

Tumours in the bone are usually the result of the spread of cancer from another part, such as the breast. However, cancer does sometimes start in the bone, particularly in children. Cancers of the soft tissue are usually recognized as a painless lump which can generally be removed.

CANCER OF THE BRAIN
Warning signs: Severe headaches over a long period, sometimes causing vomiting and disturbance of vision and personality; interference with speech or movement, or double vision.

Some tumours of the brain are benign but cause trouble as a result of pressure on the brain. Once they are removed, much of the trouble may disappear. Others can be more troublesome and the results achieved by surgery or irradiation depend on the type. The new X-ray brain scanners have made it much easier to locate difficult brain tumours.

HODGKIN'S DISEASE
Warning signs: Lasting enlargement of the glands, particularly in the neck, armpits or groin, which does not disappear as in a passing illness; tiredness, itching of the skin, loss of weight and fever may also be signs.

This disease used to be rapidly fatal but now the large majority of people are cured. Radiotherapy and drugs are the usual treatment. The cause is not known.

HOW TO AVOID CANCER

Scientists are still labouring to produce cures for cancers. It is difficult to identify all the possible causes because of the long delay that sometimes exists between cause and effect. Exposure to some noxious substance such as asbestos dust may cause cancer many years afterwards. This delay may be anything from five to fifty years. However, scientists estimate that 80 per cent of cancers are caused by something in our everyday pattern of life – the air we breathe, the food or water we drink, or chemicals or infections to which we are exposed – and these cancers are all in principle preventable.

Studies lasting many years have been necessary to establish the dangers of certain substances used in industry. And laborious studies of the changes in lifestyle and health of migrants from one country to another have established that diet can be an important cause of cancer. Nevertheless, the causes of many cancers remain completely unexplained. These are the latest clues to the causes as presently understood, and suggestions as to how you can endeavour to avoid some cancers.

RISKS AT HOME
Reduce the amount of fat you eat in your diet: The fatty diet of affluent countries appears to be linked with bowel and breast cancer. Bowel cancer is uncommon in Japan but common in the USA. When Japanese migrate to the USA they begin to suffer from bowel and breast cancer; one prime suspect is the change from a diet of rice and fish to a more fatty, meaty diet. To reduce fat in your diet, take the same measures as are taken to prevent heart disease (see Diet, pages 76–87). Try not to eat more than one meat meal a day. Cut out butter and cream. Reduce cakes, pastries, ice-cream and chocolate. Limit cheese and eggs. Do not be afraid of eating the staple starchy foods such as bread, potatoes, spaghetti and rice.

Eat plenty of fresh fruit and vegetables: People who eat plenty of fresh vegetables seem to be less likely to get cancer. Lettuce, celery, cabbage, Brussels sprouts, turnips, cauliflower and broccoli are all good for stimulating the production of enzymes (biological catalysts) in the liver which help to destroy poisons and cancer-causing chemicals in food. Oranges and lemons are not only effective in stimulating these enzymes but also contain vitamin C, which may protect against chemical reactions in the stomach that produce cancer-causing chemicals.

Eat wholemeal bread and wholemeal breakfast cereal: Lack of cereal fibre (bran) in our diet is blamed as a contributory cause of bowel and rectum cancer. Although this theory is not proved, it is likely to benefit your health in other ways if you eat wholemeal bread. Eat wholemeal cereals or add All-Bran or natural bran to other cereals.

Avoid eating mouldy food: Mouldy food does not usually cause any immediate stomach upset, as would food spoiled by bacteria. However, one of the most potent cancer-causing chemicals known – aflatoxin – is found in mouldy peanuts. Aflatoxin causes cancer in animals and is suspected of causing cancer in man although this has not yet been strictly proven. Many moulds produce potent biologically active substances and so it seems wise either to throw away mouldy food or to cut off the mould with a generous amount of the food. Improved preservation of foods by the

THE MAJOR HAZARDS/CANCER

food industry and increased use of refrigerators may be responsible for the decline in stomach cancer in the Western world. There is no evidence that cheeses ripened by introduction of moulds – such as the blue cheeses – are bad for health and so there is no good reason to forgo them.

Beware of food additives and seasonings: Only in recent years have food additives begun to be systematically screened for their cancer potential. Some three thousand food additives are used in food in Western countries, many of them flavours which have never been tested for any cancer links. Tests are still in progress on the much smaller number of food *colours* (now twenty-eight). It is only sensible to restrict the amount of synthetic and processed food eaten at home. Restrict the amount of ham, bacon, corned beef and frankfurters eaten: the nitrite preservatives which give these meats their pink colour may cause the formation of nitrosamines in the body. Nitrosamines cause cancer in animals but have not yet been shown to cause cancer in man.

Drink only in moderation, especially if you smoke: The risk of cancer from alcoholic drinks is greatest among heavy drinkers who also smoke. The risk that they will get cancer of some kind is up to fifteen times higher than for those who neither smoke nor drink. They are more vulnerable to cancer of the mouth, throat, oesophagus, larynx and liver.

Do not smoke: One in ten of all men in Britain dies of lung cancer, and the proportion of women is increasing rapidly.

RISKS AT WORK (see also Hazards at Work, Chapter 7). A relatively small proportion of all cancers, less than 3 per cent, are suspected of being caused by exposure to substances in the workplace, according to Dr John Higginson, director of the International Agency for Research in Cancer at Lyons, France. These are the cancers caused by substances such as asbestos, vinyl chloride and naphthylamine, which is used in the rubber industry.

The cancer-causing potential of some chemicals has only been noticed because they induce a cancer which is otherwise extremely rare. Vinyl chloride increases the risk of dying of a very rare type of liver cancer (*angiosarcoma*) some four-hundred-fold but the average worker in a vinyl chloride factory is still ten times more likely to die of lung cancer and five times more likely to die of bowel cancer. There may be many other chemicals which cause cancer rarely that go unnoticed. Cancer of the scrotum was first observed in 1775 as a disease of chimney-sweeps by the English doctor Percivall Pott. Today the same disease still causes the deaths of some sixty men a year. Mineral oils used in industry and the motor trade cause irritation of the skin and warts on the scrotum which may eventually turn into cancer. This cancer can be completely avoided by using clean overalls, not putting oily rags into the pocket, and regular bathing after work.

About two hundred substances are suspected to cause cancer in man. Another one hundred are known to cause cancer in animals and many more are under suspicion. The number of substances which have actually been *proved* to cause cancer in man is quite small (see table). Even everyday substances such as wood-dust can cause cancer if people are exposed to it regularly over a period of years. (Dust given off during the machining of wood was responsible for the deaths of about one in every thousand woodworkers every year before controls were introduced.)

Each industry and each process in industry has to have its own special equipment and routines to prevent the escape of chemicals in hazardous quantities. Workers are also obliged by law to take the safety measures required. A major cause of skin cancer is ultra-violet light from the sun. Most skin cancers are slow-growing and present no threat to life provided they are caught early. However, others such as melanoma can be more difficult and worth taking simple measures to avoid. A hat provides valuable protection.

Avoid unnecessary X-rays: Survivors of the atomic bombs exploded over Hiroshima and Nagasaki have to face increased chances of getting leukaemia, breast cancer and cancers of bowel and brain. Each X-ray causes a tiny amount of damage to body cells and carries a minute risk of starting a cancer. Generally you can only rely on the doctor's judgement of whether an X-ray is necessary. Bear in mind that this may be a factor in a doctor's decision not to X-ray you.

Five-point safety programme

1. Ask for a copy of your firm's safety policy and study it.
2. Treat chemicals, dusts, mineral oils and smokes with suspicion. Avoid inhaling dusts and fumes. Always wear protective clothing and breathing apparatus when advised, as failure of an employee to do so can lead to prosecution of the employer.
3. Do not eat food in the place of work. Remove dirty outer clothing and wash thoroughly before handling food, so as to avoid eating chemicals and dusts.
4. Protective clothing and overalls are best laundered by the employer and not taken home if dangerous materials and dusts are handled.
5. If you work outdoors all day, wear a hat.

Industrial substances known to cause cancer in man

Substance	Hazard	Cancer
4-aminobiphenyl	rubber industry	bladder
arsenic	vineyards, miners, copper smelters	lung and windpipe
asbestos	insulation, brake lining workers and handymen; also in air and water	lung
auramine	manufacturing industry	bladder
benzene	shoemaking	leukaemia
benzidine	dye and rubber manufacture	bladder
bis (chloromethyl) ether	industrial intermediate	lung
cadmium oxide	industry, food, cigarettes	prostate
chromate	production of chromate pigments	lung
hematite	mining	lung
2-naphthylamine	rubber manufacture	bladder
nickel	refining	lung, nose
tars, oil, soot and smoke	industry metal working	skin, scrotum
vinyl chloride monomer	production of PVC	liver

Many other substances are suspected of causing cancer in man, and many more are known to cause cancer in animals.

Drug Dependence

Drug dependence in Britain is a largely hidden problem. Junkies, glue-sniffers and pot-smokers hit the headlines. But there is also an unknown number of perfectly respectable women and men who are dependent upon drugs. These are the people who have become dependent either upon the legal drugs in tobacco and alcoholic drinks, or those who are dependent upon tranquillizers, sleeping pills, slimming tablets or other medicines like cough mixtures.

Some people argue that all mood-altering chemicals are potentially addictive. Certainly, many of them are. But only *some* individuals become hooked. Just as many people drink alcohol but only a proportion become alcoholics, so many people have mood-altering drugs prescribed for them, but only a proportion become dependent on these. Some people may be especially vulnerable to drug dependence.

The history of mood-altering drugs in Britain has followed a pattern. At first, new drugs in this field are thought to be non-addictive. Later, as they come into widespread use, it becomes clear that *some* individuals become dependent. Amphetamines and barbiturates were both thought to be non-addictive originally. Today, most doctors are wary about prescribing them except for specific medical conditions (see Sleep, pages 70–1).

Till recently, the benzodiazepine drugs – tranquillizers like Valium and Librium and sleeping tablets like Mogadon – were thought to be non-addictive. In 1979 some thirty million prescriptions for these drugs were handed out by British doctors. Yet, as Professor Malcolm Lader of the Institute of Psychiatry points out, 'We do not know the long-term effects of these drugs.'

SIGNS OF DRUG DEPENDENCE

If *any* of the following six statements applies to you, then you may have become dependent upon tranquillizers.

1. You have been taking tranquillizers for six months or more.
2. You are taking more than 20 mg daily, or 30 mg, if the original anxiety was extremely severe.
3. You have asked your doctor to increase the dose; you are taking larger doses than instructed; you are getting extra pills from elsewhere.
4. You are mixing your drugs with alcohol or other drugs. (If in doubt, ask your doctor again about exactly what other drugs or drink you may take.)
5. The drug is interfering with your life in some way, causing difficulties in family relationships, social life, work or housework, or any other activity.
6. You get withdrawal symptoms when you do not take your normal dose. These include feeling ill (like a bout of flu); being jumpy, irritable, sleepless; having muscle aches and pains; sensitivity to lights and sounds; feeling unsteady or seasick; sweating, palpitations, nausea; anxiety.

If *any* of these six danger signs apply to you, you should consult your family doctor about coming off the drug. Since it is your doctor who originally prescribed the drug, he or she may be reluctant to acknowledge your dependence. Thus, if *you* feel you are dependent (though he dismisses your fears), ask for a second opinion.

Stopping tranquillizers can be confusing. One of the withdrawal signs is anxiety, yet benzodiazepines are often prescribed *for* anxiety. Thus withdrawal anxiety can be confused with a return of the original anxiety. If you stay off the drug for three weeks, withdrawal anxiety will die down. So it is important to wait for at least this period before concluding that you still need the drug. You may find help from some of the organizations listed in Appendix Three.

ILLEGAL DRUGS

Among the illegal drugs, the most commonly used is cannabis, pot or hash. One conservative estimate puts the number of current pot smokers in Britain at more than a million. Then there is a proportionately diminishing number of people who take amphetamines, LSD, sedatives and finally drugs like heroin. The downward progression, in which soft drugs lead to hard drugs, does exist for a small number of individuals. But at every stage there are a large number of people who do not go further down. Thus it is true that a heroin addict probably started by smoking pot, but it is *not* true that a pot smoker will necessarily become a heroin addict. Most pot smokers will stick to pot and the legal drugs like alcohol and tobacco.

Using any kind of recreational drug – including the legal ones like tobacco and alcohol – carries some risks to health. It is sometimes claimed that pot, in particular, is safer than alcohol. This has not been proved either way. However, cannabis *is* harmful to health in much the same way that tobacco is, and, indeed, it is usually combined with tobacco when smoked. Apart from legal problems, it would be inconsistent to avoid the dangers of tobacco yet continue smoking pot.

In general, a lifestyle that includes heavy drug use carries considerable risks to health. Apart from the side-effects of the drugs themselves, there are obvious dangers in being stoned out of your mind or intoxicated – road accidents, accidental falls, choking and other hazards. Some people just cannot handle drugs. They cannot use them in moderation; their behaviour under their influence is unacceptable; or they become dependent upon them. The development of dependence in cigarette smoking can also apply to other drugs – first you take them because they are offered to you; next you buy your own; then you make sure of a regular supply; finally you suffer withdrawal symptoms when supplies run out. Experimenting with illegal drugs has risks. If you do *not* experiment, then you avoid these risks altogether.

Parents or relatives often worry when they discover that a family member has taken or is taking illegal drugs. If they feel they cannot ask that person directly and believe in their answer, then it probably is true that there is not much they can do. If they decide that they *can* talk about it directly, then it will be worth their while taking expert advice beforehand. There are organizations which can give information about illegal drugs and some guidance to anxious relatives (see Appendix Three).

Alcoholism

Alcoholism has long been portrayed by red-faced comedians as something of a joke. Or it has been associated with the stubbly-bearded casualties of society seen swigging their meths in TV documentaries about the slums. But the vast majority of alcoholics are also businessmen incapable of useful work in the afternoon, housewives not really up to preparing an evening meal, and people kept from work by a wide range of illnesses that have the common factor of striking the sufferer down on a Monday. Alcohol, unlike smoking, is not necessarily bad for you. A little can often be beneficial. But when a little becomes a lot, drinking can cease to be a pleasure and becomes an addiction. As many as seven hundred and fifty thousand people in England and Wales alone have been estimated to have a serious drinking problem. An even higher proportion of people drink excessively in Scotland and Ireland.

Although precise estimates about the extent of alcoholism vary, experts agree that the figures are rising dramatically. Admissions to British hospitals for treatment of alcoholism and alcoholic psychosis rose by more than 600 per cent between 1959 and 1978; if the trend continues for a further decade, alcoholism will account for 20 to 25 per cent of all psychiatric admissions. Convictions for alcohol-related offences have also soared.

Since it is quantity which causes the problems, one reason is certainly the comparative cheapness of alcohol nowadays – or at least the increase in affluence. However horrific the price of a bottle of Scotch may seem today, it still costs less than 20 per cent of the average man's disposable weekly income: twenty-five years earlier it cost 45 per cent.

This relative cheapness goes some way to explaining a fourfold increase in the total volume of alcohol consumed between those years. But it is not the only factor. Alcoholic drinks are more readily available, notably in supermarkets. Women in particular are more likely to buy alcoholic drinks in supermarkets than if it needed a special visit to an off-licence. The growing number of women who go out to work has also increased their exposure – and therefore vulnerability – to alcohol. Social attitudes have made alcohol more acceptable; foreign travel has given more people a taste for more exotic drinks.

The result is that more alcohol is consumed in Britain today than at any time in the last sixty years. What is all too easily forgotten is that alcohol is a dangerous drug. The evidence of its dangers, when misused, is sadly all too apparent – not only in the direct and often lethal effects of alcoholism itself but in the side-effects of family and work problems associated with the condition.

WHAT IS ALCOHOL?

If natural fruit juices are kept warm for a few days and exposed to the air, the sugars in them will usually ferment to form alcohol. Starches – grains, potatoes – can also with no great difficulty be persuaded to ferment. Alcohol, to the chemist, is a rather general name: the alcohol we drink is strictly speaking called ethyl alcohol. Ordinary beers contain between 2½ and 4 per cent of this alcohol by volume: 'special' strong beers may have as much as 8 per cent. Wines generally range between 8 and 12 per cent, and fortified wine (e.g. sherries and aperitifs) contain added spirits which bring the alcohol content up to about 20 per cent. To make spirits, the fermented liquors must be distilled. Most distilled liquors – whiskies, brandies, gins, vodkas – have about 40 per cent of alcohol in them, but their strength is usually described in terms of proof spirit. This, in historic testing, was an alcohol that when mixed with gunpowder produced a mass that could still be ignited: it contains about 57 per cent alcohol. Alcohol acts as a depressant rather than a stimulant and can interact dangerously with quite ordinary medicines such as aspirin or antihistamines prescribed for conditions such as hay fever.

WHAT IS ALCOHOLISM?

Alcoholic drinks provide a source of energy for the body but contain relatively few nutrients and vitamins. Those who drink them moderately, in company, are 'social drinkers'. Some social drinkers become heavy drinkers, and may develop, without necessarily recognizing it, into excessive drinkers. These are people whose drinking leads to social, economic or medical problems, or a mixture of all three. An excessive drinker does not automatically become an alcoholic, and many people do not continue down this path. If they recognize that alcohol is the source of their problems, they can cut down, or stop drinking. Many do not have such insight. An alcoholic is someone who cannot stop drinking without help, and who drinks without control, although many seldom show visible signs of drunkenness. The World Health Organization defines alcoholics as: 'Those excessive drinkers whose dependence on alcohol has attained such a degree that it shows a noticeable mental disturbance or an interference with their bodily or mental health, their personal relations and their smooth social and economic functioning or who show the prodromal [early] signs of such development.'

Alcoholism is a self-inflicted condition but its effects are not confined to the individual drinkers. It breaks up marriages, alienates children and loses people their jobs. Physically the effects can be disastrous. It is thought that around 70 per cent of chronic alcoholics suffer from fatty infiltration of the liver, about 10 per cent from cirrhosis of the liver – the death-rate from this went up by over a third between 1969 and 1979. There has also been an increase in recent years in cirrhosis among women.

Many alcoholics have peptic ulcers, but whether this directly results from alcoholic abuse is not absolutely certain. Regular drinking causes chronic inflammation of the stomach which in turn causes most alcoholics to lose interest in food. As a result of eating a small amount of convenience food, alcoholics often consume a diet low in vitamin content. They may nevertheless maintain a normal weight or increase in weight because alcohol substitutes for carbohydrates in the diet.

Excessive alcohol may also weaken the heart muscle, causing the heart to enlarge and reducing the efficiency of the pumping action. Eating a balanced diet may protect a heavy drinker from some of these effects, but not all. Another effect is the nerve damage described as polyneuritis – a tingling in the hands and feet, and cramps in the legs, are among the symptoms – which may affect a fifth of all alcoholics.

Some of the neurological complications, such as the 'shakes' and delirium tremens (hallucinations), are 'with-

ALCOHOLISM/THE MAJOR HAZARDS

drawal symptoms', and alcoholics who have reached this stage need hospital treatment under special care. Others – severe memory loss, for example – may be permanent. Nobody who has ever drunk more than modestly needs to be told that heavy drinking reduces dexterity. Alcohol is very rapidly absorbed and begins to act on the brain in about ten minutes. Co-ordination of hand and eye begins to fail, as does the ability to judge distance – precisely the brain-functions required to drive a motor car or operate powered machinery safely. But although these kinds of co-ordination fail – and sometimes brain damage can be permanent – verbal skill usually remains unaffected. So do not regard your ability to talk coherently as proof of your ability to drive safely. Drinking is also an important cause of accidents (and violence) at work and home.

However, these physical and mental effects are complications of alcohol misuse and generally arise only years after the sufferer's personal, social and professional life has been destroyed. Alcoholism itself is the underlying factor that must be treated.

The peculiar nature of alcoholism is that it starts as a pleasure. But like any drug that makes you 'feel good' alcohol can be addictive. Our diagram shows how this can lead to trouble. Occasional drinking, because it relaxes tensions, frequently becomes 'relief' drinking. Because the body accommodates many of the burdens we thrust upon it, heavy drinkers grow tolerant of 'heavy' amounts of drink. They then need more alcohol to get the effect they seek. The difference between a healthy drinker and a problem drinker is the element of compulsiveness, and the diagram shows how the compulsion develops.

ARE YOU A POTENTIAL ALCOHOLIC?

Some people are more at risk than others. Among national groups, the Scots and Irish have a high incidence of alcoholism, the Jews a very low one. Some occupations are associated with increased risk: actors, travelling salesmen, barmen, waiters, company directors and journalists, for example. It is unlikely that these have some genetic characteristic in common, because drinking habits are characteristic of cultures rather than races. All the evidence suggests that alcoholism is thus preventable.

The first problem in treating alcoholism is early recognition. Potential problem drinkers are not easily identified, least of all by themselves, while alcoholics are often as compulsive in their insistence that they don't need help as they are in their drinking. The diagram should tell you your position – or that of a friend – in the alcoholism spiral.

The heavy drinker is in the interim phase when social drinking slips towards addiction. Judge if it applies to yourself or your nearest-and-dearest by answering honestly:

1. Do you drink for the effect rather than because you like the taste of the stuff?
2. Do you slip away from work for a morning drink or drink at work before lunchtime?
3. Are you fairly frequently the worse for drink in mid-week?
4. Do you get drunk alone?
5. Do you have memory lapses about the time spent drinking?
6. Do you find that the people you are drinking with are rather slow in drinking up and buying their rounds?
7. Do you usually have at least a couple of drinks to help you face difficult problems?

If your answer is 'yes' to more than one, beware. You are probably drinking too much and you now need that amount to be satisfied. But your body cannot adapt to it in the sense of resisting alcohol's attack on its vital organs. You must seek help and stop drinking for a longish period – say, six months – so that your body can recover, and you must never start drinking heavily again.

The alcoholic is someone with an addiction that he or she is unlikely to recover from unaided. Yet no one can ever recover from alcoholism against their will, so it often falls to others to convince alcoholics they need help. Again, here are a series of questions to ask either yourself or others to gauge the extent of alcoholism:

1. Do you need a drink first thing in the morning?
2. Do your hands tremble until you have a couple of stiff drinks?
3. Do your friends frequently 'joke' about your drinking?
4. Have you started to drink in less pleasant pubs and bars than you once used to?
5. Do you get moody as you continue drinking?
6. Have you noticed over the last couple of years that you have become less ambitious?
7. Do people complain about the quality of your work?

Many affirmative answers indicate addiction. You *must* seek help: alcoholism is an illness. Consult your GP or you may prefer to contact one of the organizations listed in Appendix Three.

TREATMENTS

It may take an average of ten to fifteen years of drinking to become an alcoholic, but people who start to drink heavily in their teens often become alcoholics much more quickly. Once a person has admitted the need for treatment, the chances of recovery are good. People who have been heavy drinkers tend to relapse; there is no such thing as a cure. Treatment may differ in detail, and organizations may vary in their approach, but all those who treat alcoholism agree that a recovered alcoholic must never drink again. It is possible that there may be a few who can become controlled drinkers again, but this is a controversial point. No alcoholic should believe that he or she is one of them.

In almost every case, recovery begins with an immediate and complete end to drinking. This, and the subsequent treatment of malnutrition and other physical damage, needs expert supervision. The most immediate needs are usually vitamin supplements and short-term use of tranquillizers to help through the initial difficulties of withdrawal. The long-term treatment must help the patient to live without seeking refuge in drink or, of course, in tranquillizers.

DRINKING AND THE FAMILY

Alcohol dependence develops insidiously. But the casualties of addiction are not only the people consuming the alcohol. Family and social life also suffer. Someone who regularly drinks heavily is more likely to experience a violent marriage, separation and divorce, or have children who suffer from neglect or abuse. Work problems pile up, too, and as money worries grow so again do the pressures on family life.

THE MAJOR HAZARDS/ALCOHOLISM

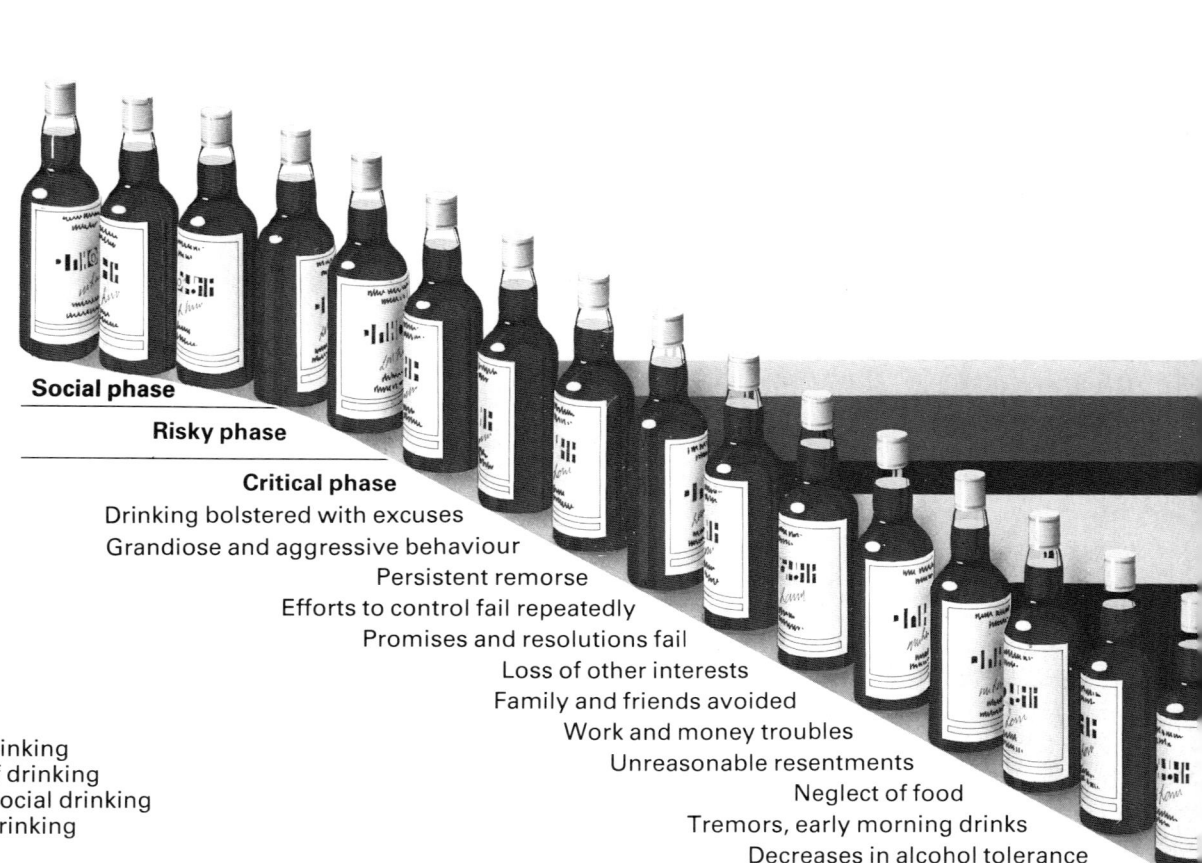

Social phase
- Normal social drinking
- Occasional relief drinking
- Heavy habitual social drinking
- Constant relief drinking

Risky phase
- Increase in alcohol tolerance
- Onset of memory blackouts
- Surreptitious drinking
- Increasing dependence on alcohol
- Repeated 'under influence' driving
- Urgency to consume first drinks
- Feelings of guilt about drinking
- Unable to discuss drinking problem
- Memory losses increase
- Decrease of ability to stop drinking when others do

Critical phase
- Drinking bolstered with excuses
- Grandiose and aggressive behaviour
- Persistent remorse
- Efforts to control fail repeatedly
- Promises and resolutions fail
- Loss of other interests
- Family and friends avoided
- Work and money troubles
- Unreasonable resentments
- Neglect of food
- Tremors, early morning drinks
- Decreases in alcohol tolerance
- Physical deterioration
- Onset of lengthy intoxications

Alcoholic

As if all this was not bad enough it is worth remembering that, as alcoholism may start as a psychological attitude to drinking, so it is possible for children to learn this attitude from their parents: children of alcoholics have a higher risk than average of themselves developing a drinking problem. Children naturally imitate the example set by their parents. If drinking is forbidden in the home and yet the children know that their parents go to drink in pubs and clubs, then the children are likely to imitate this pattern as soon as they are able. Probably the safest pattern of drinking is found among Italians and Jews, who introduce their children to alcohol in the home as part of normal family life. Young people may then be taught by parents to enjoy alcoholic drinks in moderation at mealtimes. Teenage children may then cautiously learn the effects of alcohol in the safety of the home.

Recent findings also make it clear that even unborn children can suffer permanent damage from alcohol. They themselves consume none, of course, but it is the drinking mother who puts her baby at severe risk. Alcohol abuse is an important cause of damage to unborn babies. According to one estimate, one in three alcoholic mothers must expect her child to be born handicapped. (It is worth stressing that this applies to *alcoholic* mothers, not simply mothers who drink alcohol.)

Researchers in the United States, headed by Dr James Hanson of the University of Washington, put the figure still higher, at somewhere between 30 and 50 per cent. The blood of some babies is so rich in mother's alcohol that the child would fail a breathalyser with his or her first breaths. And if they are born with the 'shakes', damage can prove to be permanent.

ALCOHOLISM/THE MAJOR HAZARDS

The alcoholic abyss
The stages by which some heavy drinkers sink into alcoholism, and the possible escape routes.

Decline
Addiction may take from 5 to 25 years to develop. The average is 10–15 years.

Recovery
Once started rehabilitation and cure in a well-motivated person normally takes a few months to achieve; in others it may take years

Social phase
Risky phase: the beginning of dependence
Critical phase: dependence well established
Bridge to recovery. At any point down to Alcoholic phase. The victim will cross the bridge if he stops drinking

Normal life restarts
Confidence of employers returns
Increased tolerance to frustration
Contentment in abstinence
First steps towards economic stability
Rationalizations recognized
Increase of emotional control
Return of self-esteem
Facts faced with courage
New circle of stable friends
Adjustment to family needs
Care of personal appearance
Natural rest and sleep
Desire to escape diminishes
Realistic thinking
Fears of future diminish
Possibility of new way of life appreciated
Onset of new hope
Regular nourishment taken
Start of group therapy
Stops taking alcohol
Told addiction can be arrested
Learns alcoholism can be cured
Honest desire for help

Moral
deterioration
Indefinable fears
Obsession with drinking
Complete defeat admitted

Vicious circles of obsessive drinking

HOW TO DRINK HEALTHILY

To some extent society needs to change. Hostesses should perhaps offer more non-alcoholic drinks at parties, for instance. Missing out on a round in a bar or ordering a small glass or a non-alcoholic drink should not be regarded as a reflection on a man's virility. Alcohol itself should be deglamorized. But in the meantime:

1. Avoid drinking alone.
2. Do try to eat at the same time as you drink. Avoid eating salty snacks such as pretzels and nuts, which have no bulk and increase thirst. Eat bread, cheese, creamy spreads and dips, meatballs.
3. Always provide such food for guests when offering drink. Serve food first, then drink.
4. Always measure the alcohol in a drink. Use the conventional size and shape of glass. Serve cocktails and spirits in small-diameter glasses. Only fill wineglasses half full.
5. Always dilute alcohol, preferably with water. Alternatively ask for a separate glass of water, so that you are not always sipping the alcoholic drink without thinking.
6. Avoid bars with loud music, which increases anxiety level (see Hangovers below), where you are likely to drink more before you begin to feel relaxed.
7. When hosting, limit drinking to one hour before serving the meal.
8. Try to limit wine to two half-filled glasses, and only serve brandy or other after-dinner drinks when the meal has lasted more than an hour and a half.
9. Serve your guests so that the pace of drinking is unhurried.

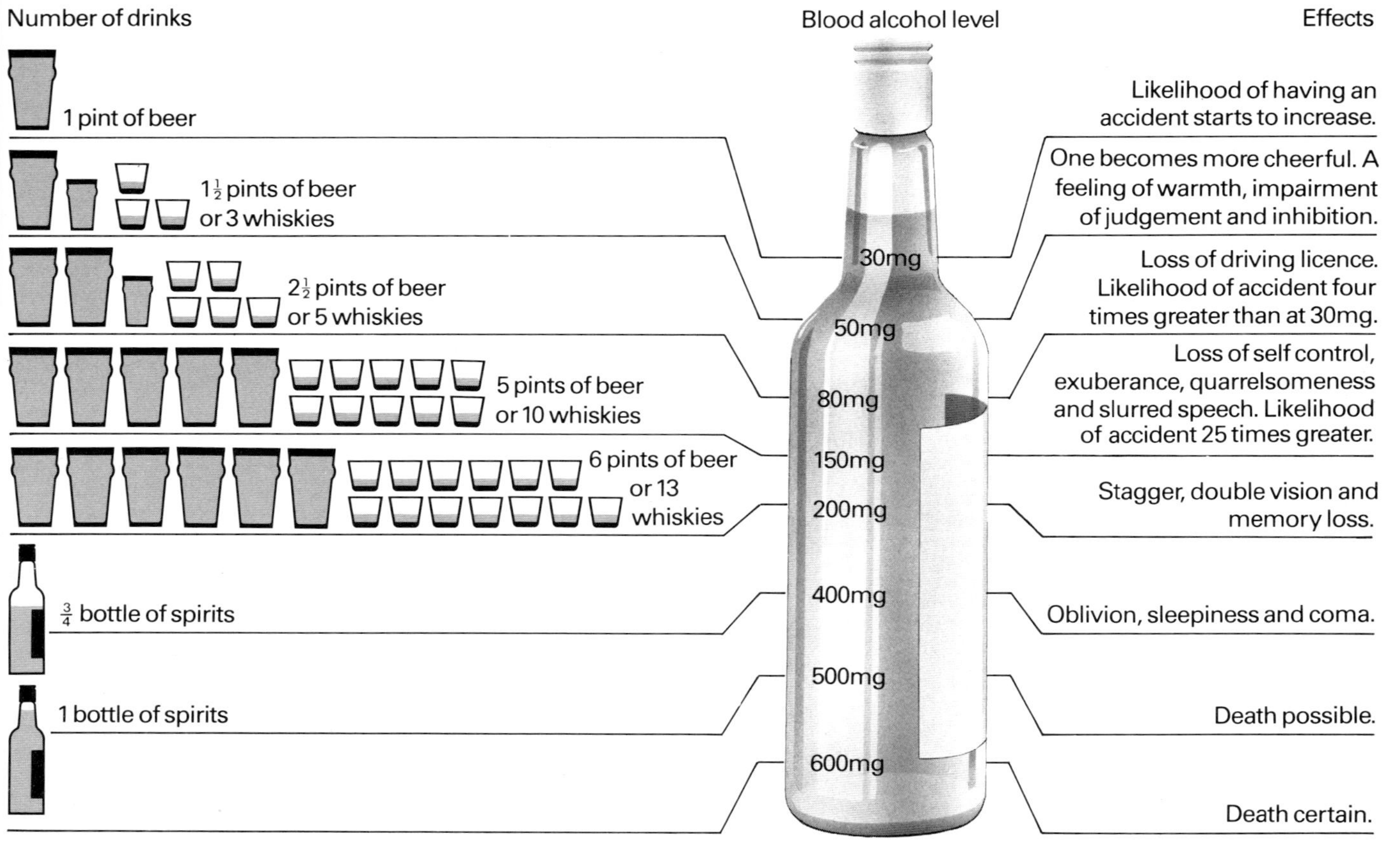

THE MAJOR HAZARDS/ALCOHOLISM

Number of drinks	Blood alcohol level	Effects
1 pint of beer		Likelihood of having an accident starts to increase.
1½ pints of beer or 3 whiskies	30mg	One becomes more cheerful. A feeling of warmth, impairment of judgement and inhibition.
2½ pints of beer or 5 whiskies	50mg	Loss of driving licence. Likelihood of accident four times greater than at 30mg.
5 pints of beer or 10 whiskies	80mg	Loss of self control, exuberance, quarrelsomeness and slurred speech. Likelihood of accident 25 times greater.
6 pints of beer or 13 whiskies	150mg / 200mg	Stagger, double vision and memory loss.
¾ bottle of spirits	400mg	Oblivion, sleepiness and coma.
1 bottle of spirits	500mg	Death possible.
	600mg	Death certain.

How drinks tot up: the alcohol levels and the physical and mental effects.

10. If a guest is drinking too much, actively offer food and only top up the drink with half portions.
11. Do not thrust drinks on people. Make it easy for them to refuse by saying, 'Would you like something to drink?' rather than, 'Come on, have a drink.'
12. If you find it difficult to refuse a drink when you don't want one, or have had enough, ask for a drink which looks as if it is alcoholic. For example, a Virgin Mary, tonic water and lime, or straight bitter lemon.

A safe level of drinking is not more than 1½ ounces of alcohol a day; that is, about half a bottle of wine, or two pints of strong beer, or three and a half measures of well-diluted spirits. This quantity was first recommended by a Scotsman, Dr Francis Anstie, in 1864 and is still known as 'Anstie's limit'. An official US Government report, *Alcohol and Health*, has since endorsed Anstie's advice.

KNOWING YOUR DRINKS – AND YOURSELF

Because drinks do vary in alcoholic content, it is important to know the differing potencies of various drinks. The diagram above shows how four different drinks equate in alcoholic content. Yet the effect of these drinks will also vary from individual to individual according to the weight of the person drinking and whether or not the stomach is empty. Alcohol in the blood is measured in terms of the number of milligrams of alcohol per 100 millilitres of blood; the alcoholic content of your blood rises more slowly if the stomach is full. Young people are also more vulnerable to the effects of alcohol in the sense that the aggressive or foolish side-effects of drinking are triggered by fewer drinks than among older people.

ALCOHOL AND HANGOVERS

You get drunk when sufficient alcohol from the drink is absorbed by the blood and carried to the brain, where the alcohol interferes with normal brain activity. First to go are the critical faculties, which is why everyone, including you, seems wittier as you drink. This is also why the drinker is the last person who should decide if he should drive; he isn't up to decision-making. The rules that govern how quickly you get drunk are complex. If you want to relax, and lose your inhibitions quickly, the first essential is to join a group of people who have the same aim, because behaviour is affected by atmosphere and suggestion. If you can arrange things so that your early party-guests are lively extroverts, only a little alcohol will be needed, cutting back on your drinks bill and reducing the number of hangovers.

The alcohol-derived effect of drinking depends on its concentration in the blood-stream. The basic rule is that the stronger the drink, the more quickly the blood-stream takes up its load. Thus a pint of wine obviously gets you more drunk than a pint of beer. However, drink stronger

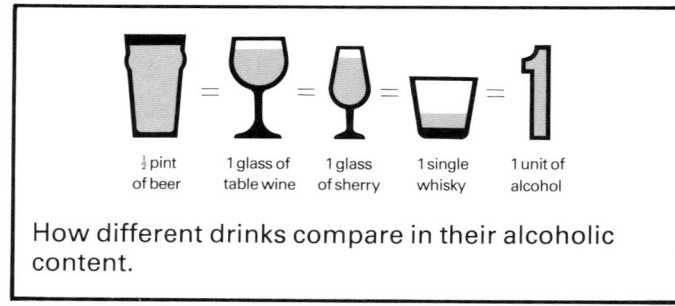

How different drinks compare in their alcoholic content.

ALCOHOLISM/THE MAJOR HAZARDS

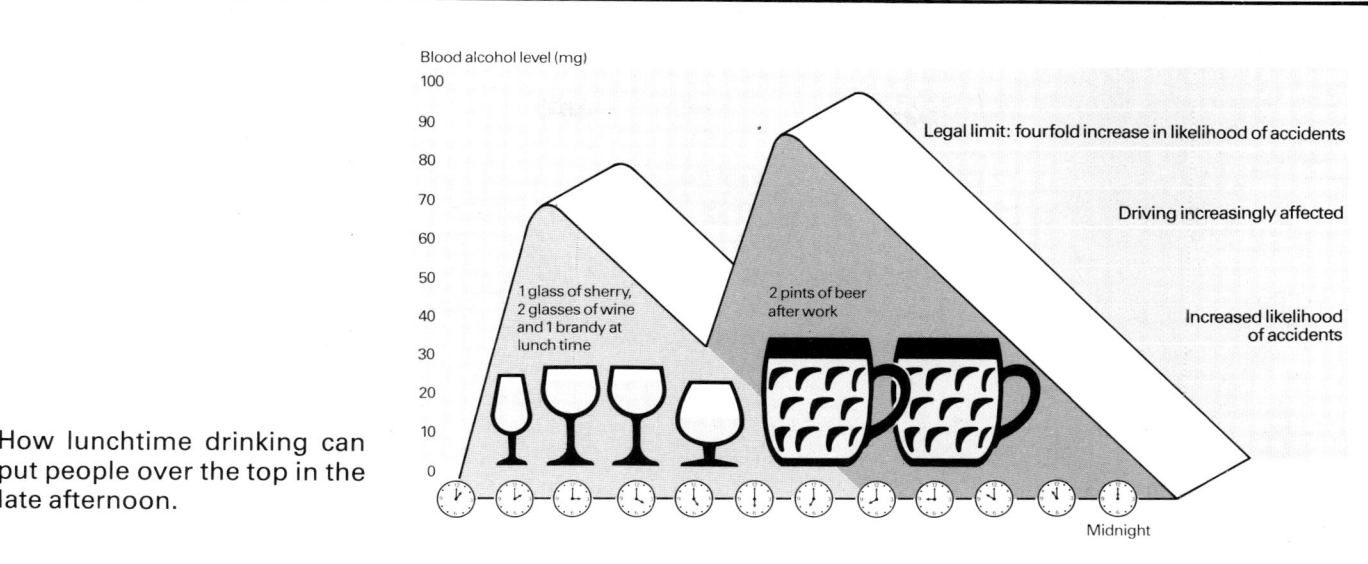

How lunchtime drinking can put people over the top in the late afternoon.

than about 18 per cent alcohol has less immediate effects than weaker drinks. It remains largely in the stomach and cannot pass into the duodenum and small intestine, where 80 per cent of alcohol absorption takes place, until it is diluted. The dangerously unexpected result of this quirk of physiology is that you can pour down a lot of brandy, say, at the end of a party, and continue to feel many of the effects next day after your morning coffee.

Food in the stomach also helps to delay alcohol absorption, and slower absorption is safer. You can reduce the risk of getting drunk by eating while, or shortly before, you drink. Nuts and crisps do not usually provide enough bulk; a sandwich or pie is more likely to help. Those who drink with meals are therefore less likely to get dangerously drunk than those who drink without eating anything.

Sobering up (removing alcohol from the blood-stream) is done almost entirely by the liver. Only a small amount of alcohol is excreted in urine although, as a matter of all-too-frequent observation, some is also exhaled. The liver works steadily at its task, removing a single whisky or half a pint of beer an hour. The process is essential because even tee-totallers have alcohol to the equivalent of a couple of pints of beer a day in their blood, as the result of fermentation in the gut. The healthy liver's inexorable cleansing action can be very slightly enhanced by taking fruit-sugar (fructose), but not sufficiently for this to be a useful way of sobering up.

Those who eat rather fatty meals hinder the liver in its task. Dr Gaston Pawan, of the Middlesex Hospital Medical School in London, has discovered that hangovers, although potentially caused by the alcoholic content of the drink, can be made worse by other substances that are present. These are known technically as 'congeners', and are the by-products of fermentation or distillation or both. Some congeners give different drinks their characteristic taste; the ones that produce hangovers are mainly amyl alcohol, methyl alcohol and acetaldehyde; a measure of only these congeners would give a direct 'hangover index'. Other congeners are contained in red wines (tannin) and beers (a rich variety of nutritious substances). This explains the apparent anomalies in our Hangover Chart.

To avoid the worst hangover many people stick to vodka, gin and white wines. Whatever you drink, keep track of what and how much you are drinking. There is a popular notion that hangovers are caused by mixing drinks. If this does often result in disaster, it may be because mixing happens most often when drinking is heavy anyway. A feeling of thirst may be part of a hangover, because alcohol is a diuretic: it encourages the removal of water from the body and the production of urine. The thirst can be simply cured by drinking water. Rest is the best cure for a hangover. A bad headache may be treated with paracetamol, but not aspirin (acetyl salicylic acid) or tablets containing aspirin, which cause stomach irritation, particularly if the stomach is already irritated by alcohol. Occasionally the combination of alcohol and aspirin causes a dangerous bleeding of the stomach.

The 'hair of the dog' remedy is not recommended. Another drink is extremely risky; it is easy to spend two or three days in a rather drunken haze, during which time the drinker is a potential danger to others; on the roads, for example. You are certain to be over the breathalyser limit if you have more than the equivalent of three drinks active in your system, and you may be betrayed by fewer. There is *no* way you can drink and drive safely.

A contributory factor towards a hangover is tiredness. Alcohol depresses parts of our brains and prevents us from appreciating signals from our muscles and nerves which tell us we are exhausted. So we continue in a stressful way, and when the effect of the alcohol finally wears off we are left extremely tired. The nausea, stomach inflammation, headache and anxiety are extreme responses to stress which can be tolerated while the alcohol works on the body but are only felt with greater intensity when the alcohol wears off. A person who is tense and uptight tends to drink more and is thus more disposed to have a hangover. If you find that anxiety combined with excessive drinking is your problem, try to learn a method of relaxation (see pages 69–70) as well as changing your drinking habits.

An habitually heavy drinker has a hangover problem of his own. He may wake, suddenly, in the small hours, frightened by he knows not what. If this happens frequently it is a powerful danger-sign: the wakening and the fright are withdrawal symptoms. The liver has reduced the blood-stream's burden to an uncomfortable but still high level. Anyone who experiences this often should take warning: almost certainly, it is a sign of alcoholism and time for expert help.

7: STAYING HEALTHY AT WORK AND PLAY

Colds and Flu

Few people escape colds. On average, an adult catches between two and five a year; teenagers catch more, and children most of all. As symptoms include coughing and sneezing, people correctly assume that colds are spread through the air to be inhaled by others. But recent research shows that in addition cold-bugs can survive for three hours on a variety of surfaces, including human skin. So they may also be transferred by touching or shaking hands.

The only efficient way to avoid spreading a cold is to isolate yourself. The best advice is to go to bed and keep away from others. Smoking may make people more vulnerable to colds and make colds – and particularly coughs – last longer.

What is certain is that there are hundreds of different viruses responsible. Rhinoviruses are the largest group and although scientists have identified more than one hundred so far, there may be as many as two hundred. The other main group are the Coronaviruses, probably fewer in number but difficult to isolate in the laboratory. Despite the common belief that colds are caused by chilling of the body, scientists at the Common Cold Research Centre at Salisbury, Wiltshire, and elsewhere have been unable to induce colds in people by putting them in cold conditions with the minimum of clothes. However, these were healthy volunteers who may not be vulnerable to infection. Other experts who have studied sickness reports find that more people report sick after sudden snaps of cold, damp weather, probably because the virus survives better in the cold and damp.

There are very few drugs which are effective against viruses and none which are of any practical use against the cold viruses. Sometimes a cold may be made worse by a secondary infection with bacteria, in which case a doctor can usefully prescribe an antibiotic drug which will attack the bacteria. Other drugs may be prescribed to relieve the various symptoms of colds such as headache, fever, cough or blocked nasal passages. Doctors often do prescribe antibiotics for colds, partly due to pressure from patients, but this is bad practice since it may simply induce bacteria to become more resistant and put the patient in a worse position should he or she genuinely need antibiotics. However bothersome colds are, they rarely last more than seven to ten days, which is all the time required to produce enough antibodies to overpower the infecting virus.

Nevertheless, Dr Linus Pauling, with two Nobel prizes to his credit, suggests that vitamin C, in large doses, can prevent colds and, if caught early enough, cure them. He argues that early man lived on an entirely vegetable diet providing up to three grammes of vitamin C a day, about three times the normally recommended daily intake today. Pauling suggests that we make up this deficiency, equivalent to around sixty oranges a day, but more easily consumed in the tablet form available at chemists. However, several experiments have now shown that vitamin C does not prevent colds and may only ameliorate the symptoms. Large doses of vitamin C for short periods will do no harm, but are not advisable for a long period. The best way to take vitamin C is as orange juice. The frozen type is best.

Influenza is also caused by a virus. There are two main types: influenza A which causes world-wide epidemics and influenza B which tends to cause more localized outbreaks in schools, factories or offices. Influenza A regularly changes its type and so evades the immunity which people develop against it. Many other viruses also cause flu-like illness. The flu virus is spread, like the cold virus, by contact and by coughs and sneezes. The virus concentrates its attack on the membranes of the nose, throat and lungs where it destroys cells. The destruction of the tissue causes a fever. The only protection against flu is vaccination. Vaccines are now available which are fairly effective. During any flu epidemic thousands of people die from the illness. The majority are old people who are in a poor state of health, people who suffer from heart or chest trouble, and especially those who suffer from chronic bronchitis, which is caused mostly by smoking. These vulnerable people stand to benefit most from vaccination against flu. Flu vaccination must be repeated every year. A vaccine against the common cold is not a feasible proposition because there are too many different types of cold viruses.

WHAT TO DO WHEN YOU GET A COLD OR FLU

It is not necessary to see your doctor when you have an ordinary cold unless you have a persistent high temperature which lasts for several days, or if after three or four days you feel you are getting worse rather than better. Children who have a cold lasting more than five days should be taken to the doctor.

The best treatment for a cold is to go to bed early and rely on standard medicines to relieve the symptoms: soluble aspirin or Paracetamol for headaches, for instance. Although cough mixtures can help relieve irritating coughs for a while, it is essential to cough so that infected mucus does not remain in the chest, where the infection will multiply. Also be wary of relying too much on medicines which are prescribed to shrink the blood-vessels or dry up secretions. These may have undesirable side-effects, particularly in old people, and they prevent the body getting rid of germs in the mucus.

Flu is altogether nastier. Your temperature is up over 38 degrees centigrade (100 degrees fahrenheit), your limbs ache, you feel weak and shivery, you probably have a headache, you're sweating a lot and you feel sick. But it is still rarely a case for the doctor: only those people described earlier as especially vulnerable to influenza should always tell their doctor.

Otherwise, stay indoors, keep warm and rest in bed if you can. Have plenty of cool drinks such as fruit juices or water – between four and six pints a day if possible. Cool drinks are refreshing if you have a fever; hot drinks are good when the nose and surrounding passages are blocked, because the heat increases the blood supply, and water vapour loosens mucus. Take soluble aspirin if you feel feverish or your limbs ache. Don't force yourself to eat – and *never* mix spirits with aspirin even if a little whisky does help you sleep. Stay away from other people as much as possible and make sure cutlery, plates, etc., are well washed so you don't pass on the infection. If the nose or chest feel raw, sore or blocked, it may help to inhale steam from a jug with a towel over the head. It can be more pleasant if you add Friar's Balsam or menthol to the water.

Sore throats are often caused by virus infections which cannot be treated very effectively by drugs. However, a sore throat may also be caused by infection with bacteria called streptococci, in which case a doctor may prescribe antibiotics. If a sore throat is more than mild you should see your doctor. Gargling with plain water or an ordinary gargle mixture may bring some relief.

Hazards at Work

Each year in Britain about fifteen hundred people die as a result of work activities – half from injuries, half from occupational diseases. Another six hundred thousand are injured seriously enough to keep them away from work for at least three days. Sometimes the deaths and injuries are dramatic and instantaneous, as in accidents; on other occasions death may be the result of long-lingering illnesses such as pneumoconiosis (black lungs) in coal-miners. Some jobs are intrinsically more dangerous than others, notably coal-mining, shipping and construction or demolition work. But accidents happen wherever people are working. Life down on the farm may be more peaceful than in the factories but it is not necessarily safer, as our league table of injuries shows opposite. Even pedestrians are at risk as they walk under the scaffolding of building-sites.

Occupational hazards have become so much part of our everyday lives that the very phrase has become a cliché. The worst conditions of the Industrial Revolution have generally been eradicated by tougher legislation and more sophisticated industrial processes. But some remaining old hazards, such as the dust that clogs the lungs of miners, quarrymen and cotton-workers have been joined by newer ones often involving chemicals which were unknown a few years ago. And there are always accidents.

The cost to the community is quite astonishing. If you add together the cost of compensation payments, insurance claims, damage to plant and equipment plus lost working time, the total is around £4,000 million a year.

Nowadays, Britain, like most Western countries, has an elaborate hierarchy of committees and specialist bodies devoted to occupational safety. In a general book of this kind it is impossible to give detailed advice about every known hazard. There are, for instance, fifty-four categories of industrial diseases for which UK injuries benefits are payable, and more than six hundred chemical substances which are subject to varying degrees of control. But before discussing the most common causes of occupational hazards it is important to stress that most illnesses and, indeed, most accidents can be prevented, although it usually costs money. So no matter what kind of work you do, whether it be indoor or outdoor, in a factory or in an office, be militant about your own health and safety:

1. Discover the potential hazards in your work.
2. Make sure all safety measures are enforced – and, of course, that you follow them yourself. More injuries are

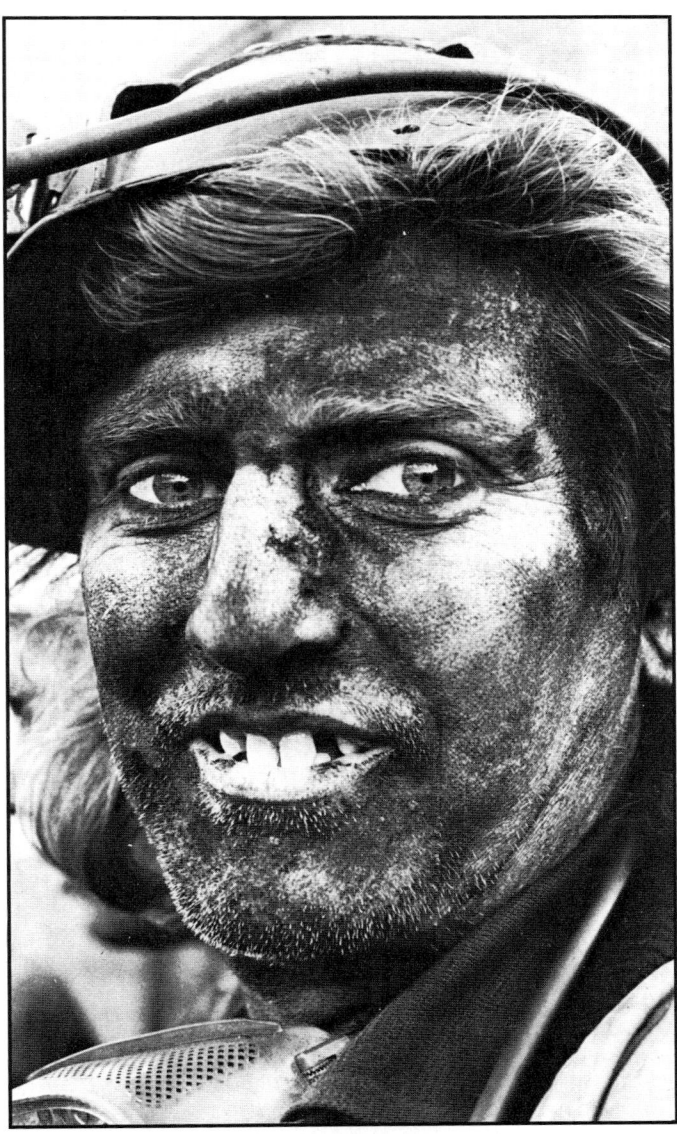

caused by a moment's forgetfulness – the safety-hat left in the cloakroom, the routine safety-check that is skipped – than occasional publicized 'disasters'.

3. If you believe there is a health or safety risk, stop work and ask for the hazard to be measured. First inform your safety representative, union official or management superior. Make sure that they take the matter up and have it rectified. If all else fails, contact the Health and Safety Executive (find them in the telephone book) or, if you work in an office or shop, your local council's environmental health department.

4. If you have to go to your doctor, tell him what kind of work you do and what materials you handle. They may be the cause of the problem.

The safety league table overleaf shows clearly the varying dangers of different types of jobs in terms of *accidents*. Occupational injuries, however, are much more susceptible to statistical identification than occupational illnesses or diseases. But it would be unwise to underestimate the dangers of work-related illnesses: many take years to develop and because of this 'time-bomb' effect may never be recognized as a consequence of work. **Official figures thus do not fully reflect both the number and severity of occupational illnesses and the league table omits work-related illnesses. If you work in one of the high-risk occupations at the top of our league table of injuries, however, naturally take special care.**

Shipping: Falls or blows from ship's tackle; accidents generally; skin diseases in fishermen, caused by allergies.

Coal-mining: Bronchitis; accidents; respiratory tuberculosis; and pneumoconiosis, a crippling and often fatal disease caused by the accumulation of mineral dust in the lungs.

Railways: Accidents involving trains, men working on the line or engineering equipment; falls from platforms, trucks, etc.

Agriculture: Accidents involving tractors, falls and animals, notably bulls; infections such as anthrax, tetanus and brucellosis; farmer's lung, an allergy caused by inhaling mouldy dust, usually from hay; and eye injuries.

Construction: Accidents, in particular falls from scaffolding or ladders and the collapse of foundations or other building materials. The machinery and transport vehicles associated with construction (and demolition) sites also cause innumerable accidents.

Deep-sea oil exploration, such as that in the North Sea, is even more dangerous than the occupations at the top of this league table. Such dangers are thankfully remote indeed for most of us. The hazards below are less dramatic but more common.

Noise: Damage to hearing is not only caused by loud bangs; most comes with prolonged exposure to noise which is not so loud that you cannot get used to it. This is now recognized as a major industrial health hazard. Noise is measured in decibels on a scale based on powers of ten: 10 decibels (dBAs) is ten times as intense as the quietest sound you can hear, 20 dBAs is a hundred times, 30 dBAs a thousand times as intense. Each increase of 3 dBAs doubles the sound intensity. In Britain the recommended legal limit for noise is 90 dBAs. Above that, protective equipment must be provided. For levels up to 105 dBAs this means properly fitted earplugs of plastic, rubber or glass down; up to 115 dBAs, ear-muffs; and for levels over 115 dBAs, protective helmets. (The EEC proposes an 85 dBA limit.)

Machinery: Accidents resulting from faulty, or improperly used, machinery are a continuing problem. Safety laws are specific on guarding moving parts and inspecting unguarded machinery. Guards should provide positive protection without discomfort to the worker, and prevent all access to the danger areas during work. If they don't and are in need of replacement or repair, work should be stopped.

Hand-tools: More than ten thousand accidents in factories every year are caused by common hand-tools. Use only the right tool for the job. Where there is a risk of an explosive atmosphere, use non-sparking tools. Use only tools in good condition. Stow all tools safely, particularly at heights. Wear eye-goggles when provided.

Lifting: Most spinal injuries result from incorrect lifting techniques and from carrying weights that are too heavy. Damage may be cumulative and not necessarily immediate. Many trade unions have agreed on limits between 45 and 60 pounds, but even this is far more than most men can manage. The International Labour Office approves of 80 to 110 pounds, depending on age and physique. The nearer the body is to an upright position when lifting, the less work is required from muscles and the less strain imposed on spinal discs. Keep arms close to the body, chin tucked in and place feet a hip-breadth apart to give a stronger base and balance. Most important of all, keep a straight back (see pages 106–12).

INTENSITIES OF TYPICAL NOISES

Approximate sound-pressure level (in dBAs)	Source and location
200	Moon rocket at lift-off, 300m away
160	Peak level at the ear, of 0.303 rifle
140	Jet aircraft taking off at 25m
120	Submarine engine-room
100	Very noisy factory
90	Heavy diesel lorry at 7m
	Road drill at 7m (unsilenced)
80	Ice-cream van at 3m
	Ringing alarm clock at 1m
75	Inside railway carriage
70	Inside small saloon car, 50 kph
	3m from domestic vacuum cleaner
65	Busy general office with typewriters
	Normal conversation at 1m
40	Quiet office
35	Quiet bedroom
25	Still day in the country away from traffic

Source: Noise, by Rupert Taylor, pp. 55–6. Reprinted by permission of Penguin Books Ltd. Copyright © Rupert Taylor, 1970.

HAZARDS AT WORK/**STAYING HEALTHY AT WORK AND PLAY**

Chemical hazards and dusts: Almost every working process uses chemicals in the form of oils, solvents, metals, gases or resins. There are 'threshold limit values' (TLVs) for over six hundred substances, and management must inform workers using these and monitor work-areas regularly.

Most diseases caused by chemicals in fact start with either their inhalation, which affects various parts of the body, including particularly the lungs, or their ingestion through the skin and blood-stream. Coal-miner's pneumoconiosis is the best known, often fatal and caused by coal-dust clogging the lungs. Asbestosis is also particularly toxic and notorious but silicosis, byssinosis (from cotton, flax or hemp dust) and bagassosis (from sugar-cane fibre) can all be fatal and cause chronic bronchitis and emphysema. Any kind of dust (including sawdust) is a potential hazard to health. Oil mist, caused by mineral oil vaporizing, can cause dermatitis and cancer; mercury and lead vapours are particularly dangerous.

Ideally dangerous substances should be prevented from entering the air at all – by fitting effective exhaust ventilation to machines, for instance. If this is not possible, suitable breathing apparatus *must* be worn, especially if working in confined spaces.

Not all substances stop short at the lungs. Cadmium can affect both the liver and kidneys; vinyl chloride affects the bone structure – thickening of the fingers, for instance – and can also affect the liver, causing cancer. Lead and benzene both affect bone marrow, and some substances affect the haemoglobin in the blood – carbon monoxide being the most lethal. Three particular substances cause the overwhelming majority of skin disorders: epoxy resins, mineral oils and solvents. They are widely used in industry. Protective clothing, thorough washing and medical attention for any skin rashes or injuries is essential. Chemicals should not be allowed to come into contact with the skin, because even if they do no immediate harm they can be absorbed through the skin into the body.

The scale of the threat posed by chemicals – the invisible contaminants – can be indicated by a few figures. More than thirty thousand individual chemicals were manufactured in Britain in 1980 in quantities of more than 1 tonne. The total production of chemicals increased in twenty years from 7 million tonnes a year to 63 million. No fewer than a thousand of these chemicals have been suspected of causing cancer.

Radiation: There are several types of electro-magnetic radiation, some harmless like radio-waves, some lethal like gamma-rays. Microwaves will 'cook' any exposed part of the body, with severe physical and possibly mental effects.

Infra-red radiation can come from any red-hot material. Strong radiation produces burns, and long exposure can produce cataracts in the eye. This means the lens in the eye begins to go opaque and you start to go blind. Safety glasses with special filter lenses should therefore be worn and eyes examined regularly.

Ultra-violet radiation: the sun is the biggest source of this. Sun-tanning is the skin trying to defend itself by developing brown pigmentation. Ultra-violet radiation can dry and wrinkle the skin, produce localized skin sores and – in certain rare cases where there has been years of open-air work on farms or building-sites – skin cancer. The commonest occupational sources of this radiation are arc-welding and sterilizing-units. Protective clothing and masks must be worn.

Radiation is one of the most insidious of all occupational hazards. Except in cases of severe over-exposure it can be neither seen nor felt at the time, but its effects can include burns, cancer, leukaemia, sterility and infertility. The most commonly used are X-rays and gamma-rays. Anyone whose work involves either form of radiation must by British law wear film-badges or other dosometers in radiation areas to monitor their annual dosage.

Accidents: Accidents are usually the result of lack of training – especially in the construction industry – and neglect. Noise, vibration, high and low temperatures, stress, fatigue and narcotic fumes can all increase 'accident-proneness'. Usually, though, some additional hazard actually delivers the injury, such as poor lighting or oil on the floor causing someone to slip, or trip over some waste. If standards for lighting, ventilation, cleanliness and overcrowding are low, the accident-rate is likely to be high.

There are so many other minor causes of occupational illness that whole books have been written about them (see Appendix Three). Many, for instance, are forms of allergies which were covered earlier in the chapter. If you suspect that you may be suffering from an occupational disease, consult your doctor – both your family doctor and, if there is one, the works doctor, who may have more specialist knowledge. If the doctor confirms that you are suffering from such an illness, investigate your liability for compensation; trade unions are a great help here. But many diseases, such as asbestosis and scrotal cancer, are not sudden illnesses which the layman or sufferer can detect; their incubation periods can take anything from ten to thirty years. So always be vigilant in taking all possible precautions. In the UK the factory inspector will advise on any potential hazard, and has the power to force employers and employees to make the workplace safe.

THE SAFETY LEAGUE

Latest annual statistics of injuries per 100,000 workers in large-scale occupations

Industry	Fatal	Serious
Shipping	67	1,800*
Coal-mining	19	16,800*
Railways	17	2,800*
Agriculture	12	1,400*†
Construction	12	500
Metal manufacture	10	930
Bricks and cement	5	590
Chemical	5	510
Food, drink & tobacco	3	750
Timber and furniture	3	550
Paper, printing & publishing	3	360

*all injuries with at least three days off work
†excluding farmers and their families

Sources: Health and Safety Executive; Ministry of Agriculture; National Coal Board; British Rail; Council of British Shipping; Dept. of Trade; RoSPA.

STAYING HEALTHY AT WORK AND PLAY/PREVENTING INFECTIONS

Preventing Infections

Infections of the body are caused by many different types of organisms: viruses, bacteria, fungi and protozoa such as amoeba. These infectious organisms enter the body in contaminated food or water; droplets carried in the air we breathe; direct contact on hands, lips, or in sexual intercourse; and as a result of animal- or insect-bites. It is common sense to avoid spreading infection by observing the usual rules of hygiene (see page 163) and by avoiding contact with people when they are ill. Nevertheless, infectious organisms invade the body all the time and the body is equipped to defend itself.

The first line in the body's defence against infection is the skin, which is impervious to most assaults. Tears, saliva and the secretions of the stomach and the bowel all contain substances which attack stray bacteria, viruses or any foreign organisms. If an attacking organism does penetrate the body, then it will be attacked by antibodies and white blood-cells which digest and kill any foreign substances they come across. These are the defences of the body which are stimulated by vaccination in order to prepare the body in advance for a potential invasion.

Resistance to disease may be lowered by illness or the way we live. During convalescence, people are more vulnerable to disease, which is why they must rest. An inadequate diet with a shortage of essential vitamins will make a person more vulnerable to infection. So will smoking, excessive drinking, drug addiction, overwork, excessive worry, insufficient sleep and exercise. More information about these topics can be found elsewhere in this book.

An individual can protect him or herself from infection not only by high standards of hygiene (see above) and avoiding other people when ill but also through vaccination (see page 32). Elsewhere in this book we advise readers on how to protect themselves against the cold, how to avoid sexually transmitted diseases and how to protect your health while on holiday abroad. But it is impossible to give detailed instructions on avoiding or preventing *all* diseases. Ask your doctor about quarantine measures which may be advisable in any individual case. In this section, however, we give the basic information about infectious conditions most common in temperate climates. Prompt recognition and careful quarantine measures can do much to prevent the spread of illness. Few drugs are effective against virus diseases, which are caused by germs which can only grow inside the living cell. Most, but not all, bacterial or fungal diseases can be treated effectively with antibiotic drugs.

BRUCELLOSIS, also called undulant fever, Malta fever and mountain fever.
Mode of infection: Caused by a bacterium, brucella, transmitted by drinking or eating unpasteurized raw milk or dairy products, or by contact with infected cattle. Most common among farmers and butchers but rarely transmitted from one person to another.
Symptoms: Exhaustion and weakness at the least exertion, irritability, alternating chills and fever, headache and pains in joints and back. Glands may become enlarged in neck and armpit. May last for months but rarely fatal.
Treatment: Rest in bed. Vitamins and antibiotics.
Prevention: Never drink raw unpasteurized milk or eat raw cheese except from an attested brucellosis-free (and tuberculin-tested) herd. Avoid contact with sick animals.

CHICKENPOX, also called varicella.
Mode of infection: Caused by a virus, spread by contact or by breathing in droplets coughed out by infectious person. One infection usually gives lifelong immunity.
Symptoms: Symptoms appear ten to eighteen days after exposure to infection. Fever, discomfort, loss of appetite. Rash on back and chest spreading to face, scalp and arms. Rash consists of separate red spots which develop into a blister, fill with a clear fluid that becomes cloudy later, and finally form crusts which fall off after about two weeks.
Treatment: Rest in bed while feeling ill. Personal hygiene is important to prevent secondary infection. Avoid scratching; cut fingernails and keep them clean to avoid infection of spots. Use medicated shampoo for spots on scalp.
Prevention: A person with the illness should be kept isolated until the crusts have gone, which is usually about twelve days from the start. The same virus which causes chickenpox also causes shingles (see below), so an adult with shingles can give a child chickenpox. Although the illness is generally not serious, special care should be taken to avoid exposing infants to infection.

CYSTITIS
Mode of infection: Bladder inflammation, often an infection caused by bacteria which may come from the kidney or, most often, travel up the urethra (the tube down which the urine passes). Most frequent in women.
Symptoms: Pain in the bladder area, tiredness, fever. Desire to pass urine frequently. Urination accompanied by burning sensation.
Treatment: Antibiotic drugs, rest, drinking large quantities of water – two or three times normal intake – which literally flushes the bacteria from the bladder.
Prevention: Keep the genitals clean. Wipe anus from front to back. Avoid alcoholic drinks and highly seasoned foods which may irritate the bladder. Women should empty the bladder after intercourse.

DIPHTHERIA
Mode of infection: Caused by a bacterium which enters the body through the windpipe or lungs. The bacterium is coughed into the air by an infectious person. Milk or other food may carry the infection.
Symptoms: These may appear within twelve hours of infection. Similar at first to those of common cold, sore throat, weakness and fever. But the illness rapidly becomes serious; breathing and swallowing become difficult. A poison produced by the bacterium paralyses the heart and nerves. Untreated, the disease is often fatal. Medical help should be sought urgently.
Treatment: Antitoxin, penicillin and bed rest.
Prevention: Diphtheria is spread by apparently healthy people (carriers) as well as by those suffering from the illness. The disease is now rare because of vaccination. Ill people should be isolated until tests show that the infection

PREVENTING INFECTIONS/**STAYING HEALTHY AT WORK AND PLAY**

The body's defences against infection.

Lymph glands throughout the body produce scavenging white blood-cells which defend the body against infection. The lymph glands also produce antibodies which are secreted into the blood and which attack any foreign substances entering the body. These are the immune defences of the body. Lymph glands near the surface (shown in white) may be felt with the fingers, especially if they become swollen when defending the body against local infection.

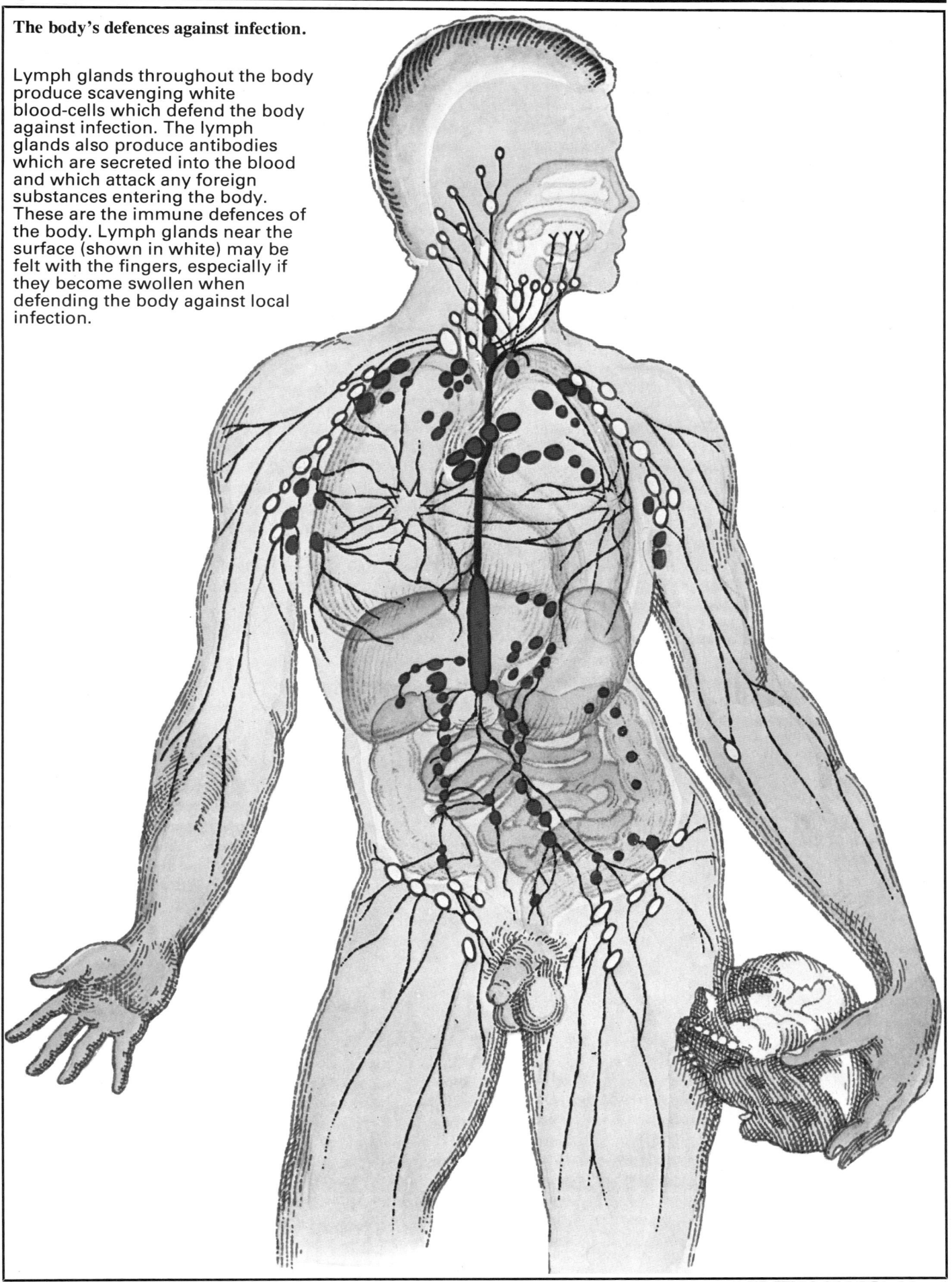

STAYING HEALTHY AT WORK AND PLAY/PREVENTING INFECTIONS

has gone. Anyone exposed unwittingly to infection should seek vaccination, if not already vaccinated, and report any suspicious symptoms to a doctor at an early stage so that preventive treatment can be given.

ERYSIPELAS
Mode of infection: Caused by a bacterium (streptococcus) infecting the skin, and spread by contact or by touching some object which has been in contact with an infected person. Extremely infectious.
Symptoms: Inflammation of the skin appearing in dark red patches with swollen, raised border, particularly on the face and legs. Fever and headache. Commonest in middle and old age.
Treatment: Antibiotics. Paracetamol for pain.
Prevention: Avoidance of contact with someone who has the disease. Bacteria may enter any small crack in the skin. If caring for someone with the illness, scrupulously wash with soap and water. Scrupulous personal hygiene and washing of food dishes.

GASTRO-ENTERITIS, also called food poisoning, gastritis.
Mode of infection: Stomach and bowel upsets with vomiting or diarrhoea can have many causes – one of the commonest is over-indulgence in alcohol or food. They may also be caused by infection of bowel by viruses or bacteria, or by allergy or food poisoning. Food poisoning should be suspected when several people eating the same food all become ill at about the same time – usually within about twenty-four hours. Its commonest causes are:

1. Eating food contaminated with bacteria called salmonella which are common in sewage. If they enter the bowel they increase in number, causing infection.
2. Eating food which has been spoiled through infection by staphylococci, another type of bacterium. These bacteria do not invade the bowel themselves but a poison (toxin) produced by them in the food causes the familiar symptoms. Another type of food poisoning, botulism, is caused by inadequate preservation of food. Food poisoning is also occasionally caused by eating poisonous plants.

Symptoms: Diarrhoea, vomiting, nausea, pain and tenderness of bowel.
Treatment: Consult doctor; some drugs are available which may relieve symptoms but avoid unless prescribed by doctor. Most important, drink plenty of water, fruit juices or squash to restore fluids; add a level teaspoon of salt per pint of water and a generous teaspoon of honey or sugar. Drink at least 2½ pints a day. Rest.
Prevention: Washing hands after going to toilet and before preparing or eating food. Do not store cooked food at room temperature. Avoidance of unhygienic eating places. Care in preparing and preservation of food. (See also Holiday Health, Chapter 9).

GERMAN MEASLES
See **Rubella**

GLANDULAR FEVER, also called mononucleosis.
Mode of infection: Believed to be caused by the Epstein–Barr virus and to be transmitted by close contact such as kissing. Common in residential institutions such as colleges, military bases, etc.
Symptoms: Fatigue, fever, headache, sore throat, swollen glands in neck, armpit and groin. Blood-test shows abnormal number and types of certain white blood-cells. May last for weeks or months and is associated with depression.
Treatment: Rest and well-balanced diet. No drug treatment is available.
Prevention: Avoidance of close physical contact with anyone known to have the illness until symptoms have cleared.

HEPATITIS
Mode of infection: Liver infection generally caused by a virus. Two main types: infectious hepatitis, spread by contaminated food or drink in areas where hygiene is poor, symptoms appear two or three weeks after infection; serum hepatitis, spread in blood from unsterilized syringes or by blood-transfusion.
Symptoms: Headache, loss of appetite and fever. Followed by jaundice – that is, skin and whites of eyes become yellow. Liver and spleen enlarge and become tender; pain below right rib margin.
Treatment: Rest in bed while jaundiced. Convalesce for at least two weeks. Eat whatever food is most appetizing. Avoid alcohol, which may delay recovery of the liver, for at least a year after the illness. If jaundice does not clear up rapidly, a specialist opinion should be sought.
Prevention: Take care when travelling always to drink sterilized water. Passive immunity against hepatitis can be given by injection of an extract of blood serum – worth having if travelling in areas with primitive sanitation, or if someone in the family gets the illness. Isolate patient until one week after jaundice has disappeared. Take great care in disposal of wastes and in washing of clothes and dishes.

IMPETIGO
Mode of infection: Caused by bacteria – usually staphylococci but sometimes streptococci – which invade skin, particularly the face.
Symptoms: Skin turns red; pus blisters form which burst and make a weeping sore with yellowish, crusty scabs. Highly infectious, spreads quickly, especially to children.
Treatment: Application of antibiotic ointment, and antibiotics by mouth. Apply warm compresses of salt and permanganate solution to remove crusts.
Prevention: Anyone with the condition should have their own towels and avoid skin-contact with others. Cut nails, scrupulous washing. Avoid scratching sores.

INFLUENZA (see also pages 154–5)
Mode of infection: Caused mainly by two different types of viruses. One of them regularly changes, causing widespread epidemics. Infection by inhaling airborne droplets.
Symptoms: Weakness, chills, fever, loss of appetite, headache and general aches and pains, inflammation of nose and throat.
Treatment: Bed rest, plenty of fluids.
Prevention: Vaccination. Avoidance of people who have symptoms, avoidance of crowded places in winter.

MEASLES, also called rubeola, morbilli.
Mode of infection: Caused by a virus spread by droplets in the air which are released when someone with the illness coughs or sneezes. One infection usually gives lifelong immunity.
Symptoms: First symptoms similar to cold: sore eyes, run-

ning nose, coughing and sneezing. Raised temperature. Rash of many small red spots does not appear until three to five days after start of illness. Rash usually starts behind the ears and often spreads to whole body, disappearing after about a week. First signs of measles other than illness are Koplik's spots – red with white centres – which appear in the mouth and inside the cheeks about two days before the rash. Symptoms appear ten to fifteen days after exposure.
Treatment: Bed rest in well-ventilated room until temperature returns to normal. Avoidance of anyone with colds or other illness. Consult doctor, because complications – particularly infection of the ear – can occur.
Prevention: Vaccination. Avoidance of anyone with the illness until a week after disappearance of rash.

MENINGITIS
Mode of infection: Caused by several different types of bacteria, particularly the meningococcus, which enter blood-stream through nose or mouth and reach the nervous system. Also caused by viruses.
Symptoms: Shivering, temperature, severe headache, vomiting, fever, stiffness of muscles of neck and back, rash. Person may become unconscious.
Treatment: Prompt medical treatment vital. Antibiotics are effective against bacterial forms of illness. Some virus forms of the disease can also be treated with drugs.
Prevention: Close contacts of anyone who gets this illness should be observed for any early signs of the disease, and these should be reported to a doctor. Work is in progress on a vaccine. Patient should be isolated.

MUMPS
Mode of infection: Caused by a virus which appears in saliva and is spread in air-droplets. One attack usually gives lifelong immunity.
Symptoms: Headache, fever, vomiting, swelling of the salivary glands on one or both sides of the face just below the ear. In men, mumps sometimes also involves the testicles, and in women the ovaries, but seldom causes sterility. Illness appears two to three weeks after infection.
Treatment: Consult doctor, since similar symptoms are sometimes caused by other illnesses. Bed rest and plenty of fluids if feverish. In mild cases, rest at home until swelling goes down. A simple mouthwash occasionally, and paracetamol tablets for pain.
Prevention: Avoidance of person with illness for three weeks after onset. Avoidance of towels, etc., used by infected person. Vaccination of young adults who have not had the disease.

PNEUMONIA
Mode of infection: Caused by bacterial infection, particularly by the pneumococcus which is present in all healthy mouths and throats. When resistance is lowered by colds, flu or ill health, then this or other bacteria may invade the lungs. Another type – viral pneumonia – is caused by a virus infection.
Symptoms: Sharp pains in the chest, a sharp dry cough, fever. Coughs up a rusty-coloured spit which may also contain blood or pus.
Treatment: Consult doctor. Antibiotic drugs and oxygen.
Prevention: Proper convalescence after colds and flu. Avoidance of hurried eating, which results in inhalation of food. People who are bedridden should sit up as much as possible or change position frequently to prevent accumulation of fluid on lungs. Perform coughing and breathing exercises after an operation.

POLIOMYELITIS, also called polio, infantile paralysis.
Mode of infection: Caused by a virus which enters the body through the nose or mouth and attacks nerves.
Symptoms: May be mild, resembling flu. Otherwise, headache, fever, vomiting, drowsiness, stiffness of head and back. Muscle weakness and paralysis of shoulder or hip may develop within a week.
Treatment: Skilled nursing in hospital. May spread to muscles controlling breathing so that a respirator may be necessary. Moist-packs relieve muscle spasms.
Prevention: Vaccination, particularly of people going abroad.

PSITTACOSIS, also called parrot fever, ornithosis.
Mode of infection: Caused by inhalation of a virus transmitted to people by birds such as pigeons, parrots, budgerigars, chickens and ducks.
Symptoms: Vary from mild flu-like illness to pneumonia.
Treatment: Antibiotic drugs.
Prevention: Avoid sick birds. Bird-fanciers should destroy sick birds.

RABIES
Mode of infection: Caused by a virus carried in animal saliva entering through a break in the skin. Commonly carried by dogs, cats, foxes and bats, but can be transmitted to man by almost any animal – for example, a cow bitten by a fox may then bite a man, so transmitting the disease. The disease is increasingly common in Europe but does not occur in the British Isles.
Symptoms: Convulsions, muscle spasms, hydrophobia – fear of water – develop because any attempt to swallow causes painful contractions of the larynx. Death inevitable if victim is not vaccinated after the bite. Symptoms first appear from a few days to months after a bite.
Treatment: When bitten by an animal, wash the wound with soap and warm water and go to a doctor. Ideally the animal should be shot so that it can be tested for rabies. Immunization should begin immediately if the bite is on the face or neck; if the bite is further from the brain, then the animal may be tested for rabies first.
Prevention: Quarantine of animals entering Britain. When in other countries, avoid any animal you do not know well. Do not let animal saliva enter any break in the skin. Avoid stroking all stray animals, especially on holidays abroad.

RINGWORM, also called tinea.
Mode of infection: Caused by a fungus which is highly infectious. It may be spread by direct contact or by using infected linen, combs, etc.
Symptoms: An itchy eruption of the skin, especially of groin and toes, and scalp or nails.
Treatment: Antibiotic drugs such as griseofulvin. Must be taken by mouth until new nails have grown if nails affected, and anti-fungal ointment used.
Prevention: Prompt treatment of infection. Scrupulous hygienic measures, and avoid contact with victim.

RUBELLA, also called German measles.
Mode of infection: Caused by a virus which gives rise to

STAYING HEALTHY AT WORK AND PLAY/PREVENTING INFECTIONS

symptoms two to three weeks after infection. One infection usually gives immunity for life. Virus spread by infected droplets from coughs and sneezes.
Symptoms: Pink rash on face and body which fades after three or four days. Symptoms usually mild. Major risk is to foetus in the first three or four months of pregnancy.
Treatment: No special treatment necessary. If infection occurs in first three months of pregnancy, there is a possible ground for abortion.
Prevention: People with the illness should stay at home in order to minimize the risk of infecting a pregnant woman. Vaccination available to girls before puberty.

SCARLET FEVER, also called scarlatina.
Mode of infection: Caused by the bacterium streptococcus which also causes sore throats; close physical contact. Food contaminated with nose discharge. Infected droplets from sneezes etc.
Symptoms: Nausea, vomiting, headache, fever, sore throat and widespread red rash. Thickly coated tongue with raw red edges.
Treatment: Used to be a dreaded disease but can now be treated very effectively by antibiotics such as penicillin. Bed rest for ten days. Paracetamol for pain relief.
Prevention: Isolation from family. Clothing, dishes must be disinfected. Patient no longer infectious when rash fades and skin starts to peel about two weeks after.

SHINGLES, also called herpes zoster.
Mode of infection: Caused by the same virus as chickenpox.
Symptoms: Fever and pain for a few days. Many small blisters in lines along the back following the path of nerves, and extremely painful. The virus inflames the nerves, causing pain which may last for weeks or even months after the rash has cleared up.
Treatment: Pain-relieving drugs, drugs to prevent eye complication. Rest. Seek medical advice.
Prevention: Shingles is almost certainly caused by activation of viruses which have lain dormant in the body since a childhood infection with chickenpox. It does not seem to be caused by adults coming into contact with children with chickenpox. No means of prevention available.

TETANUS, also called lockjaw.
Mode of infection: Caused by clostridium bacteria from the soil and faeces. The bacteria invade the body through wounds contaminated by dirt. Deep, dirty wounds caused by nails or bullets are particularly vulnerable.
Symptoms: Spasm of muscles, convulsions which may be so bad that the whole body arches backwards.
Treatment: Clean and dress wounds. Seek medical advice over any dirty wound. Booster immunization with tetanus toxoid, and penicillin to kill bacteria. Tranquillizing drugs. Muscle-relaxing drugs may be given and the patient put on a respirator.
Prevention: Vaccination, which gives protection lasting many years. Careful cleaning of wounds with soap and warm water. Professional care for deep wounds.

THRUSH, also called moniliasis, candidiasis.
Mode of infection: Caused by a yeast-like fungus called candida albicans. Exacerbated by irritation. Diabetics are particularly vulnerable. The fungus often lives in the bowel and so infection does not necessarily come immediately from another person, but can come by contact.
Symptoms: A wet eruption of the skin with extremely unpleasant itching, which breaks out in any of the skin-folds, the nails, the anus, vagina or the mouth. The term thrush strictly refers to an infection of the mouth, where it causes white patches inside the cheeks, but is often used to refer to infection in other places. Candida may also infect the lung.
Treatment: Fungicidal drugs such as nystatin, tablets or pessaries. Also rinses and ointments.
Prevention: Scrupulous personal hygiene. Wash with soap and water only. Do not add perfume or bubble mixtures to baths which may cause irritation and provoke infection. Always wipe anus from front to back.

TUBERCULOSIS
Mode of infection: Caused by a bacterium, mycobacterium tuberculosis, which may be inhaled or swallowed in food. The bacteria most commonly invade the lungs but may attack many other parts of the body. The germs used to be spread in infected milk but this is now rare in the UK because cows are tested for tuberculosis and most milk is pasteurized.
Symptoms: Infection with tuberculosis often causes a mild illness which gives immunity to the disease. Pulmonary TB – that is, infection of the lungs – causes loss of weight, weakness, fever, and bloodstained sputum. TB may also infect bones, joints, lymph glands, intestines, kidneys and the nerves.
Treatment: Drug treatments introduced in the 1950s have conquered what used to be a killer disease. The three most effective drugs are: Streptomycin, isoniazid and para-aminosalicylic acid.
Prevention: Vaccination. Never drink unpasteurized milk. Milk is likely to be safe in Western countries, but beware in less developed countries.

WHOOPING COUGH, also called pertussis.
Mode of infection: Caused by bacterial infection, usually of a type called bordetella pertussis, which infects the body in droplets entering the lungs. Highly infectious. One infection usually gives lifelong immunity.
Symptoms: Begins as a persistent cough and heavy cold with fever. This lasts a week and then for about another three weeks the victim suffers a barking cough which is very debilitating. This is an extremely serious illness in babies. Symptoms take up to two weeks to appear after infection.
Treatment: Rest. Food in small, frequent amounts if patient is liable to vomit. Drug treatment not very effective. Hospitalization is often necessary for infants.
Prevention: Vaccination, but this is controversial because it may cause damage in rare cases (see page 32). Avoid anyone who has had the illness for at least four weeks from the start of the illness or until the cough entirely subsides. Close contacts who were exposed before the illness was diagnosed should also be kept in quarantine for two weeks until it is known if they have caught the infection. Babies under one year who have been in close contact with someone who develops the illness may be given antibiotic drugs to prevent the infection – at an early stage drug treatment may be effective.

Rules of Hygiene

1. Buy only from clean places. Get the food home clean.

2. Use clean containers in your home.

3. Keep family foods away from food for pets. Use separate utensils and crockery.

4. Wash your hands always before preparing food, always after using the WC. See your children do too.

5. Cover cuts and sores with waterproof dressings. If you are not well with no one to take your place in the kitchen then be extra careful about personal cleanliness.

6. Keep food clean, covered and either cool or piping hot.

7. Reheated leftovers must be made really hot right through. Do the same with ready-packed foods intended to be eaten hot.

8. Keep working surfaces clean. Use really hot, soapy water. A wipe with a dish cloth is not enough.

9. Stack washed and rinsed crockery and pans to drain. If you use drying cloths be sure they are clean.

10. Keep the lid on the dustbin.

REFRIGERATOR RULES

1. Allow food to cool at room temperature before putting into the refrigerator.

2. Do not attempt to keep cooked food or meat for more than three days in the refrigerator.

3. Keep raw and cooked food separate and covered so that drips from meat, for example, do not contaminate other food.

4. Do not overload. Allow space for air circulation so that it can work efficiently.

5. Ensure it is cooling to 3–5°C. Defrost regularly for efficiency. Keep clean.

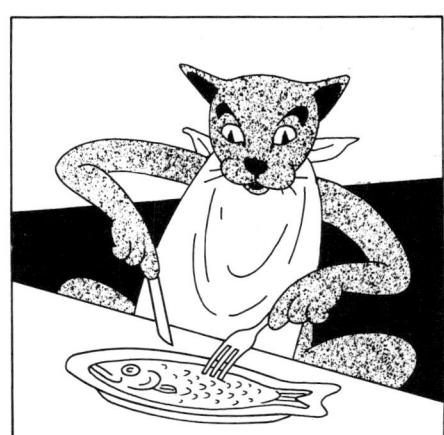 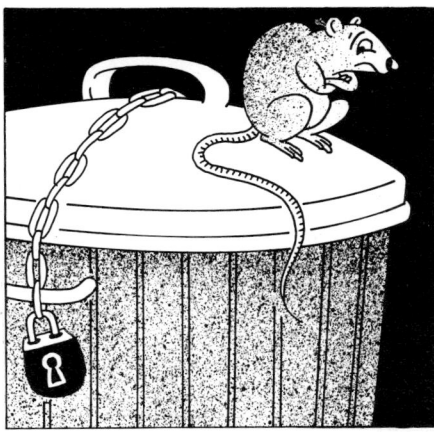 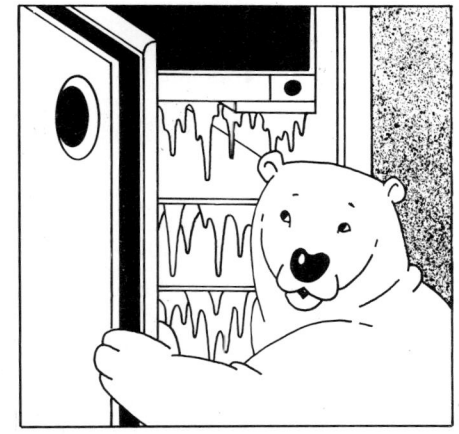

Reproduced by kind permission of the Health Education Council

Allergies

Do you feel ill when you smell paint, become breathless in front of a birdcage at the zoo, or develop severe stomach pains and wind on eating onions? If so, you may be suffering from an allergy. Allergies can make people extremely ill with asthma, eczema or bowel troubles. In rare cases, allergies can be life-threatening. But they are also a form of illness which the patient can often avoid, once the allergy has been identified.

Allergies take so many unusual forms, however, that the causes often go unrecognized by those who suffer. Or, if a person does recognize the substances which make them ill, he or she will often get little sympathy from friends who too often consider the story an unlikely one, like the girl who was allergic to beer and came out in spots if only a few drops were spilt on her feet. But if the cause of the allergy can be identified and the person can learn to avoid it, then the illness may miraculously end. Sometimes it is easy, sometimes very difficult, to identify the problem.

Allergies occur because in some people the body's defence against infection is over-sensitive. When foreign substances such as bacteria, dust or some foods enter the body they react by producing antibodies which attack the bacteria to prevent infection. Some unfortunate people make antibodies against normal, harmless substances in their environment like grass pollen. It is not surprising that when a mechanism evolved to protect us against a few bacteria reacts with the relatively enormous quantities of pollen which we inhale, the body's response can be devastating.

When an allergic substance combines with antibodies in a person's body, excessive quantities of histamine and other irritating substances are released in the body, causing certain tissues to swell: especially vulnerable are the skin, the delicate lining of the nose, the windpipe and the intestines. This produces a spasmodic contraction of the tubes of the windpipe and bronchi, causing asthma in some people. But everyone produces their own type of antibody, which is located in different parts of the body so that the same substance from, say, cats might cause one person to develop asthma and another to develop a skin rash. Most people who are allergic to grass pollen suffer from hay fever in their eyes and nose, but in a few people only the chest reacts, causing asthma without any symptoms elsewhere.

The main types of allergy are discussed below.

HAY FEVER

This only occurs when plant pollen and mould spores are present in the air in large numbers. There are three million sufferers in Britain: nine out of ten are sensitive to grass pollen. However, a wide variety of pollens or mould spores may cause 'hay fever' in some people.

Victims of hay fever suffer a running nose and sneezing, itching eyes and an itching throat. This dulls mental processes so that at times it becomes extremely difficult to concentrate. There is no easy escape from pollen. It is carried everywhere on the wind into the heart of cities and inside air-conditioned buildings. A modern air-conditioned building may provide the best respite because less pollen penetrates it.

People with mild hay fever may find that a drug prescribed by the doctor is sufficient to prevent the worst symptoms and they may then be able to play golf or watch a cricket match. Treatment with eyedrops and aerosols containing disodium cromoglycate or locally acting steroids such as beclomethasone are more generally effective than antihistamine tablets and have fewer side-effects. Disodium cromoglycate is exceptionally safe. However, severe sufferers must so far as possible stay indoors during the pollen season. They should keep doors and windows closed as much as possible. If extra air is needed in the room, then a frame covered with two or three layers of butter-muslin can be constructed to fit into a window. If the muslin is kept damp it acts as an excellent filter, but it must not be allowed to go mouldy.

Perhaps the best cure is to go for a month's holiday at the start of the pollen season to an area where the pollen is out of season, either north where it has not started or south where it has finished. It is an advantage to go to the coast, where sea breezes are relatively free of pollen, or to the mountains where the air may again be clearer. For those who can afford it, a sea cruise is ideal.

If these measures do not work, the hay-fever sufferer should try desensitizing injections of the pollen which is the cause of the allergy. The injections, which must be taken during the winter, cause the body to produce another antibody. This new antibody blocks the reaction of pollen with existing antibodies which are attracted to certain parts of the body, for example the nose or lungs, and cause the irritating symptoms of hay fever. It used to be necessary to have twenty injections, but now a modern injection is available which releases the pollen slowly in the body and has the same effect after nine injections. A newer 'depot' formulation requires only three injections but it has not yet been proven to be equally effective. A single year's course of injections is unlikely to give long-lasting protection and it is usual to give treatment for three years in succession. Then many of the patients will never relapse.

ALLERGIC RHINITIS

Allergic rhinitis (constantly runny nose and sneezing attacks) may be caused by all sorts of things from cats to scrubbing new potatoes. Mice, monkeys, face-powders, feathers, certain fabrics and upholstery, fungal spores in damp houses, detergents and aerosols can all cause the condition. But the commonest cause is house dust. This consists of small pieces of dirt, fibres from material, hairs and minute scales of skin which have worn off the surface of the body. The skin-scales are one rare cause of allergies but there is another cause which escaped detection until recently, when it was discovered that house dust contained thousands of minute mites, about a third of a millimetre long, which are invisible to the naked eye. These mites live by eating the scales of human skin and are found everywhere that people are found. Bedding and upholstery are particularly full of them. They are quite harmless for people who are not allergic to them.

A great deal can be done to free a house from dust and mites (see panel). Desensitizing injections to house dust are available but there is some controversy over how effective they are.

'INTRINSIC' ALLERGY

There is another type of allergic rhinitis which is not caused by inhaled particles. Some doctors call this 'intrinsic' allergy. It usually affects people over thirty-five years old and is characterized by nasal obstruction and running of the nose, but not by sneezing. The patient loses his sense of smell and may develop polyps, which are small lumps of jelly-like material that hang in the nose. Food allergy is sometimes found to be the cause (see below). A few patients have nasal polyps and sneezing attacks as well. They are likely to sneeze because of allergy to inhaled particles, but if this is dealt with, the polyps will not disappear. Nasal polyps are usually treated by surgical removal – a minor operation – but it may have to be repeated every few years. Alternatively, a nasal spray containing a steroid drug may be found effective, but this must be used only under the supervision of a doctor.

ASTHMA

Asthma, which simply means difficult breathing, can be a most serious complaint. There are one million sufferers in Britain and the number is increasing. Although an allergy is often the main cause of asthma, infection and psychological stress are also important. However, it can be extremely difficult to sort out which factor is most important.

The difficulty in breathing experienced during an asthmatic attack is the result of swelling of the membranes and constriction of the muscles in the breathing tubes, the bronchi, which lead to the lungs. The victim is then forced to wheeze, in attempts to get air into the lungs. The swollen membranes then produce a sticky liquid which further increases the difficulty in breathing.

Any of the dusts, odours or animals capable of causing hay fever or allergic rhinitis can also cause asthma. A great deal can be done to relieve the condition in some people by looking for the factor which triggers the attack and eliminating it from the house, or by general measures to make the house allergy-proof.

However, asthma does not always have an identifiable airborne cause. It is then called 'intrinsic' (see above).

The psychological factor in asthma seems to be secondary; a child, for example, may find that it can manipulate its parents by having an attack. Stress makes any allergic condition worse, but the most important factor is often simply fear of the asthma itself. But asthma should always be taken seriously because when it gets severe it can kill. Any attack which does not respond to the drugs which a person usually takes requires medical attention. With modern drugs it is always possible to relieve asthma, provided treatment is started early enough.

Asthmatics are also prone to bronchitis and should avoid people suffering from influenza or colds. These infections tend to aggravate the condition and set up a vicious cycle of repeating infections and asthmatic attacks. Asthmatics should avoid smoky rooms, as irritation from tobacco smoke usually makes asthma worse. Alcohol can also upset many people with asthma, and social drinking is likely to cause trouble from both smoke and alcohol.

The asthmatic may find it easier to breathe in bed if propped up on a lot of pillows. Most asthmatics are worse at night or in the early morning, even if the thing which caused the allergy was encountered many hours earlier. (For example, about one third of hay-fever sufferers are at their worst when they wake up, although they encountered grass pollen the previous afternoon.) These night-time attacks often mislead people into concentrating on possible causes of allergy in the bedroom, when in fact the rest of their environment is equally important.

Asthma attacks often follow a definite pattern like this, and can be forestalled by taking an appropriate drug before the expected attack. A variety of different drugs and inhalers are available for asthmatics, and finding the right treatment is a matter for professional advice.

People who suffer from asthma will have to choose carefully the types of sports they pursue. Asthma is usually made worse by exercise, but movements which cause vibration in the chest like running, jumping or boxing will provoke wheezing far more readily than 'smooth' exercises such as swimming, cycling or even rowing. Many distinguished athletes have suffered from asthma, so someone who suffers from it should not necessarily curb their ambition to succeed in sport. Exercise, short of that which provokes wheezing, can do an asthmatic nothing but good.

Breathing exercises for asthma: These can help to teach an asthmatic to expel the air from his lungs and so be in a better position to take the next breath. These exercises should be done if an attack of asthma threatens, as well as first thing in the morning and last thing at night, in order to clear the chest.

Blow the nose to clear the upper passages as far as possible. If producing a lot of spit on coughing, do the following exercise to drain the lungs. Lie flat on the bed, with head and shoulders supported on a chair or stool at a lower level. Cough repeatedly to clear the passages. Then lie first on one side and then on the other, coughing again to clear each lung in turn. (Coughing can make asthma worse in some people, in which case this exercise should obviously be avoided.) When the breathing passages are clear, practise diaphragm breathing as follows: breathe in slowly without raising the chest, using the belly muscles and diaphragm; breathe out slowly, taking as long as possible and emptying the lungs as fully as possible. Children may be helped by being given candles to blow out or ping-pong balls to blow across a table.

Any asthmatic can bring on an attack voluntarily by increasing their rate of breathing, and the onset of many attacks is a consequence of an unconscious rise in the rate of breathing caused by emotion – often simple fear that an attack is developing. An exercise which controls the rate of breathing by humming while the breath is slowly exhaled may be practised and then used to nip an attack in the bud. A physiotherapist can give guidance on suitable exercises and can train a patient to perform them correctly.

NETTLERASH (URTICARIA)

Nettlerash is an extremely itchy raised rash, very similar in type to the rash produced by nettle stings except that in some cases it may cover large parts of the body. Heat, cold or pressure of any kind makes the irritation worse. Certain foods, colouring matter or preservatives, and drugs, especially aspirin, laxatives, sleeping tablets and antibiotics are often responsible. Urticaria is also sometimes a reaction to vaginal thrush or, rarely, other disease.

To discover the cause, make a list of all the foods, drinks or medicines taken in the twenty-four hours preceding an attack. Foods commonly causing this allergy are: eggs, fish (especially shellfish), pork, strawberries and some other fruits, nuts and pips. After two or three attacks it should be

STAYING HEALTHY AT WORK AND PLAY/ALLERGIES

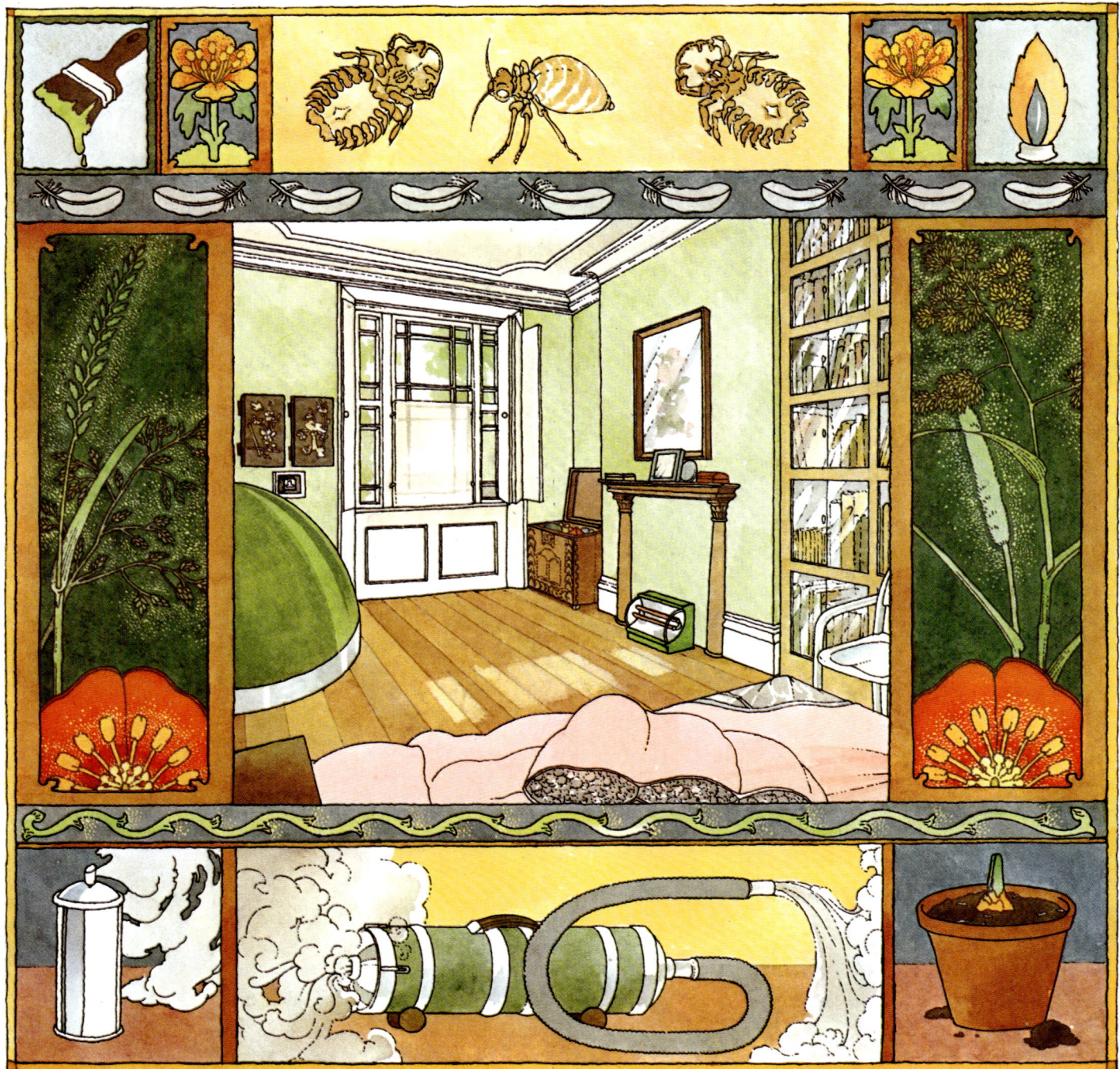

HOW TO MAKE AN ALLERGY-FREE HOME

If you want to try to make your house less likely to induce allergy, these are some of the things you might do, beginning with the bedroom.

First take out all unnecessary furniture to make the room as easy as possible to keep clean and dust-free. Remove all carpets and have a tiled, linoleum, or polished-wood floor. If you need a bedside rug, choose the washable type. Furniture should be plain wood, plastic or metal. If upholstered it should be plastic, cotton or nylon and the stuffing should be synthetic.

Walls should be plain wood or paint so that they can easily be wiped clean every two or three months. Windows should always be kept closed and should be covered by easily washable curtains. If windows need to be opened in the summer, then a filter frame consisting of several layers of butter-muslin can be made for placing in the window; moisten it for best results. All beds in the room must be fitted with a rubber mattress or the ordinary mattress covered with plastic sheeting, selotaped together to make it inpenetrable to dust and mites. However, polyurethane and rubber can have an irritating smell for some asthma sufferers. The mattress can be covered with several cotton sheets to prevent the discomfort of sleeping on plastic. Box springs should also be entirely enclosed in plastic as this is a favourite place for house mites to live. However, another school of thought recommends *not* enclosing the mattress in plastic, which may make it damp and encourage the growth of mites and mould, but alternatively vacuuming the mattress regularly to remove mites. Pillows should be made from synthetic material and washed every few weeks. Bed coverings should be made from cotton or synthetic material. Wool, hair, kapok or feathers should be avoided. Bookshelves should ideally be closed with a sliding-glass door. Toys should be kept in a box. Clothes and shoes should be stored outside the room.

The room should be cleaned from top to bottom every three months, as well as dusted, and the floor cleaned regularly. Dusting should be done with a wet or oiled duster, and floor cleaning should be done by a wet or polish method. If you use a vacuum cleaner, make sure that it is the type that is fitted with a special renewable filter and dust-collection bag. If possible the allergic person should not be present while the dusting is done, or for forty minutes afterwards while the dust settles. A nylon floor-duster is useful because it attracts dust electrostatically which must then be washed off.

Aerosols and strong-smelling substances should not be used when cleaning since these often cause irritation to the lungs of allergic people. Do not have any house plants in the room as these will contain fungi which shed spores. Even fresh flowers are best avoided, because they shed pollen.

Some people who suffer from allergies find that air-purifiers which remove dust-particles produce a dramatic improvement in their condition, while others find it makes them worse. Make sure you try before you buy. Air-conditioning does not always help hay-fever sufferers much, because they can be so loaded up with pollen while outside the house that it can take more than a week for it to be eliminated from the body.

possible to pinpoint the suspect substance or at least narrow it down to a short list, but identifying 'delayed' food allergies of this kind is often not so simple (see below).

To complicate matters, many sufferers from urticaria will not develop their rash after they have been exposed to the thing to which they are allergic, unless a second factor is brought into play. This may be exercise, psychological stress, a hot bath, or pressure on the skin. One patient, for example, only developed his rash if he played tennis within twelve hours of swallowing aspirin.

It is not always possible to identify a definite cause. Psychological stress has been suggested as a cause in some cases. When no cause can be found, anti-histamine drugs can help to make an attack bearable, while rough or tight clothing, and overheating, should always be avoided. People who suffer from urticaria caused by cold should be warned that they may suffer a general collapse if they expose themselves to severe cold, while swimming in the sea for instance.

ECZEMA

Eczema is not always caused by an allergy, and expert help is needed in diagnosis. Eczema can be particularly distressing in childhood and it is often difficult to find any cause. If the baby is breast-fed, something in the mother's diet may be a cause and with careful observation it may be possible to eliminate it. Fish, eggs, citrus fruits or chocolate are possible causes and should be eliminated from the mother's diet for two weeks at a time to see if it makes any difference (see also under Food Allergy for further ideas).

If the baby is bottle-fed, it is possible that the eczema is caused by an allergy to cows' milk. Several artificial milks are available which either have allergic materials removed from the cows' milk or which are made from plant substances; not all of these are suitable for infant feeding; ask your doctor or pharmacist for details. In severe cases of eczema children may have to wear gloves and face-masks to prevent them from scratching and making the condition worse. Bedclothes should be light to prevent overheating. Cotton should be worn next to the skin, and nappies should be washed in mild detergents or soap powder. Non-perfumed soap such as Simple Soap should be used sparingly, or an emulsifying ointment can be prescribed by the doctor for use in the bath. The child's skin should not be exposed to direct sunlight for any length of time. The child should not be vaccinated against smallpox because it may cause aggravation of the eczema.

Eczema in adults must be dealt with similarly. The cause may again be food or contact with some material (see below). Medical treatment with ointments and creams can often prevent the problem or at least control it. But care must be taken with the use of some creams, particularly those containing fluorinated corticosteroids which may permanently thin the skin if used on the face.

CONTACT DERMATITIS

This is caused by some object or substance touching the skin and causing local allergy which may then spread. Detergents, for example, may start to cause an irritation on the hands which later spread to other parts of the skin. Other common causes are metals, especially nickel and chrome, dyes and chemicals. The first clue to the cause usually comes from the part of the body affected. If, for example, it is the scalp, then the cause may be a shampoo or anti-dandruff lotion, hair dyes or rinses, curlers, combs, wigs or even a hatband. If it is the feet, then rubber or leather shoes may be responsible, or dyed socks. The eyelids may react to mascara, but also the sensitive skin of the lids may react to something rubbed on them from fingers before the thicker skin of the hands has time to react. Once the cause has been found, a change of detergent or cosmetics may be all that is needed. Several firms now make cosmetics which are less likely to produce allergy. It is possible to test for allergy by placing a little of the substance on the skin of the upper arm or back and covering with a plaster or tape which is not allergic. If there is no reaction after forty-eight hours the substance is probably safe.

FOOD ALLERGY

Food allergy is much commoner than is realized because people simply learn to avoid foods which they know upset them. However, many people with chronic allergic diseases are suffering from unrecognized food allergy. It can cause urticaria, eczema, intrinsic asthma or rhinitis, diarrhoea, constipation, pains in the belly, swelling of a part of the face or tongue (so-called 'angio-neurotic oedema') and migraine. It now seems likely that rheumatoid arthritis may be triggered by food allergy and there is a body of opinion which even attributes some forms of mental illness to food allergy, though this is still highly controversial.

A diet diary which records everything eaten and drunk sometimes helps to spot the offending food, but this simple system usually fails for two reasons: first, the allergic response to a food is frequently so delayed and prolonged that it is difficult to spot a relationship; second, most people with delayed food allergy are sensitive to several different commonly eaten foods, and reactions overlap.

Most experts in the field agree that an 'exclusion diet' restricted to foods which are less common causes of allergy offers the best chance of improvement. In extreme cases an artificial diet called 'vivonex' may be used. This was developed for use on space flights, and is very unlikely to provoke allergy. The disadvantage is that it is so expensive that its widespread use is totally impracticable. Of course, after a person has lost their symptoms on an exclusion diet, all the foods which have been left out must be eaten one by one to see which cause symptoms.

Foods likely to cause allergy can be divided into groups. For instance, a person who is allergic to a nut such as hazel-nut is likely to be allergic to all the nuts, pips, peas and beans in their diet, even chocolate and coffee. However, the factory preparation of foods often in some degree destroys the allergy-causing part of the food, so that this person could probably drink powdered instant coffee (not the freeze-dried granules), and could also eat margarine made from nut-oil after it had been altered to make 'solid' fat. Again, heat often destroys the allergy-producing chemicals in food, so that someone allergic to milk and yeast is likely to be able to eat ordinary bread (which may contain both).

Foods suggested as the basis of a simple but practical exclusion diet – those which are least likely to cause allergy – are shown below. Beneath them is a list of groups of foods to test, one at a time, for allergy. Remember, the exclusion diet is not intended to be nutritionally balanced, and once it has been tried for a month it should be abandoned if there is no improvement. If it is obvious that the allergy has disappeared when the exclusion diet alone is being eaten, then the other food 'groups' should be started again, one by one, at weekly intervals. Any food which causes no ill-effect can then be included in the diet while the next one is being tested. Keep a diary of your diet and symptoms each day. This will make interpretation much easier.

Foods to eat on basic exclusion diet
1. Beef or mutton.
2. Green vegetables (not cauliflower, which is a 'pip' allergen). Potatoes.
3. Tea, sugar, but no milk or lemon.
4. Rice is a possible substitute for wheat but sago is better. (Grain allergy is different from gluten sensitivity which is the cause of coeliac disease and dermatitis herpetiformis.)
5. Butter. Syrup for flavour but no jam.
6. Rhubarb.
7. Cook with lard or corn oil.
(See Appendix Three for source of further information on this diet.)

Foods to test, one group at a time
1. Egg, chicken, sponge cake, mayonnaise.
2. Milk, ice-cream (but most milk-allergic patients can eat butter).
3. Nuts, pips and all fruit, peas and beans, cauliflower, chocolate, fresh coffee, tomatoes, sweets, preserves, and drinks made from fruit or nuts (wines and cola), 'soft' margarine, mustard, curry and all spices.
4. Fish.
5. Cheese (separate cause of allergy from milk).
6. Yeast in flavourings and drinks (most important are gravy browning and Marmite).
7. Onion.
8. Mushroom.
9. Pork and all liver.
10. Wheat (bread, biscuits, cakes, beer and many other foods).
11. Chemical food additives (colours, flavours, preservatives) found in manufactured foods.
12. Chewing gum and toothpaste.

Foods likely to cause attacks of migraine fall into two groups. First, the foods causing allergy – identify them as described. Second, there is a list of foods which contain a substance called tyramine which may provoke an attack of migraine without an allergic mechanism. These foods include: cheese, wine (especially red), chocolate, broad beans, Marmite, bananas and tinned fish. Coffee and tobacco may also trigger migraine.

DRUG ALLERGIES
These are also quite common. There are two sorts. First, the true allergies: many drugs may cause a rash; some such as sleeping tablets may cause a sensitivity to sunlight. Sometimes drug allergy can cause other reactions such as asthma. Allergy to drugs, particularly penicillin, can be dangerous. If you change your doctor or go to hospital, do not forget to tell the doctor about your allergy. It is a good idea in such cases to wear a Medic-Alert bracelet or necklet (see Appendix Three), which warns of your allergy in case you should be taken to hospital unconscious.

The second sort of 'drug allergy' can be equally serious: aspirin, for example, can make other allergies catastrophically worse. There need be no initial period of sensitization when the drug is being taken without causing a reaction. If a patient is aspirin-sensitive, the very first dose of several chemically unrelated drugs used for rheumatism may provoke a severe attack of the patient's usual allergic disease. What is worse, tartrazine, a yellow dye used in food manufacture, may also do the same. Strangely, a number of anti-allergy tablets are coloured with tartrazine – so beware.

OCCUPATIONAL ALLERGIES
There are a great many allergies which are suffered by individuals as a result of exposure to particular substances at work. Bakers, for example, often become sensitive to flour or to weevils and moulds which grow on the flour. These may cause eczema, a runny nose or asthma. Builders may become sensitive to sawdust or cement which cause eczema or asthma. Paints and glues may cause a runny nose, asthma or eczema. Dry-cleaners and dyers often become sensitive to dyes. Cotton-mill workers often become sensitive to dust from the raw cotton which causes an allergic asthma. Farmers may become allergic to their animals, and mouldy hay may give them a severe chest allergy called farmer's lung. Market gardeners may become sensitive to moulds which grow readily in greenhouses, causing asthma. Hairdressers and leather-workers often become sensitive to the dyes and chemicals they use in their work. Metal-workers may become sensitized to chrome, copper, nickel or oils which may all cause skin trouble. Even office workers may develop eczema, as a result of handling carbon paper or inks, or runny nose or asthma due to dust from old documents.

WHAT WILL HAPPEN IN THE END?
A small proportion of people who start any allergy will find that, as time goes on, they develop new symptoms and start to react to more allergens, but most people will grow out of their problem. An allergic episode may last for twenty years or more. However, some people only experience hay fever, for example, lasting for one or two summers. So it makes sense to see if an allergy will go away naturally before embarking upon a major course of action. Only for very few will an allergy be lifelong. It is doubtful whether the treatments used for allergy make much difference to the natural process. Desensitization, for example, seems to have a temporary effect, lasting at best five or six years. People who seem to be cured permanently may have lost their allergy naturally during the time when their symptoms were suppressed by the treatment.

8: SEX AND HEALTH

A Happy Sex Life

A happy sex life is an important part of most people's lives. Enjoyable sex with a loving partner refreshes both the mind and the body. It is both stimulating and relaxing. Good sex between people who care for each other is really making love.

In the last half-century there has been a great deal more openness about sexual behaviour. Nowadays, women's and men's magazines, paperback books, radio and even television programmes all devote a lot of time to the subject. But, despite all this publicity, individuals may still find the whole subject bewildering, embarrassing and rather difficult to discuss.

The major influence for change came with the work of Professor Alfred C. Kinsey, an American entomologist who took up the study of human sexual behaviour. He wanted to find out exactly what people did, how often and with whom. To do this, he talked to thousands of ordinary men and women about their sex lives in detail.

At the time, this kind of research was very controversial. Professor Kinsey published first a report on men's behaviour titled *Sexual Behaviour in the Human Male*, in 1948, then a report on women, *Sexual Behaviour in the Human Female*, in 1953. These reports are still used today, when people want to study sex – even though by now their statistics are about thirty years out of date.

The Kinsey reports, as they were known, startled most people. They showed that there was a lot more sexual activity going on outside marriage than had previously been thought. Masturbation, sex before marriage, sex outside marriage and homosexual sex were surprisingly common. Today many people probably know and accept just how much sex happens outside marriage, but at that time it was a bombshell.

More importantly, the Kinsey reports gave an amazing picture of the huge variety of people's sex lives. There was the most extraordinary difference between one individual and the next. Some men had sex more than twice a day; some had had perhaps only one sexual experience in a lifetime. Women's sex lives showed an even more startling difference. Some women had a huge amount of sex, while others not only had no sex at all but had never ever felt any kind of sexual desire at all.

What we should learn from this is that there can be no hard and fast rules about sex. For some people it will be natural to want a great deal of sex, while for others it will be natural to want almost none at all. Neither wanting a lot nor wanting only a little is abnormal. This means that it is pointless for anybody to compare him or herself against some kind of average. Each person needs a sex life which is happy for that individual.

There can therefore be no rule about how often husbands and wives should make love. Research into marriage shows that it does not seem to matter at all whether a couple make love only occasionally during the year or whether they make love twice a day.

What does seem to matter is that both husband and wife should be having the amount of sex they like. So, if one partner wants a great deal of sex and the other wants only a little, there may be tension. Both will need to give a little so that a workable compromise can be reached. If in doubt ask yourself, 'What is the loving thing to do?' With love on both sides most sexual disagreements can be resolved.

The next major piece of sex research came with the work of Drs William H. Masters and Virginia E. Johnson. This American couple studied sexual response in the laboratory and noted exact bodily changes of both men and women during sex. Their findings, published in 1966, were particularly interesting to women.

Until the publication of their book, *Human Sexual Response*, it had been thought that women had two different kinds of climax. One was a 'vaginal orgasm', which was felt inside the vagina; the other was the 'clitoral orgasm', which was felt round the clitoris. Some psychoanalysts thought that the only 'proper' orgasm was the vaginal kind.

From Masters' and Johnson's research, it looked as if there was only one kind of orgasm. Wherever orgasm might be felt, it seemed as if the clitoris was the organ which was most important. Sensations radiated from there, rather than starting in the vagina.

Though not everybody agrees with Masters and Johnson, their work has influenced most people to admit that any sort of orgasm is a good orgasm. Whether a woman feels her climax in the vagina or in the clitoris simply does not matter. Nor does it matter how she reaches a climax or what techniques a couple use.

While all this research was going on, there had been important developments in medicine. The discovery of penicillin and other antibiotics meant that cures for venereal and sexual infections now existed. The invention of the pill and the inter-uterine device meant that there was reliable means of contraception.

At first it seemed as if all the problems of sex had been

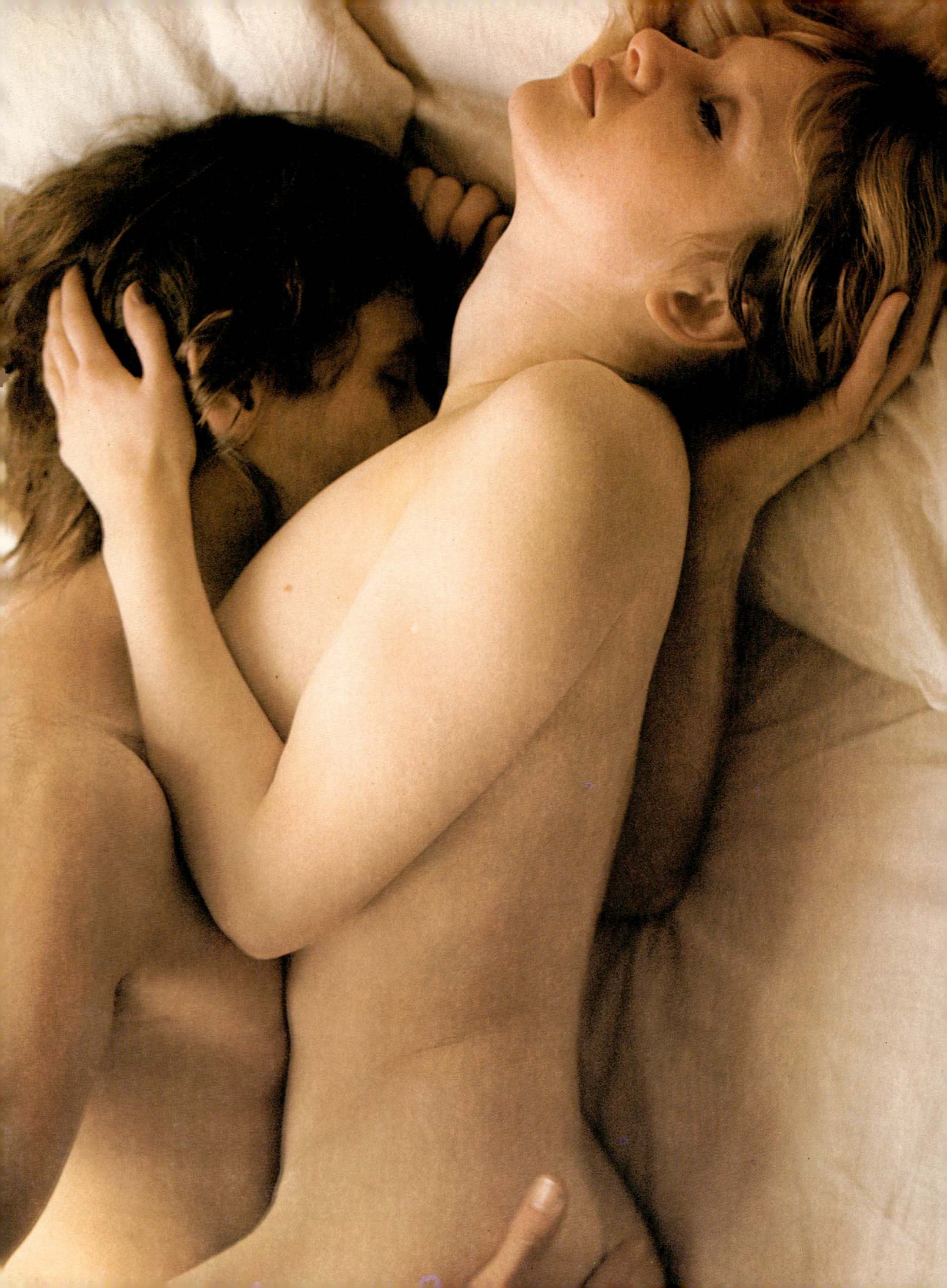

A HAPPY SEX LIFE/**SEX AND HEALTH**

solved. Nowadays, we are more cautious. Sexual infections still exist and have not been wiped out by antibiotics. Even contraception has its dangers, if it is used unwisely. But a responsible attitude to sex should mean that for most people it will be a very safe activity. However, knowing a little more about sexual activity will help most of us get more enjoyment out of our sex lives.

KNOW YOUR OWN BODY

Knowing your own bodily responses means that you must look, touch and feel. Men, since their genitals are within easy reach and vision, generally do this from an early age. Many women, however, are still amazingly ignorant about their bodies.

Some women do not even know what their sexual organs look like. Spend some time with a small mirror, and a torch if necessary, looking at your own sex organs. Most sex books provide pictures of the female sex organs. Identify the various parts from this. If your own sex organs look slightly different from the ones in the picture, do not worry. Sexual features differ, just as facial features vary.

In particular it is important to identify the clitoris. This is the small hood at the top end of the space between the large lips. The clitoris is the centre for sexual feeling. Touching it directly may not be pleasurable. But touching the area around it probably will.

Try touching it with your own fingers, and feel exactly which areas give the most pleasure – and to what kind of touching they respond best. Until you yourself know what kind of touching gives pleasure, how can you expect your partner to know?

Most men will probably have done this kind of experimenting in youth. If not, they too can profitably spend some time looking, feeling and touching. This same exercise can also be done together. It can be fun. As the military strategists say, time spent on reconnaissance is never wasted.

STOP MAKING RULES AND REGULATIONS FOR YOURSELF

There is a terrible human tendency to make up rules, regulations and categories. Consciously, or unconsciously, most of us have set ideas about how to make love and what our responses ought to be. When our personal performance does not conform to these rules, we worry.

For instance, many people believe that sex between a man and a woman is made up of loveplay, followed by vaginal penetration by the penis, followed by the male (and possibly the female) orgasm. But this order is neither necessary nor even necessarily desirable. You can start with vaginal penetration and male orgasm, if you like, then follow it with oral sex, with the man stimulating the woman. Or you need not have vaginal penetration at all. The order in which you do things is up to you and your partner.

Perhaps the most common misconception about sex is the idea that a woman should climax from the thrusting of the penis in the vagina. Many men and women still believe this is the 'right' way, and worry if it does not happen.

But a great many women do not get orgasms just from this thrusting. They need manual stimulation of the clitoris, either before, during or after the thrusting. Other women find that their partner's stimulation is somehow not sensitive enough. These women may choose to stimulate themselves during lovemaking.

Simultaneous orgasm is another myth to be found in the old-fashioned sex books. It used to be thought that coming together was somehow better than one partner's climax followed by the other's. Simultaneous orgasms are very enjoyable, but so are sequential ones. Do not worry yourself by trying to time orgasms together. It can get in the way of relaxed and enjoyable sex.

Men sometimes suffer from the idea that it is up to them to make their woman respond. In particular, they feel that it is their responsibility to produce her climax. Of course, it is wonderful to be a skilled and sensitive lover, but sex does not have to be started by the male and kept under his control all the time. The man who takes it as a personal reflection on his technique if his partner does not climax does not know enough about lovemaking.

The truth is that individual men and women vary a great deal in their sexual response. Women vary in the ease with which they have orgasms. Some women have them easily at almost every lovemaking session. But about one in three women find they have orgasms only irregularly or occasionally, and among these women are some who do not ever seem to have orgasms. These variations are entirely normal.

Of course, a skilled and sensitive lover will make it more likely that a women has an orgasm. Oral sex, clitoral stimulation and other techniques may help too. A vibrator gives some women orgasms for the first time. Sometimes a woman's sexual response varies according to the time of the month.

But orgasms are not the aim of sex. You do not have to have an orgasm to enjoy yourself. Sensuous skin contact and sexual arousal are extremely exciting and enjoyable. If you make love with the fixed idea that you must have an orgasm, you will miss out on the pleasures of other bodily responses. Disappointment, anger and anxiety are emotions which are bad for sex.

All in all, most disappointments spring from the way people impose an artificial pattern on sexual relations. If you measure your own performance or your partner's against some idea of what is 'normal' or 'sexy', then you may well be disappointed. If, however, you concentrate on what pleases you – regardless of any other ideas – then you should be on your way to enjoying lovemaking as much as possible.

SEX IS ALWAYS NEW

If you feel you would like to learn new sex techniques, there are now plenty of sex manuals in the bookshops. Some of these are rather unrealistic about people's performances, but often books are a pleasurable way of arousing yourself or your partner. Do not think a sex technique *ought* to be enjoyed just because a book says so.

Most individuals have likes and dislikes in lovemaking. They vary enormously in sexual appetite and sexual responsiveness. One person's turn-on is another person's turn-off. No book can make a good lover.

Sex, therefore, must be learnt anew for each different partner. You need to discover what your partner likes – not do what you think he or she ought to like, what others have liked, or what some book says people like.

Indeed, this information needs constant updating. People's tastes change, with age, with mood, and with situations. The ideal lover doesn't simply apply a routine of so much foreplay, say, followed by so much sexual intercourse. He or she responds to what is desired by a particular person on a particular occasion.

SEX NEEDS COMMUNICATION

It sounds obvious to say that lovers must be able to communicate in order to have good sex. How, otherwise, are they going to be able to tell each other what they like doing, how, and exactly where? Yet thousands of couples cannot talk to each other in bed because they are too shy.

One problem is that the words are difficult. The official words sound too medical and a bit of a turn-off. The unofficial words sound obscene to many.

Non-verbal communication may be a solution. Be sensitive to responses such as 'Umm' and 'Ouch' from your partner. Listen – and try to remember. It is sometimes difficult to recall exactly what turned your partner on. But only by remembering the details of successful loveplay will you be a good lover.

Sex therapists Masters and Johnson acknowledge this problem. For some of their training, they suggest that one partner places his or her hand over the other's. By this means, the hand underneath can be guided to sensitive areas, lifted away from painful activities, and encouraged by pressure to continue pleasurable activities. No words are needed.

Words, however, will be a turn-on for some people. For some individuals this will mean the use of obscenities or slang which would otherwise be unacceptable. Others will enjoy verbalizing sex fantasies, or even running commentaries on what is going on.

PRINCIPLES FOR A HAPPY SEX LIFE

There is such a thing as anti-social sex. It is anti-social to have sex that can cause an unwanted pregnancy. Men need to remember that not every woman is on the pill, and women need the courage to make sure that their contraception is organized *before*, not after, sexual activity has started in a relationship.

It is also anti-social to pass on sexual infections. If in any doubt, you should go to the nearest hospital VD clinic. You will probably be asked not to have sex while you are undergoing treatment, and you should always finish the treatment before starting your sex life again.

Nowadays, the old moral code which said that all sex outside marriage was wrong has been widely questioned. But sex does raise moral questions, even for those who do not accept the old code. Force, fraud or simply unwarranted pressure on a person to have sex, or to engage in a particular activity, are immoral. Withholding sex as a punishment is also wrong. Kindness and thoughtfulness are virtues that will help you and others enjoy sex.

The law steps in to protect children who are under age or people whose mental state means that they cannot be responsible for their actions. Homosexual activities, too, are still somewhat restricted. Most people do not realize it, but anal intercourse between a man and a woman is still an illegal act. Prosecutions are rare, but occasionally occur in the context of rape. People who want heterosexual anal intercourse should be discreet.

It is also worth remembering that sex is *not* essential for health or happiness. If you are not having sex (for whatever reason) you are not jeopardizing your health in any way. The body can survive without sex remarkably well, so can the mind. Abstinence, whether voluntary or forced, need not be feared. However, most people without a partner will find physical relief in masturbation – the natural outlet. Wet dreams may also increase in number. This is normal.

Loneliness is the other result of being without a partner. Our society seems geared to couples rather than singles. If you live alone, you will need to make positive efforts to combat isolation. Seek out friends at work, at clubs, in part-time voluntary activities, or at evening classes. Try to make both your work and your leisure interesting and rewarding so that the lack of a partner will not loom so large. If you are fond of animals, a pet may provide companionship at home. Even budgies provide a little bit of friendship in an otherwise empty flat or house.

Those who are disabled, or who live in an institution, may need further help to deal with loneliness or sexual frustration. There are now books which specifically deal with sex and disabled people (see Appendix Three). Social workers and doctors are more broadminded than they used to be, if you can find the courage to consult them.

A WORD OF CAUTION

Most sexual activities are perfectly safe. Men should remember, however, that very violent or aggressive sex can hurt their partner. Bruises and love bites are fine, if she likes them, but the female sexual organs can be hurt by an aggressive lover. Do not use your penis like a battering ram. Young men without much sexual experience may be misled by soft-porn literature which suggests women like being hurt. Most do not.

There are some individuals who find their pleasure in either inflicting or receiving pain. But sado-masochistic games carry a risk, particularly if they get out of hand. Bondage, or any kind of sex game which interferes with breathing, is highly dangerous. If you cannot do without this kind of activity, it is probably wisest to restrict them to a loving reliable partner. Have rules between yourselves about how far you will go. This kind of sex may lead to trouble if you sleep with relative strangers. For guidance about how to make such games safe, consult *The Joy of Sex*.

Anal intercourse is one other sexual technique which can produce harm. An infection can arise when dirt from the anal passage is then deposited in the woman's vagina. Do not combine both anal and vaginal penetration – unless you use a condom for one of them.

Sex with a great many partners also carries risks of sexual infections. Take precautions against these. Sex with strangers, or with people you do not know very well, can occasionally be dangerous. If your sex life involves picking up relative strangers, you will need to think out how you can best guard against an unhappy experience.

GUILT

Many people feel guilty about some part of their sex lives. Sometimes they feel guilty about something that happened in their past. Or they may feel guilty about sex longings, or perhaps some aspect of their sexual activities. Remember that the variety of human experiences is astounding. What you may think is shamefully abnormal may be a fairly common experience. A look at the two Kinsey reports will show you just how many people have engaged in the more unusual forms of sexual activity.

Guilt is corrosive, however. There are two ways to deal with it. You can try to change your thinking, so that you no longer *feel* guilty. A chat with a therapist or counsellor may help with this (see Sexual Difficulties, page 174). Or you can stop doing the things that make you feel guilty. Some individuals are happier coming to terms with their guilt in this way.

On the whole, it is usually not a good idea to burden your partner with your guilty secrets, particularly if they involve infidelity. Sometimes confessing all may be necessary, but often it simply hurts your partner without helping the relationship. Once again, consult a trusted friend or a counsellor about this. Talking to them may relieve your own guilty feelings.

MASTURBATION

Nearly all men and about two-thirds of women have masturbated at some time in their lives. Some people continue to masturbate as well as enjoying sexual intercourse with a partner regularly. Others have recourse to masturbation when no partner is available. There is absolutely nothing wrong with masturbation. Ideas that it can cause ill-health, mental disorder or acne are nonsense. On the contrary, masturbation is a pleasurable habit which harms nobody, and it is a convenient source of enjoyment.

Most men and women masturbate with the help of sexual fantasies or sometimes pornographic literature. Both are good aids to masturbation. Sometimes fantasies (which may also be used to produce sexual pleasure during intercourse with a partner) are about behaviour which would not be desired in reality. This is nothing to worry about. Sexual fantasies, whatever their content, do not have to be put into practice and are a good sex aid.

For men, it is obvious how to proceed with masturbation, since the genitals are outside the body and their response is visible. But for some women, it is not obvious how to masturbate because they are unsure how their genitals work. Though clitoral manipulation of some kind is the most common form of female masturbation, some women use thigh pressure, muscular reactions and occasionally fantasies alone. *The Hite Report* (see Appendix Three) contains detailed examples of masturbation which will be useful for women who want to know how it can be done. The purchase of a vibrator will also help women who are finding it difficult to masturbate – and may enhance the pleasure of those who already know how.

For women, masturbation may be a worthwhile path to a better sex life with a partner. There is evidence which suggests that, if a woman can produce an orgasm by masturbation, she is more likely to have one in sexual intercourse. Some sex therapists teach masturbation to non-orgasmic women, before trying to teach orgasm with a partner.

Common sense suggests that, if a woman knows exactly what gives her pleasure, she can teach a man to do this, if he is willing to learn. Sometimes, of course, this does not work. *The Hite Report* suggests that, in this case, the woman may like to masturbate in the setting of sex with a partner – thus putting the pleasure into the context of mutual loveplay.

HOMOSEXUALITY

Somewhere between one in ten and one in twenty people is basically homosexual. The latest research suggests that sexual orientation – the kind of sexual attraction one will feel in later life – may be fixed at a very early age; probably before puberty and perhaps by the age of four or five years. This sexual orientation governs a person's strongest and most common feelings.

But human sexuality does not fall neatly into categories. A large number of men and women have had a homosexual experience at some point in their lives. By their middle forties, 13 per cent of women and 37 per cent of men will have had a homosexual experience resulting in orgasm. There are many men and women who enjoy sexual contact with both sexes. Others will turn to heterosexuality after a period of homosexuality – or vice versa. In single-sex societies such as prisons and boarding schools, people who are normally heterosexual may turn to their own sex for sexual outlet.

Although many men and women will have had, if not homosexual experiences, then at least homosexual feelings, many myths and prejudices remain. Most arise from fear or ignorance. One assumption is that homosexuality is a passing phase, common in adolescence, but one which everyone can and should grow out of. This will be true for some people but, for the minority who are basically homosexual, these feelings are the beginning of their natural sexual expression. Another common slur on male homosexuals is that they are eager to seduce young boys. Most homosexual relationships, like heterosexual relationships, involve partners of roughly the same age.

It is also often believed that all male homosexuals are effeminate in their appearance and manners, and that all lesbians are mannish. Neither belief is generally true, though individuals may sometimes conform to this pattern – as may heterosexuals. Most gay men and women look and behave like heterosexual members of the community – except in the sexual side of their lives.

Although the law in Britain places some restrictions on the expression of love between male homosexuals, nowadays homosexuality is increasingly accepted. Most reputable psychiatrists and therapists will try to help women and men who are oriented towards their own sex to accept and be happy with their sexuality. It is now usually accepted that it is as impossible to change or 'cure' someone who is homosexual as it is to turn a heterosexual into a homosexual.

Most of the distress felt by homosexual women and men is due either to their fears of rejection by parents, friends or society, or to their being already involved in a relationship such as marriage. Some homosexual men and women marry before they are aware of their true feelings or in the hope that they may be able to suppress those feelings in a 'normal' marriage. As some men and women are 'bisexual', attracted to people of either sex, not all marriages are fake just because one partner has formed a strong homosexual attachment.

However, if the person has had homosexual feelings throughout their lives, it is unlikely they will be able to abandon them for ever. Both partners in such a marriage need sympathetic and supportive counselling while they determine what course to take. There are organizations which can help with this. For homosexuals coming to terms with their sexual orientation, the love and support of parents and friends will be extremely helpful. Parents who discover a child is homosexual can be helped too (see Appendix Three).

If you are worried by your own homosexual feelings, it will probably be worth contacting a homosexual organization which can offer advice and support. Finding others who share your feelings and experiences may calm your anxiety and help you to cope with social problems. Alternatively the organization may help you choose a sympathetic and up-to-date therapist or counsellor (see Appendix Three).

SEXUAL DIFFICULTIES

Sexual difficulties can arise from time to time between the most well-matched partners. People are not machines, operating with well-oiled efficiency. One cannot, therefore, expect one's sex life always to be highly competent or highly responsive.

Bodily tiredness, sickness or ill health will affect one's sexual appetite and response. So will mental preoccupations. A looming anxiety, worry about work or feelings of anger are likely to lower sexual desire and competence.

The occasional episode of sexual difficulty is therefore no cause for anxiety. When health or happiness is fully restored, one's sexual desire and response will also be. A weekend away from the troubles of ordinary life, a holiday, or just a relaxing evening out may help a couple to rediscover the old magic.

However, if sexual difficulties persist you may want to get help. Quite often the chance to talk absolutely freely to a sympathetic counsellor will clear up worries. Sometimes people are anxious because they are expecting too much from their lovemaking. But a sexual difficulty is something that makes you or your partner feel bad about it; if both of you are happy, then you do not have difficulties.

The most common worries in men are impotence or ejaculation difficulties:
Impotence: Occasional episodes of impotence happen to all men. Tiredness, ill health, too much alcohol and some kinds of prescribed drugs can all produce temporary impotence. If impotence is the rule rather than the exception, then it may be helpful to seek advice.
Ejaculation difficulties: Some men ejaculate too soon, and some men cannot ejaculate at all into the vagina. If this worries you or your partner, then seek help.

The most common worries of women are about orgasm or painful intercourse:
Orgasm difficulties: Some women do not have orgasms at all. Others do not have orgasms when they want them, usually after traditional sexual intercourse alone. Expectations are sometimes too high among women, but advice will help you decide whether you can do something about this problem.
Painful intercourse (also known as dyspareunia): There is a condition known as vaginismus, when the muscles round the entrance to the vagina go into spasm during penetration. Occasionally, marriages remain unconsummated because of this. Seeking help from a doctor can usually put this right.

It takes courage to ask for help with sexual difficulties, but it is better to ask for help than to continue to suffer anxiety. The first place to start is your family doctor's surgery. People's sex lives can be affected by illness, and also by prescribed drugs. Check with your doctor that you are in good health, and ask him about the side-effects of any drugs he may have prescribed. If the woman suffers from painful intercourse, she may have a vaginal infection. She should ask for a gynaecological examination. A high alcohol intake can also affect your sex life. Cut down the amount you drink, or stop it altogether.

Having checked that there is no physical cause for your sexual difficulties, you may decide you need further help. Occasionally family doctors can provide sexual counselling, or they may know of a reliable sex counsellor.

Just having the chance to talk things out openly can do wonders. Some sexual anxieties arise simply because people expect too much from themselves or their partners. Reassurance from an expert will help. Sometimes it is possible to get sex therapy, which trains people to make love in a more pleasurable way.

If your doctor does not know of a sex therapist, ask your local Marriage Guidance Council to help. There are sex therapists among their counsellors, and, if they do not have a local therapist, they may be able to suggest somebody.

It is also worth seeing whether a good book can help you. There are now one or two do-it-yourself books upon the market. In particular, these may help some women with orgasm difficulties and men with ejaculation difficulties.

Sex therapy is occasionally available from other sources. Insist upon knowing the therapist's qualifications, which should be either in medicine or psychology. Any therapist without such qualifications should be attached to a respectable institution or hospital.

Girly magazines sometimes have advertisements for sex therapy. Treat these with caution. It is wiser to avoid unusual encounter groups or therapists who seem to have no particular training.

Perhaps the only exception is women's liberation groups. If you are happy with a feminist atmosphere, this kind of group may help. But remember that they are amateur self-help groups in the main. Anybody with severe distress should concentrate on finding help from more official sources.

Menstruation

Menstruation starts in most women between the ages of eleven and eighteen, around the time that the outward signs of puberty are appearing – developing breasts and body hair. For the next thirty to forty years, women will menstruate monthly except during pregnancy. Menstruation is the shedding of the womb lining after the female egg has descended into the womb, but has not been fertilized.

Failure to menstruate may be a sign of pregnancy or some disorder. When menstruation first begins, periods may be irregular. But after they are established any major change in their occurrence may be cause for medical advice. Shedding blood between periods should be reported to your doctor, even though it may have a harmless cause.

Two different aspects of menstruation can cause difficulties. One is pre-menstrual tension, a physical and mental disorder, which occurs before the first shedding of blood. The other are the period pains associated with the beginning of menstruation. These two disorders need different treatment.

About four out of ten women who are not on the pill suffer from some degree of pre-menstrual tension. The physical signs are breast discomfort, headaches, backaches or stomach cramps, skin disorders and swollen body. The mental symptoms include tension, irritability, depression, clumsiness, lethargy, lack of concentration, lack of confidence and a feeling of worthlessness, loss of sexual desire, and illogical reactions.

It is always helpful for every woman to keep a diary record of her periods, with some kind of record of when the next is expected. For those who have only mild pre-menstrual tension, this will be reassuring. If you feel bad during this period, you will know why. Important occasions or decisions can be postponed.

About one in four pre-menstrual-tension sufferers have severe symptoms. For some, this can disrupt their lives, causing difficulties at home and at work. Simple measures help many women to avoid or reduce symptoms. Be sure to eat something at least every three hours during the critical days. Low blood sugar seems to be a cause of the aggressive and emotional behaviour that occurs sometimes in pre-menstrual tension. It may also help to cut down on fluids and salty foods at this time.

Another easy self-help treatment is to take Vitamin B_6, known as pyrodoxine, three days *before* the onset of pre-menstrual symptoms. Start by taking 40 mg twice a day, and increase the dosage if necessary, up to 75 mg twice a day. Continue the tablets until two or three days after the period. The only side-effect may be mild stomach upset. Opinion differs about the effectiveness of this treatment but it is worth trying.

If this is doing no good, you will need to consult your doctor. Take along any written records you have of period onset and symptoms. He or she may need to be convinced that your problems are linked with menstruation.

Old-fashioned doctors are still handing out tranquillizers and diuretics for period problems and if your doctor is one of these you may have to ask for referral to a specialist. There were only eleven pre-menstrual tension clinics in England in 1981. Try Women's Health Concern if you have difficulty getting help (see Appendix Three).

The modern treatment is to use progestogens, one of the hormones contained in the birth-control pill. 'This should not be a life-long treatment,' says Dr Michael Brush, of the pre-menstrual clinic at St Thomas's Hospital. 'It's highly unlikely that very long-term treatment will be needed. A good time to re-assess treatment is nine months after it's been started. Have a gap then and see how you get on. Some women, of course, will need to go back on treatment.'

However, Dr Katharine Dalton, a London doctor who has made a lifelong study of pre-menstrual tension, believes that the synthetic hormones in the contraceptive pill may make pre-menstrual tension worse. She prescribes natural progesterone (Cyclogest), which can only be taken in the form of suppositories. This drug cannot be taken by mouth because it is broken down in the liver.

Period pains are not helped by hormones or Vitamin B_6. The traditional remedy is aspirin, a hot-water bottle and rest. If you suffer severe pain, it is worth asking your doctor if she or he can prescribe either anti-spasmodic drugs or anti-prostaglandin drugs. It is worth trying to get help for severe period pains *before* such crises as examinations or important work. Otherwise, menstruation need mean no change in daily life. It is quite acceptable to take baths or go swimming at these times and there is no reason (other than personal preference) why you should not have sex. Some women find sexual desire is at its peak during a period. Place a towel under the body, or have one handy, if it is likely to be messy. The diaphragm helps hold back menstrual blood during sex.

Tampons used to absorb the menstrual blood have been found in very rare cases to be associated with a serious disease called 'toxic shock syndrome'. The symptoms of the disease are high fever, headache, sore throat, diarrhoea and reddening of the skin. If you have these symptoms consult a doctor. The disease is caused by infection of the vagina and subsequently the rest of the body by a particular bacterium. Although this disease is rare, milder disease associated with use of tampons may be more common. When flow of blood is impeded by tampons, bacteria are able to multiply abnormally. The drying of the vagina by a tampon may also make the membrane more vulnerable to infection. If you suffer from illness with fever, or even malaise, at the time of your period it is worth trying sanitary towels as an alternative. Tampons should not be used if you are suffering from any infection of the skin such as pustules, boils, abscesses or impetigo, or infections of the nailfold, as these infections are caused by the bacteria which can cause toxic shock syndrome if they get a chance to multiply undisturbed.

Contraception

Birth control is now the rule rather than the exception. Yet many women and men remain ignorant of the relative merits and disadvantages of different methods. Which is best for your particular needs? What are the medical pros and cons of the various ways of preventing conception?

At the heart of the matter is the individual couple's own priorities. Some people are cautious in their approach to life, wishing to reduce risks rather than maximize pleasure. They may be happy to make extra effort to avoid risks. Others will be happy to run slight risks in return for the most convenient method of birth control.

Using no contraception at all has risks. A million young women having a regular sex life without using birth control would produce about six hundred thousand babies yearly. Of those births, about fifty-three would result in the death of the mother. So pregnancy itself has a potential, though slight, risk to life.

The most efficient forms of contraception for women are the pill, the intra-uterine device (IUD) and female sterilization. All of these carry slight health risks. It is a question of balancing these risks against the risk of pregnancy.

The pill is the most efficient and easily reversible method

SEX AND HEALTH/CONTRACEPTION

of contraception. Judgements about its safety have varied over the last generation. At first, it was considered almost completely safe, then doubts set in and there was a swing back to greater caution. At the time this book was written, 1982, the Family Planning Association felt that the pill was safe in the early years of fertility.

In deciding what method of contraception to use, a woman needs also to take into account her attitudes to abortion. From the statistics, an American contraception expert, Dr Christopher Tietze, has shown that the safest method of birth control for women of all ages is the diaphragm or condom, backed up by early abortion under proper conditions. However, this calculation leaves out the feelings of women towards abortion. Some may feel that it is entirely wrong under all circumstances, and even those who are in favour of abortion being available may feel that it would be an upsetting experience for them.

Contraception also varies with the individual. Some women, for instance, find that they can use the diaphragm efficiently and easily. Others find it difficult. So it is of great importance to find a contraceptive method which *you* find easy. If you are happy with your contraceptive method, it will become habitual and therefore more effective. Once again, the statistics conceal a wide variety of individual reactions.

All in all, the pill will probably have a place in most people's contraceptive strategy. It is most useful for the young, the unmarried who are anxious not to get pregnant, women who are opposed to abortion, or couples who are determined against a pregnancy. But some women who try the pill do not like it. For these, the diaphragm or the condom is the best method of contraception in the early years. Used carefully and habitually, these are quite effective. Couples who intend to have a family and who would not mind the early arrival of a baby might also use these.

But, as a woman's fertile years draw towards their end, a switch of contraception is usually advisable. The risks of taking the pill become noticeable in later years, and seem especially to affect those women who smoke. If you must smoke, then stop taking the pill after the age of thirty. Women who do not smoke should start thinking of changing from the pill in their late thirties. An IUD might be the answer for the woman who does not want further children. For couples who have completed their family, the man should think of a vasectomy. Female sterilization, which is slightly riskier than vasectomy, is a possibility if he does not like the idea of vasectomy.

THE PILL

The pill is now the most popular method of contraception. In 1980 there were three million British women using it. This means that four out of every ten fertile women choose this method. Most use the combined version.

History: The combined pill contains synthetic versions of the two female hormones – oestrogen and progesterone – which control natural ovulation. These two hormones in combination manage to prevent the ripening of an egg in the woman's ovary. In the 1930s it was confirmed that injections of natural oestrogen, progesterone or the male hormone testosterone would successfully prevent ovulation. But it was not until 1940 that a cheap and universally available oral contraceptive pill became a possibility. In 1955 a progesterone-only pill taken daily went on trial in Puerto Rico, but it was soon decided that a 'combined' pill was better for most women.

How it works: By altering the natural hormone balance of the body, the pill does three things. It alters the mucus at the neck of the womb, making it hostile to sperm; it prevents the ripening and release of the female egg; and it alters the lining of the womb so that a fertilized egg would not be accepted there.

Effectiveness: In theory the pill is virtually 100 per cent effective. It will usually only fail if the woman forgets to take it, or if the drug is not fully absorbed because of vomiting, diarrhoea or interaction with some other drug. A course of antibiotics can have this effect.

Advantages: It is the most reliable form of reversible contraception. It is easy to take and does not interfere with lovemaking. It can help menstrual disorders and pre-menstrual tension. Because it cuts down blood loss, it may help women with iron deficiency (anaemia). It prevents ovarian cysts and certain benign breast lumps, and modifies acne and sebaceous cysts. It reduces the risk of endometrial cancer.

Disadvantages: It is now known that the pill makes the blood clot more easily and can therefore lead to thrombosis and other circulation problems. It makes women more vulnerable to heart disease and strokes. In a few women the pill produces high blood pressure. These risks start taking effect with age, and become serious more quickly for women who smoke. There are also some mild side-effects such as headaches, nausea and vaginal discharge, but these may disappear after persisting or changing the brand. A few women also experience depression. Women who stop the pill in order to conceive may find there is a delay before conception.

Advice: Women cannot conceive during the week in the monthly cycle in which they are not taking the pill: it is perfectly safe to have sex then. With some kinds of pill, you can avoid a period by just taking the pills during that week – check with your doctor that you have the right brand.

If you forget your pill, take it as soon as you remember. If your pill is more than twelve hours late, conception may occur in highly fertile women, so take other precautions as well for fourteen days. If two or more of the following apply to you, you should think hard before going on the pill: age over thirty; overweight; smoker; anyone in the immediate family died of heart disease under the age of fifty-five (count father, mother, brother, sister); any personal history of heart disease, diabetes or high blood pressure. In general, women who are heavy smokers should stop taking the pill at the age of thirty; women who do not smoke should stop taking it by the age of forty. Make sure you tell your doctor if you suffer from epilepsy, jaundice or vaginal discharge. Anyone opting for the pill should have regular blood-pressure check-ups and, ideally, stop smoking. Women who want a baby should stop the pill at least three months before trying to conceive. Use other methods in the mean time.

Check with your doctor urgently if you experience any of the following symptoms while taking the pill: severe pain in the calf of one leg; severe chest pains; unexplained breathlessness or blood-stained cough; severe stomach pains; severe or long headaches; fainting or loss of consciousness; marked numbness, sudden weakness or severe tingling on one side or one part of the body; sudden disturbance of eye-sight or speech; severe skin rash or jaundice.

A progestogen-only pill, sometimes known as the mini-pill, is used for women breast-feeding and for others for whom the combined pill is not suitable.

THE SHEATH

Before use of the pill became so widespread, the contraceptive sheath – also known as the condom or French letter – was the most common method of birth control. In Britain about 2.8 million women rely on their partners' use of condoms to avoid pregnancy.

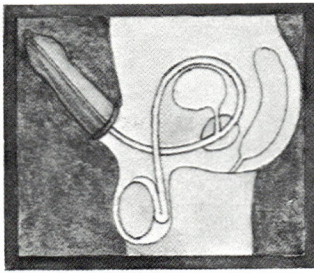

History: The ancient Egyptians seem to have been the first to use some kind of sheath. In Europe a linen version was in use in the sixteenth century, and in the next two hundred years it rapidly gained popularity. There were sheaths made of gut and even of soft leather, decorated with ribbons. Not everybody was enthusiastic. Madame de Sevigny coined the famous remark that the sheath was 'armour against enjoyment and a spider's web against danger'. Till the last century, however, sheaths were used primarily as a protection against venereal disease, with birth control as only a secondary consideration. For the same reason the British armed forces are also still issued with sheaths.

How it works: The sheath puts a barrier between sperm and female egg, and keeps all the sperms within itself. Leaving aside such curiosities as washable rubber sheaths and odd designs to enhance sexual pleasure, sheaths are mainly distinguished by shape and colour. There are sheaths made out of plastic or animal gut for those men and women who are allergic to rubber. Most sheaths nowadays are also lubricated for extra comfort. This lubrication does not usually have any contraceptive effect, though a few sheaths are specifically lubricated with a spermicide.

Effectiveness: If a hundred women used condoms for birth control for a year, on average four would become pregnant. As with other methods of contraception, regular and practised use would probably mean a slightly lower failure rate.

Advantages: There are no physical side-effects. Sheaths guard against venereal disease, and are useful for occasions when sex was not anticipated or planned. They can be obtained without a doctor's prescription in chemists, hairdressers and sometimes from slot machines. It is sometimes claimed (but unproven) that they lower the risk of cervical cancer.

Disadvantages: They dull male enjoyment. Couples may find them off-putting in loveplay. They can be an expensive method of contraception.

Advice: Make sure you have a reputable brand. Do not use them after the date marked on the packet. Read the instructions, and use them before any genital contact. The Family Planning Association recommends using a spermicide with the sheath, to make extra sure. But do not use Vaseline or grease as a lubricant, as these destroy the rubber.

THE DIAPHRAGM

Before the advent of the pill and the IUD, the only reliable contraception which allowed women to control their own fertility was the diaphragm, and other similar caps. Today nearly two hundred thousand women in Britain use this.

History: Although the ancient Egyptians may have used some kind of vaginal cap, it did not reach Britain until the nineteenth century. Before the cap, women had used vaginal sponges, tampons and douches. In the last century, spermicide creams, jellies and suppositories had also been invented, and with the cap these proved efficient.

How it works: Like the sheath, the diaphragm or cap puts a barrier between sperm and egg by covering the cervix, the entrance to the womb. There are two main types of cap: the flat dish-shaped diaphragm sometimes known as the Dutch cap and the much smaller high-domed cervical cap. The diaphragm covers the cervix, reaching back to the end of the vagina and forward towards the pubic bone, under which it lodges. The cervical cap does not cover the same amount of vaginal wall as the diaphragm. Instead it fits neatly over the cervix itself.

Effectiveness: If a hundred women used the diaphragm and spermicides as birth control for a year, about three of them would become pregnant. Regular and practised users have the lowest failure-rate.

Advantages: There are no physical side-effects. It is often used as a stop-gap between the pill or the IUD. During menstruation it holds back the flow of blood, thus making intercourse less messy. Diaphragms with spermicide offer partial protection against sexually transmitted infections.

Disadvantages: They may be off-putting in some forms of loveplay. Women who dislike touching their genitals may find them distasteful to insert. There is the danger that women in a hurry may insert them incorrectly. Cervical caps can be difficult to put in and take out.

Advice: Diaphragms and caps must be carefully fitted by an expert and checked at regular intervals. Since not all doctors are experts, get a diaphragm or cap from a clinic. Check that it remains in good condition, with the rubber still supple and shaped. Failures often occur because a diaphragm has become too old or misshapen. Do not use Vaseline or grease as a lubricant, because it destroys the rubber.

Diaphragms must *always* be used with spermicide, and indeed fresh spermicide must be added after three hours. They should be left in place for at least six hours after the last sexual intercourse. Cervical caps must be taken out after twenty-four hours.

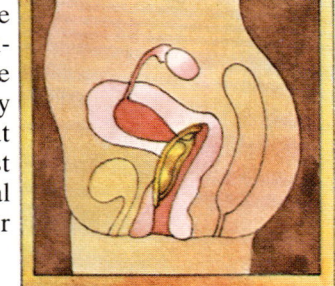

The Family Planning Association recommends spermicide with cervical caps to make doubly sure pregnancy does not occur.

THE INTRA-UTERINE DEVICE

About four hundred and ninety thousand women – nearly half a million – in Britain rely upon an intra-uterine device to prevent pregnancy. Intra-uterine devices are also known as IUDs or coils.

History: Nineteenth-century European doctors occasionally fitted women with intra-uterine devices. These were known as stem pessaries and they were fitted to deal with gynaecological problems. The idea was that they supported the womb after a number of pregnancies. This century, the IUD was rediscovered, this time as a contraceptive.

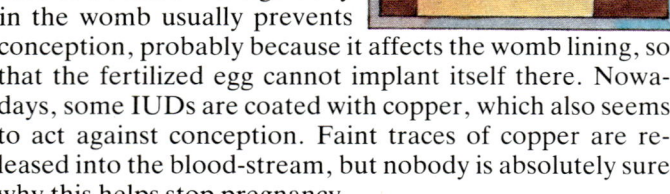

How it works: A foreign body in the womb usually prevents conception, probably because it affects the womb lining, so that the fertilized egg cannot implant itself there. Nowadays, some IUDs are coated with copper, which also seems to act against conception. Faint traces of copper are released into the blood-stream, but nobody is absolutely sure why this helps stop pregnancy.

The IUDs that are approved by the Family Planning Association are: Lippes Loop, Saf-T-Coil, Copper 7, Copper T, the Multi-load Copper 250 and Novagard.
Effectiveness: If a hundred women wore IUDs for a year, two or three would become pregnant, but much depends upon who fits the IUDs.
Advantages: Once inserted, an IUD can be left in place for two years or more. Devices which carry copper can be left in for much longer. The woman does not have to remember to take it or insert it. Sex can be had at any time without preparations.
Disadvantages: Skill is necessary in fitting to ensure that the device is correctly placed in the womb. Though pregnancy chances are small, if it does occur there is a high risk of miscarriage or ectopic pregnancy. Some women find IUDs painful or suffer heavy periods; some automatically expel them and occasionally women suffer from a discharge. IUD wearers are at a greater risk of pelvic inflammation, which may affect future fertility.
Advice: Make sure you get your IUD inserted by a doctor

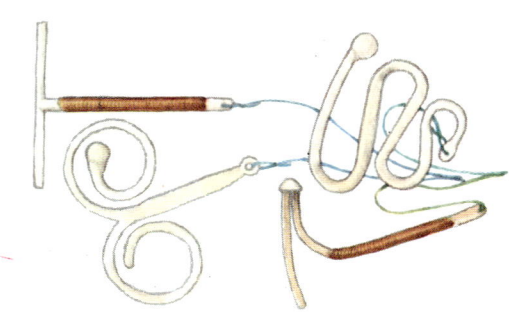

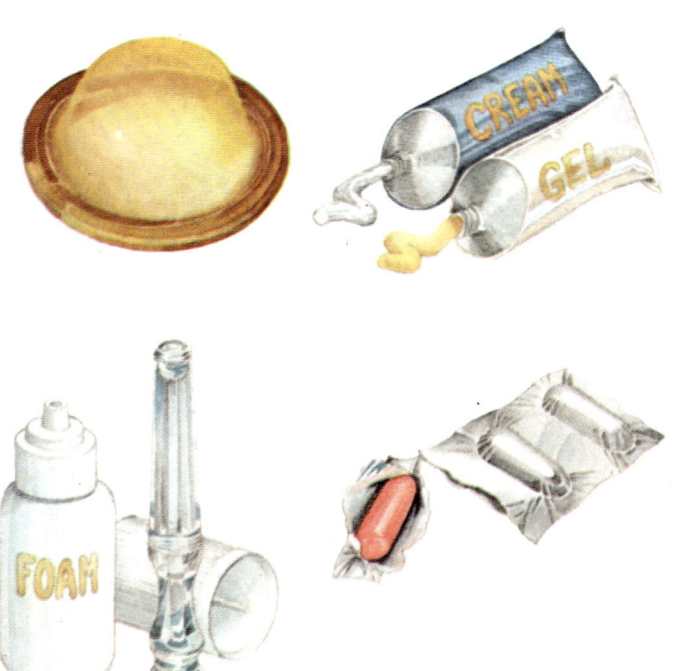

who is practised in the technique. It is probably best to go to a family planning clinic where you know the doctors will have had plenty of practice. Women who have not had children, or who know that they want further children, should use other methods if possible.

COITUS INTERRUPTUS
It is not known how many British couples still rely on coitus interruptus, or the withdrawal method, for birth control.

History: The Biblical story of Onan, who spilled his semen on the ground rather than impregnate his brother's wife, indicates its early origins.
How it works: The man withdraws his penis from the woman's vagina just before ejaculation, in an effort to keep sperm away from the female sex-organs.
Effectiveness: There are no reliable figures for its efficiency, since so much depends on the individual self-control and skill of the man. But it is rarely efficient.
Advantages: It can be practised when no other form of contraception is available. It has no physical side-effects.
Disadvantages: Semen can be released into the vagina before ejaculation. Sexual satisfaction is often impaired.
Advice: Better than no precautions at all, but it cannot be relied upon as a method of contraception.

STERILIZATION
Every year, about a hundred thousand women are sterilized to prevent further pregnancies.

How it works: The principle is to cut or block off the Fallopian tubes, down which the female egg travels from the ovary to the womb. Several different techniques are available. The tubes may be cut (tubal ligation), sealed (diathermy) or blocked by clips or rings. The tubes are usually reached by a small cut in the stomach wall.
Effectiveness: Tubal ligation is more than 99 per cent effective, though very occasionally the Fallopian tubes rejoin automatically. Sterilization by clips and rings has a failure rate of up to 2 per cent.
Advantages: It ends worry about pregnancy permanently.
Disadvantages: The menstrual cycle may be disrupted, and for a time sexual intercourse may have to be avoided. Some disorders, possibly psychological, like backache, headache and depression have been reported. As with any surgical operation, sterilization carries a slight health risk. Should circumstances change, fertility cannot normally be regained.

Advice: Because of the permanent loss of fertility, this is not an operation to be undertaken lightly. A woman should think carefully before taking the decision, for she must assume that it will end all chance of bearing further children. It is not a good idea to combine sterilization with abortion, because a woman wanting an abortion may be too upset to make a balanced decision about sterilization. If your doctor says he will only give you an abortion on condition you are sterilized at the same time, contact another doctor or a charitable abortion agency for help (see Appendix Three).

VASECTOMY

Between fifty and a hundred thousand men in Britain have a vasectomy every year.

History: Vasectomies only really caught on in Britain in the early sixties, though they had been common in India before then. In 1972 they were made available on the National Health Service, if the local authority opted for providing this service.
How it works: Vasectomy is the male equivalent of sterilization. The operation involves cutting and tying the two *vas deferens*, tubes which carry sperms from the testicles to the penis. Since these are just under the skin, usually only a local anaesthetic is needed.
Effectiveness: One in every thousand vasectomies is a failure. The other possible cause of post-vasectomy pregnancy is that it takes three or four months before the sperm-flow disappears. Sperm tests are necessary to check that all the sperms have disappeared.
Advantages: It ends worry about pregnancy permanently. It does not in any way affect male virility. It is a much easier and less serious operation than female sterilization.
Disadvantages: Should circumstances change, fertility cannot normally be regained.
Advice: Make sure that all the sperm tests have proved negative before giving up other methods of contraception. Because of the permanent loss of fertility, this is not an operation to be undertaken lightly. A man should think carefully before taking the decision, for he must assume that it will end all chance of fathering further children.

SAFE PERIOD

About four hundred thousand British women practise the safe-period method, sometimes called the rhythm method or natural family planning.

History: Up to the end of the nineteenth century, doctors did not know about the female cycle. In the 1920s, medical researchers Ogino and Knaus showed that ovulation occurred about twelve to sixteen days before the next menstrual period – thus providing the basis for the calendar method.
How it works: All safe-period methods are based on the principle that sexual intercourse must be avoided around the time when the female egg is released into the Fallopian tubes. This means a minimum period of five days, to cope with the seventy-two-hour life of the sperm and the twenty-four-hour life of the female egg (with a possibility of a double ovulation as in the case of non-identical twins). Some sperm live for five days.

With the **calendar method** the woman keeps records of the last six to twelve cycles, noting the length of the shortest and the longest cycles; she then makes calculations to predict the fertile phase. This method, which did not allow for unexpected irregularities or irregular cycles, is no longer recommended by natural family planning organizations. Instead, the new methods use signals which a woman's body provides during each menstrual cycle.

The **temperature method** relies on the charting of a woman's daily waking temperature. When an egg has been released, the woman's temperature rises to a higher level. After three consecutive daily temperatures at this level (a full forty-eight hours), the ovum – or even twin ova – will no longer be capable of fertilization. From then onwards, the woman is infertile. With this system, abstinence must be maintained until the third high temperature.

The **mucus method** relies on a second signal: the changing consistency and appearance of the cervical mucus and the sensations it offers at the entrance to the vagina. A woman can be taught to recognize her own mucus pattern with the help of a qualified instructor. This is known as the Billings method, because colour charting and rules for determining fertile and infertile phases were initiated by Dr Billings of Australia. It is also known as the ovulation or cervical mucus method.

The **sympto-thermal method** uses both temperature and mucus signals of fertility. It is also known as the muco-thermic or double-check method. Temperature and mucus are recorded on a combined chart. This offers the reliability of the post-ovulatory temperature method, while allowing some sexual intercourse in the pre-ovulatory phase, where mucus gives a warning signal of approaching ovulation.
Effectiveness: If a hundred women use the temperature method for one year, with intercourse confined to the time after the third high temperature, up to six pregnancies can be expected, allowing for user failure. International figures for the mucus-only method range from fifteen to twenty-five pregnancies per hundred users, but a large proportion of these pregnancies are due to failure to abstain from intercourse during the fertile time. Sympto-thermal figures vary in many surveys, but fall mainly into the five to nine pregnancies per hundred women per year range.
Advantages: Natural family planning is acceptable to the Catholic Church. There are no physical side-effects. It is a shared method of contraception, involving both husband and wife. Timed differently, it can also be used as an aid to conception.
Disadvantages: It limits sexual intercourse and requires abstinence. In the temperature method, couples must abstain until the third high temperature; with the sympto-thermal method intercourse is allowed in the pre-ovulatory phase but only on alternate days. The couple must be in agreement and well motivated to make the system work. Some women may find charting irksome; some may find body secretions distasteful.
Advice: Those trained in other methods of family planning are not always competent to teach natural methods. A qualified instructor who offers full clear explanations and follow-up support is needed. You will get information from your local Catholic Marriage Advisory Council (see Appendix Three). There are trained instructors in many areas of the country. For those who are not within reach of an instructor, a correspondence service operates from the Catholic Marriage Advisory Council in London.

Sexual Infections

Each year two hundred and fifty thousand men and women in Britain receive treatment at VD clinics. Yet because sexual diseases and infections are rarely openly discussed, there is great ignorance about their nature and symptoms and the sensible precautions you can take to avoid infection. There are only two major diseases which can be strictly defined as venereal: syphilis and gonorrhoea. This is because they are always caught by sexual contact with an infected person. Exceptions are exceedingly rare. There are, however, several other illnesses and infections which are known as sexually-transmitted infections (STI). Some are not the result of sexual intercourse, but they are still treated by VD clinics. Some clinics, recognizing this, run housewives' sessions, or call themselves genito-urinary clinics. 'We deal with anything between the hips and the knees,' says a venereologist in London.

SYPHILIS

The disease with all the horror stories. Fortunately it is so rare that some doctors train without ever seeing a case. It *is* increasing, though, among homosexual men. It is easily cured at any stage with penicillin, but because it is such a serious disease doctors perform tests over several months to make sure it has really disappeared.

The first symptoms are sores, usually round the genitals, sometimes round the back passage or the mouth. They look like little craters, the size of a pinhead to a pea, with a shiny red centre. They do not hurt and disappear without treatment. The second stage appears weeks or months later with a rash. This does not itch or hurt and indeed it can be confused with other illnesses. But if you have been taking chances with your sex life and had sores earlier, then it may be syphilis.

GONORRHOEA

This is far more common than syphilis. It can be serious if untreated. Women, particularly, risk infertility. The cure is with antibiotics, but repeated tests may be needed. Doctors will probably want patients to take a syphilis blood-test later, to check that they do not have both sorts of VD at the same time. Symptoms in men are easily recognized. There is a burning sensation during urination. There is also a greenish-yellow discharge from the tip of the penis. In women, symptoms are less obvious. It may hurt to pass water and there may be a vaginal discharge; but for almost two out of three women there are no symptoms at all, except an infected boyfriend.

NON-SPECIFIC URETHRITIS (NSU)

NSU is the illness most on the increase. It is sometimes called non-specific genital infection (NSGI) or non-gonococcal urethritis (NGU). Symptoms are as in gonorrhoea: an inflamed urethra (the tube through which the urine passes); pain in passing water; and a discharge. Cures are not always easy; antibiotics are given, but relapses are common. Some men get Reiter's syndrome, which can cause the joints to be painful and swollen. NSU can occur without sexual intercourse. On the other hand, much NSU is sexually transmitted, so doctors usually investigate partners, who might be carriers without symptoms.

Women, in particular, can carry the infection without knowing it since they may not have recognizable symptoms. It is important that women whose husbands or boyfriends have NSU should have a check-up themselves. It can lead on to pelvic inflammatory disease which in turn makes some women infertile.

TRICHOMONIASIS

This is caused by a single-celled organism in the female vagina. It has been found in virgins, but it can also be passed on by sex. Some men may be carriers. The cure is usually easy – just taking metronidazole tablets – but partners must be seen and checked to cut the risk of re-infection. Symptoms are a vaginal itch and sometimes a smelly discharge. In severe cases this can make the genital area red and sore. Occasionally, men have irritation in the penis from the same organism.

THRUSH

Thrush is another female infection of the vagina, caused by a yeast-like organism which grows when the natural bacteria in the vagina are upset: by antibiotics, by the pill, diabetes or even by an emotional upheaval. It may be aggravated by sex and can be occasionally passed on to men. Female symptoms are an itch in the vagina, especially at night, and sometimes a creamy white discharge. Men may get irritation at the tip of the penis. Thrush is cured by pessaries for women and ointment for men.

Women who are suffering from thrush may find sexual intercourse painful. Occasionally even when the thrush has cleared up, this pain continues because the vagina fails to lubricate or the muscles tense in *anticipation* of pain. 'Phantom thrush' one VD specialist calls it. If all infection has ceased, then what is needed is treatment for the sexual difficulty (see page 174).

HEPATITIS

Hepatitis is sometimes spread by sexual contact, and evidence of this disease is found among one in twenty male homosexuals who attend VD clinics. If untreated it can develop into serious liver disease in some people. An obvious attack produces yellowing eyeballs and skin, but there may be no symptoms in a mild attack. Symptomless carriers can remain infectious for months.

GENITAL HERPES

There are two kinds of herpes viruses – the mild form which produces cold sores and a severer form usually found on the genitals. Symptoms are burning, little itchy blisters which produce shallow sores. In the first attacks there may also be headache, raised temperature, backache and a general feeling of illness. The virus persists in the affected person for the rest of their life, and from time to time may set off another attack of sores. For a small proportion of those women who get genital herpes, there is a link with cancer of the cervix. This type of cancer is easily cured and detected in the early stages. All who have had genital herpes should have *yearly* cancer smears to check up, from the onset of their herpes onwards. If your family doctor will not give smears that often, get them done at a family planning clinic or a VD clinic. This is a very important measure of health protection and you should insist upon its being done.

GENITAL WARTS
These appear about three months after intercourse with an infected person, and tend to spread. They do not do any harm, except for looking unpleasant and itching slightly. Occasionally, they form large masses of warts on some individuals. Get them treated at a VD clinic.

PUBIC LICE
This is also known as crabs. It is mostly spread by sexual contact, but can also be acquired from infested bedding and even (very occasionally) from lavatory seats. It can be treated with a lotion from the chemist, but it is best to go to a VD clinic in case other infections have been acquired at the same time.

Other sexually transmitted infections include a skin rash called scabies and a very rare tropical venereal disease called chancroid, which produces small ulcers on the genitals. Occasionally the hair follicles on the genitals become infected and produce boils which give the impression of being some kind of sexual infection.

CUTTING THE RISK
If you sleep with only one person, and you are both faithful, you should avoid both gonorrhea and syphilis. 'A loving, caring partner is the best protection against venereal disease' is how one VD specialist puts it. Fidelity, however, does not rule out some of the other infections, which can be – but are not always – spread by sexual contact. You should not assume your partner has been unfaithful, if you catch one of these.

Sexually transmitted infections are no respecters of persons. It is wrong to assume you will only catch an infection from layabouts or prostitutes. However, one-night stands, sex with strangers and partner-swapping increase the risks. If you are taking risks, try to take other precautions:

1. Use a condom, or get your boyfriend to do so. Condoms protect against gonorrhea and NSU, though not against syphilis. Using a sheath, even when other contraceptive precautions are being taken, is probably the best protection against sexual diseases.
2. Women can use a spermicidal pessary. Spermicide kills some, if not all, of the sexual infection bugs. If you dare not ask the man to use a condom, use a pessary yourself. He need not even know.
3. Urinate and wash the genitals after intercourse. Some people say that this can flush out the germs. It is worth trying.
4. If you have any doubtful symptoms whatever, go to a VD clinic or doctor. Clinics are much friendlier places than most people expect, and you will find a non-judgemental staff and doctor there. Because they have specialist facilities, VD clinics are rather better at dealing with sexual infections than are ordinary family doctors. Even infections like thrush which may have nothing to do with sexual intercourse may get better treatment at a clinic than in an ordinary doctor's surgery.
5. Women and homosexual men, who may have no symptoms at all, should have regular check-ups if their lifestyle involves lots of different partners. If there is any possibility of infection, check with a clinic. Homosexual men should avoid amyl nitrate 'popper' which some doctors now believe may be associated with infection. It is also worth bearing in mind that partner-spacing may help avoid sexual infections. Heterosexual men, whose symptoms will normally show up in about ten days, could leave a ten-day interval between partners. If you are being unfaithful to a regular partner, this would help protect her against infection.
6. Finish any treatment. Many patients do not bother to get the clinic's all-clear, because the symptoms vanish. Despite the symptoms' disappearance, *you may not be cured*. Keep all clinic appointments until you are given a clean bill of health.

Menopause

Somewhere between the age of forty and sixty every woman faces the menopause, the time when periods stop and pregnancy is no longer possible. It is also known as the change of life or the climacteric, names redolent with the gloom and mystery with which it has been surrounded. But this need not be so. Indeed, one in four women experiences little or no difficulties at all.

THE SYMPTOMS
Strictly speaking, the menopause simply describes the end of a woman's periods, but it is often used loosely to cover the time before and after this event when some women – but not all – experience a range of symptoms. These can occur just before the periods begin to change their frequency, and can last for some years after. The menopause seems to be a variable phenomenon and doctors do not all agree on what the symptoms include. Some doctors think that symptoms like pins and needles, constipation and flatulence are part of the menopause. Others disagree. But five major symptoms, most doctors agree, are common. These are: hot flushes, depression, vaginal dryness, insomnia and palpitations. A very few women also experience an itching skin sensation.

Unpleasant though they may be, these symptoms are not the sign of some dangerous affliction. The menopause is not such a fearful event. It need not just be endured; sensible health rules and a good doctor's help can reduce problems to a manageable minimum; and for some women it is a chance to rethink their lives and start a vigorous new career.

HORMONE REPLACEMENT THERAPY
Perhaps the single most important choice that faces the middle-aged woman is whether to ask for hormone replacement therapy over the menopause. Doctors disagree fiercely over HRT (as it is known for short). Almost every article or book is either for or against it. But does it really work? And is it really safe?

Hormone replacement therapy is based on the idea that during the menopause a woman's ovaries stop making the female hormone, oestrogen. The lack of oestrogen causes many unpleasant menopausal symptoms. By giving a woman oestrogen tablets, this makes up the natural lack of

SEX AND HEALTH/MENOPAUSE

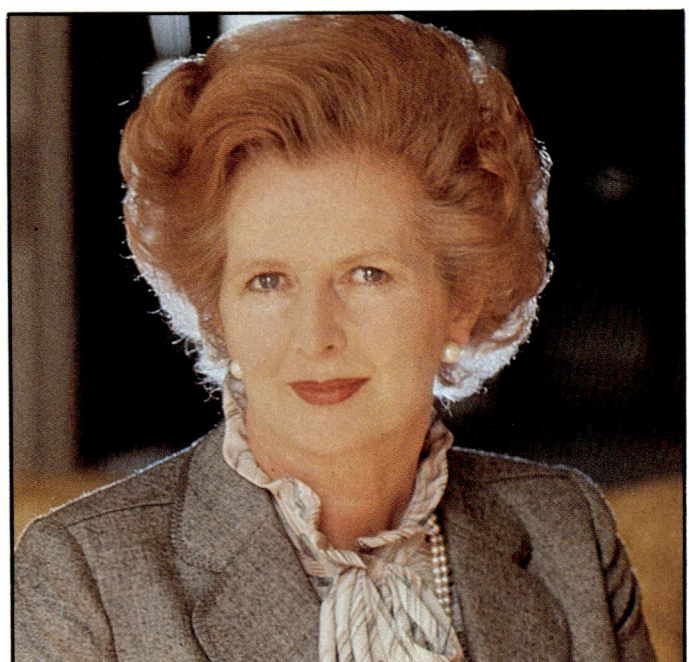 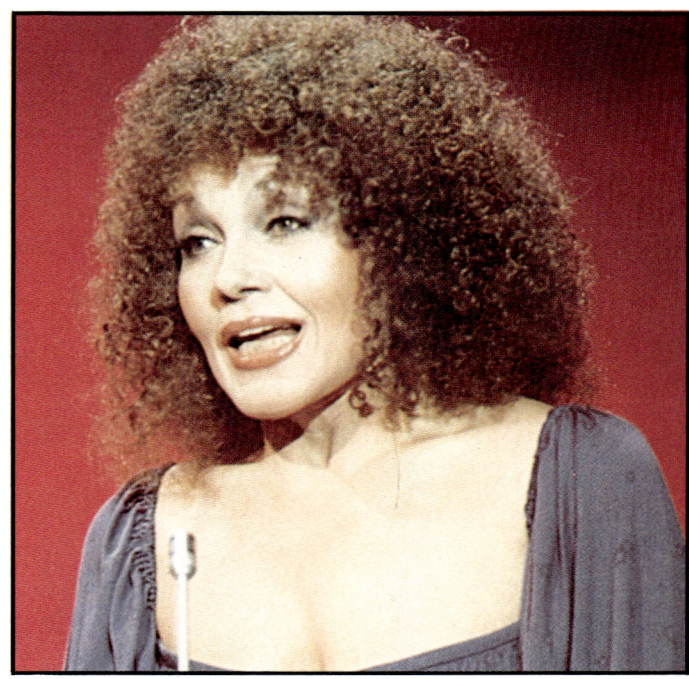

Women can be at their peak during the middle years. Margaret Thatcher became Tory party leader at the age of 49 and Prime Minister four years later. Cleo Laine, the singer, won the Variety Club of Great Britain Show Business Personality Award at the age of 50.

hormones and her symptoms vanish. That is why it is called hormone *replacement* therapy.

The history of hormone replacement therapy has been rather like that of the contraceptive pill. At first, it was hailed as a major breakthrough, particularly in the USA. Doctors there argued that *all* women should automatically be put on hormones when they reached middle age. It was even claimed that HRT was a kind of youth pill.

This wild enthusiasm was succeeded by serious criticism in the 1970s. Dangers were perceived in the way women were given just oestrogen by itself. And as the research findings began to mount up, it was clear that the old way of giving HRT was not suitable – but new kinds of HRT did not have its dangers.

Opinions are still divided in the 1980s. Some family doctors take the view that the menopause is natural and women who complain of the symptoms are just making a fuss. Others are so enthusiastic that they may hand out HRT to women whose problems are not connected with hormone deficiency. However, HRT is only worth considering for a minority of women who have really distressing symptoms.

Most doctors, however, agree that HRT does cure the major symptoms. It is the best treatment so far for stopping hot flushes, night sweats, and for preventing vaginal dryness. Because it cures night sweats, it helps insomnia and the general feeling of tiredness that some women feel at this time. It reduces palpitations, too. But it does not have any effect on serious depression.

The other success of hormone replacement therapy is its effect on osteoporosis, the bone thinning that sets in at the menopause and that causes fractures and dowager's hump some twelve to twenty-five years later. Osteoporosis in women costs the National Health Service about £67 million in fractures, and among women over the age of sixty-five one in four has a crush fracture of the vertebrae, which, in its severest forms, can lead to loss of height and dowager's hump. Hormone replacement therapy stops bone thinning for as long as it is taken.

If the effectiveness of HRT is no longer doubted, its risks are still questioned. The old HRT was simply regular oestrogen tablets, taken continuously or with a mere week's break. Oestrogen given in this way by itself stimulated the womb lining and could produce uterine cancer.

The new method of giving hormones gets over this problem. Oestrogen is given for sixteen days, followed by twelve days of oestrogen with added progestogen. The progestogen produces three or four days' bleeding, like a period – but the woman is not fertile since no ova are shed. On this kind of HRT, with regular bleeding, women are *protected* against uterine cancer.

The old-fashioned HRT produced a higher risk of coronary heart disease, high blood pressure, strokes and thrombosis troubles. This was because early HRT used synthetic and very powerful oestrogen. When natural oestrogens with added progestogen are used, this risk may be reduced or abolished.

Doubts remain over another risk – breast cancer. So far, research has produced conflicting results. We do not know for certain whether HRT protects against breast cancer, or whether it produces it. There is also a possibility that HRT causes gallstones. Indeed, new findings may still emerge about HRT so we cannot entirely pronounce even the new HRT 100 per cent safe (few medical treatments are). At the time this book was written, 1982, the main possibility of risk with the new HRT was that of breast cancer.

So how should a woman decide? There are two main reasons for wanting HRT. The most obvious reason is that HRT will cure hot flushes, night sweats, vaginal dryness or atrophy, and some other minor menopausal symptoms. One out of four women does not have these symptoms and therefore does not need HRT. Of those women who do have such symptoms, only one in four seems sufficiently troubled to seek medical treatment anyway.

MENOPAUSE/SEX AND HEALTH

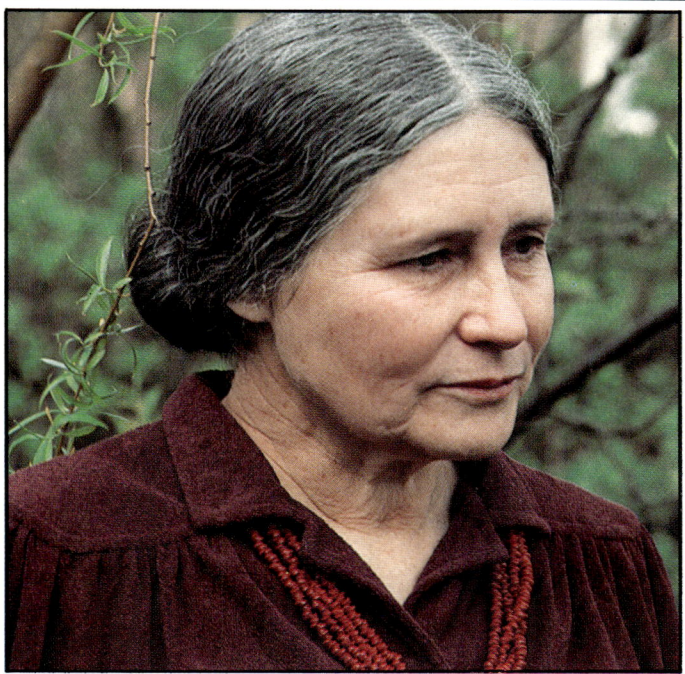

At the age of 60, novelist Doris Lessing published her first science fiction novel.

The other reason for HRT is to prevent bone-thinning. Unfortunately doctors still cannot tell in advance which women are going to suffer osteoporosis in their sixties and seventies. 'Those who should take HRT to prevent osteoporosis are women with a family history of osteoporosis; women who have had a fracture under the age of sixty because of thin bones; women with a premature menopause before the age of forty; and small, thin white women who seem to make less natural oestrogen,' says Dr Malcolm Whitehead, lecturer at King's College Hospital Medical School.

Once you have decided that you may need hormone replacement therapy, it is vital to get the correct kind of treatment. Family doctors cannot always keep up to date with new research, and so it is probably best to ask your GP if she or he will refer you to a menopause clinic. If you meet a refusal, you can get a list of clinics from Women's Health Concern (see Appendix Three).

If your family doctor decides to give you HRT, it should be the combined hormone treatment, which produces three or four days of bleeding. If he is giving you oestrogen by itself, without any progestogen added, then you should change to a menopause clinic.

You should also be given natural oestrogens. Brand names include Harmogen, Hormonin, Ovestin, Premarin and Progynova.

HRT needs to be properly supervised. You should have six-monthly checks on blood pressure, weight, an annual breast check and an annual pelvic examination. Any bleeding outside the time of the progestogen-induced bleeding should be reported to your doctor, and should be followed by a d-and-c operation. Again, change to a menopause clinic if you are not getting this kind of supervision.

Some women should never have HRT – women who have had breast cancer, womb cancer or endometrial hyperplasia. Other women should only have HRT if they badly need it, and are getting expert supervision – women who have had strokes, heart attacks, thrombosis, liver disease, benign breast lumps, high blood pressure, obesity, heavy smoking, or who have a family history of strokes and heart attacks in blood relatives at a young age. Any woman who continues to smoke while having HRT is taking an unnecessary risk. Stop immediately.

HOT FLUSHES

Hormone replacement therapy is the most effective treatment for hot flushes. But, if you have only occasional flushes, you may not need this. Flushes are sometimes brought on by alcohol, hot curries, embarrassment or too much tea or coffee.

Hot flushes respond well to placeboes, pills that contain no drugs but which the taker believes will cure her. So, if you think something helps your flushes, you may be right.

If you are a woman who cannot have normal HRT, then it is worth asking if you might have progestogen on its own. This will help flushes. 'Hypnotics, sedatives and tranquillizers are no good at all for flushes,' says Dr Whitehead. There is a drug called clonidine which is worth trying, if HRT is ruled out for you.

DEPRESSION

This hits many women during the years before and after the menopause. They feel weepy, lethargic, irritable and unreasonably gloom-ridden. Indeed, because of old wives' tales about the climacteric, some women fear they may be heading for mental breakdown. In fact, this fear is exaggerated. Though many women feel depressed in middle age, there does not seem to be any greater risk of really serious mental illness. Those women who *are* admitted to mental hospital are usually the ones that have some kind of history of mental problems. The menopause has not caused their illness; it has just been the last straw.

Yet even a mild bout of depression is horrible for the sufferer and bad for her family. It is difficult to know how far, however, these feelings are due to the physical changes of the menopause, or how far they are due to the problems of middle age, 'the empty nest syndrome' as it is sometimes called. At this time, children are leaving home, women are worried about growing old, and a marriage may be running into difficulties. If this is the case, a marriage guidance counsellor may be able to help as much as a doctor.

So women should possibly try to take a look at their lives to see if anything in them needs changing. Is this the moment to go back to work? Or to opt out of a tiring, boring job for something more fulfilling? Or might evening classes, voluntary work, or even a local protest-group help your morale? This advice sounds trite, but it can work. Dr P. A. Van Keep, a Belgian gynaecologist, surveyed a number of middle-aged working women. He found that for well-off women, a job seemed to ward off the unpleasant effects of the menopause. But it was just the opposite for the women at the other end of the social scale. For them a job, perhaps because it was boring, ill-paid and taken only because the money was needed, seemed to increase the unpleasant side-effects of the change of life.

It is still disputed whether hormone replacement therapy helps the milder forms of depression. Women who have hot flushes, vaginal trouble or thinning bones as well as depression, should certainly try it. The depression may clear up when the other troubles are dealt with. Even if you do not have these other symptoms, it may be worth trying

HRT. Try it for a short time and see if your depression lifts.

In general you can help yourself by making sure you are in good physical health. Put your eating habits right. Avoid getting overweight. Take regular exercise. Tranquillizers really do not help with depression, and an overprescribing doctor can give you a bad drug habit (see Drug Dependence page 147).

For serious depression, you need anti-depressants and it will probably be worth getting help from a psychiatrist rather than merely your GP. Severe depression needs expert help, and the sooner you get it the better (see Depression, pages 73–4). Hormone replacement does not help severe depression.

SEX AND VAGINAL DRYNESS

Vaginal dryness sometimes sets in after the menopause. The vagina loses its flexibility and its usual moist surface. Sex may be painful and unpleasant. In due course, unless treatment is given, this dryness leads to vaginal narrowing in some women.

Hormone replacement therapy does seem to cure vaginal dryness. Family doctors sometimes recommend merely a hormone cream to be put on the genitals. But nowadays we know that the hormones from the cream go into the bloodstream, so that it is probably safest to take your hormones by tablet. In cream alone, you will not be getting the progestogen you need.

There are other ways of coping with vaginal dryness, if you do not want or cannot have HRT. KY jelly will make sex less unpleasant. Emulsifying ointment from a chemist can be used as a moisturizing agent, or as a way of cleaning the genitals. Test with just a little cream first to make sure you are not allergic.

There is no truth in the old wives' tale that your sex life is bound to diminish in middle or even old age. Indeed an active sex life may help to keep the vagina in working order. Some women feel a new enthusiasm once the fear of pregnancy is lifted. But, if you have had several weeks of vaginal dryness, you may find that painful sex continues even after hormone replacement therapy has restored the vaginal lubrication. This is probably due to muscle-tensing in fearful anticipation (see Sexual Difficulties, page 174).

Menstrual irregularities can be confusing during the menopause. Some women have increasingly heavy periods. Sudden floods should always be reported to your doctor, and a d-and-c operation should follow just to make sure nothing is wrong. For those whose periods get heavier there are drugs which cut down the flow of menstrual blood and which do not contain hormones: ask your doctor to recommend one. Check, also, that you are not anaemic: look out for pale gums and pale corners of the eyes, as these could be a sign. Again, your doctor can test for anaemia and prescribe iron tablets.

For most women, however, the periods phase themselves out by becoming either more scanty, or by occurring less frequently. This means that you may find it difficult to know whether bleeding from the vagina is an irregular period or a sign that you need a doctor's check-up. Keeping a record of your periods, to see what their pattern is, is a good idea. Any bleeding that does not seem to fit this pattern or that looks different in consistency, flow or colour from normal menstrual bleeding, should be reported to your doctor. You are not wasting his time, but just keeping a reasonable check on your health.

There is nothing particularly dangerous about the menopause itself, though cancer risks increase with age. Older women should remember to keep doing their regular breast-examinations (see page 142) and they should also have a regular cervical smear taken. Doctors will do this, but so, too, will family planning and VD clinics. And don't forget that contraception should be continued for a year after the last period. If an unplanned pregnancy occurs at this stage and is unwanted, an abortion can usually be obtained in Britain on the grounds that the risk of having a mongol (Down's syndrome) baby is at its highest. The first step, though, would generally be an amniocentesis (see Chapter 1).

INSOMNIA

Being unable to sleep quite often causes a lot of unhappiness and worry, which in turn makes it more difficult to sleep! However, if you do find you have a sleep problem, it is worth analysing why. If you are suffering from hot flushes, these probably include the so-called night sweats, when you wake up bathed in perspiration. In this case if you deal with the hot flushes by hormone replacement, the sweats will also go and your sleeping pattern should be restored.

If, however, your insomnia is nothing to do with sweats, it may be that you are one of those people who has always had a sleeping problem. The menopause, after all, is another stressful experience, like adolescence, illness, losing a job, and so forth. If you have had sleep problems before, you will probably have worked out your own system of coping by now. But before getting addicted to sleeping pills, don't despise the homely remedies of exhausting physical exercise and hot baths. It is also generally true that, as we move towards old age, sleeping may become more difficult. However, we do not need that much sleep. Rig up a small lamp by the bedside (so as not to wake your sleeping mate) and if you cannot sleep, read, knit or do anything so that you do not get into the vicious circle of not sleeping, panicking and then being even more unable to relax. For some people, relaxation classes may help (see Chapter 3).

ITCHING SKIN

Itching in the genital area is probably a sign of vaginal dryness. For this and for any other skin irritations, consult your doctor. Skin irritations may be some form of disease, so it is worth making sure. Alternatively, it may just be one of the signs of menopausal 'nerves'. One form of this is the sensation that hundreds of ants are crawling about under the skin. This is extremely unpleasant, but do not panic. If you have checked with the doctor that it is not a skin disease, then it is just one of the eccentric ways in which the human system copes with the change. If you can cope with your other more serious physical and mental symptoms, this should go away too.

PALPITATIONS

This is another of the 'nervous' symptoms women can experience. It is as if the heart beats like thunder or jumps out of the breast. Again, this is a symptom you should check with your doctor just in case there is a serious cause other than the menopause. But it is more likely that it will be simply due to the change, a nervous reaction which is frightening *but nothing else*. Alas, the more you worry about palpitations, the more likely they are to occur, so try not to panic. Mental quietness will help. Try hormone replacement therapy, if it persists.

BRITTLE BONES (Osteoporosis)
In general, though the bones start thinning at the menopause, the consequences do not show up until about twelve to twenty-five years later. But, if you have a fracture after the menopause and X-rays suggest that osteoporosis is setting in, it may be worth going on to hormone replacement therapy in your sixties. This decision is a complicated one. Ask your doctor to refer you to a menopause clinic. They will then decide whether the benefits will outweigh the risks.

Other measures may also reduce bone-thinning. It may help to take a calcium supplement to the diet – available as pills from your doctor. Or you can make sure that you drink milk, at least half a pint, daily. Drink the semi-skimmed fresh milk (stripey top) to avoid gaining extra weight or increasing risk of heart disease. Regular exposure to sunlight helps the skin to make Vitamin D, which is also good for bones. It is not necessary to strip down to bathing gear just to try to get out of doors and get the sun on the face, hands, arms and legs. Regular exercise is also important to prevent bone-thinning – astronauts lose calcium from the bones and this has been attributed to the almost total lack of exercise in their regime.

Age and Sex

Growing old does not mean that sex has to come to a full stop. Elderly men and women can enjoy active lovemaking right into their seventies and eighties, if they desire to. Indeed, the occasional nonagenarian, according to a Danish survey, is still leading an active sex life.

Age, however, does affect sexual response. The process is not a sudden one, nor does it occur after a set number of years. It is rather a very slow decline over a long period. If men and women have led an active sex life for a long time, they will find this can continue right into old age.

The research of Masters and Johnson has shown the principles of sexual response are the same in youth and in old age. But age slows down sexual arousal in men, and may diminish the intensity of sexual response in both sexes. In particular, women may suffer from a lessening of vaginal lubrication. The vaginal walls thin with age, and the whole vagina can shrink. Sometimes the thrusting of the penis in the vagina irritates the bladder. Older women may find they have to urinate after sex, and that a long sex session can cause cystitis (see page 158).

Women who are suffering with vaginal difficulties should try KY jelly, or emulsifying cream. If neither of these help, then hormone replacement therapy or a hormone cream may be the answer. But for both of these, you need proper medical supervision (see Menopause, page 184).

It has been suggested that women who have regular sexual activity have vaginas that stay in better condition. If this is so, then sexual intercourse may have a protective effect. If you have no partner, or if your partner's sexual appetite is not strong, you may like to try regular masturbation with a vibrator. Stretching the vagina by vaginal penetration seems to keep it exercised.

The ageing male will probably find that it takes longer to get an erection, and that this erection is only at full height just before ejaculation. Intervals between erections will be longer, and ejaculation itself may be more of a leaking than a spurting sensation. But – as compensation – he will probably be able to hold his erection longer, and have better control of ejaculation.

Older men who want to have a lot of lovemaking sessions may find that this can be achieved by *not* ejaculating in every session. Saving up the ejaculation may mean they can manage lovemaking more frequently.

Old age is also a good time to reconsider sexual habits. Oral sex, manual stimulation by both partners, even 'heavy petting', can replace the traditional way of making love with the penis thrusting in the vagina. For those who are happy with the idea of sex aids, a vibrator can be used to stimulate both women and men.

If either lose the desire for sex, this may be the effect of ill-health. Similarly, many drugs given to combat disorders of the elderly can have this effect. Elderly men and women may also be more susceptible to alcohol.

If in doubt, check with your doctor. Sometimes people give up sex because they think it is dangerous – for instance, people with a heart condition. This is rarely so. Ask your doctor and insist on a detailed answer. If he or she still thinks that the elderly should not need sex, it is time to educate your medical adviser.

If your sex life does seem to be waning, this need not mean an end to your love life. A hug, a kiss, hand-holding and other caresses are the language of love. There is no need to give these up. A kiss and a cuddle, and a long warm hug in bed at night, remain among life's most heart-warming pleasures.

9: HOLIDAY HEALTH

Vaccinations

We all take sensible measures to protect our health every day in our own familiar environment, but when we travel we are exposed to a new set of hazards. Wise travellers can do a great deal to protect their health. The necessary knowledge can come either from bitter experience or through careful planning. Here we examine the unfamiliar dangers of travel and foreign lands so that the traveller can take all precautions and enjoy the journey. Do not forget to insure yourself against medical expenses which may arise from illness or accident while abroad. It is also worth insuring for the increased air fare which you will have to pay if you have to return home as a stretcher-case occupying three aircraft seats, particularly if you are going on a skiing holiday where you may break a limb. Insurance of £10,000 is advisable to cover all contingencies, and substantially more for the USA and Canada.

If you fall ill *after* your return home, tell the doctor that you have been abroad and where you have been. Otherwise he is not likely to consider the possibility that you have contracted an unusual disease.

It is important to have the correct vaccinations for foreign travel not only in order to prevent ill-health but also to prevent a great deal of bureaucratic inconvenience. For instance, you might be diverted or have an unscheduled stop-over in a neighbouring country. Cholera and yellow fever are the subject of strict international regulations and the vaccinations which you are required to have depend on the country you arrive from, not your nationality. For detailed information, consult *Vaccination certificate requirements for international travel*, published by the World Health Organization (WHO) and available in Britain from Her Majesty's Stationery Office. Or ask the embassy of the country you are going to visit; do not rely on tourist offices, since they are likely to tell you only the minimum requirements.

The most important vaccinations for your personal safety are polio, typhoid, tetanus and, if you are going to certain countries outside Europe, yellow fever, although others may be legally required in addition. Check that children are up-to-date with the usual childhood vaccinations. Diphtheria and whooping cough are very common in some African and other third-world countries. Vaccination against whooping cough may be advisable in these countries when the balance of risks does not make it automatically advisable in Western countries. It is common to feel feverish after certain vaccinations and best to have an early night and avoid drinking alcohol, otherwise you may feel very ill.

Polio: Vaccination against polio is advisable for all holidays abroad except those in Northern Europe, USA, Canada, Australia or New Zealand. People going to Spain, Turkey or North Africa are particularly advised to have polio vaccination. It is just as important for adults to be protected as children. Protection starts almost immediately and lasts for five years.

Typhoid: Although this vaccination is not required officially, it is the most important vaccination for British holiday-makers going abroad. It should be routine for all countries except North-West Europe, North America, Australia or New Zealand. Protection lasts one to three years.

Tetanus: Vaccination is advisable for everyone except for children who are up-to-date with it. The booster for adults lasts five years.

Yellow fever: This disease occurs in parts of equatorial Africa and in Central and South America. Yellow fever is a mosquito-borne disease but vaccination against it is very effective. In Britain, vaccination can only be done at one of about sixty special centres which usually charge a small fee – ask your local doctor. Protection lasts for ten years.

Smallpox: This disease was eradicated in 1977 and vaccination against it is not medically necessary. At the time of going to press, Chad is the only country demanding a certificate of vaccination against smallpox.

Cholera: Cholera outbreaks are likely in parts of West, Central and East Africa and in the Middle and Far East, and occasionally occur in some Mediterranean countries such as Portugal. There is disagreement over the effectiveness of this vaccination and WHO has expressed no confidence in it. Nevertheless, vaccination may be required for entry into certain countries, although sensible hygienic precautions are the most important preventive measures. A certificate is valid for six months after a six-day waiting period.

Hepatitis: Passive immunity can be given against this disease, which can cause serious illness lasting several months, with an injection of human immunoglobulin (an extract of blood). This measure is well worth taking when travelling to Africa or the Middle or Far East or any country where sanitation is poor. It must be given after the other vaccinations, and lasts for up to five months, depending on the size of the dose given.

THE JOURNEY/HOLIDAY HEALTH

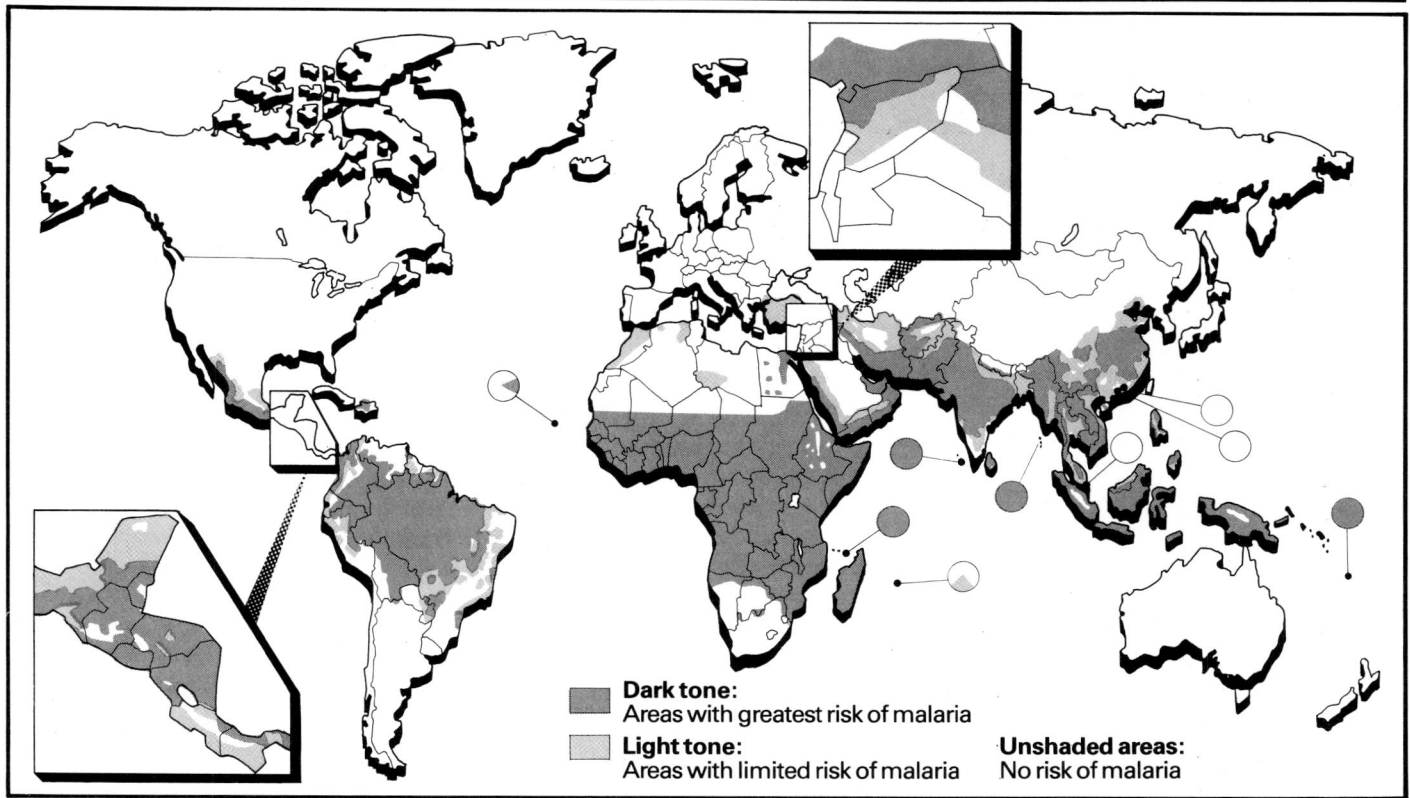

Dark tone: Areas with greatest risk of malaria
Light tone: Areas with limited risk of malaria
Unshaded areas: No risk of malaria

This shows the areas of the world where malaria is still a problem.

Rabies: A new vaccine has been developed which may be life-saving for a person who has been bitten by an infected animal. Immediate treatment should then be sought. It is also recommended as a preventive measure for veterinarians and people who work with them. Rabies is becoming increasingly common and spreading across Europe. Take care to avoid stray dogs and cats.

Malaria: If you are going to a country where there is malaria (see page 191 for important details), you should make sure you obtain drugs to prevent the disease before you leave, and continue to take them for at least four weeks after you have left the malarial area.

The Journey

MOTION SICKNESS

It has long been known that car drivers seldom suffer from motion sickness while passengers, especially those in the back seat, often do. This difference gives clues to the understanding of motion sickness and suggests ways in which we can control or prevent it. Dr James Reason, reader in psychology at Leicester University and an expert in motion sickness, recommends that a person who is vulnerable should imitate the movements of the driver, even to the extent of pretending to drive with a toy steering-wheel. However, it may not be necessary to go that far.

It appears that there is a natural position for the head when it is moving normally with the body, as in running around a bend: the head and body lean into the bend. This rule is broken when the body is moved artificially, and the head is thrown into unnatural positions. Drivers, or sailors occupied on the deck of a boat, are inclined to steady themselves by leaning into the motion and so maintain a more natural posture, while passengers are much more likely to allow their body to be moved passively and so are thrown into an unnatural posture. When the head is in an unnatural posture, there is a discrepancy between the information a person receives in the brain through the eyes about their bodily position and that received through the balance organs in the ear. This is what causes sickness. Dr Reason suggests two strategies for minimizing travel sickness:

Active strategy

A. If possible sit in the front seat and imitate the driver leaning into bends. If necessary use a toy steering-wheel. Alternatively, restrict head movement by using a head rest.

B. Look ahead at the road. If forced to sit sideways, still look ahead and change seats from time to time to avoid a crick in the neck. Don't turn round to talk to passengers in the back seat.

C. Do not think about your stomach even if you start to get the first signs of queasiness. Talk or listen to talking on the radio (not music), or do mental arithmetic – anything to engage the mind.

D. Don't read, because this takes your eyes off the road. If you must read maps, ask the driver to slow down or better still stop, especially if the road has many bends.

E. If badly affected, try drugs such as Kwells, Stugeron, or Marzine, though Stugeron and Marzine should not be taken in pregnancy. The Victorians believed that bubbly drinks such as champagne helped, but too much alcohol, which prevents the eyes from concentrating on the road ahead, is almost certainly self-defeating. Passengers going on a long journey are best advised to stick to the limit of one or two small drinks.

HOLIDAY HEALTH/THE JOURNEY

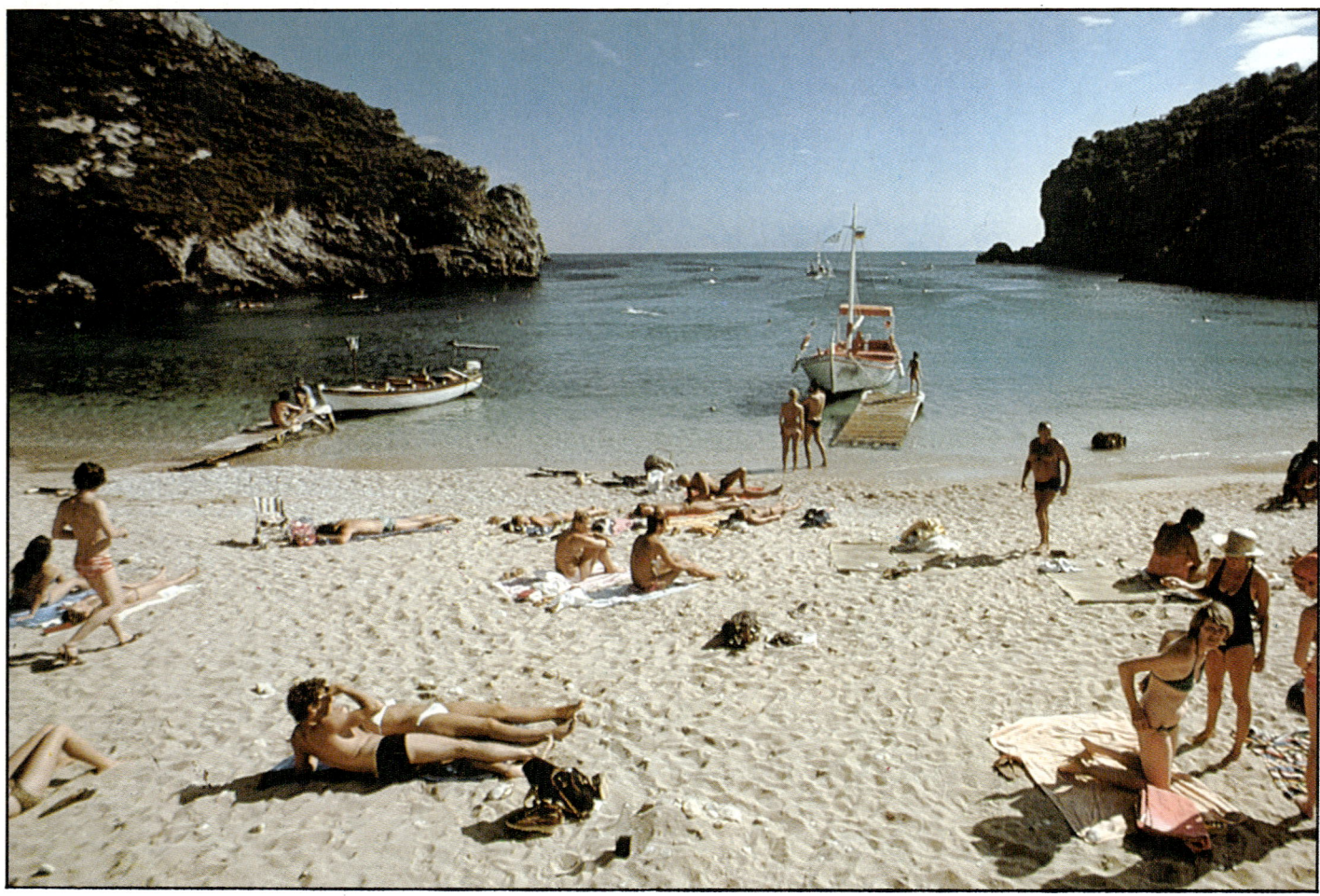

A dream holiday, such as that suggested by this beach scene in Corfu, can become a nightmare if hygiene precautions are neglected

F. On boats, walk around on deck and scan the shore, the horizon or the sky – the only stable reference points – and lean into the motion of the ship. Do not watch seagulls or waves which are moving irregularly.

G. Provide children with special car seats so that they can see out of the window. These are also safer.

Passive strategy

This is the only possible strategy on aeroplanes, unless you have a window seat on a clear day, and the only strategy on ships at night, unless you want to stay on deck and look at the stars.

A. If possible, lie down on your back with face upwards. This limits head movement and puts your balance-organ (otolith) in the most neutral position.

B. Shut your eyes: this reduces conflicting signals reaching the brain. Listen to the radio or talk if you cannot sleep.

C. Anxiety is often an additional cause of travel sickness. Yoga, meditation or other established methods of relaxation should help if you are familiar with them (see Chapter 2).

Especially for children

Children under twelve are particularly vulnerable to travel sickness, perhaps because they cannot so easily see out of the window and are not so interested in scenery. Get special car seats for young children. Play games such as counting horses or buses ahead (it does not count if it is behind). Open windows to provide some wind on the face: no one knows why this works but it may be by providing the body with another sense of movement, or by reducing stuffy car smells which may cause nausea.

JET-LAG

The body has a regular daily rhythm in its temperature, sweating and pulse-rate. When you fly north or south and do not change time-zones, these rhythms are not interrupted; but when you travel east or west the rhythms of sleeping and waking are altered and it may take days for the body to adjust. After travelling across time-zones, normally simple actions take place out of time: a person may want to empty their bladder several times during the night or move their bowels at a time they never would usually.

To minimize jet-lag try to have a good night's sleep before you go, and try to plan your journey so that you arrive near your normal bedtime and are able to sleep when you arrive. Keep alcohol down to a minimum while travelling, especially if you are travelling to a warm country, because it will delay your acclimatization. It is vital to allow time for rest after arrival and not attempt to go straight into an important meeting. If you do, you may make a wrong decision. It is best, if possible, not to travel at night.

The pressure in the cabin is reduced during flight in even the most modern aeroplanes, and this often gives rise to a distended feeling as gases in the bowel expand. It will help to eat sparingly on the aeroplane. The atmosphere in an aeroplane is comparatively dry and people generally lose a lot of fluid. Soft drinks and water will help, but avoid fizzy drinks, which are likely to add to the distended feeling. Wear loose-fitting clothing and shoes, because the legs are likely to swell during the flight as a result of the restriction of movement which prevents a full return of blood to the rest of the body – so walk about the aircraft when you can.

Your ears
Diving under water, especially with an aqualung, and also high flying, may produce sharp changes of pressure in the ear. Anyone who has difficulty in equalizing the air pressure behind the drum should seek specialist advice before diving or flying. In flying, the main problem is coming down to land. Although all commercial flights have pressurized cabins, repressurization may happen quite sharply. When coming down in a plane it is always advisable to swallow at regular intervals, waggle the jaw, and if necessary pinch the nose and blow down it. This allows the air pressure to equalize on both sides of the eardrum by allowing the passage of air through the Eustachian tube, which connects the middle ear to the back of the throat. People who have special difficulty may find additional benefit from using decongestant nose-drops or nasal sprays for two days before flying. Where possible, do not fly when you have a cold.

The commonest complication of air travel is a conductive deafness caused by blockage of the Eustachian tube, preventing pressure equalization. However, sudden changes in pressure may occasionally affect the inner ear as well, and cause rupture of a small membrane covering the entrance to the cochlea. Fluid may leak out, producing deafness and giddiness. As this is treatable by operation, it is vital to seek specialist advice as soon as possible. Delay may result in irreversible deafness, but this is very rare.

When You Arrive

HYGIENE

The commonest source of illness among travellers is diarrhoea caused by eating food contaminated by bacteria. Several more serious diseases, such as cholera, typhoid, paratyphoid, bacillary dysentery, hepatitis, amoebic dysentery and other parasitic diseases, are caught from food prepared without sufficient regard to hygiene or from contaminated water. But most common of all is travellers' diarrhoea, also known by various picturesque names such as Rangoon runs, Delhi belly, Gippy tummy and Turista, which is often caused by exotic local varieties of the common colon bacillus. People who come from Western countries with high standards of hygiene are vulnerable to these diseases, because they have not developed immunity over the years, unlike residents of countries where standards of hygiene are lower.

It is vital in countries where the general standard of hygiene is low to maintain the highest personal standard of hygiene, in order to avoid unpleasant and debilitating diarrhoea. Vaccinations will protect against typhoid and paratyphoid but there are other serious diseases which can only be avoided by hygienic measures. And there seems to be an endless variety of travellers' diarrhoea.

We recommend the following strict hygienic measures, which should be taken in any non-European, non-Western country. People going on package tours to Russia have contracted an unpleasant parasite called *Giardia* simply by brushing their teeth in tapwater. Care must also be taken in Mediterranean countries. The more insanitary the conditions in the country you are visiting, the stricter your personal hygienic measures should be.

1. Always used bottled water for drinking and for cleaning teeth. Alternatively sterilize water yourself. Boiling is best but filtration with special equipment is effective and so is sterilization with chlorine tablets (Halozone or Steritabs) or iodine drops. Iodine tincture is more effective against amoeba than chlorine tablets: add two drops of 2 per cent tincture of iodine to a litre of uncloudy water, and leave for half an hour. Remember that however high you are in mountain areas there is almost certainly someone else higher up putting their wastes into the water. If you have to drink unsterilized water, try to make sure it comes from a deep well with a wall around it to prevent surface water draining in.
2. Be cautious with shellfish – try to see them alive first. Avoid cold, cooked food.
3. Make sure food is well cooked and has not been standing.
4. Make sure all fruit and tomatoes are peeled, or immerse in iodine water for half an hour.
5. Sterilize lettuce and unpeeled fruit with chemically treated water.
6. Only drink milk if it has been boiled, and do not eat raw cheese unless foreign residents tell you it is reliable. You can always cook it.
7. Do not eat left-overs or local ice-creams.
8. Drink mineral waters made by reputable firms. Coca Cola, Pepsi Cola and other internationally licensed brand names can usually be relied upon and so can other soft drinks made in the same factories by the same local operator.
9. Avoid any food which may have been visited by flies.
10. If specially vulnerable to stomach complaints, consult your doctor about taking a preventive drug such as Streptotriad but do not relax the hygienic measures. Enterovioform and other types of clioquinol drugs such as Mexaform have been suggested as the cause of extremely serious side-effects on the nervous system. These drugs, which are also sold under many other names, do not necessarily prevent diarrhoea and in Britain are now only available on doctor's prescription. Lomotil and drugs containing morphine simply paralyse the bowel and do not actually reduce the infection or poisoning – in fact, they may make it worse. Much better to use the natural measures described below.

How to cope with diarrhoea
Rest as much as you can and be sure to take plenty of fluids such as orange squash, soft drinks or fruit juice. Potassium is lost from the body when a person suffers diarrhoea, and it is important to replace this as much as possible. It may be best to eat nothing for the first twenty-four hours, or if the attack is not too bad and you feel hungry eat a bland, starchy diet such as plain boiled rice which seems to help settle the stomach. It is best to avoid milk, which may make

HOLIDAY HEALTH/WHEN YOU ARRIVE

the bowel irritation worse. Diarrhoea is the natural reaction of the bowel trying to expel invading organisms or irritating poisons, and so it is best not to try and prevent this with antispasmodic drugs such as Lomotil.

Drugs such as Streptotriad which attack the invading organisms may also help, although some diarrhoeas are caused by viruses which will not be stopped by any drugs. If the diarrhoea becomes acute, worsens or has not gone away after two or three days, then it is best to consult a doctor if you can. Stay indoors out of the sun if you have diarrhoea, so that you avoid any unnecessary dehydration through sweating.

HEAT AND SUN

It takes a few days to acclimatize to a hot country, and some people may take a week or more. During this period the body increases the flow of blood through the skin, and more sweat with a lower salt-content is produced. Sometimes the ankles swell up. It is important during this time to take things easily and rest indoors in the middle of the day, take plenty of fluids, eat extra salt, wear light clothing, and avoid drinking excessive amounts of alcohol.

If these precautions are not taken, you may suffer from heat exhaustion caused primarily by lack of salt and water in the body. The symptoms are lethargy, giddiness, headache, and sometimes muscle cramps and nausea. In some cases, a person may suffer from vomiting and collapse. The best treatment is rest in a cool room and plenty of fluids such as squash or fruit juice containing a pinch of salt.

In cases of severe exposure to heat, a person may suffer from heatstroke. Their temperature rapidly rises, their skin is dry, they vomit, collapse and go into a coma. This is caused by a failure of the body to control its temperature by sweating. The victim must be cooled by continuous spraying with cool water and vigorous fanning. Once the temperature is controlled, the victim can be treated as for heat exhaustion. Basic rules to avoid heat exhaustion are:

1. Avoid physical fatigue during the first few days in a hot climate.
2. Each day drink one pint of water for every ten degrees fahrenheit outside temperature, or two litres of water for every ten degrees centigrade plus another litre.
3. Take extra salt with food.

Prickly heat

This is the name of an irritating rash which is common in hot climates. It is caused by the blocking of sweat-glands through the formation of very itchy red pimples. It often occurs in the armpits, around the waist, and over the breastbone and forearms, where there are clefts in the skin and where clothes rub against the body. It can be prevented by wearing loose clothes which allow the sweat to evaporate more easily. Always wear cotton in hot climates; avoid nylon or any man-made fibre. Wash frequently and apply talcum powder to the sore area. If the rash becomes infected, consult a doctor since an antibiotic cream may be necessary.

Sunburn

This can be extremely unpleasant but there is no need for anyone to suffer from it. In extreme cases, sunburn may cause a person to feel generally ill with headache, nausea and vomiting and high fever. But it is entirely preventable. Anyone going to a Mediterranean country in the summertime should only spend half an hour in the sun on the first day, unless they have already had exposure to the sun at home, and not more than fifteen minutes in a tropical country. Each day the length of time in the sun can be roughly doubled, but be careful that areas such as shoulders and nose which tend to catch the sun do not burn. A cream such as Uvistat, which blocks ultra-violet radiation, is useful to protect exposed areas.

However, a cream does not give complete protection from exposure to the sun, and if you want to spend more time on a beach it is better to put on a shirt and wear a hat and thin trousers. It can also be a good idea to wear an old shirt while swimming and playing in the water. It is important not to forget the power of reflected light. People with fair skins need to be specially careful, since they may burn without even leaving the shade of a beach umbrella. Fair people are advised to take all precautions, and to wear

A tan makes a holiday for many people, but too much sun too quickly can lead to pain and illness

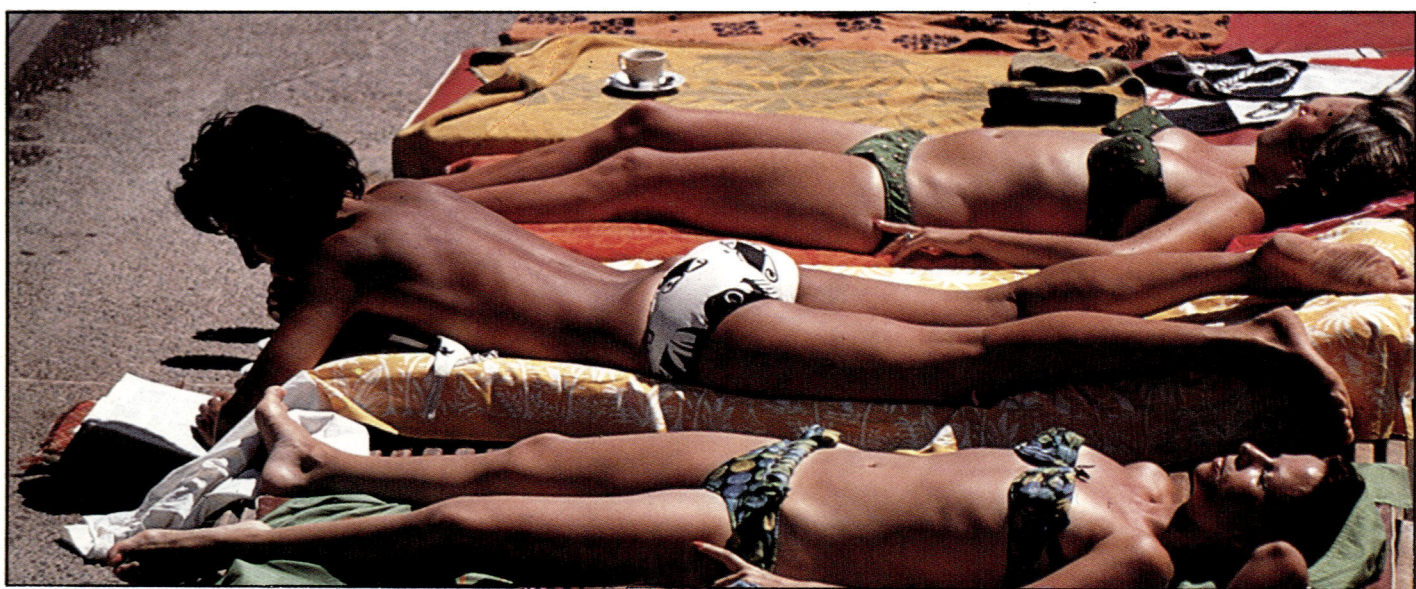

WHEN YOU ARRIVE/HOLIDAY HEALTH

long-sleeved clothing; wear a broad-brimmed hat and swim with an old T-shirt on. They may also need to use protective cream at least for the first few days of the holiday. Some doctors recommend vitamin A and calcium carbonate tablets (Sylvasun) to prevent burning, but trials showing them to be effective have not been controlled according to the strictest criteria and they may not be so effective as manufacturers claim.

If you do suffer from sunburn you may find that calamine lotion is soothing. Do not burst any blisters if you can help it. If blisters become infected, consult a doctor. Antihistamine tablets may help if irritation is intense.

It is best to get polaroid sunglasses because they cut down on light evenly across the spectrum; cheap sunglasses may let light in at some wavelength and damage the eyes.

ON THE BEACH

One of the commonest hazards of the beach – particularly those of the Mediterranean – are sea-urchins. It is good sense to wear sandals or plimsolls while bathing in rocky areas frequented by sea-urchins. If you stand on a sea-urchin, remove as many of the spines as you can with your fingers and use tweezers (eyebrow-tweezers are ideal) to remove any awkward ones. If you cannot remove a spine yourself, go to a doctor, who will do it for you. Leaving a spine in is sure to cause infection.

Jelly-fish are another common hazard and are best given a wide berth. They can give an extremely unpleasant sting which can cause acute shock or collapse. The worst type is the Portuguese man-of-war, which is bluish-purple in colour and has many tentacles. They go around in shoals and it is advisable to keep well out of their way. If stung by a jelly-fish, apply soothing calamine lotion. If a fever follows or the pain is intense, consult a doctor. Sea-anemones and sting-rays can also give an unpleasant sting, and so can weevil-fish if you stand on them when they are hiding in the sand. Treat them as for jelly-fish stings.

MALARIA AND OTHER INSECT-BORNE AND PARASITIC DISEASES

In many tropical and sub-tropical countries precautions must be taken to prevent **malaria** and other insect-borne diseases. Travellers are often given insufficient warning about these hazards. Malaria is caused by a parasite which is spread from one person to another by mosquitoes. The mosquitoes breed in wet, swampy areas and are active at night. Malaria is an extremely serious disease, killing more than one out of every hundred visiting Europeans who get it. However, it is possible to live perfectly safely in malarial areas if simple precautions are strictly adhered to.

The most important precaution against malaria is to take tablets of a drug such as proguanil (Paludrine) or chloroquine, which prevent the malaria parasite from growing in the blood if you are bitten by an infected mosquito. As mentioned in the Vaccination section, these tablets should be taken while in the malarial area and for a month after leaving it. Paludrine tablets must be taken every day but chloroquine tablets need be taken only once a week. However, it is safer to take a daily tablet than a weekly one. Another drug (pyrimethamine) is available which is more suited to children because it does not have a bitter taste. In some areas (parts of Brazil, Southern Tanzania and everywhere east of India where there is malaria) the parasite is resistant to proguanil and chloroquine, so Malaprim or Fansidar should be taken. Up-to-date details of the position in a particular country and the best drugs to take can be obtained from the Ross Institute of Tropical Hygiene, Keppel Street, London WC1. It is most important because of the parasite's resistance to drugs to adhere strictly to routine procedures to avoid being bitten (see below). It is not sufficient to rely on the tablets.

Routine procedures are based on the knowledge that the malaria-carrying mosquitoes bite between dusk and dawn. After dusk, wear long trousers and long-sleeved shirts. Use an insect-repellent on the exposed skin areas. Those based on diethyl toluamide, such as Flypel and Skeet-o-Stick, are probably most effective, although others based on dimethylphthalate or indalone are also efficient. These applications only last up to about four hours, and less if you are sweating. If possible, make sure that all windows are covered with mosquito-netting, and use a mosquito-net over your bed. Check that there are no holes in the netting; if there are, the mosquitoes are sure to find them. Another useful measure is an aerosol spray to kill any stray mosquitoes which penetrate the room. Do not give any reliance to 'electronic' buzzers which are said to repel mosquitoes. They do not work.

In Mediterranean countries, where malaria is not a threat but mosquitoes are still a nuisance, basic precautions can be simpler. Do not open the shutters at night until you have put the light out, inspect the room killing insects individually with swotter or sprays, and, if necessary, use the patent insect-repellent spiral taper – usually obtainable locally – which smoulders through the night.

Kala-azar is an unpleasant and debilitating fever spread by sandflies. It occurs on some Mediterranean shores, including those of Greece, Yugoslavia, Southern Italy, Sicily, Spain and North Africa, and even on parts of the western end of the French Riviera. Fortunately, the disease is relatively rare. The sandfly is so small that a mosquito-net will not keep it out, and the only precaution is insect-repellent.

Filaria worms which cause **elephantiasis** – a gross swelling of the lymph-glands – are carried by mosquitoes in various parts of the tropics. Other filaria worms which affect the eyes are carried by forest-flies and buffalo-gnats. These are rare in towns. Nets and repellents will protect against them in the countryside.

Sleeping sickness is spread by the tsetse fly in Gambia, Sierra Leone, Ghana, Nigeria, Cameroon, Zimbabwe and East Africa, but is only a serious hazard in rural areas which include game parks. Several other diseases such as **dengue** and **yellow fever** are carried by insects in tropical and sub-tropical countries.

If you are travelling rough and staying in local houses, take DDT powder to prevent attacks from fleas and ticks. Do not go about barefoot in underdeveloped countries, except on the beach, or you may be invaded by hookworms, which bore into the foot and then move to the bowel, causing debilitating disease.

A parasite called **bilharzia** – known to soldiers during the war as Bill Harry – lives in freshwater snails and as a parasite in man. It is most common in North, Central and parts of South Africa, but is also found in Brazil, Venezuela, the island of St Lucia, Iran, Iraq and isolated parts of Spain and Portugal. It can be completely avoided by not bathing in infected water, because the parasite can burrow into the skin, and by always drinking clean water.

10: A HEALTHY OLD AGE

Starting to Live

More people are living longer than ever before. A century ago people over the age of sixty-five comprised around 5 per cent of the total populations of most Western countries; today the proportions range from 15 per cent in the UK to 20 per cent in the USA. Both the numbers and proportions will probably grow as living conditions – notably sanitation and housing – and medical practice improve. This greater longevity will increase demands on medical and social services. It will also increase obligations for looking after ageing parents or other relatives. But growing old does not mean that people are unable to help themselves. Nor does it mean that people are inevitably condemned to poor health.

Nobody in fact dies just of old age itself. A majority of even those who survive into their eighties or beyond still die of the same diseases as the rest of us: heart disease, cancer and strokes. Although older people become ill more easily than younger people and take longer to recover, generally they need to take the same measures to conserve and promote health as everyone else: eat a balanced diet, take regular exercise and stop or restrict smoking. Growing old gracefully also involves remaining mentally active since this will help maintain a full social life to replace that based on your work or family.

However, there are some health problems which are a particular consequence of growing older or, at least, more likely to occur among older people. There are also some universal problems which manifest themselves in different ways among the ageing. This chapter is devoted to these problems so that older people may help themselves – or children help their parents – to enjoy their later years.

Think of your life as having four distinct periods. The first twenty years or so are spent getting under way – childhood, schools, adolescence, further education and first jobs. During the next twenty years or so comes setting up homes, bringing up children, sorting out jobs and careers, deciding on what kind of a life you want and doing something to try to achieve it. During the third twenty years or so, you consolidate and enjoy the pattern of your life; for most of the time, at least, your children have taken responsibility, or some responsibility, for their own lives. Then come twenty or thirty years or more of a new life, retired from the job that has occupied much of your attention and emotions for so long and with almost unrestricted possibilities of development. If you get it right, this can be the most satisfying period of all.

But if you are going to get it right you would do well to spend some time thinking about it before you reach it. Investment in health pays off later so prepare for retirement by establishing sensible patterns of exercise and diet as intrinsic elements of your daily life. This will make it much easier to continue the good habits later. If you look around, you will find plenty of examples of those who didn't get it right. If you intend to make the most of the opportunities in the last decades, however, it is also worth looking at what produces unhappiness in this period.

A cause of frequent rage and bafflement is that you should be retiring at all. People working in large companies often see their seniors collect watches and leaving presents, and yet still manage to feel that an exception should be made for them. Anyone who talks to recently retired people will be surprised at the way that virtually every one of them feels they still have plenty to offer. Yet it is as unreasonable to get upset about retirement as to get irritated about a rainstorm: both will turn up at some time or other. You need only to be ready, and what you need to avoid is a querulous, ill, self-pitying old age.

It is quite certain that shutting your mind to novelty is also bad, and so dismissing the modern social scene, the political parties and the lively arts should be avoided. Remaining mentally active will enhance your social life and help give you the feeling of being *wanted* that overcomes the loneliness and isolation which can be such problems in old age. What this means is that you must not choose your friends and companions from only your own age group.

The first decision, probably, that this affects is where you are to live. The choice is yours, but think very carefully indeed before you move. You may want to spend the rest of your life among those of your age and older, but be sure; leaving your old home can also mean leaving your old friends. It is usually best for elderly people to stay in their

Martha Leitch was sixty-six when she took up swimming at a London pool. She learnt to swim on her second lesson though she admits she has developed her own rather unusual style of breaststroke. Miss Leitch remembers when as a rather delicate child she was not even allowed to go in the sea with her brothers and sisters. Since she joined an old people's centre she has never been lonely and rarely inactive. She joined because she thought she would like to learn something such as painting. But there were so many other classes available that she has taken nine subjects – and is the star pupil in yoga.

STARTING TO LIVE/**A HEALTHY OLD AGE**

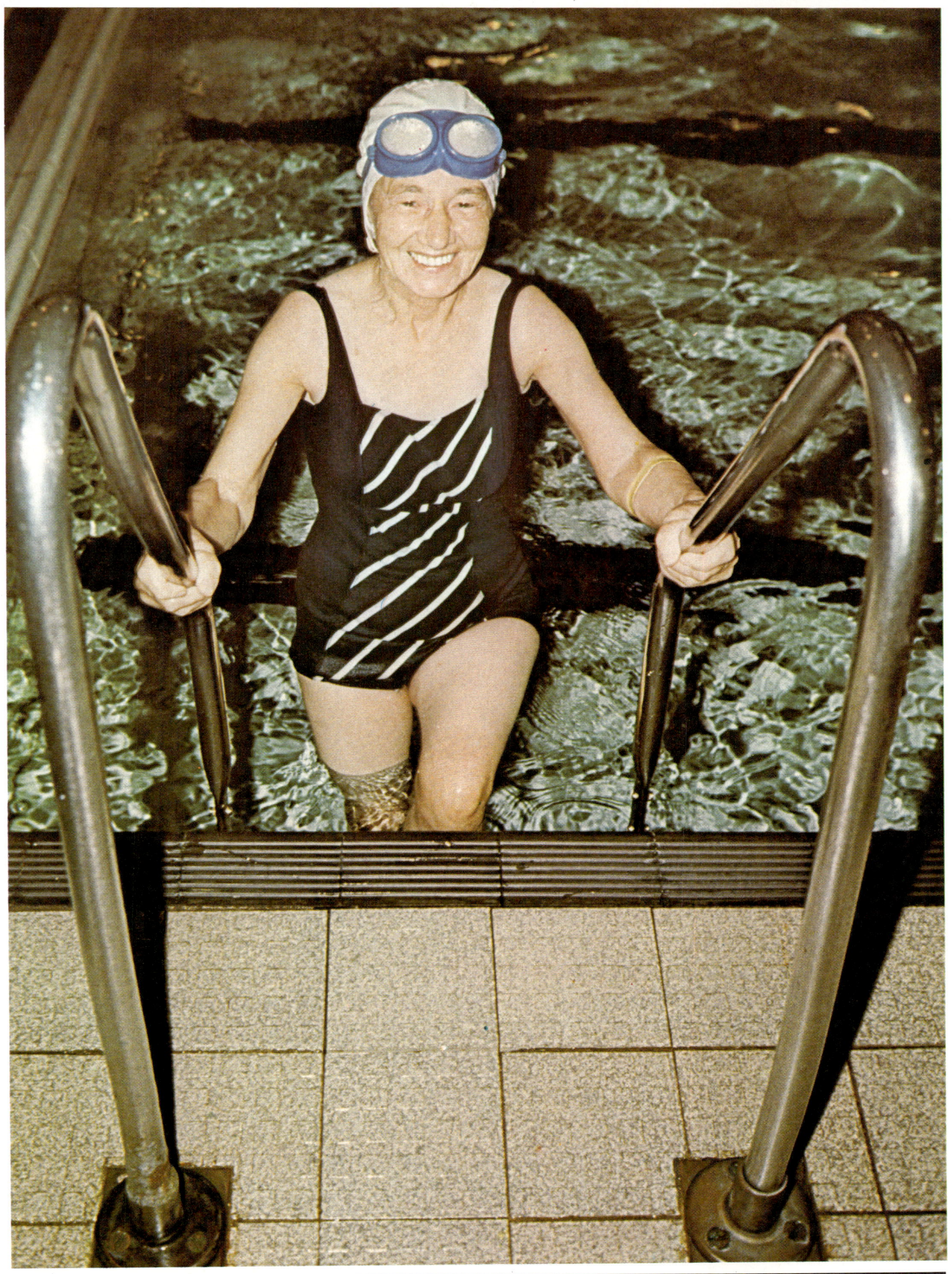

A HEALTHY OLD AGE/STARTING TO LIVE

own community, where they are known. If you do move, make sure that your new home is reasonably accessible if you want people to visit you, especially your children and other relatives. The bowls and bingo may be better but a society formed merely of one age group can be not only confining but also more limited in the range and adequacy of its medical and social services. Consider, too, the availability of public transport; many old people have neither the money nor the health to drive their own cars for very long.

During planning, you have to give some thought to money. First, you need to make the most of your opportunities for saving and investment: bank managers and Citizens' Advice Bureaux can help. Don't forget, too, that you may be able to make, as well as save, money. You may not be wanting to make a living from anything, but if you look around you will be surprised both by the opportunities and by what elderly people are actually doing. They are doing odd-jobs, helping out as part-time book-keepers or working in supermarkets on Saturdays. You can even run a small shop of your own, which brings not only trade but also people into your life. The possibilities of surveying opportunities in advance is another reason for continuing to live in the same area. But always treat any investment involved with the care it warrants. There are plenty of crooks around only too eager to exploit old people. If you have had enough of work but want to do something, think about voluntary work. A wide range of skills or willing help is always required, and this way you will help others as well as, perhaps, yourself.

One very sharp change that the husband and wife should prepare for occurs where both spend the day about the house. For a long time one or both has been going out to work, and the effect on the household has been to allow them some relaxation from continuous company. Each has been able to meet others. With retirement, it suddenly becomes possible for them to spend a solid twenty-four hours cluttering up the house, creating an obligation to provide an extra meal a day, and quickly exhausting any repertoire of interesting events and people to talk about. It is extremely important to maintain a lively mind in retirement. Going out to work and voluntary activities open windows on what could otherwise be a claustrophobic world.

You can also use these retirement years to enrich your mind. A worryingly large number of people start, in old age, to regret the education they missed when young. Education the first time around, however, tends to lead to a career; the second time, it can really be for its own sake. There is a wide range of evening classes, weekend schools and summer schools, and they all have the advantage of mixed age groups and mixed social backgrounds. For the determinedly academic there is the Open University; apart from degrees there are extra-mural classes. In some areas, courses preparing for retirement (as well as other subjects) are organized by the Workers' Educational Association.

Naturally this advice applies throughout to men and women equally, and the choices made must allow for the preferences, or at least balance the preferences, of husbands and wives. Women have a possible advantage because if they have been 'only' housewives the transition to pensioner status can be less abrupt.

The whole quality of your life will depend on your health. You are bound to suffer minor afflictions, and it is important to get advice from your doctor while they are still

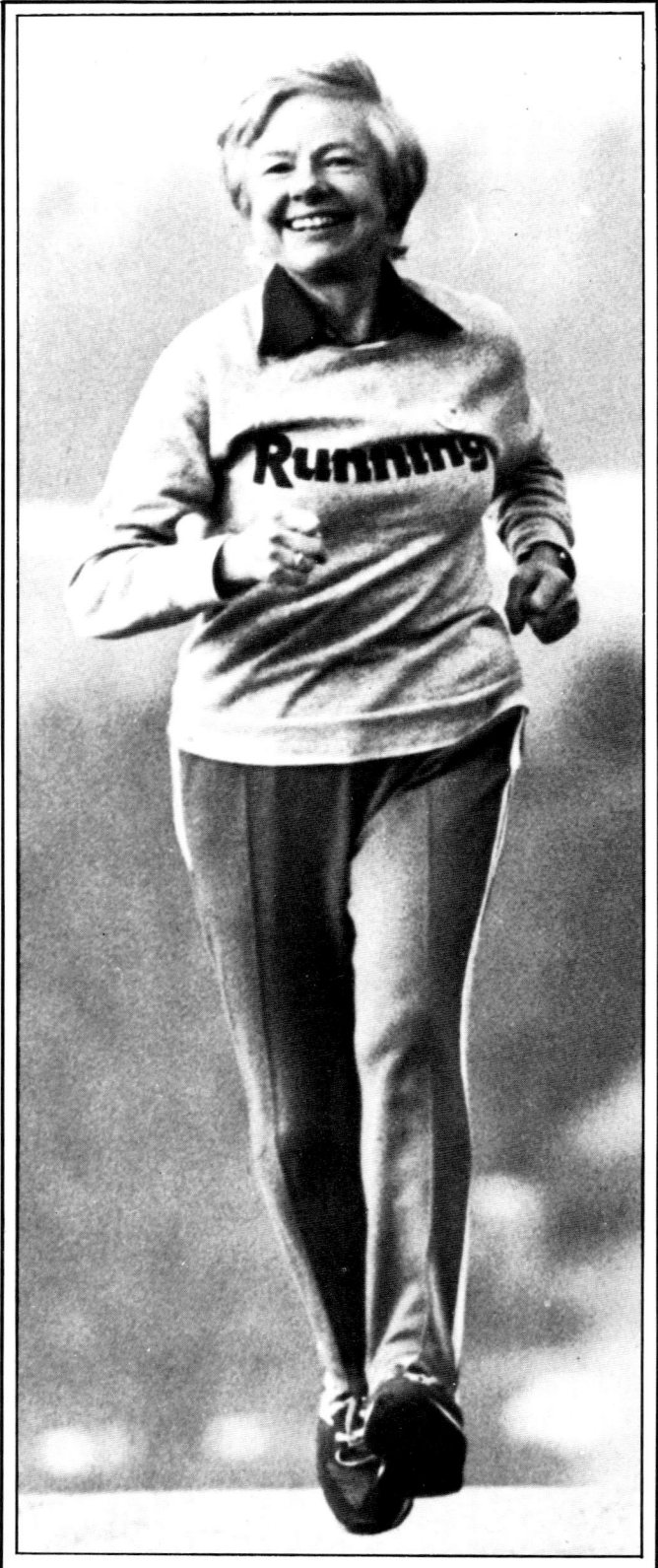

Madge Sharples, from Winchester, was 64 when she competed in the first London Marathon in 1981. Her determination to finish – she succeeded – and her good humour won her considerable fame including an invitation to compete in the New York marathon later that year and a starring appearance in BBC Television's Sports Review of the Year. Now she is a well-known figure on the marathon circuit and leads rambling tours in many countries.

STARTING TO LIVE / A HEALTHY OLD AGE

minor: don't put off the visit because you feel it is simply a matter of 'getting old'. Many of the afflictions of old age are debilitating because the sufferers do not have much to do except think about their health. Being busy in mind is, as ever, a good piece of preventive medicine. But make sure that you are also being practical about, for example, diet and avoiding accidents to which the old become increasingly liable. The following pages spell out in some detail how elderly people can help themselves, and how children can help their ageing parents.

CARING FOR AN ELDERLY PARENT: 12 RULES

1. **Loneliness:** One of the greatest problems of old age. Visit your parents regularly, and remember their anniversaries and special days. Try to get them out of the house for regular commitments such as a lunch or social club. Do everything you can to keep them in touch with their own community where they have their friends. If possible, install a telephone and call them often. Encourage them to try a sport or do voluntary work.

2. **Warmth:** Help them to reorganize their house so that in the winter it is possible to live in one bed-sitting room. Insulate the house and provide safe extra heating to protect them against hypothermia during a cold spell. Check to see they are getting all the help to which they are entitled from social services and social security.

3. **Diet:** Make sure they are eating a varied diet and that they are not having difficulty in shopping. Don't just ask them what they eat; look in the cupboard. Consider meals-on-wheels or lunch clubs at day centres.

4. **Eyesight and hearing:** About one in seven people have such inadequate glasses that they cannot easily read the newspaper. Better lighting helps and large-type books are available from most libraries. Annual eye check-ups are advisable. Make sure your parents also have regular hearing tests.

5. **Teeth:** Many elderly people suffer unnecessary discomfort. Check that dentures fit properly and that your parents have regular dental care.

6. **Mobility:** It is vital for old people to keep moving and, if possible, to get out of the house every day. Make sure they are getting the chiropody they are entitled to from the Health Service or local authority. Ask the doctor for names of chiropodists providing NHS treatment.

7. **Benefits:** Make sure the local health visitor knows about your parents and that they are taking advantage of all the local facilities (see Appendix Three for examples).

8. **Incontinence:** Look for any signs that your parents are having trouble with incontinence. Simple practical measures may solve the problem (see pages 202–3), but don't be shy about seeking medical advice.

9. **Bereavement:** When one parent dies the other will need you to share their grief. It is necessary to work through grief before a new life can be started. Remember they will want to talk about the dead person: this is natural and healthy. Tranquillizers cannot do more than provide a temporary relief, and are probably best avoided because they interfere with the normal process of sorting out and understanding of feelings. Try not to let the surviving parent make any irrevocable decisions such as moving house until a year has passed.

10. **Drugs:** Many old people have trouble with their medicines. Make sure they understand when each tablet has to be taken, and help them work out a timetable system. If in doubt, do not hesitate to telephone the doctor or the chemist to check. Make sure that your parent asks to see the doctor when he or she gets a repeat prescription. Warn them about the dangers of taking too many drugs or mixing drugs that may conflict with each other.

11. **Depression:** Watch for the following signs: loss of appetite, disturbed sleep, and general loss of vigour and interest in life. Depression can often be successfully treated with drugs, so take your parent to the doctor.

12. **Accidents:** Do all you can to make the house secure against accidents (see page 196). Secure loose carpets, avoid long electrical flexes, make sure there is lighting in cupboards and dark passages, provide bannisters on both sides of the stairs.

LONG LIFE AND HEALTH

Although nobody dies just of old age itself, there are medical consequences of the ageing process. The arteries slowly harden in old age and this process is aggravated by atheroma, which causes blood-vessels to silt up and can lead to strokes and heart disease. Cells throughout the body are replaced by inactive supporting tissue. Specialized cells slowly die in various organs of the body, making the body much less adaptable to sudden stresses. The cells of the skin, the intestine and the blood usually continue to be replaced in the normal way, but the fibrous tissue supporting the skin changes so that the skin wrinkles and becomes less elastic. It is likely to become covered with areas of pigment and the flesh is easily bruised, particularly the backs of hands. Muscles waste slowly and bones become thinner and more brittle. An old person often shrinks in height because of thinning bones and permanent changes in posture. The brain itself also loses cells which are irreplaceable. This may affect an old person's intellectual powers but most commonly affects their ability to remember recent events. The older person should feel fit and happy, and only under the stress of sudden physical exertion should there be any difference between an old person and a younger. The body's ability to adapt to ageing is remarkable.

Because old people become ill more easily than young people and take longer to recover, they often suffer from several disabilities or illnesses at once. This creates special difficulties for doctors in diagnosing their illness and in treating it. Old people are often slow to recognize the importance of symptoms of illness in old age and too ready to put up with them, partly because they attribute these symptoms to ageing. In the panel at the end of this chapter we list a number of important symptoms which old people should not overlook and which should lead them to consult their doctor.

Do not, however, be unduly depressed by this recital of the consequences of ageing. Innumerable men and women remain vigorous, active and healthy through their seventies, eighties and even nineties. In our researches for this book we met an eighty-seven-year-old cyclist, an eighty-five-year-old dancer, a ninety-two-year-old runner and a sixty-seven-year-old swimmer. But you do not have to be particularly athletic to enjoy your later years. At evening classes throughout the country old people are learning new skills and hobbies. Some are even reading for university degrees. Should anyone discount the qualitative contribution of older people to our way of life, they should re-read their history books.

Conserve Health and Fitness

Old people, as has been said earlier, need to take the same measures to conserve health as younger people. You must take care to eat a balanced diet, take exercise and stop or at least cut down on smoking. It also helps to remain active mentally, socially and sexually. Confusion, forgetfulness and other mental disorders are neither inevitable nor untreatable. Consult your doctor for help in containing mental as well as physical problems. But here, in alphabetical order, is more specific advice.

ACCIDENTS

A major threat to the aged, but a great deal can be done to make an old person's house safer and to prevent falls and burns. Although most accidents occur in the living room, most falls occur on the stairs. Make sure that the carpets are securely fixed on the stairs and that corridors and stairs are well lit. Remove clutter. If there is a step in a difficult place, mark it with bright paint and a special light. Carpets and rugs should have non-slip backs and floors should not be polished underneath them. Put a non-slip mat in the bath and install a grab-handle. For someone who is very infirm, a walk-in shower with a flexible shower-hose and a stool to sit on will be much easier than a bath. If possible, obtain a non-slip bathroom-floor covering. Try to get rid of uneven surfaces and replace any defective tiles or linoleum.

To avoid burns, the most important measures are not to smoke in bed and to make sure that any paraffin heater is one of the modern self-extinguishing kind which can be tipped over with safety. Be sure to use a fire-guard around an open fire or the electric type with a red-hot element; many old people suffer dreadful burns from night-clothing catching fire. Woollen, nylon and terylene fabrics are safest. Hot-water bottles should be renewed regularly because an old bottle can split and cause a bad scald. Electric blankets should be serviced annually; remember there is a danger if they get wet. (Special electric blankets for incontinence sufferers are available.) For old people, electric cookers are safest.

BED

It is best for old people not to spend too much time in bed as this can cause muscle wastage, bedsores, congestion of lungs and the clotting of blood in leg veins. Simply the weight of blankets on the feet over long periods can cause foot-drop. If you have to spend a long time in bed, obtain a cradle to lift the weight of the blankets off the feet and provide bedclothes which are as light as possible yet provide all necessary warmth. To prevent bedsores, don't stay in one position all the time in bed as the pressure on the skin cuts off the blood-supply and damages the skin by pressing it against the bone. Also, lie propped up with pillows, with a protective pad under the legs to take the weight off the heels. Sheepskin bootees are an alternative way of protecting the heels from bedsores. If a person cannot move they should be lifted into another position once every hour. If an old person is bedridden, it is advisable to ask the doctor whether a district nurse can visit regularly.

BOWELS

It is not necessary to have a bowel motion every day. Some people go on average every three days and are still not constipated. A person is only constipated if the faeces are hard, not simply if the bowels have not moved for forty-eight hours. To prevent constipation, eat a diet with plenty of roughage, wholemeal bread and wholemeal breakfast-cereal, and drink at least four or five pints of liquid a day (more in hot weather). It is also important to go to the toilet when the need is first felt and not delay. Regular exercise helps to strengthen the abdominal muscles which help in bowel movement. Constipation can have serious consequences in old people by interfering with the emptying of the bladder and causing mental confusion. If it does not respond to increased roughage in the diet or mild laxatives, it should be treated by the family doctor.

DEAFNESS

This is extremely common in old age but often goes unnoticed or is accepted because it comes on so gradually. Loss of hearing should be reported to the doctor. Quite often it is simply due to an accumulation of wax which can be syringed out. If this is not the explanation it may be necessary to see a specialist. Many people who would benefit from a hearing aid do not have one simply because they have not had their hearing investigated. When talking to deaf people, do not automatically shout. It may be that their problem is in interpreting the sounds they hear rather than in actually hearing them. Try to talk slowly and distinctly, accentuating consonants. Talk face to face so that they can lip-read or at least get cues by watching your mouth, and make sure that your face is in a good light. Ask your GP or social services about NHS-provided hearing aids.

DIET

Eat a varied diet to ensure that you get all the necessary vitamins and minerals (see Chapter 3 for fuller details). Old people often become deficient in certain vitamins or minerals simply because they lose interest in food. If this happens, ask yourself why. Is it because of illness, loneliness, unhappiness, depression? The solution may be to seek medical treatment, to go out once a week to a luncheon club, to cook for a friend now and again, or to find someone who will help with the shopping. Keep an emergency store-cupboard of favourite and staple foods, including tins of fruit and vegetables, so that you do not have to worry if you cannot get to the shops for a few days.

Watch your weight. It is important to keep weight within the normal range in old age. Excess weight puts more of a strain on joints, reduces mobility and makes operations more of a hazard. If weight is a problem, cut down on sugary foods, cakes and biscuits rather than bread and potatoes, which contain vitamins and minerals.

Ageing kidneys require more rather than less fluid. Elderly people with weak bladders tend to cut down on fluids but this can be dangerous, especially in hot weather.

CONSERVE HEALTH AND FITNESS/**A HEALTHY OLD AGE**

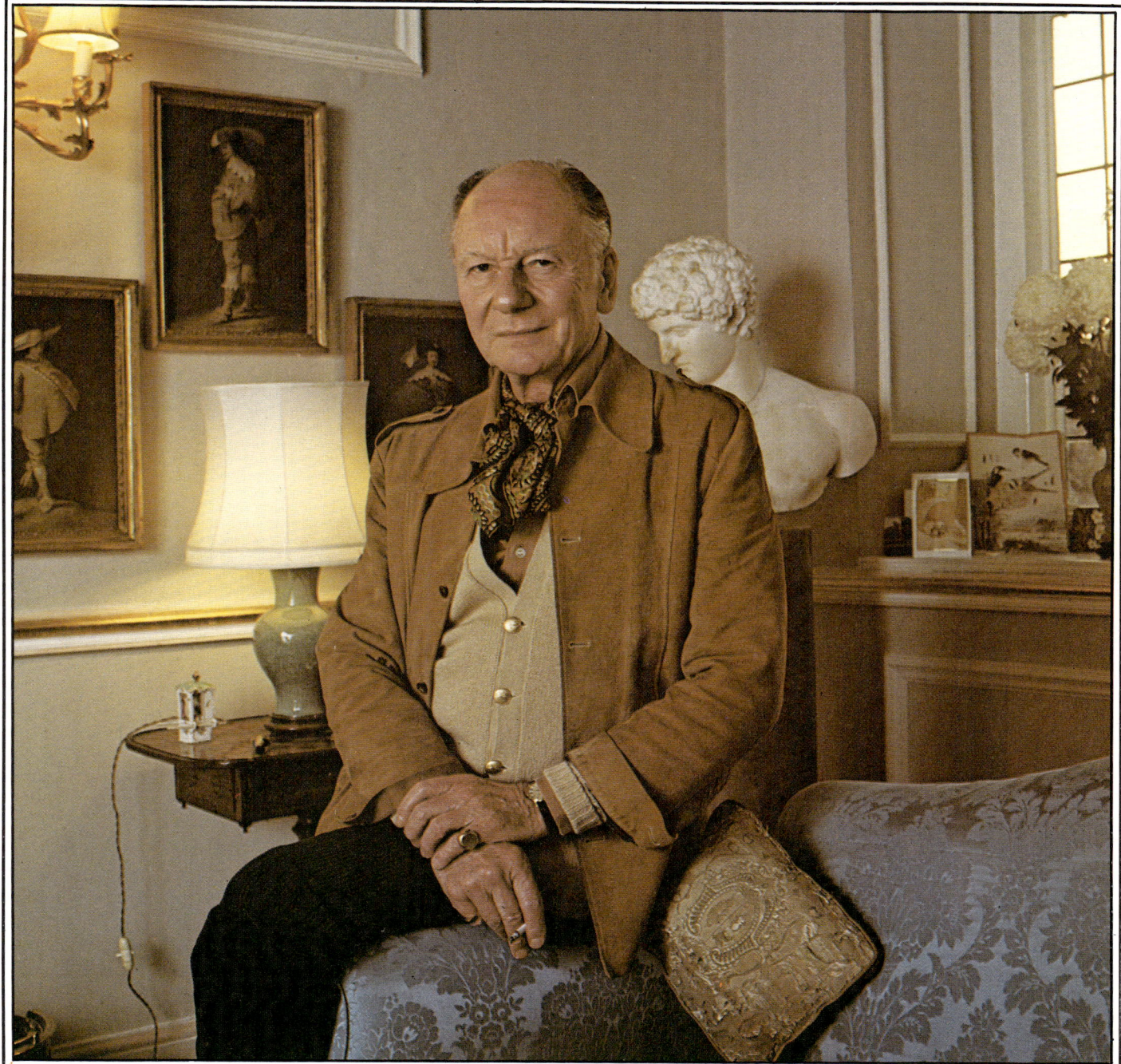

Sir John Gielgud. Still a star of theatre and films in his seventies. The variety of his career is undiminished by age – movies, Shakespearean parts, modern drama, television. One month in *Julius Caesar* the next in Waugh's *Brideshead Revisited*; has age had any effect at all? 'I find that you are treated very politely and called "Sir" rather than "John",' he says. 'I also think one can interfere with a little more authority at my age and with a little more tact.' What is only to be recommended on stage, though, is the use of the cigarette.

DRUGS

Old people respond more idiosyncratically to drugs than younger people; sometimes very small quantities which would have no effect on a younger person are too powerful for an old person. Do not hesitate to report any disturbing symptoms which start after taking a new set of tablets. The doctor may then adjust the dose or perhaps prescribe a different drug. Quite often, old people are given too many drugs, which make them confused and ill. Then when another doctor takes them off all the drugs they show a miraculous cure. But more frequently, old people are to blame for not taking the tablets prescribed for them or not taking them according to instructions. Many old people have to take four or five tablets at various times of the day. It may help to work out a drug time-table, or to put aside all the tablets to be taken each day in a separate container. Sleeping tablets should not be kept beside the bed, because an old person may easily wake in the night and think they have not taken their tablets and by mistake take another dose. If they have difficulty in understanding the instructions on a bottle, they should ask the chemist to repeat them or to write them out on a separate sheet of paper in large letters. Some older people are incapable of taking

A HEALTHY OLD AGE/CONSERVE HEALTH AND FITNESS

their own medicines by themselves, and an informed relative or neighbour, or perhaps a district nurse, may have to give the drugs. Old medicines should not be kept but given back to the doctor, nurse or chemist, and the doctor seen every month or two rather than taking repeat prescriptions automatically. Chemists can dispense tablets in ordinary bottles on request if an elderly person has trouble opening childproof containers.

EXERCISE

Elderly people do not have the same reserves of strength as younger people but they, too, can improve their physical fitness through exercise. Although the nature of the exercise will be less rigorous, the potential gains are just as great. In fact, the rewards of physical fitness in retirement are probably greater than at any other period of your life.

Yet it is also the period when people are most reluctant to take exercise. To some extent this is understandable. After a hard working life it is nice to take things easy. It is also true that certain bodily strengths do decline with the years. Muscles grow weaker and the joints tend to lose their mobility. But this ageing process should be a reason for *more* not less exercise.

The retirement years should be ones of fulfilment: an opportunity to do things for which you may not have had the time during the busy years of building a career and raising a family. However, you need energy if you are to use the retirement years to the full – and energy begets energy. More specifically, studies have shown that the decline in bodily strength can be arrested through exercise. One Soviet exercise programme involved a group of men and women aged between fifty-four and seventy-one. Over a ten-year period the programme prevented any deterioration in their physical abilities.

The benefits of fitness for elderly people are very much the same as those for everyone else, described in Chapter 2, although increasing mobility of joints is of particular significance for older people. However two indirect benefits of fitness are possibly even more important.

First, fitness will enable you to live a more active life. You will be able to get out and about, meet people and take up hobbies. All this will keep the mind lively as well as the body. Second, the more active you are the more independent you can remain. Many old people's homes are run with love and care but the loss of independence can be a personal tragedy. Such a problem can often be avoided by maintaining a reasonable standard of fitness.

As ever, therefore, it is *unfitness* that poses the problems rather than exercise. The best preparation for retirement is to be fit when you retire. But it is never too late to improve your physical fitness. A study of exercise funded by the British Sports Council concluded:

❛ It has been shown many times that the capacity of elderly people for physical exercise can be improved with training just as with young people. Muscle power, tendon strength and the economy of the cardiovascular system can be restored and maintained with exercise. These beneficial effects have been demonstrated for both the aged in the community and geriatric patients in hospital. The amount of exercise required to have a training effect is within the reach of elderly people. Walking at 3 to 3.5 m.p.h. will produce improvement except in those who are already used to walking a good deal. ❜

What exercise?

Simply walking more, as stated above, is a start on the road to fitness. But walking by itself is insufficient to improve all-round fitness: it will not, for instance, improve joint mobility. And it will need to be brisk walking to have a significant effect on the heart and lung system. Chapter 2 details a number of routes to fitness – and on page 43 there is a safety check about when to see a doctor before or during an exercise programme.

Exercise should begin gradually whatever form it takes. Don't try too hard too soon. If you have difficulty in walking far, go for short walks several times a day with rests in between. The desirability of 'warming up' gently is even greater for elderly bodies than it is for more youthful ones. Generally, however, the advice on exercise offered in Chapter 2 holds good for older people.

Many elderly people feel self-conscious about exercising in public, particularly if they haven't taken any exercise for a number of years. One answer to this worry is to start some keep-fit exercises at home. The loosening-up exercises shown on pages 54–5 are a good introduction, especially if you add on some running on the spot to develop stamina. Otherwise look for activities tailored to your own age group.

Many education authorities run keep-fit classes especially for elderly people. So do some sports centres and gymnasiums. Look out for advertisements in local papers, ask your doctor or contact one of the organizations listed in Appendix Three. Some sports are particularly suitable for older people – not merely golf and bowls but tennis, too, if your opponent is much the same in age and ability. Aerobic activities (see pages 48–52) such as running, swimming and cycling have the advantage that they don't need opponents and so can be done at your own pace.

Swimming is an excellent activity since it promotes strength and suppleness in all the body's major muscle groups. The nature of the exercise can also be adjusted from the mild to the strenuous. And the buoyancy of the water makes it easier for people with foot or leg problems to undertake exercise. Rambling is also popular with many old people and, when done as part of a group, can enhance social life as well as physical fitness. Dancing also offers this dual attraction.

Above all, try to build exercise into your daily routine. Walk or cycle to the shops. Walk down stairs instead of using the lift; walk *up* the stairs when you are fit. Look around for projects that will keep you busy and active: change the garden around, redecorate a room, etc. One problem might be to resist the help offered by well-meaning friends or members of the family. Don't let them do everything for you. It is not impolite to say, 'Thank you, but I'd rather do it myself. I *can*, you know.' (Ironically, some good intentions can do a disservice to old people. Putting shelves, drawers or switches where they can be reached without bending does nothing to keep joints flexible or muscles supple.)

Gardening is a particularly good way to get exercise and enjoyment. If you have difficulty with heavy digging, buy one of those gadgets that fit onto a spade to lift the soil, or

Putting life into their years (opposite): in America jogging is no longer the preserve of the young.

CONSERVE HEALTH AND FITNESS/**A HEALTHY OLD AGE**

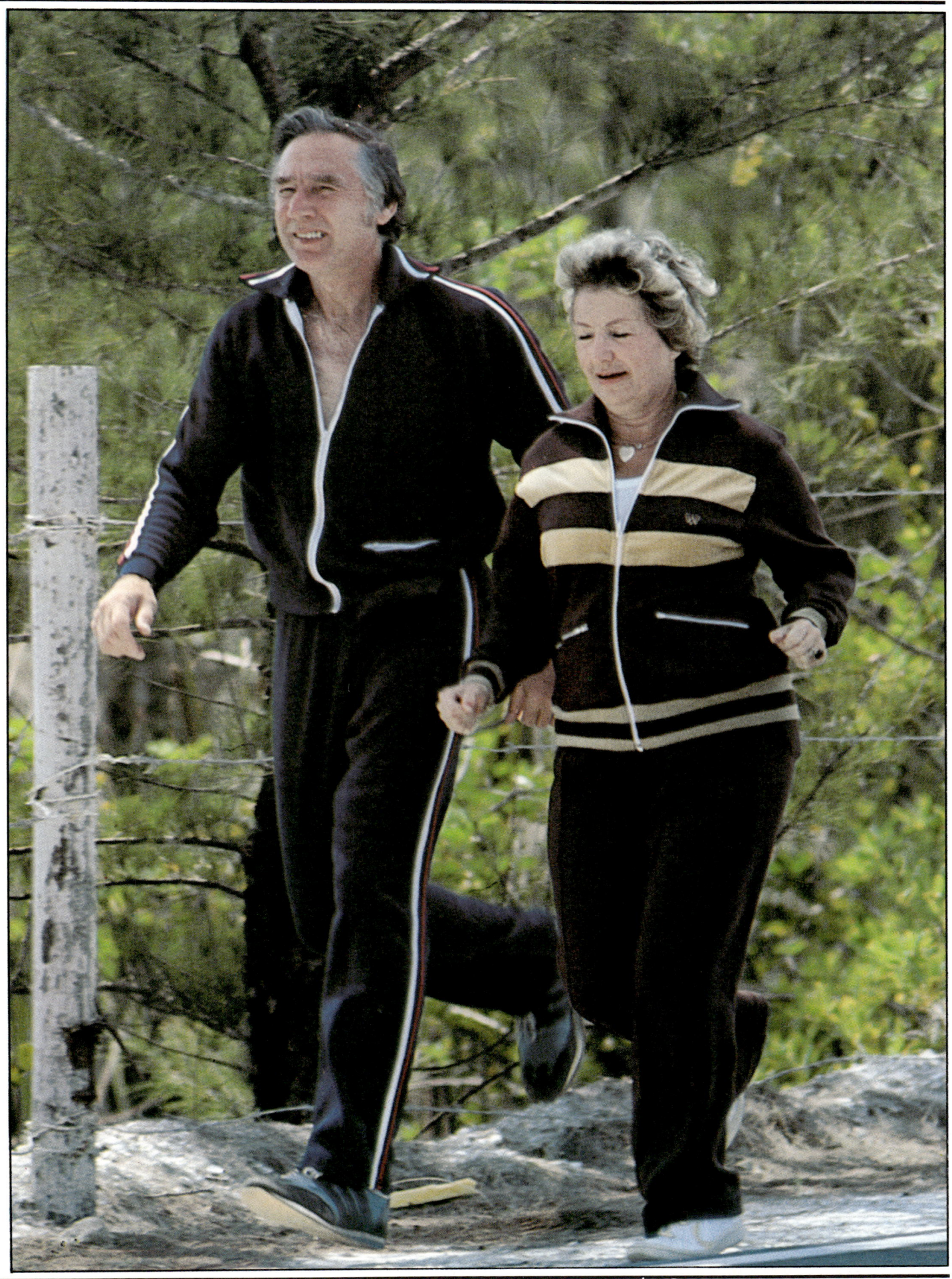

A HEALTHY OLD AGE/CONSERVE HEALTH AND FITNESS

invest in an electric digger. If you cannot afford these, rearrange the garden so that you do not have to do so much. Raised flower-beds will take away the need for stooping. And if you cannot manage a garden, you will still probably be able to get a lot of fun out of a little greenhouse. It is a tribute to the way gardening helps keep you young that the great British gardener Fred Streeter was still doing a weekly BBC radio programme at the age of ninety-eight.

No age is too old to begin some gentle exercises. Even the simplest stretching may help: on waking, open the mouth in a wide yawn and move each part of the body through its full range of movement. From such small beginnings, the potential gains are enormous. But don't imagine it will be easy. It will need will-power both to get started and to keep going in the initial stages, especially if you have neglected fitness for any length of time. Take encouragement, however, from the fact that the greater your unfitness, the greater will be your improvement and your renewed zest for life.

EYES

Many old people have sight problems, which can be put right by the correct glasses. Eyes should therefore be examined annually by an optician. Specialist advice from hospital eye-departments is available for the partially blind. Much can be done to help partially blind people with magnifiers, correct lighting and large-type books. Ageing eyes need more light anyway, so try to read where the light is good to minimize strain.

FALLS

In old age, when bones do not mend so easily as in younger people, a fall is a serious matter, and the person may find it difficult to move normally afterwards. Older people have inefficient postural mechanisms, and are liable to be unsteady. Once they start to fall they are often unable to correct their balance. Even getting out of a chair can sometimes be hard and often leads to falls. This is the recommended technique: first, sit on the edge of the chair, rest a moment then hold onto the arms of the chair. Then, tightening stomach muscles and keeping head in the air, rise to the standing position. On rising, old people often feel light-headed as the blood-supply to the brain is temporarily diminished. After a few moments, though, this feeling should wear off.

Some old people suffer from 'drop attacks', in which they fall suddenly to the ground. The attacks have many causes, one being a sudden drop in blood pressure similar to that commonly experienced by other old people on rising from a chair or when a person of any age gets quickly out of a hot bath. These can be very frightening and give an old person a fear of going out alone. Drop attacks are sometimes caused by a certain type of neck movement and it is possible to get a special collar from the doctor to prevent this happening. If it does happen you may have difficulty in finding your feet again once you have lost the normal standing posture. It may be helpful to wriggle around until the feet can be placed against some solid object; when pressure is felt on them again it should be possible to rise. It is best to rest after a drop attack, and it is essential to notify the doctor and be checked up after this experience.

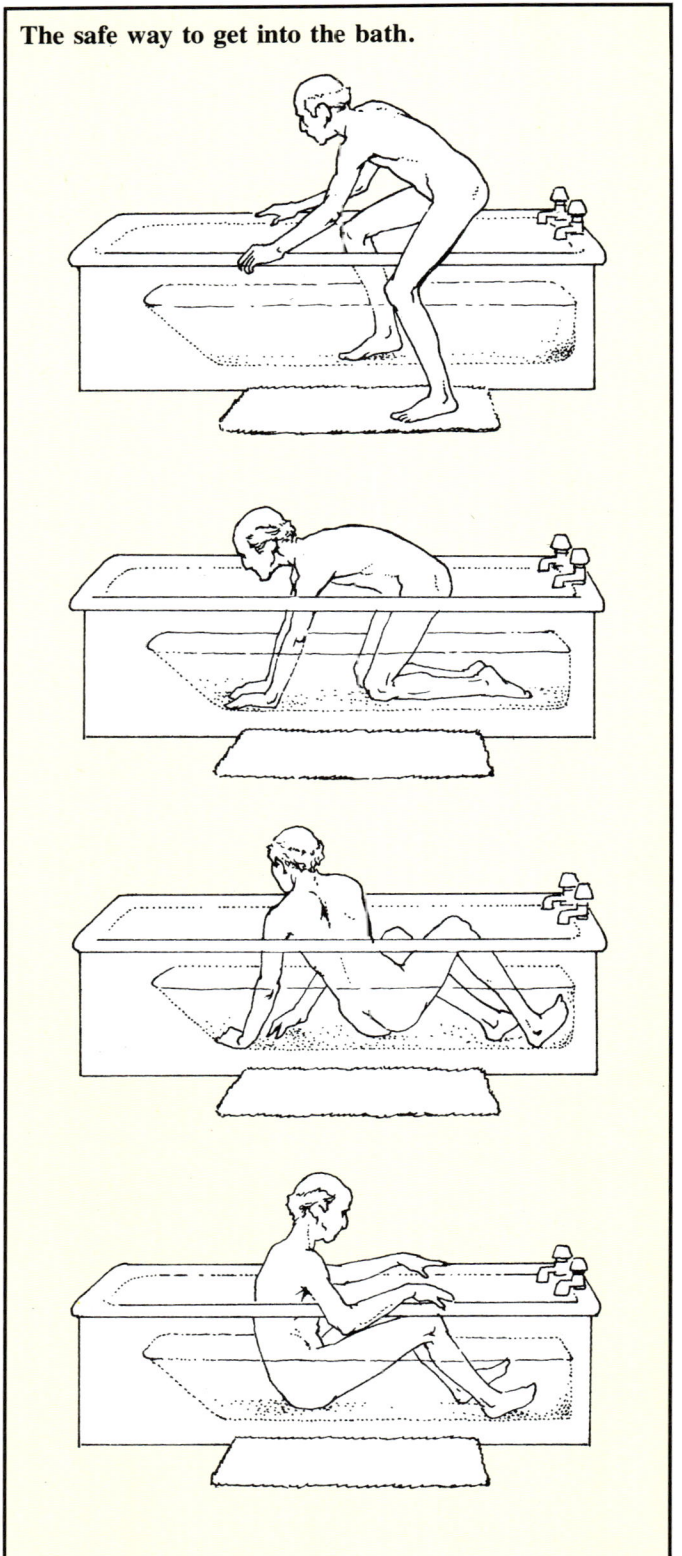

The safe way to get into the bath.

FEET

Mobility in old age is of great importance. Lack of mobility can lead to loneliness, depression and isolation. Consult your doctor for advice and visit a chiropodist. Some voluntary agencies organize nail-cutting services.

THE HEART AND BLOOD-VESSELS

These are neither so strong nor so adaptable in old age. To keep them working well it is necessary to continue with regular exercise and as far as possible avoid smoking or eating a fatty diet. However, it is also wise to avoid putting sudden strains on the heart and circulation. For example, it is unwise to take either vigorous exercise or a hot bath after a meal because the heart must then circulate blood to the muscles or skin as well as the digestive organs. It is not good to sit for long periods with crossed legs because this presses the knee into the back of the other leg, interfering with the flow of blood. You must also be careful to wear shoes which do not pinch the feet and restrict circulation, because this can cause injury to the tissues, particularly around the toenails. Thick woollen socks and soft shoes keep the feet warm and encourage the circulation.

Old people are particularly vulnerable to angina, coronary artery disease and heart failure. A severe pain in the chest when exercising should be reported to the doctor; similar pain which cannot be relieved by rest may be the sign of coronary heart disease but may only be a form of indigestion. In old people, heart disease is not always signalled by this type of pain but any discomfort in the chest indicates the need for consultation with a doctor. Shortness of breath, palpitations, mental disorientation or physical collapse can also be signs. If you suffer such an attack, lie down and move as little as possible until the doctor comes, and loosen tight clothing around the head and waist. Do not attempt to go upstairs to bed.

Although a heart attack need not be fatal, it is a warning that too much strain is being put on the heart. Readjustment to life by improving diet, reducing stress and taking moderate exercise often makes people who have had a heart attack feel much better afterwards than they did before.

In old age the heart sometimes becomes less able to pump blood around the body and begins to fail; when this begins to happen a person usually feels a shortness of breath and a feeling of fatigue. The ankles also begin to swell, particularly at the end of the day, and the person often feels the need to pass water once or twice during the night. The seriousness of these symptoms may not be realized until the person wakes up in the middle of the night gasping for breath and coughing. The condition – called heart failure – can be treated by drugs, so consult a doctor. However, rest is also important. It may therefore help to have your bed brought downstairs so that you can easily rest during the day and not have the difficulty of stairs. It is also important to give up smoking, reduce the amount of salt taken with food and to eat a light diet. Similar symptoms may be due to anaemia, and so the advice of the doctor is necessary to exclude this illness.

HYPOTHERMIA

Old people are much more vulnerable to cold than young people because reduced blood supply and lowered skin insulation renders the body's natural thermostatic control less reliable. This makes old people vulnerable to hypothermia, a gradual cooling of the body below normal temperature (37°C). A 1972 survey in London showed that one in ten people over sixty-five had deep body temperatures at least 1.5°C below normal – that is, on the borders of hypothermia. A cold spell together with a failure of the heating would put their lives in danger. In very cold weather an old person with inadequate heating will gradually cool down, and when their temperature goes below 35°C (95°F) their body-movements and speech become slow. They usually do not realize what is happening, become drowsy

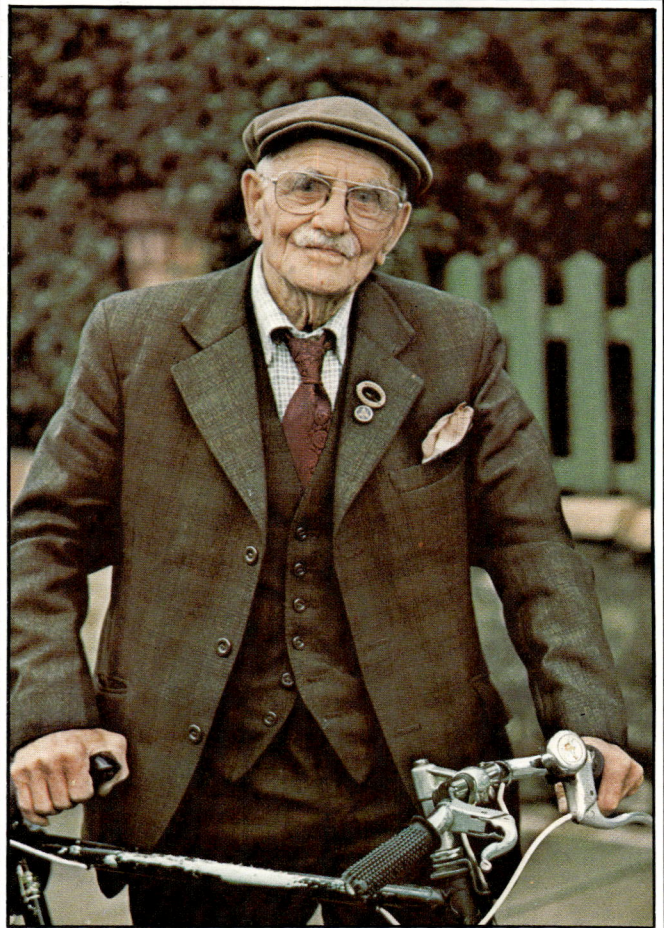

Frank Armond at eighty-seven had been riding a bicycle for seventy years. In 1920 he held the Land's End to London record of 19 hours 46 minutes and in his late eighties was still an enthusiastic member of the Fellowship of Cycling Old Timers, which is open to anyone over fifty. 'If it wasn't for my bicycle I wouldn't be able to do all the things I can otherwise do,' says Frank, who lives in south London and has been governor of seven local schools, all of which he visited by bike. 'Bicycling has definitely helped to keep me going.'

and finally unconscious. You can tell when anyone is suffering from hypothermia because the whole body is cold, even their armpits and their abdomen. Mild hypothermia sufferers should in the first instance receive medical treatment at home. Wrap the person in blankets, warm the room, provide warm (but not hot) sweet drinks, but ensure hot-water bottles are well wrapped. (Direct heat can be dangerous and unwrapped hot-water bottles warm the skin but take heat away from vital internal organs.) Investigation into the cause of hypothermia is essential, as it is commonly associated with other diseases which should be treated. Severe cases of hypothermia should be treated in hospital.

Try to avoid becoming a victim of cold in the first place by keeping one room of the house really warm. You can even turn it into a mini bed-sitter. Keep windows and doors shut, especially at night and in unused rooms. Place the bed and armchair against an inside wall but remember that sitting still for too long can be dangerous. Keep on the move by

A HEALTHY OLD AGE/CONSERVE HEALTH AND FITNESS

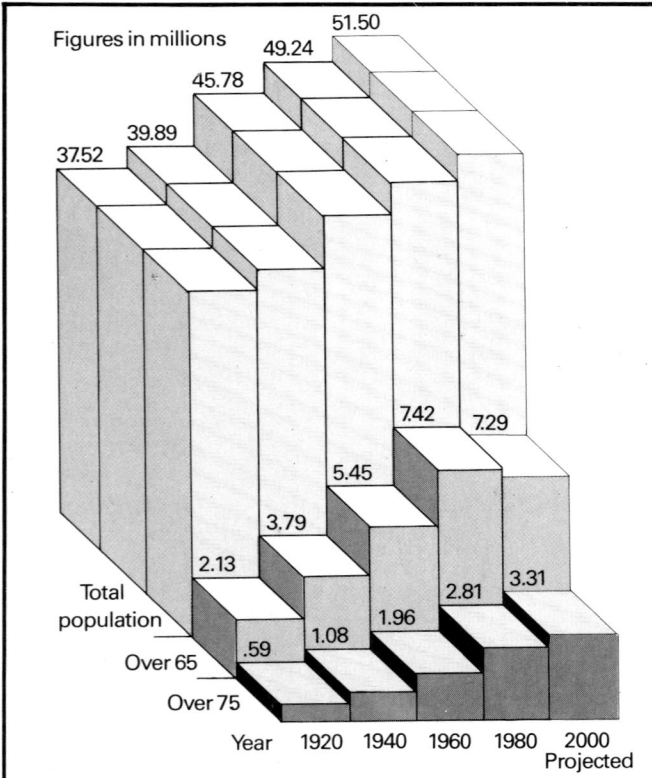

The chart shows how improved health has resulted in larger numbers of people living well beyond retirement.

spreading jobs about the house through the day. Wear warm clothes. Several layers are better than one thick layer; wear them indoors, too, if necessary and wear gloves, socks and even a woolly hat in bed if that helps.

Ask your family, neighbours or friends to help you insulate the house. Draughts around windows can be easily sealed with tape, and block off gaps around doors or skirting boards. Ask your social services department or one of the voluntary agencies listed in Appendix Three about help with fuel costs and grants to cover the insulation of lofts and hot-water tanks.

INCONTINENCE

One of the commonest reasons why elderly people have to go into geriatric wards is incontinence of urine – the inability to manage the bladder adequately. It is a problem fraught with such shame and embarrassment for the sufferer that people won't ask for help. Yet much can be done either to cure or to control incontinence in a way that means sufferers can continue to lead an independent life.

The word 'incontinence' covers a lot of different problems, but all have in common urinating at unexpected or inconvenient times. Rather than total loss of control, it can be a series of sudden leaks, the need to go frequently by day or night, the urge to go immediately, or just a problem about getting to the lavatory easily. Other symptoms which should lead to a medical consultation are dribbling after urination, leakage when coughing or laughing, pain or 'burning' while urinating, difficulty in starting, dribbling or difficulty in forcing the urine out, blood in the urine or bad-smelling urine.

At the first sign of any of these it is crucial you should see your doctor. Even though it is an embarrassing subject to mention, it is worth acting fast. Incontinence is more easily helped at its onset, while delay often exacerbates problems. Explain in detail to the doctor exactly how, when, how often, and with what physical sensations the attacks of incontinence occur. Mention, too, if there is any change in your life which you think might have brought it on. The doctor will probably want to examine you.

Sometimes incontinence in women occurs because the muscular valve which controls the flow of urine fails to work. Your doctor may think this could be cured by a local operation, or he may decide a physiotherapist could help with exercises. This is a topic where increased knowledge is constantly being gathered, and if you feel that your own doctor's advice and treatment is not helping, then it is worthwhile to ask for a specialist opinion by either a urologist, a gynaecologist or a physician practising geriatric medicine.

The essential problem in urinary incontinence is for an exact diagnosis to be made of the cause of the trouble. Once this is done, many methods of treatment are available, for example a course of drugs like antibiotics for cystitis or specialized drugs to control urination.

Drugs need your doctor's prescription, but there are things you can do to help yourself. It is important, first of all, to keep on drinking normally. Some people hope they can beat their problem by drastically reducing their liquid intake. That only increases the chance of complications. However, you may find it is worthwhile to drink more in the morning and less in the evening, so as to have less need to pass water during the night.

Keep your bowels moving regularly. This is extremely important, since constipation alone can create incontinence of the bladder, and occasionally of the bowel, too. A doctor will treat this with enemas, but a healthy diet with lots of roughage such as bran is needed to make sure it does not recur. Sedentary people are more likely to get constipation, so do take exercise.

One in three women, either when elderly or before, suffers at some point in their lives from 'stress incontinence' – they 'leak' at physical moments such as lifting, coughing, sneezing, or sometimes just turning over in bed. See a doctor about this. It is also worth seeing whether exercises worked out by a physiotherapist might help. Here are some you can do by yourself at home.

1. Sit or stand comfortably without tensing the muscles of the bottom, tummy or legs. Imagine you are trying to control the onset of diarrhoea by tightening the ring of muscle round the back passage. Do this several times until you can make the correct movement.
2. Sit on the lavatory and start to pass water. Try to stop the flow in mid-stream by tightening the muscles round the front passage. Do this on several occasions until you get the feeling of conscious control.
3. Now that you have identified the muscles, do the following exercise: you can do it quite unobtrusively sitting, standing, or lying down. Tighten first one set of muscles, then the other; then both together. Count four slowly, then relax. Do this four times. Repeat the sequence every hour you are awake, if possible, and keep it up over a three-month period.

CONSERVE HEALTH AND FITNESS/A HEALTHY OLD AGE

How people cope with incontinence depends on the way it affects them. For instance, many elderly people who are slow or handicapped in their movements wet themselves just because they cannot get to the lavatory in time. A commode, disguised as an armchair in the living room or in the bedroom, may cut accidents like this to the minimum. There are also heightened lavatory seats and grab-rails available for people who find using a lavatory difficult. The problem of dribbling can often be made tolerable for men by gadgets that fit onto the penis with a bag concealed in the trouser-leg. Bedridden people can be helped by special easy-to-use urinals or bottles.

There are protective knickers, pads, mattress covers, bed-pans, special clothes, neutralizing deodorants and various other gadgets. There is a much wider choice than is generally known, so if one idea is not effective, ask for something different. A bit of persistent self-help – instead of giving up in despair – can make the management of incontinence much easier.

Before you spend a fortune on aids, make sure you are getting what you are entitled to from your doctor, the state health and social services or voluntary agencies. There may be free laundry services, home-helps or grants to improve the house. You must overcome your reluctance to ask for help; it is nothing to be ashamed about. Incontinence is a difficult and complex problem and very occasionally is a cry for help when people are in situations which have become unpleasant or intolerable for them. It often happens when a person is moved from one institution to another, or from their own home to a hospital.

JOINTS

These begin to wear out as people get older and are subject to attacks of osteo-arthritis, rheumatoid arthritis and gout. A doctor should be consulted about painful and swollen joints. Tendons and ligaments become weaker in old age and old people easily damage them, possibly by a sudden movement. This can cause a complete break such as commonly occurs in the Achilles tendon, or it may cause an incomplete tear which is the cause of tennis elbow or frozen shoulder. These conditions usually cure themselves in the end but medical treatment can speed it up.

The cause of osteo-arthritis is not known. It often develops in the joints which do most of the weight-bearing – that is, the knees and the hips. The lining of the joints becomes worn away and they can be felt grating together. Reduction in weight can help halt further damage. It is also important to exercise the muscles around the joint to maintain strength. Physiotherapists will advise on the correct exercises, but a lot more can be done by choosing forms of exercise which do not involve putting all the weight on the legs. For an old person who is otherwise fit, swimming, cycling, rowing and horse-riding are possibilities. A walking stick held on the opposite side to an affected limb can also be a great help and reduce the weight on the limb to a quarter. For a person who is generally infirm, a tripod stick or walking frame is the best aid, and a rocking-chair can be a great help in keeping limbs mobile while keeping weight off them.

Rheumatoid arthritis is a different illness from osteo-arthritis, and may actually be caused by an infection, although researchers have so far failed to identify an organism causing it. A person may suffer from rheumatoid arthritis at any age but it is most common in late middle age and after. Sometimes an attack starts with a fever but more often it begins insidiously. Pains in the joints may begin first or the initial signs may be loss of appetite, loss of weight and tiredness. Inflamed joints should be rested as much as possible and the doctor may decide that it is best to splint them. It is important to seek medical treatment at the beginning of the illness. Drug treatment is available which controls pain and reduces inflammation. In severe cases of

FLEXIBILITY EXERCISES

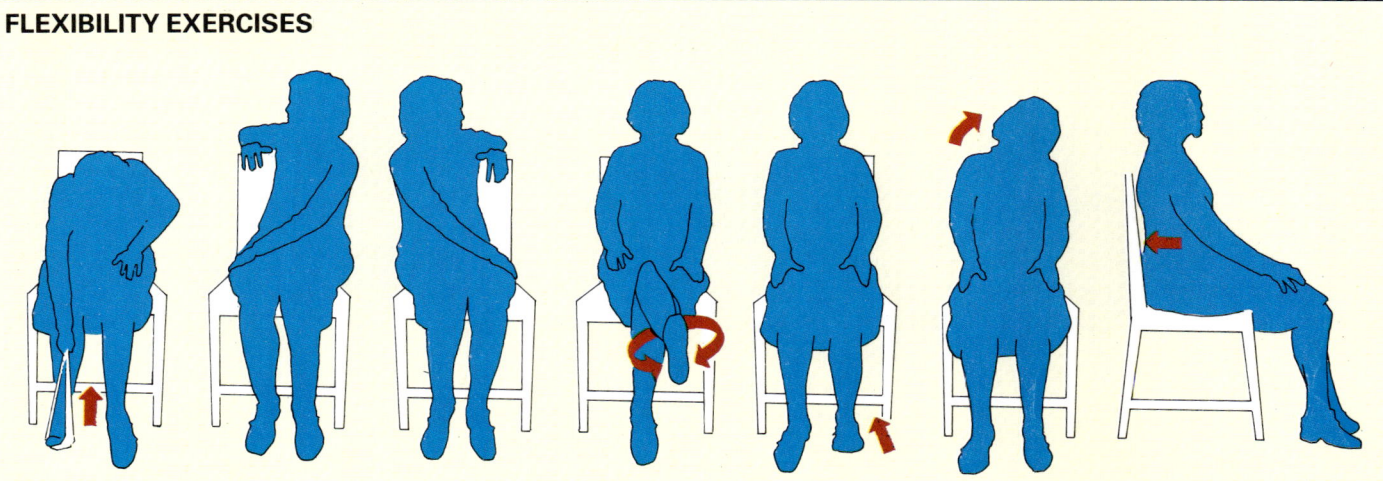

These exercises need an upright chair. If you can't make a movement, don't. Never strain yourself.

With a scarf under the shoe, using it as a lever, gently pull each toe up several times.

For waist mobility, start with your hands on either side of the chair and swivel round.

For swollen ankles, hook or cross one leg over the other. Press toes up, down, out, in, then circle round one way and the other.

Keeping feet on the ground, lift up heels then toes. Do with each foot, then both together.

For neck flexibility, let the head sag forward (don't push), then lift it up. Let it fall to the side, then bring it up. Do this both sides.

Sit in the chair, bottom right at the back and spine touching the chairback all the way up. Draw yourself up – chest out, head up.

either type of arthritis, an operation to replace a knee- or hip-joint may ultimately be the best answer. Such operations have a very high success rate (more than 90 per cent) and the new joint is absolutely pain-free and as good as new. There are many gadgets such as raised lavatory and bath seats which can make an enormous difference to everyday life for people disabled by arthritis.

MOBILITY

Mobility is the key to staying young, or, to put it another way, nothing makes you grow older faster than immobility. So the rule is to keep moving. This applies as much to the bedridden or partly immobilized as to the really fit. There is a widespread assumption that, as you grow older, the less physical activity you should take. Often without any prompting either from people or from illness, older people start cutting down on their activities. But when you stop doing something, you soon find that you *cannot* do it. A vicious circle sets in.

The other assumption is that physical fitness will decline with age, and that therefore it cannot be improved – only, as it were, kept at a static level. A British study of a group of elderly people, however, showed that an extensive programme of physical exercise left them fitter aged seventy than at the start of the experiment ten years earlier; physically they had improved and were 'younger' at seventy than at sixty.

Even a little movement helps. Another British study involved twenty-five elderly men and women doing exercise for just twelve weeks. They only exercised twice a week, with fairly gentle exercises worked out under medical supervision. After this twelve weeks, they were examined again by a heart consultant. He found that their blood pressure had dropped, their resting pulse-rate was lower, and their blood-fat levels had improved.

In order to keep mobile, it is important to use all the limbs that can be used. 'Use it or lose it' is not far from the truth. Even if you are in a wheelchair, you can do arm-and-shoulder exercises. In general, though, it is wise to check with your doctor before taking up a new kind of exercise. And don't push yourself to the limit. 'If you ache the following day, it's a sign you have worked too hard' is the rule that a British physical education teacher, Mrs Jackie Billis, lays down for her pupils. They include a lady of 102 and several wheelchair participants.

Elderly people with severe handicaps, of course, will need more than a few exercises. The important thing is not to assume that a physical disability puts an end to mobility. There is always something that can be done to make life easier. Nowadays there is a wide range of disablement aids, ranging from the simple walking stick to elaborate electronic wheelchairs. For example, an elderly woman with a severely arthritic hip could get either crutches or a walking-frame to help her get about. Inside the home, grab-rails at various important junctions would help her move from room to room, and work in the kitchen. The bathroom could be fitted with a specially high lavatory seat and a shower with a seat, instead of a bath.

One warning: do take expert advice on what aids to get. Doctors or social workers will be able to advise you about what you can get free from the social and health services. Occupational therapists can advise you about what aids you need. Never buy elaborate and expensive equipment without taking this advice first. You may be buying what you could get free, or it simply may not be the right aid for your particular disability. Unfortunately, there are a few unscrupulous operators about who will try to sell you costly hearing aids, elaborate armchairs, or expensive walking devices. If you really think it might be worth it, take the literature to an expert for advice. Never, never let a salesman talk you into buying without doing this, and be especially wary of salesmen who visit you at home. The best way to choose disablement aids is to go, preferably with an expert, to a centre where several can be tried and tested.

Finally, you can increase your mobility by changing your house or where you live. If you do not have a car or find you cannot afford one, move house to wherever there is a good bus service. In the same way, moving from a large house with many stairs into a one-level flat or bungalow might help – bearing in mind that for some people stairs provide good exercise!

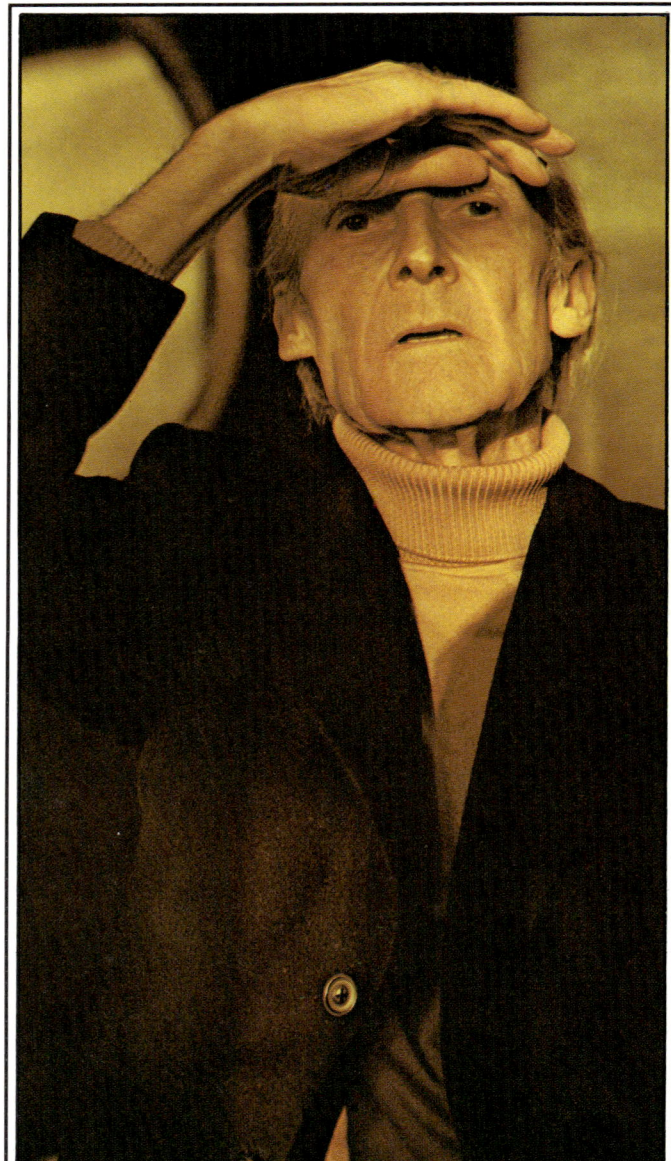

Bill Brandt, the photographer who recorded the social contrasts of the thirties, was still working in the seventies. In the fifties he began producing startlingly original nude studies, while in his seventies he began branching out again to make collages of driftwood and jetsam.

SEX

Many old people continue to enjoy sex in their eighties and there is often no reason why sex life should not continue at this age. The exercise is good for the heart and lungs, quite apart from the pleasure which sex itself brings. However, interest in sex tends to decline in both men and women. Women sometimes get a dry vagina after the menopause, although this can be considerably helped by the use of jelly or cream and sometimes by hormone treatment (see section on the menopause, pages 181–3).

SLEEP

Old people often require less sleep at night but worry when they cannot get it. The sleep-rhythm becomes upset, and frequently an older person tends to have little cat-naps during the day, particularly if he or she wakes early. A daytime nap does often make an older person livelier in the evening – which may be important when living with the family but if you doze after lunch you cannot expect to sleep as long or perhaps as deeply during the night. If you take too little exercise you may not be sufficiently tired to sleep well at night; it can be a good idea to take a walk before retiring to bed. Other important factors are:

1. A comfortable mattress: some old people use broken mattresses on which anyone would find it difficult to sleep.
2. Do not drink tea or coffee late at night as they are stimulants which keep you awake. A warm milky drink, a glass of wine or a drop of brandy are excellent ways of promoting sleep.
3. Try to avoid worrying about problems just before going to bed, because you may stay awake all night thinking about them.

If sleep is impossible it is probably best to walk about or read a book to try to break the train of thought. But do try to avoid sleeping tablets. They interfere with normal sleep and dreaming and sometimes make older people confused. The effects of the drugs may persist the next day, and getting up in the middle of the night when under the influence of the drug may lead to a fall. Sleeping tablets may also prevent an old person from getting up in the night to pass water, thus making them wet the bed. If failure to sleep is due to pain or depression, a doctor may be able to help by relieving these causes.

STROKE

This occurs when the blood-supply to the brain is interrupted by a blood clot in a vessel, or by the rupture of a blood-vessel. The result is damage to the brain which may result in paralysis of half of the body or in loss of some faculty such as speech. Old people often have little strokes which are sometimes barely noticeable except to someone who knows the person well. Minor strokes may impair mental ability or ability to walk or talk. They may even produce an apparent alteration in character such as loss of interest in life or in personal appearance. When a person ages rapidly, begins to walk unsteadily or develops a slight droop at the corner of the mouth they may have had a minor stroke. A person may suffer many minor strokes over a number of years. These should always be reported to the doctor.

Major strokes are much more serious and can involve paralysis or loss of speech. If a right-handed person has a stroke which paralyses their right side, they also lose the ability to speak; and for a left-handed person paralysis on the left side also goes with loss of speech. But a great deal can be done to rehabilitate a person who has had a stroke, by the doctor working in co-operation with a speech therapist, occupational therapist and physiotherapist. Remember, though, that someone who has had a stroke and cannot speak can often hear perfectly well and can be extremely upset when friends fail to realize that they can understand everything that is being said. Communicate by asking questions which can be answered by yes or no, and by saying, 'Squeeze my hand' or 'Blink once for yes'. The brain in any case has surprising powers of recovery. Old people are often able to relearn how to feed themselves, to walk and to speak. For further information on help available to stroke victims (and their families), see Appendix Three.

TEETH

Many elderly people have lost their natural teeth, have uncomfortable dentures (or none at all) and consequently adopt unhealthy diets. All necessary treatment is available on the NHS and old people should make regular visits to their dentist. People on low incomes are eligible for free treatment.

Checklist of Symptons

If an elderly person has the symptoms below,* they should see their doctor. The cause will often be simple and put right quickly, but it might be serious.

Eyes: Flashes of light before the eyes; seeing double; failing sight; seeing haloes around objects; pain in the eye or above the eye.
Hearing: Loss of hearing; reduced effectiveness of hearing aid; ringing in ears.
Skin: Spots or sores on skin which enlarge or bleed; irritation or sudden dryness of skin; a lump anywhere, particularly in the breast; widespread itching.
Feet: Pain or discoloration of the toes or forefoot; pins and needles or numbness.
Legs and arms: Loss of power in an arm or leg; persistent trembling or shaking; pain, swelling or stiffness in a joint or bone; pain in the calf.
Chest: Breathlessness; pain in the chest, arm or throat; persistent cough or hoarseness; coughing blood.
Bowels: Loss of appetite; difficulty in swallowing; dry cough or excessive thirst; unexplained loss of weight; persistent indigestion; vomiting blood; altered bowel habit; persistent constipation or diarrhoea; passing blood from the bowel; black faeces.
Bladder: Blood in urine; difficulty in urinating; increased frequency and urgency of urination.
Genitals: Itching around genitals; bleeding from vagina.
Feelings and behaviour: Falling or unsteadiness; giddiness, unnatural tiredness; marked deterioration of memory; feelings of despondency, hopelessness or persecution.

*Symptom table adapted from *Health for Old Age*, published by the Consumers' Association.

EMERGENCY

Alphabetical Guide to Emergencies

These guidelines tell you what to do in a crisis when someone may be seriously ill or hurt. If in doubt, always call a doctor. He or she will decide if medical treatment is necessary and may give advice over the telephone. However, it may save vital time to take the injured person to the nearest major hospital casualty department. It may help if someone else can telephone the hospital to say that you are coming – do not waste time doing this yourself. Remember, the injured person will be less frightened if you remain outwardly calm. Reassurance is important, as it will reduce the physical and emotional shock. This is especially important with children.

Applying Bandages

Slings: to support and protect the arm

1. arm sling.

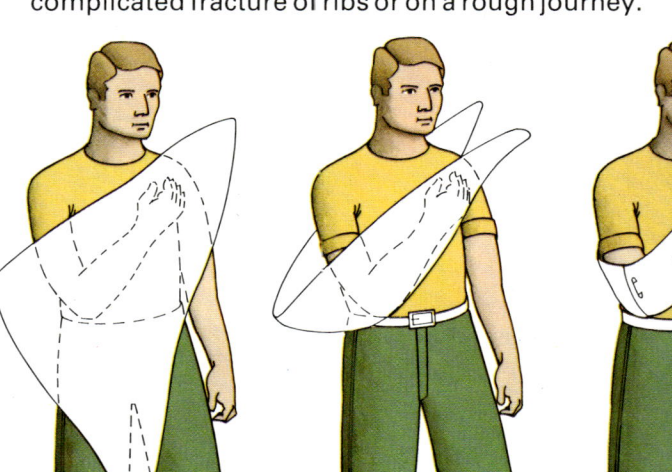

2. triangular sling – supports hand and forearm in raised position. Particularly in case of hand injury, complicated fracture of ribs or on a rough journey.

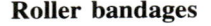

Roller bandages

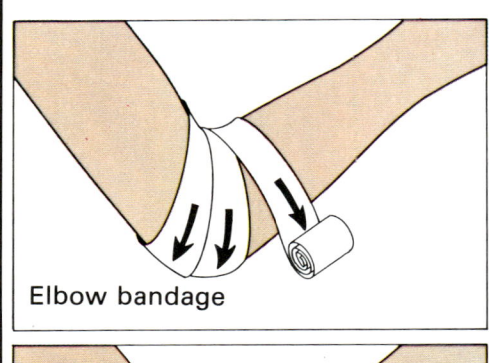

Elbow bandage

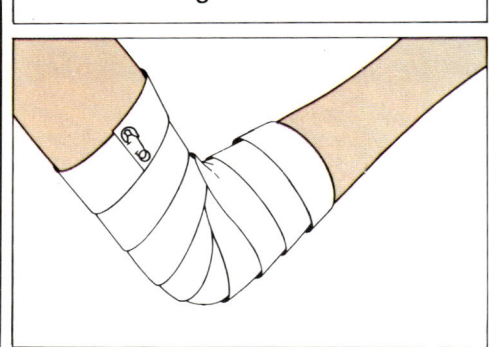

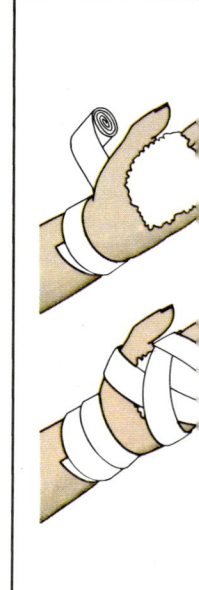

A two-inch

Fractures

Do not move unless absolutely necessary. If the injured person must be moved, immobilize the injured part as shown below but do not attempt to correct any deformity. Treat for shock. Check bandages every half hour, and loosen if the limb is swelling. Seek expert help.

Broken finger

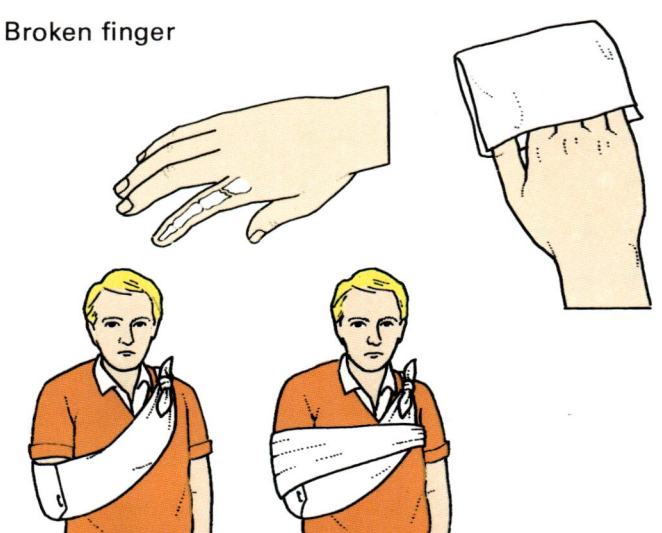

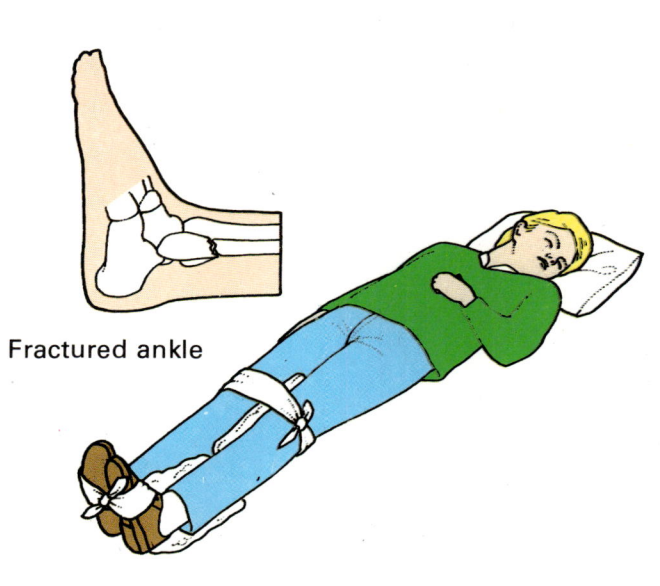

Fractured ankle

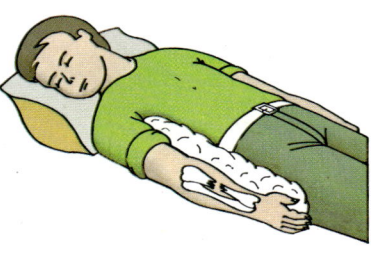

Broken arm: support, using plenty of soft padding, in an arm sling

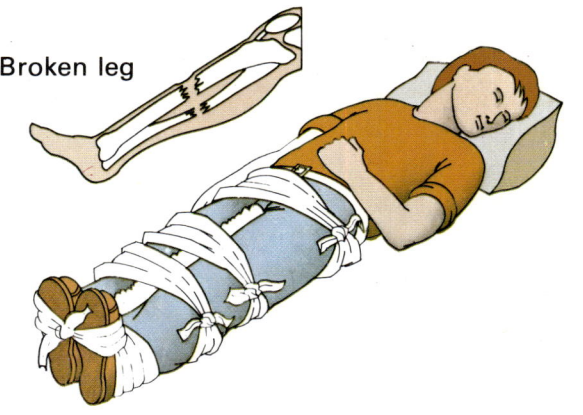

Broken leg

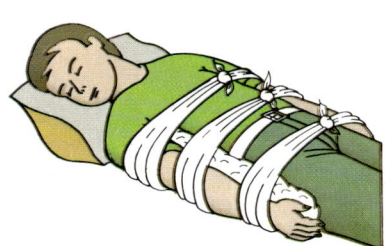

Broken elbow: this shows the treatment for an elbow that cannot be flexed; if arm can be flexed, follow instructions for broken arm

Fractured wrist: make sure wrist is supported in position most comfortable to casualty at all times. Support forearm with a flexible book or magazine and then put in an arm sling

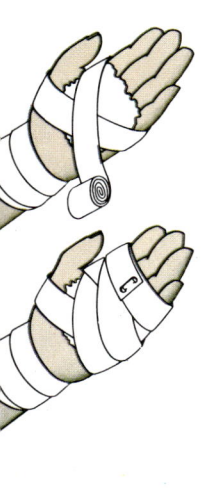

or the hand

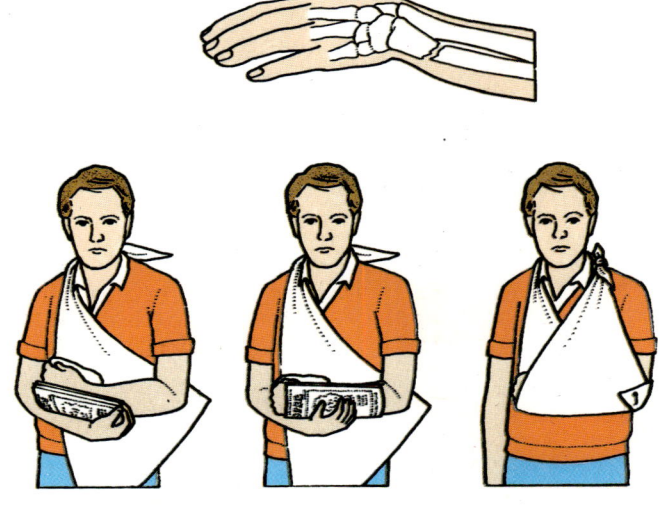

EMERGENCY!/ALPHABETICAL GUIDE TO EMERGENCIES

Artificial Respiration

Mouth to mouth (mouth to nose)
This is the most effective method and should be used except where there is severe injury to the face and mouth; where the casualty is trapped face downwards; or if the casualty is vomiting.

Positioning the head (tilted back) to open airways

closed airways

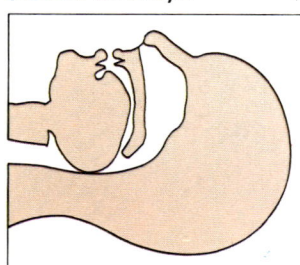
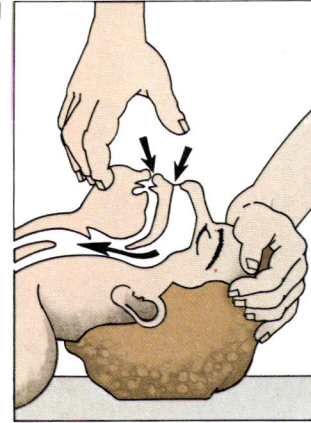

1. Lay casualty on his back. Extend head backwards. Remove obvious obstructions from the mouth. Loosen clothing.

2. Position of head and hands.

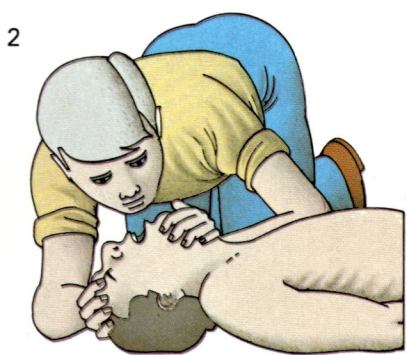
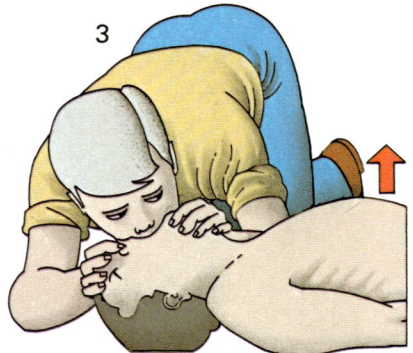
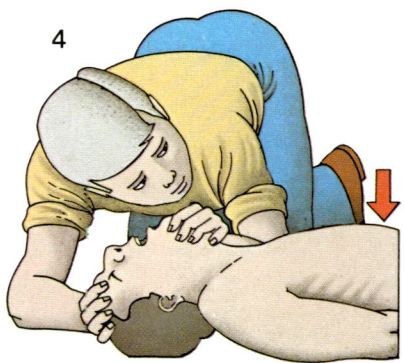

3. Seal nose by pinching, blow into mouth and watch chest rise.

4. Give four quick inflations.

5. Remove your mouth, watch chest fall.

6. Continue to inflate every 4–5 seconds until natural breathing is restored and then place casualty in recovery position (page 213). Send for medical aid.

NB: With a baby or young child, seal lips round mouth and nose and blow gently into lungs until chest rises.

Revised Holger Nielson

This should be used if the face is damaged or the jaw fractured, making mouth to mouth resuscitation impossible.

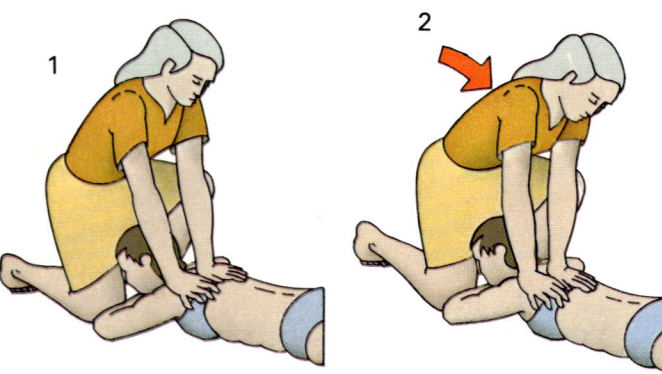
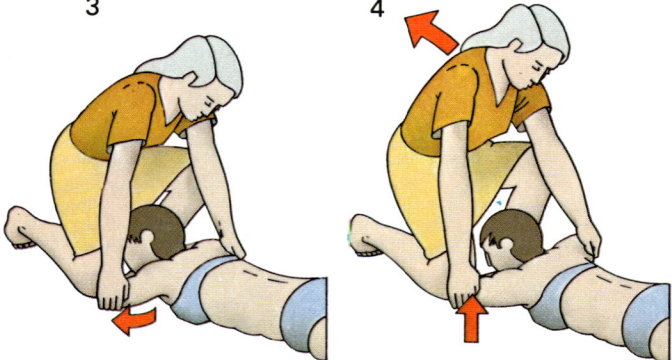

The casualty lies on his front with head facing forwards, hands under his chin and his elbows out. The mouth and nose must be clear of obstruction. Loosen clothing.

1. Kneel in front of casualty with hands flat on his back just below shoulder blades.
2. Rock forwards, keeping your arms straight until they are vertical over the body. Exerting a steady pressure let the weight of your body be the force.
3. Slide your hands past his armpits and along arms to grasp them firmly just above elbows. Rock backwards until body is vertical, raising elbows until resistance and tension are felt.
4. Drop elbows and return to picture 1 position.

Repeat as necessary, keeping all movements continuous and smooth.

ALPHABETICAL GUIDE TO EMERGENCIES/**EMERGENCY!**

Bites and Stings

Insect-bites and stings are not often serious. Very rarely, a person may have a severe allergic reaction, go into shock, and possibly have difficulty in breathing, or the heart may stop. If this happens it will develop over the first one to twenty minutes following the sting; seek medical help and give artificial respiration and heart massage if necessary. Normally, bites and stings are only serious when received in large numbers or in awkward places such as the mouth. Remove stings if left in the skin and soothe with surgical spirit or a *weak* ammonia solution or a solution of bicarbonate of soda. If the sting is in the mouth, give a mouthwash of one teaspoonful of bicarbonate of soda to a tumbler of water. If there is difficulty breathing, give an ice-cube to suck.

Snakebite: The viper or adder is the commonest poisonous snake in Europe and North America. It has a triangular head with a V-shaped mark and has zigzag markings on the body. Adder-bites are seldom fatal in adults but are more serious in children. Do not cut the wound. Reassure the victim convincingly and keep them at rest. Wash the bitten surface with plain water without rubbing, and wash away the venom; support and immobilize the limb. Seek help as soon as possible. If the bite is in the limbs, carry the child, if possible, to the nearest telephone or send for help.

Dog or cat bites: Treat as for a wound. Use a disinfectant wipe to cleanse wound. An anti-tetanus injection is advisable. If the animal is behaving oddly in any way suggestive of rabies, report it to the police and seek expert advice as quickly as possible. The animal should be shot and examined for rabies infection; if positive, anyone who has been in any physical contact with the animal should be given anti-rabies vaccine.

Bleeding

Press the edges of the wound together firmly for a few minutes, put on a sterilized dressing, then pad and bandage. If the bleeding continues, raise the limb, if possible, and put on more pads and bandages. Never remove the bandages; if bleeding continues, add more. **Do not use a tourniquet.** If there is a foreign body in the wound, only remove it if it is obviously on the surface. Otherwise, cover a wound containing a foreign body lightly; use of a ring pad will avoid pressure on the foreign body. Seek expert help. Small wounds should be washed before bandaging. Stab-wounds may cause internal damage even if the actual entry is small and should always be taken to a doctor.

Varicose veins: Bleeding from burst varicose veins is serious and you should act quickly to prevent the rapid loss of blood. Apply immediate, direct pressure with the hand to the bleeding point. Remove anything from the leg which could impede circulation. Lay casualty flat on his back and raise the leg up. Seek medical aid.

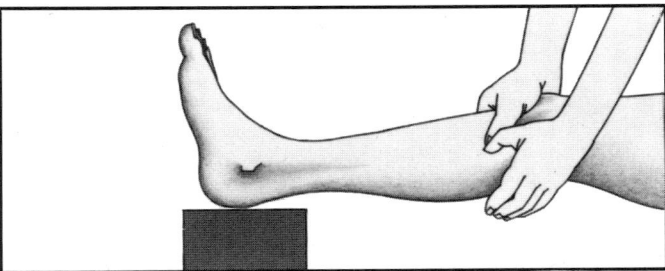

Internal bleeding: If internal bleeding is suspected it is important to get medical help immediately. Meanwhile, make casualty lie down with legs raised (see foot of previous column). He should be kept quite still. Loosen all clothing, and check for other injuries. Keep him warm and watch his breathing and pulse-rate.

Burns or Scalds

Fire: Smother flames with a coat or blanket. Cool the burnt area with cold water for at least ten minutes or until the pain ceases. Cover with dry, clean dressing. If an arm or hand is burnt, and you are at home, place arm in freshly laundered pillow case. If large areas are burnt, wrap the person in a sheet and get him to a casualty department. Do not use creams or ointments and do not remove burnt clothing next to the skin.

Corrosive chemicals: Speed is essential. Flood the affected part with running water for at least ten minutes to dilute the chemical. Remove contaminated clothing under the water if possible. Seek medical attention.

Eye injury from chemical: Urgent treatment required to prevent permanent damage. Flood eye immediately and copiously with nearest available bland liquid – water or clean milk. Continue for at least ten minutes. Take the casualty quickly to hospital.

Chemical taken by mouth: see Poisoning.

Sunburn: Rest in the shade. Give cold drink. If sunburn is severe, seek medical help. (Skin lotions are available for mild sunburn.)

Scalds: Caused by moist heat such as boiling water, steam, hot oil. Place affected part under slowly running water or immerse in cold water for at least ten minutes. Reduction of heat is essential. Remove clothes and anything of a constricting nature (rings, belts, etc.). Treat as for a burn and take to hospital if badly scalded.

Remember:

DO NOT burst or break blisters.
DO NOT apply any lotions or grease.
DO NOT breathe over burnt area.
DO NOT touch the burnt area, as this will spread germs.
DO NOT remove clothing or handle the casualty more than necessary.
DO NOT remove dressings once they have been applied.
DO NOT put fluffy or hairy materials (e.g. cotton wool) onto burnt area.

Choking

If the victim is still able to breathe effectively do not interfere with his attempts to remove the foreign body. The symptoms of choking are readily confused with heart attack or stroke but can be distinguished in the following way:

(a) The victim will usually have been eating immediately prior to the incident and suddenly is unable to breathe or speak, and unable to answer questions.

(b) The victim may make the distress signal of choking: holding the hand to the throat.

(c) The victim may turn a bluish colour and make exaggerated breathing movements.

If the victim is conscious but unable to breathe at all:

• Give three or four sharp slaps between shoulder blades with the victim bending over. If the victim is lying down roll

EMERGENCY!/ALPHABETICAL GUIDE TO EMERGENCIES

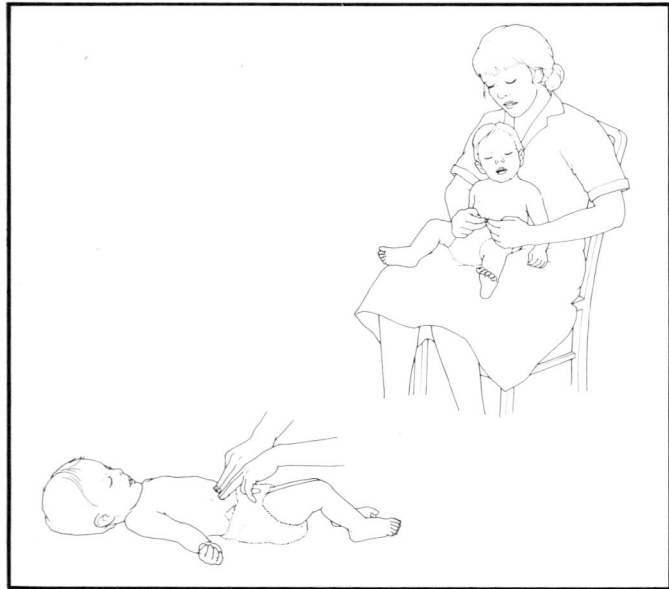

him onto his side facing you and, supporting his chest with your knee, deliver rapid blows to the back between the shoulder blades. In the case of an **infant or child** hold upside down by legs and deliver sharp blows to the back; if the child turns blue, attempt mouth-to-mouth resuscitation, then rush to hospital.

• If obstruction is not removed, as a last resort attempt abdominal thrusts (also known as the Heimlich Manoeuvre). Stand behind the victim and join hands round the waist (or chest in the case of a fat or pregnant person). Place the fist slightly above the belt but below the ribs. Rapidly thrust into the abdomen with a forceful movement. If the victim is lying down: place him on his back, kneel astride the hips, place hands one on top of the other just above the navel and below rib cage. Thrust into the abdomen with hands forcefully. In the case of an **infant or small child:** either hold the infant on lap or place face up on a firm surface with first-aider at infant's feet (see diagram). Place index and middle fingers of both hands on child's abdomen, slightly above navel and well below the rib cage, and press into abdomen with a quick upward thrust. Several thrusts may be necessary to expel the object.

• If these actions do not work repeat and rush to hospital.

If the victim is unconscious:

• If it is possible to give mouth-to-mouth respiration do so – see the instructions above. If there is no pulse, an experienced first-aider should give heart massage – see instructions page 212. Forceful respiration may keep the victim alive if the foreign body is partially dislodged.

• If it is impossible to give artificial respiration then roll victim onto his side and, supporting his chest with your knee, deliver rapid slaps to the back between the shoulder blades. In the case of a child hold upside down by legs.

• As a last resort, perform abdominal thrusts (see above).

• If a foreign body can be seen in the mouth and it is possible to grasp it easily then remove it. But beware of pushing the object further into the throat especially in the case of a small child. That is why other procedures are recommended first. Finger probing should only be attempted when the victim is unconscious and other attempts have failed. This is what to do:

• With the victim on his back grasp the tongue and lower jaw between the thumb and fingers and lift. This draws the tongue away from the back of the throat and may help to relieve the obstruction. Insert the index finger down the inside of the cheek into the back of the throat and attempt to hook out the foreign body or ease it into the mouth by pushing it against the opposite side of the throat until it is possible to dislodge it. In the case of a child use a small finger. The risk of pushing the object further down the throat is much greater with a child so use extreme caution.

• If necessary repeat the procedures above:
1. Attempt artificial respiration.
2. Perform four back slaps.
3. Perform four abdominal thrusts.
4. Probe the throat.

• After removing the object perform more mouth-to-mouth respiration if necessary and heart massage.

• When the victim recovers he should be seen by a doctor. (Not necessary if the victim recovers fully without any period of unconsciousness.)

Prevention

The causes of choking in adults are often excessive alcohol intake, dentures or large, poorly chewed pieces of food. Every year people die as a result of choking. To prevent:

• Cut food into small pieces and chew slowly and thoroughly, especially if you wear dentures.

• Do not laugh and talk while chewing and swallowing, and avoid excessive intake of alcohol.

• Restrict children from walking, running and playing while they have food or other foreign bodies in their mouths, and keep small objects such as marbles, beads, or thumbtacks out of reach of infants and small children.

Cold Injury

Old people, babies and mountaineers are most vulnerable to hypothermia – a cooling of the body below normal temperature. If the person is cold to the touch – even their armpits – and appears dopey and confused, then seek expert help. Hospital admission may be necessary. In the meantime, take all possible measures to warm the person up. Remove any wet clothing and dry the sufferer. Cover with blankets and provide warm food and drink (not scalding) but not alcohol. Warm the room. Mild cases will recover by these measures alone. Do not use hot-water bottles or electric blankets since warming the skin takes heat away from vital internal organs.

A baby suffering from cold will be pink, with swollen limbs and a very cold skin. It will be lethargic and unwilling to suck. The body temperature will be below normal. Re-warming must be very gradual – increase the room temperature and put more coverings over the baby. Cold injury can be dangerous and hospital treatment is advisable.

Convulsions

Remove the victim from danger. Guide their movements to prevent injury; do not try to stop them. Do not force the mouth open, but if possible put something, such as a knotted handkerchief, between the teeth to prevent the person biting their tongue. On recovering, they will probably not remember what has happened; reassure them and consult a doctor.

Babies and young children may have convulsions, or momentary loss of consciousness accompanied by a tremor, as a result of a high fever. Call the doctor and give the baby a tepid sponge with warm water to bring down body temperature. Whether the convulsion is serious or more like a faint, make sure the child has a medical check-up following upon it.

Drowning
Give artificial respiration and heart massage if necessary. Arrange the victim's urgent removal to hospital. There are many recorded cases of people surviving after twenty-five minutes or even longer under water: give artificial respiration even if the person appears completely lifeless, and continue until expert help arrives.

Electric Shock
Switch off the supply, pull out the plug or tear the cable free. If this is impossible, stand on a dry insulating material such as wood or newspaper and push the person away from the supply of current. Be careful not to touch any conducting material with the other hand while doing this. Give artificial respiration and heart massage if necessary. Treat for shock (see below).

Electric shocks may have greater effects than most people expect, since there may be little external signs of damage. Medical advice should always be sought after a serious electric shock. Burns must be treated.

Faints
These are common in illness or when standing in a crowd, and caused by a temporary drop in the blood-supply to the brain. There is often some warning: the person may sway, become giddy, white-faced and break out in a sweat.

Urge him to breathe deeply and flex his muscles to aid blood circulation. Loosen clothing and lay him down in a current of air with his legs above his head until colour returns. If this is not possible, sit him down with his head between his knees. As he recovers, give him sips of water.

Foreign Bodies
In the ear: An insect in the ear is very distressing; pour in tepid water or olive oil and it should float out. (Do not poke the ears to remove a foreign body: consult a doctor.)
In the nose: Tell the person to breathe through their mouth and consult your doctor or, if possible, rush to the nearest hospital casualty department.
In the eye: Tears may wash the object into the corner of the eye so that it can be removed with a clean cloth. Never use a hard object to remove something from the eye. Try lifting the upper lid by the lashes over the lower lid; this draws the lashes of the lower lid over the inside of the upper lid and may brush the object out. Look under the lower lid, and remove any object with a clean cloth or tissue.

If these measures fail, the upper and lower lids may in turn be rolled back over a match, and any grit gently wiped off with a cloth. Never attempt to remove any object from the coloured part of the eye (the pupil and iris), but go to major hospital casualty department.

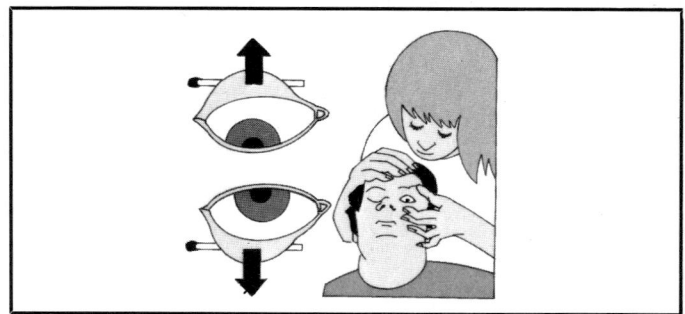

Inhaled: If a foreign body is inhaled it is advisable to consult a doctor without delay.

Gas and Exhaust-fume Poisoning
Carbon monoxide gas from the domestic gas supply, from a car engine left running in a garage or in fumes coming out of a cracked stove can be lethal. However, natural gas, owing to its lower carbon monoxide content, is much safer than the old coal gas. If the victim is in an enclosed room, take a deep breath before going in and carry them out immediately. The victim may be confused or in a coma. Provide fresh air and give artificial respiration if breathing has stopped. Call a doctor or ambulance; these will provide oxygen if necessary.

Head Injuries
In the case of an injury to the head from a sharp blow causing a wound or any temporary loss of consciousness, consult a doctor. Rest for forty-eight hours after any head injury unless told not to. Report any abnormal drowsiness, persistent vomiting or disturbance of behaviour to the doctor. Persistent headache after forty-eight hours which cannot be relieved by aspirin should be reported to a doctor.

Heart Failure
(see overleaf)

Heat Stroke
The body can no longer control temperature by sweating. Signs are a high temperature and pulse; hot, dry skin; noisy breathing; unconsciousness. Strip casualty and wrap in wet, cold sheet. Keep wet until his temperature has gone down. Place in recovery position. Fan casualty from above. Send to hospital.

Nose-bleed
Only rarely serious. Ask the sufferer to sit down with their head forward and to breathe through their mouth. Pinch firmly the soft part of the nose for ten minutes. Loosen clothing at neck, chest and waist. Put a bowl or pad under the nose to catch the blood, and place an old towel or sheet around the shoulders to take care of any mess. Seek medical advice if the bleeding is severe or does not stop in an hour. When the person, naturally enough, wants to spit, do not discourage this; but try to discourage sniffing, which will dislodge the blood clots forming over the injured blood-vessel.

EMERGENCY!/ALPHABETICAL GUIDE TO EMERGENCIES

Heart Failure
(See also Artificial Respiration)

When the heart stops, the victim turns a blue-grey colour, has no pulse at wrist or neck and the pupils of the eyes are dilated (large).

1. Give artificial respiration (see page 208). If the heart does not start, an *experienced* person can begin external heart massage while continuing artificial respiration. An inexperienced person is not advised to try this as it may cause injury if done incorrectly. Should heart massage prove impossible due to obstruction, or difficult due to inexperience, keep the artificial respiration going as first priority until help arrives, giving any heart massage you are able.

2. Heart massage. With the injured person on their back, place the heel of the hand (use two fingers only for babies) over the breastbone where the ribs meet. Place the other hand over the first hand. Press down on the lower half of the breastbone sufficiently to move the chest down 1½ inches or 4 cm, depending on size or age of casualty. Repeat every second for five seconds, then inflate the lungs; repeat this cycle to the ratio of fifteen compressions to two quick inflations until the patient recovers or help arrives.

3. When breathing begins again, lay the person in the recovery position and treat for shock.

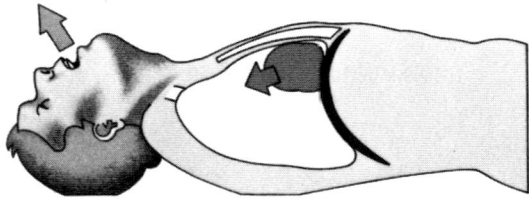
Striking of victim's breastbone induces a cough; diaphragm relaxing forces blood out of heart.

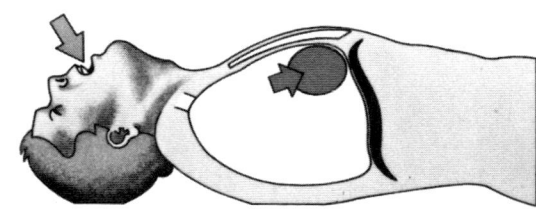
On breathing after cough, diaphragm takes pressure off and blood goes back into heart.

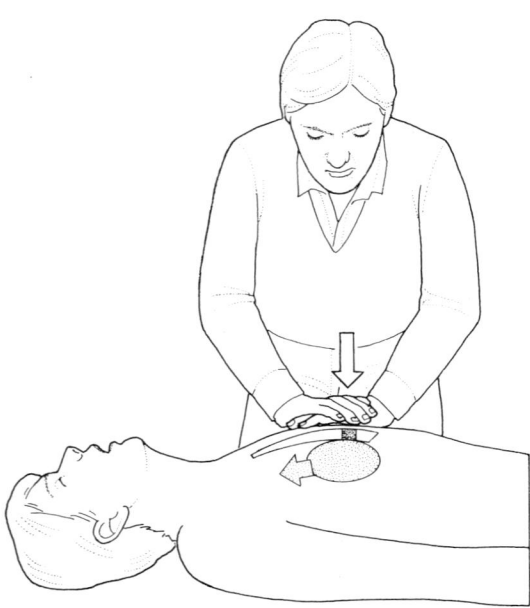
Pressing on indicated part, halfway between middle and end of sternum, expels blood. It is important to keep hands on the same spot.

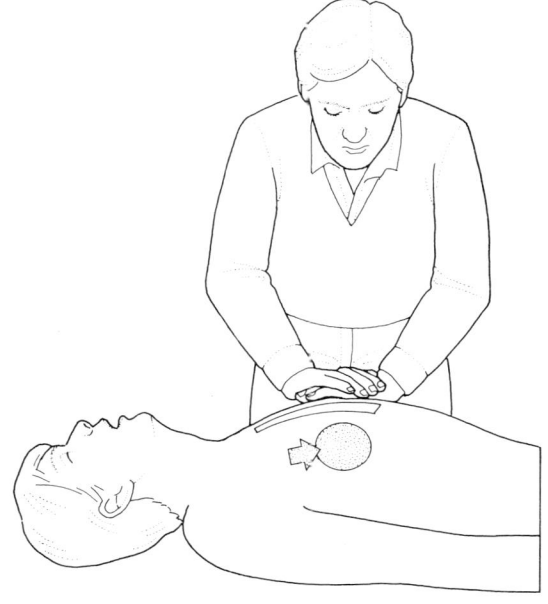
On release, blood goes back into heart.

Poisoning

Ask the person, if conscious, what they have taken. Also, remember that many poisons can be identified by smell.
Non-corrosive poisons such as medicines, weed-killers, cigarettes, poisonous plants: Do not give the person a drink, and particularly do not give them a salt-water drink; this can be dangerous in itself. Seek medical advice.
Corrosive poisons such as disinfectants, cleaning fluid, caustic soda, paraffin, petrol or insect spray: dilute the corrosive by giving milk or water to drink. Do not make the person vomit, as this may lead to more burning. Yellow, grey or white burns around the mouth may betray a corrosive poison – wipe any poison away and rinse out mouth. Seek help urgently. Phone your doctor or take the person to the casualty department of the nearest hospital, even if the person appears to have vomited the poison. Some poisons, e.g. aspirin, have serious delayed effects. If the person is unconscious and not breathing, give artificial respiration and, if necessary, heart massage. If unconscious but breathing, lay them on their side in the recovery position. Send any particulars of the poison to the hospital with the victim, including any remaining poison, its container or any vomited matter.

Recovery Position

This position should be used with unconscious casualties where internal injuries and fractured bones are not suspected. The casualty is kept stable and comfortable, and the position of the head allows any fluid or vomit in the mouth to drain out. Never use a pillow, but the head *can* be placed on a thin cloth or handkerchief. If the casualty is left on his or her back there is a danger of the tongue falling to the back of the throat thus blocking airway. The only time *never* to put a casualty in the recovery position is in cases of suspected neck or back fracture. If internal injuries are suspected, place casualty gently in the recovery position on uninjured side.

Red Urine

Usually due to beetroot, blackcurrant, red wine or sweets. Blood in the urine gives it a smoky appearance. This may not be an emergency if the person is otherwise well, but seek medical advice.

Shock

Recognized by rapid pulse becoming weak, cold and clammy skin, profuse sweating. It may be caused by bleeding, burns, or injuries, loss of body fluid, a burst appendix, or even by a cut, bad news or fright. Check on bleeding. Send for help. Lay casualty down and treat the cause of shock if possible. Keep head low and raise lower limbs. Loosen tight clothing at neck and at waist; protect if necessary with blanket or coat. Keep the person warm with blankets and heat the room if cold. Do not give hot-water bottles and warm drinks, and do not move more than necessary.

Stupor and Coma

If the stupor is not deep, the person may be roused by pressing firmly upwards on the ridge beneath the eyebrows at a point where there is a small dent in the bone. This will cause sufficient pain to rouse the person without hurting them. If the person will not be roused (coma), check that the air-passages are free from any obstruction such as vomit and, if breathing, lay them on their side in the recovery position. If the person is trapped and cannot be moved, keep the airway clear by tilting the head back. Call the doctor; be ready to give artificial respiration and heart massage. Check that the person is not wearing or carrying any identity discs or cards, which may explain the cause of the coma (diabetes, epilepsy, etc.) and give instructions about what to do and whom to contact.

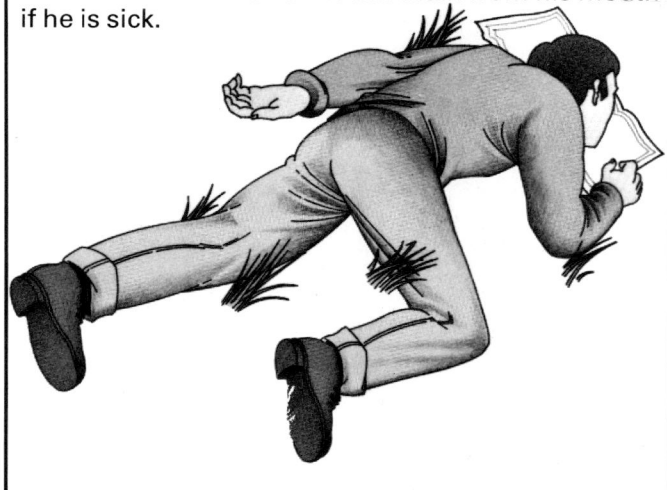

Recovery position
Casualty lying on his side with one knee drawn up and one arm out, bent at the elbow. His head is on one side so that the vomit will drain from his mouth if he is sick.

Suffocation

Remove the obstruction, lift the person up, and cut or loosen cords, ribbons, etc., if hanging. Give artificial respiration and heart massage if necessary.

Swallowed Objects

Smooth or round objects such as coins, marbles, buttons or plum stones seldom cause trouble when swallowed. Do not worry unless the person complains of pain, in which case consult the doctor. Pins, needles, safety pins and other sharp objects can be dangerous and you should *call the doctor at once*. But do not panic: many frighteningly sharp objects have been found to pass through the bowel harmlessly. Eat a bulky diet and examine the stools carefully for five days until the object has been passed. X-rays are not generally justified except in an emergency, or if the object cannot be found.

Unconsciousness

First check airway and remove any obstacle. If not breathing, give artificial respiration. Once normal breathing resumes, lay casualty on side to ensure that vomit is not inhaled. Keep the person quiet and warm, and consult the doctor. If the person recovers, it is quite safe to let them fall asleep provided they remain in the recovery position. Loss of consciousness may be caused by a blow to the head severe enough to shake the brain (concussion).

EMERGENCY!/ALPHABETICAL GUIDE TO EMERGENCIES

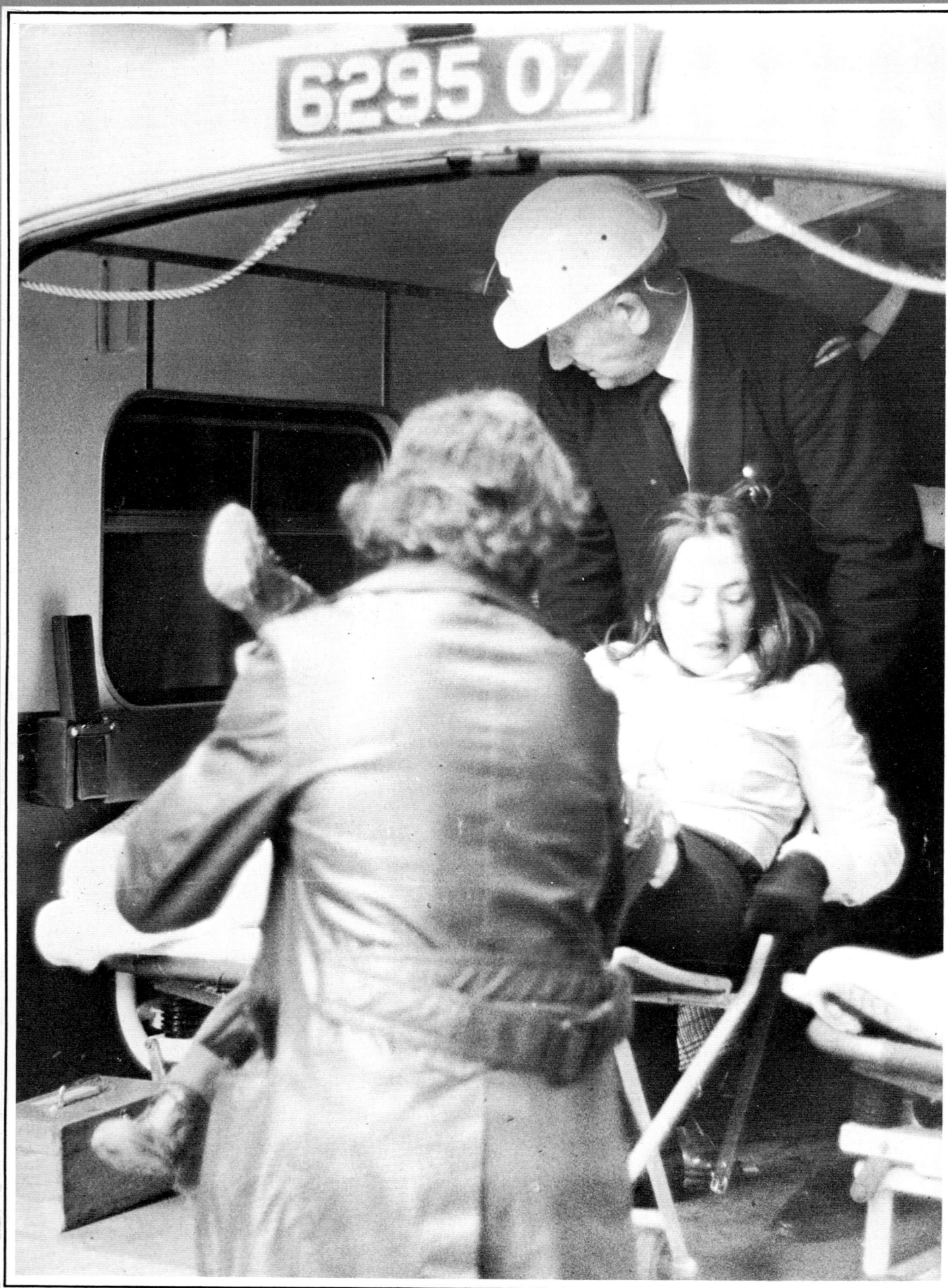

When to Call the Doctor

Whenever possible, go to see your doctor in his surgery. But do not hesitate to call a doctor in the evening or at night if someone is obviously seriously ill or there has been a serious accident. In an emergency you can call on any doctor, but try your own doctor first. Or you can take the ill person to a hospital casualty department.

It is impossible to give a comprehensive list of circumstances when a doctor should be called in an emergency at night. A high temperature or fever is not normally sufficient reason to worry the doctor. However, if the fever is accompanied by other symptoms such as a severe headache it may be wise to call the doctor, even though all that he may be able to do is to give advice on the telephone. Coughing a small amount of blood, blood in motions or urine are not usually sufficient reason to call a doctor at night unless accompanied by severe pains or other symptoms. However, a doctor should be called when a woman bleeds from the vagina during pregnancy, especially if it is accompanied by pain.

A doctor should be called if someone has difficulty in breathing, or has an unexplained severe and continuous pain in the abdomen – or anywhere else – which does not go away after half an hour, or has a severe, constricting chest pain, especially if accompanied by sweating, or when someone collapses or loses the ability to move limbs or to speak.

Parents should call a doctor to their child if the child suddenly becomes ill or feverish and lies still without the energy to move. Children cry differently when ill and a mother usually knows when something is seriously wrong; if the child does not have the energy to respond in the normal way, then that is a good indication that something is wrong and the doctor should be called.

Copious diarrhoea in babies is an emergency and the doctor should be called. An epileptic attack in a child lasting more than ten minutes, or recurring attacks, should be treated as an emergency. Rashes are hardly ever an emergency and are best taken to the doctor the next day so that the rash may be examined in daylight.

There is no need to call the doctor if your child vomits once, cries for half an hour or so, or misses a meal, provided that they are otherwise happy and gaining weight and sleeping well. Call your doctor if the child looks odd – pale, blue or yellow; if the child appears to be in pain and will not be comforted – the legs may be drawn up and fists clenched; if the child has a persistent cough, persistent diarrhoea, or persistent vomiting; if a baby misses two or more feeds or a child does not eat for twenty-four hours; if the child has convulsions; if there is blood in the urine, faeces or vomit; if there is any injury to the head and the child does not recover in fifteen minutes. Odd behaviour such as drowsiness, listlessness or irritability may also be reasons for seeking medical advice.

Earache is a common cause of doctors being called by parents at night but there is not much that can be done until morning, when a course of antibiotic drugs may be started. The best remedy for earache or any pain is a small dose of paracetamol or other simple pain-killer. Panic or conflict in the family when illness is recognized is often the reason for calling the doctor. Pause for a moment to ask yourself if it is a genuine emergency: if you are really worried, especially in the case of a child, do not hesitate to call the doctor.

Appendix One: Good Food

The following recipes have been chosen to show that a good meal does not need to have a large meat or fat content to be delicious and attractive. Many of them have been contributed by Caroline Conran. Additional recipes have been selected from *The Sunday Times Guide to the World's Best Food* by Michael Bateman, Caroline Conran and Oliver Gillie (published by Hutchinson). Others have been contributed by Claudia Roden, Robin Howe, Julie Jordan, Anna McMeádhian and Maria Lourdes. The recipes are for dishes eaten every day by people in the healthiest parts of the world – and so we believe are the healthiest food that anyone might eat. (Salt and pepper are not included in the lists of ingredients.)

SOUPS AND STARTERS

Indonesian soup (serves 4)
This is simply a rich vegetable soup, nutritious but satisfying in its range of flavours: hot, sweet, sour and spicy. The basic flavour is due to the combination of chicken stock and an infusion of coconut milk.

4 tablespoons desiccated coconut	1 teaspoon turmeric
½ pint boiling water	2 pints home-made chicken stock
1 large onion, very finely chopped	2 teaspoons brown sugar
oil (sunflower or olive)	2 large carrots
1 clove garlic, crushed	2 sticks celery
1 slice of fresh green ginger, the size of a marble (optional)	1 small leek
1–2 chilli peppers (green, or dried and pounded), finely crushed	handful of green beans
	juice of 1 lemon

Make the coconut milk by steeping the desiccated coconut in the boiling water and straining after 15 minutes.

Gently fry a tablespoon of the onion in a very little oil until soft; add garlic, ginger and chillies (or powdered chilli or chilli sauce) and the turmeric. Heat through without burning until it is a sticky paste, stirring with a wooden spoon.

Heat the stock with the coconut milk and the spicy paste, add sugar and the remaining vegetables, which should be cut thinly but not quite so small as Julienne matchsticks. Simmer slowly for 30 minutes. Check for seasoning. You can add soy sauce instead of salt for a more characteristic flavour.

Before serving, stir in lemon juice.

Onion soup (serves 2)
Here is a traditional dish in which the vegetables themselves, in this case onions, can be made to exude their own juices to replace the usual fat. Although less rich than the usual onion soup, which is cooked with lots of lard, the flavour is equally good.

1 tablespoon oil (olive or sunflower)	1 teaspoon wine vinegar
1 lb large onions, sliced thinly in rings	1 teaspoon sugar
	2 large slices French bread, toasted
1 generous pinch of caraway or fennel seeds	2 oz Gruyère or Emmental
1 pint best stock, well skimmed of all fat	1 glass white vermouth (optional)
	a dash of brandy (optional)

Heat the oil just enough to lubricate the bottom of the pan, put in the onions and stir them round. Add the caraway or fennel seeds, cover the pan and let the onions stew in their own juice for at least fifteen minutes.

In a separate pan, bring the stock to the boil, pour it over the onions, add the vinegar and cook fairly fast for about 15 minutes. Meanwhile, caramelize a teaspoon of sugar by putting it under a hot grill in an old tablespoon and leaving it there until it is a dark chestnut-brown, then stir it into the soup to colour it. You will be needing the grill anyway for toasting the French bread. When it is toasted, cover each piece with half the grated Gruyère or Emmental.

Put the soup into bowls, float the toast on top and stick the bowls back under the hot grill until the cheese is bubbling. If you can add a glass of dry white vermouth to the stock it improves the flavour greatly, and a dash of brandy at the end is quite traditional and a great comfort to a tired person.

Borscht (serves 4)
A very filling soup, full of good nourishment. Made as it is in the Ukraine with different kinds of meat, it is almost a whole meal in itself. There are as many different kinds of borscht in Russia as there are families: with meat, pork, mutton, beef, duck; or without meat, with vegetables in every quantity and combination. There are two common denominators: beetroot is the main vegetable, and sour cream is added at the end to counter its earthy sweetness. Instead of sour cream you can use yoghurt and cottage cheese, mixed in equal parts and sieved; or add plain lemon juice just before serving.

1 lb uncooked beetroot (or 2 lb cooked beetroot)	tablespoons tomato purée (optional)
1 lb carrots	2 pints chicken stock or meat stock (preferably home-made)
½ lb turnips	
1 large onion	
2 medium tomatoes or 2	pinch of sugar

Cut the vegetables into very thin strips (so that the water can extract maximum flavour). Put them in the pan with stock, bring gently to boil, and simmer on lowest heat for 45 minutes, with lid on. You may need to add more water if it starts to boil dry. Season with salt, pepper and sugar. Strain, pressing out every bit of juice. Check for seasoning. Serve with blobs of soured yoghurt, or a squeeze of lemon juice.

Lentil spinach soup (serves 4)
This rich green soup makes a satisfying lunch when served with thick slices of home-made wholewheat bread. You can also make a good soup with Swiss chard or frozen spinach. If you are using brown or green (whole) lentils soak for 2–3 hours before cooking. Split lentils (red) do not need soaking.

6 oz lentils	1 clove garlic, crushed
2 oz green split peas	1 tablespoon finely chopped fresh dill, or 1 teaspoon dried dill
1½ pints water	
1 bay leaf	
1 potato, scrubbed but not peeled, diced	8 oz fresh spinach, well washed, stems and leaves chopped together
1 tablespoon olive oil	
1 medium onion, chopped finely	1 tablespoon red wine vinegar, or 1 teaspoon malt vinegar

Put the lentils, peas and water into a large, heavy-based pan with 1 teaspoon sea salt and bay leaf. Bring to the boil, then reduce the heat and simmer, covered, for about 1 hour. Stir occasionally to prevent sticking.

Boil the potato in a separate pan in enough water to cover, until just tender but still firm. Add the potato and its cooking liquid to the lentils and peas.

Heat the oil in a frying pan and sauté the onion in it for 1–2 minutes, then add the garlic, dill and a pinch of freshly ground black pepper, and sauté for 1 minute more. Add the spinach a handful at a time, waiting for one handful to wilt before adding the next. Cook for 2–3 minutes.

Add spinach mixture to the lentils and peas. Then stir in the vinegar and simmer for at least 30 minutes more. Remove the bay leaf, taste and add salt and pepper if necessary. Serve piping hot with plenty of bread.

Crudités – Celery with hot anchovy oil (serves 4)

The French love to offer treats of raw radishes (sometimes with butter and salt), celery and slivers of carrot, served with aioli, which is a lovely garlic-flavoured mayonnaise. Unfortunately, this is not so healthy as it sounds, because mayonnaise is an emulsion of cholesterol-rich egg yolks and oil, and it is egg yolks we need to cut down on. But there is no reason why crudités should not be served with an olive oil and vinegar or lemon dressing, or, in the case of celery, with the appetizing hot dressing described below.

1 small tin of anchovies	1 large head of celery
3–4 tablespoons olive oil	

Put the anchovies and their oil in a small saucepan and heat gently; after about 4 or 5 minutes, when they start to dissolve, pound them up. Stir in extra olive oil, beat well together. Keep hot until ready to serve.

Cut up the stalks of celery and serve with the bowl of anchovy dressing, mopping up the juice with plain wholemeal bread.

The mixture is beaten before serving because it will separate. If you like an emulsion, this one stands up to gentle heat without breaking down:

1 small tin anchovies	2 teaspoons lemon juice
2 teaspoons Dijon mustard	4 tablespoons olive oil

Put the anchovies and their oil in a small saucepan and heat gently; after about 4 or 5 minutes, when they start to dissolve, transfer them to a mortar and pound them. The bones stick to the bottom of the pestle and can be removed. Pound in the mustard and lemon juice until well blended, then drip in the olive oil, as though making a mayonnaise. Return to the saucepan, heat very gently and serve.

Aubergine purée (serves 4–6)

This is also known as caviare of aubergines.

3 aubergines	2 cloves garlic, finely crushed
1 large onion	chilli powder (optional)
juice of 1 lemon	2 tomatoes, deseeded and
3 tablespoons olive oil	roughly chopped

Grill the whole aubergines until charred on the outside and soft and pulpy inside. (Alternatively, bake them in the oven for half an hour, until they are very soft inside.) Cut them in half and scoop out the pulp; mix it with the juice of the onion, obtained somewhat painfully either by grating the onion on the coarse blade of the grater or pulping it in the liquidizer, and then by rubbing it through a wire sieve with the back of a spoon so that the juice is pressed out.

Season the paste with lemon juice, olive oil and garlic, and with salt and pepper or a little chilli powder. Stir in the tomatoes. Serve cold with home-made bread.

Houmous (serves 4)

This eastern Mediterranean dish is becoming increasingly popular as Greek restaurants continue to boom. It also happens to be particularly rich in protein, as are all dishes made with pulses; in this case it is chick-peas that are the main ingredient.

Although apparently very filling because of the olive oil and sesame-seed oil, it is very safe food. Eaten with plenty of pitta bread and followed by a Greek-style salad it makes a very good lunch. It can be made with tinned chick-peas, but if you are patient it is very easy to make from dried chick-peas. (Tahina paste is made of crushed sesame seeds and is sold in jars.)

6 oz dried chick-peas	juice of 1 lemon
4 tablespoons tahina paste	1 clove garlic, crushed
a sprig or two of parsley, chopped	olive oil to taste

Soak the chick-peas overnight. Put them in a pan covered with fresh cold water and bring them gently to the boil. Simmer for about 1½ hours or until tender – it may take as long as three hours. Put the cooked peas through a Moulin Légumes, using the coarse blade first, and then the small blade, to obtain a smooth paste; or mash, pound or beat in a liquidizer or a sieve, whatever method suits you.

Stir in the tahina paste, lemon juice, garlic, salt and chopped parsley, adjusting lemon and garlic to suit your taste. Add enough olive oil to make a smooth moist paste: be generous with everything, you are not trying to run a restaurant. Eat with hot pitta bread or wholemeal bread; you will not need butter.

Tapenade (serves 2–3)

This blackish, ugly paste is really delicious with fresh home-made wholemeal bread, but is probably best of all, if it is your day for eating an egg, with a hard-boiled egg.

4 oz black olives, stoned	squeeze of lemon juice
6 anchovies	1 tablespoon oil
1 tablespoon capers	

Put all the ingredients in the liquidizer and whizz to a slightly rough-textured paste. Serve as a very appetizing and unpretentious starter, with slices of bread and a bowl of the white-tipped radishes called French Breakfast. You can include raw garlic too, if you wish.

VEGETABLE DISHES

A healthy diet should include a high proportion of vegetable dishes. Also included in this section are recipes for vegetables and rice combined, which exploits the nutritional virtues of each.

Scalloped potatoes (serves 4–6)

One of the more demanding vegetables, as far as butter is concerned, is the potato. If it isn't being mashed with loads of butter, it is probably being fried in quantities of oil or roasted in lakes of fat. But this dish, a variation on the old Scottish stoved potato, when the onions and potatoes are cooked in water and a bit of bacon fat, is nice and creamy although it contains no cream – only milk and a teaspoon of soft margarine.

1 teaspoon soft margarine	1 teaspoon fresh chopped rosemary
1½ lb potatoes, thinly sliced	
1 medium onion, finely sliced	1–1¼ pints milk
2 teaspoons flour	

Grease a 3-pint ovenproof dish with soft margarine. Spread a quarter of the potatoes over the bottom of the dish and put a third of the onions on top. Sprinkle a third of the flour, a pinch of salt, pepper and some of the rosemary over. Repeat the layers, finishing with a final layer of potatoes. Pour enough milk over almost to cover the potatoes. Bake at Reg. 4/350°F for 2–2½ hours. Every half-hour, for the first 1½ hours, push the topmost potatoes down under the milk to keep them from browning too much. If the potatoes become dry (there should be juices about an inch below the top of the dish), add more milk. When cooked, the potatoes should be brown and crusty on top, with creamy juices underneath.

Potatoes with cheese sauce (serves 4)

By adding a richly flavoured and coloured sauce to your potatoes and serving them with marinated onion rings, black olives and hard-boiled eggs, they are transformed into a decorative and nourishing meal.

juice of ½ lemon	8 medium potatoes, peeled
3 dried hot red chillies, seeded and crumbled	3 tablespoons olive oil
	1 fresh green or red chilli, cut in ⅛-in strips.
1 large onion, sliced into thin rings	

APPENDIX ONE/GOOD FOOD

For the sauce:

6 oz coarsely grated mozzarella or Munster cheese	1 teaspoon turmeric
8 fl oz yoghurt	1 fresh green or red chilli, finely chopped.

Combine the lemon juice and dried chillies with salt and pepper in a bowl. Add the onion and leave to marinate while you boil the potatoes until cooked.

To make the sauce, combine the ingredients in a blender until smooth.

Heat the olive oil in a frying pan. Add the sauce and cook over a low heat, stirring constantly for 5 minutes or until the sauce thickens.

Arrange the potatoes in a heated serving dish and pour the sauce over them. Drain the onion rings from the marinade, and arrange them over the potatoes with the fresh chilli strips.

This dish is often served garnished with halved hard-boiled eggs, black olives and lettuce leaves.

Vegetable stir-fry (serves 4)

Using the Oriental technique of stir-frying, you can make delicious and nutritious meals very quickly. This American recipe uses broccoli, cauliflower, cabbage and carrots, but you can substitute whatever vegetables you like. Serve the stir-fry as a side dish with a quiche perhaps, or make it into a meal by serving it with a cooked grain such as brown rice or buckwheat.

about 1 lb broccoli, cut into 1 in lengths	2 sticks celery, sliced diagonally
about 8 oz cauliflower, divided into 1 in pieces	about ½ in piece fresh ginger, finely chopped
2 tablespoons oil (corn, safflower, sesame or peanut)	3 cloves garlic, finely chopped
2 medium onions, sliced and then halved to make crescents	2 tablespoons soy sauce
	2 tablespoons sherry
	about 4 oz coarsely chopped green cabbage
2 green peppers, deseeded and cut into thin strips	4 oz mung bean sprouts (optional)
2 medium carrots, cut into thin rounds	juice of ½ lemon

Put the broccoli and cauliflower into a wide pan, pour on boiling water to cover, then boil for 5 minutes. Drain off the water (keep it to use in a soup) and set aside the vegetables.

Heat a large frying pan or *wok* and pour the oil in. When it is very hot, put in the onions, peppers and carrots. Stir constantly while you fry the vegetables over a high heat for 3 minutes. Add the celery, ginger, garlic, soy sauce and sherry. Stir-fry for 2 more minutes. Add the broccoli and cauliflower and fry to heat through, then add the cabbage and fry for 2 minutes. Finally, put in the mung bean sprouts, if using, and lemon juice and stir-fry for 2 minutes.

Taste and add salt and pepper as necessary. Serve immediately while crisp and hot.

For variety add any vegetables you like, remembering to boil hard ones such as potatoes, green beans or Brussels sprouts for 5 minutes, and stir-frying first those that need the longest cooking. You can add soya bean curd (*tofu*) to the stir-fry, and toasted almonds and sesame seeds. Try adding cooked grain or pasta as well.

Spinach with black-eyed beans (peas) (serves 4)

Olive oil gives the best taste to this salad, but you can use a light vegetable oil instead when the dish is a hot accompaniment to the main course.

5 oz black-eyed beans (peas)	1 large onion, finely chopped
1 lb shredded fresh spinach, or 8 oz frozen leaf spinach completely thawed	5 tablespoons oil

Cover the black-eyed beans with water in a saucepan (they do not need soaking) and bring to the boil. Simmer until tender, generally after about 20 minutes; do not overcook or they will become mushy. Add salt to taste towards the end of the cooking time.

Meanwhile, wash the fresh spinach, the thick stems having been removed prior to shredding, and drain well. If using frozen spinach, squeeze all the water out of it.

Fry the onion in the oil until soft and transparent. Add the spinach and fry, stirring constantly, until well cooked. Season with salt and pepper, then stir in the drained beans and warm through together. Allow the dish to cool and serve as a first course at lunch, or hot as a side dish with the main course.

Stuffed tomatoes (serves 2 to 4)

These can be stuffed with almost any mixture, but to make a more filling dish use a combination of rice and meat.

1 lb large tomatoes	¼ pint tomato juice
1 small onion, finely chopped	3 oz cooked rice
2–3 tablespoons oil (olive or sunflower)	pinch oregano or basil
	pinch of coriander and cumin seed
3 oz raisins	
3 oz minced beef or lamb	squeeze of lemon juice

Cut the tomatoes in half and scoop out the centres. Sprinkle the insides with salt, and leave them upside down to drain for half an hour while you make the stuffing.

Fry the onion in half the oil until tender, then add raisins and meat and fry a few minutes more. Now mix this and the tomato juice into the rice, and season well with herbs, spices, salt and lemon juice. Stuff the tomatoes with this mixture, sprinkle with the remaining oil and bake at Reg. 3/320°F for up to an hour in an earthenware dish or baking tin. Serve hot or cold, with a generous green salad or a salad of lettuce, endive, sliced fennel and thinly sliced radishes.

Tomato tart with fresh thyme (serves 4–6)

By evaporating all the water liquid from fruits or vegetables, you can obtain the very essence of their flavour without adding butter or cream. This kind of cooking should contain lots of concentrated flavours and should never be watery.

pastry made with 4 oz flour and 2 oz vegetable fat (see pages 78–9)	2–2½ lb ripe red tomatoes
	bunch of fresh thyme
	dried thyme
dry beans for blind baking	cayenne pepper

Line a flan tin with the pastry and bake it 'blind' in a hot oven. This means putting foil or beans on greaseproof paper into the uncooked pastry case. After 10 minutes or so, when the pastry is firm, remove the foil or beans and paper and prick the bottom of the flan. Cook for a further 5 minutes or until the bottom is done.

Skin the tomatoes. Take 1–1½ lb of the ripest of them, cut them in half and squeeze out the pips, giving a shake to remove some of the watery juice. Put the dryish tomato halves in a small pan with plenty of fresh and dried thyme, a pinch of salt and a good sprinkling of cayenne pepper, and cook, stirring occasionally until all the water has evaporated and you are left with a dryish purée. Let this cool. Meanwhile slice the remaining tomatoes carefully with a sharp knife, sprinkle with salt and leave to drain on a tilted board.

When the purée is cool, spread it over the bottom of your tart and lay the sliced tomatoes, well drained, on top, as if you were making an apple tart. Sprinkle with a few drops of oil, and bake in a quick oven for 12–15 minutes or until the tomatoes are *just* cooked through. Serve hot or cold.

Stuffed mushrooms (serves 2)

½ lb large mushrooms (about 10)	2 cloves garlic
	3 tablespoons oil (olive or sunflower)
½ lemon	
1 large slice brown bread	1 oz pine nuts
2 oz ham	1 oz Parmesan, grated
4 sprigs parsley	pinch of thyme

Stalk the mushrooms, and wipe their outsides with lemon. Reserve the stalks. Make crumbs of the bread, moisten it well with water and squeeze out excess water. Chop the ham, mushroom stalks, parsley and garlic, and mix with the breadcrumbs.

Heat 1 teaspoon of the oil and fry the pine nuts in it until they have browned a little. Add the ham mixture and stir it over the heat for a few minutes. Let it cool a bit, then add the Parmesan, thyme and some pepper. Put the mushroom caps, top down, in a baking tin, heap the stuffing on top, dribble the remaining oil over them and bake at Reg. 4/350°F for 25 minutes. Serve with rice and a green salad or with stuffed tomatoes and a cucumber salad.

Leeks and egg vinaigrette (serves 4)

The main feature of this is the sauce, which can be used in several different dishes, being a very healthy hybrid – half vinaigrette, half mayonnaise – without any of the bad qualities of its parents, as it contains very little oil and no raw egg yolks. Use it with fish salads (together with capers, raw onions, black olives, prawns), with asparagus or with a salad of raw celery, cooked chicken and boiled new potatoes.

If the sauce appears granular you have curdled it, but never mind – rescue it with more mustard and yoghurt.

12–16 small leeks	1 large teaspoon Dijon mustard
2 eggs, hard-boiled and chopped	1 tablespoon wine vinegar
2 spring onions, chopped or a handful of chives, chopped	½ clove garlic, thoroughly crushed
For the salad sauce:	pinch of sugar
3 tablespoons sunflower oil	3 tablespoons plain yoghurt

Split the leeks in half if necessary. Cook them in salted water, drain and cool.

Mix oil, drop by drop, into mustard as if making mayonnaise. Thin with the wine vinegar. Season with garlic, salt, pepper and a tiny pinch of sugar. Stir in the yoghurt.

Arrange the leeks lengthwise on an oval dish. Pile the hard-boiled eggs on top. Pour the dressing over and sprinkle with spring onions or chives.

Brown rice (serves 4)

Brown rice contains natural healthy fibre which is removed from polished white rice.

The whole secret of cooking brown rice is to soak it before cooking. This makes it lighter and helps it to cook more quickly.

Soak ½ lb brown rice in cold water for a minimum of half an hour. Drain and put it into a saucepan with at least 2 pints of salted water. Bring to the boil and simmer for 40–45 minutes. Drain and rinse in warm water.

Brown rice with ratatouille (serves 4)

1 aubergine	½ tin of tomatoes
½ lb brown rice, soaked for 1 hour	thyme
	oregano
2–3 tablespoons oil	rosemary
1 onion, sliced	1 pint chicken stock
1 green pepper, sliced	grated Parmesan cheese
2 cloves garlic, chopped	
2–3 tomatoes, skinned and coarsely chopped	

Cut the aubergine in half lengthwise, then slice across into ¼-inch pieces. Sprinkle with salt if you have time, and let the pieces sit in a colander to drain for 30 minutes.

Drain the rice, rinse and cook in boiling salted water for 40 minutes. Meanwhile heat 2 tablespoons of oil in a frying-pan and fry onions and aubergines for 5 minutes. Add the green peppers, then the garlic and lastly the chopped fresh and the tinned tomatoes. Flavour the mixture with herbs – and let it simmer until just cooked, adding stock to prevent the mixture from becoming too dry.

Put the drained rice, steaming hot, in a hot bowl with a tablespoon of olive oil and a tablespoon of freshly chopped herbs. Mix round, then lightly stir in the vegetables. Serve with grated Parmesan.

If any is left over, mix it with a little garlicky oil and vinegar dressing for a very good salad or it can be reheated quite successfully.

Rice and beans (serves 6)

This is one of those traditional dishes shared by the poor of several countries: Brazil, Turkey and Italy, where this version comes from. The nutritional value of the dish, which the original makers of it can never have known, is increased 43 per cent by the complementary effect of the rice and beans in providing essential amino acids (the constituents of proteins) in the most favourable ratio.

½ lb red kidney beans	1 lb tin of (or 1 lb fresh) tomatoes
¾ lb rice	
3 tablespoons oil (olive or sunflower)	large pinch of thyme
	small sprig of rosemary
2 onions, chopped	large pinch of oregano
2 carrots, chopped	large pinch of cumin
2 sticks of celery, chopped	chopped parsley
2 cloves garlic, finely chopped	4 oz grated Parmesan

First soak the beans overnight. Next day cook them slowly until tender but not bursting, then drain, reserving the cooking liquid. Cook and drain the rice. Heat the oil in a frying-pan and soften the onions, carrots, celery and garlic; then add the tomatoes, herbs and seasoning. Stir the beans into the mixture and cook for at least half an hour, adding bean liquid if it becomes dry. When beans and sauce are nicely married, stir in the rice, heat through and serve sprinkled with parsley and olive oil. Offer the Parmesan separately.

MEAT AND POULTRY

Here we give some recipes for lean meat, game and chicken. They contain a minimal amount of the animal fats that are harmful in quantity. Don't make the mistake of adding butter or cream to game dishes – if you do, you might as well be eating beef so far as benefit to your heart is concerned. Make sure you eat these meat dishes with a generous helping of potatoes or rice, and vegetables to provide carbohydrate, vitamins and roughage.

Pork fillet, stuffed with mushrooms

Of all the pieces of a pig, the fillet is probably the leanest and most tender, but does not, alas, go very far. The stuffing makes it go further, and keeps it moist.

2 oz breadcrumbs, moistened with milk	a squeeze of lemon juice
	2 teaspoons soft margarine
2 oz onion, very finely chopped	*For the gravy*
1 tablespoon oil	juices from the pan, skimmed
2 oz chopped mushrooms, finely chopped	1 glass white wine
	1–2 tablespoons arrowroot
parsley, chopped	¼ pint good stock
½ egg, beaten	2 oz small button mushrooms, quartered
lemon rind, grated	
nutmeg	
1 large pork fillet	

Pre-heat oven to Reg. 5/375°F. Soak the breadcrumbs in milk and squeeze dry. Half soften the chopped onion in half the oil, then stir in mushrooms and cook together gently. Allow to cool. Mix bread, mushrooms, onions and parsley together, bind with half the beaten egg, and flavour with grated lemon rind, parsley, nutmeg and salt and pepper.

Make a cut the length of the fillet and flatten it out. Bang it a little with a rolling-pin, season the inside with salt and pepper, and rub it all over with lemon juice. Spread the stuffing over the centre and enclose it in the pork fillet. Roll it up and tie with string. Rub the outside with soft margarine and cover the top lightly with foil. Put in a small roasting tin with the remaining oil and roast for 45–60 minutes depending on size, removing foil to baste occasionally, and leaving it off for the last 15 minutes to allow the meat to brown.

To make the gravy: put the pork fillet on a dish to keep hot. Skim *all* the fat from the roasting tin. Stir in the white wine and deglaze the pan in the usual way. Dissolve the arrowroot in a little of the stock, add to the pan stock and arrowroot, the mushrooms and seasoning, and simmer for five minutes, adding more liquid if needed.

Serve with boiled new potatoes and vegetables.

APPENDIX ONE/GOOD FOOD

Sautéed pork fillet (serves 4)
This is an excellent way of keeping an otherwise dryish meat, calling out for a rich creamy sauce, juicy and appetizing. It would also work excellently for lean lamb such as you might use for kebabs, or veal.

2 small pork fillets, trimmed and cut into 1-in pieces	4 anchovies, chopped
1 sprig fresh rosemary, very finely chopped	2 cloves garlic, crushed
	juice of ½ lemon
3 tablespoons olive oil	1 glass white wine
1 dried or fresh red chilli (seeds removed), chopped	2 teaspoons wine vinegar

Roll the pork pieces in the rosemary. Heat the oil, add the chillies, anchovies, garlic and pork, and brown the pork. When it is nicely browned, add the lemon juice and white wine (no salt; anchovies are salty).

Cover the pan and simmer for 10 or 15 minutes until the liquid has lost the fresh taste of the wine. Add the vinegar, and simmer uncovered until the liquid gets syrupy. Serve very hot, with rice and a lettuce salad.

Greek chicken and tomato casserole (serves 4–6)
The success of this dish depends on using the rich, fleshy tomatoes that grow in Mediterranean countries. Canned Italian tomatoes make a good substitute.

juice of 1 lemon	6 tomatoes, peeled and chopped
pinch of ground cloves	
½ teaspoon ground cinnamon	2 tablespoons tomato paste
1 large chicken, jointed	1 pint hot water
4 fl oz olive oil	

Mix together the lemon juice, cloves, cinnamon, salt and pepper and rub well into the chicken pieces. Heat the oil in a large saucepan and fry the chicken in it until golden brown.

Lift out and keep hot while you stir the tomatoes and tomato paste into the oil; gradually stir in the hot water and cook over a gentle heat until the tomatoes are mushy and the sauce thick.

Return the chicken pieces to the pan, turn each piece over and over until coated with the sauce and then cover the pan. Cook over a very low heat for about 45 minutes, or until the flesh begins to fall off the bones. Serve with plain boiled rice.

Chicken with mushrooms and black pepper sauce (serves 4)
This chicken dish is for a special occasion, and takes a little trouble; but you will end up with a dish with a succulent sauce which owes nothing to animal fats or cream. Chickens, pigeons, pheasants and partridge can all be cooked in the same way to eliminate all their fat without drying them up.

3 onions, finely chopped	½–¾ lb young fresh mushrooms, chopped (the colour of the dish depends on their being pale around the gills)
1 tablespoon sunflower oil	
1 plump chicken	
½ pint very best stock (preferably made from the carcass of a previous chicken)	
	½ teaspoon black peppercorns, pounded coarsely in a pestle and mortar (mignonette pepper)

Put onions in a flameproof casserole with the sunflower oil. Put on the lid and let the onions soften over a low heat for 10 or 15 minutes. Then put in the whole chicken, nicely seasoned, and pour on the stock. Cover the pot and simmer the chicken until the leg will come away but still shows very faintly pink – about 45 minutes. Now tip the pan and skim off all fat from the juices. Add the mushrooms and cook on for a further 15 minutes or until the chicken is done.

Remove the chicken and skim any remaining fat from the juices before reducing the sauce, mushrooms and all, by fast boiling until it is just becoming slightly syrupy. Meanwhile, peel the skin off the chicken and carve the chicken into joints. Put the pieces on a dish and keep them hot.

Put the sauce in the liquidizer and whizz it to a fine texture, adding a little more chicken stock if necessary to make it light. Stir in half the mignonette pepper, reheat the sauce, pour it over the chicken in its dish and scatter the rest of the pepper over the top.

Kidneys with mushrooms and sherry (serves 4)
Offal is free of fat and, as long as you do not use it as part of a hefty mixed grill, which is bad for an overstressed heart, it is economical and nourishing. This particular dish is the recognizable cousin of a French dish, but is cooked with olive oil instead of butter. Sliced liver is none the worse for being cooked in olive oil either, and will not then need the creamy sauces offered in many Italian restaurants, but British-style braised onion instead.

2 medium tomatoes, very ripe and juicy, chopped	½ lb mushrooms (tiny button mushrooms are best), halved or quartered if large.
1 clove garlic, crushed	
1 lb lambs' kidneys (or other kidneys)	2 tablespoons olive oil
	1 sherry glass of sherry or dry white wine
flour	

Cook the tomatoes with the garlic in a small pan until they have been reduced to a dryish purée. Sieve.

Skin and quarter the kidneys, removing the core with a sharp knife. Roll them very lightly in a little seasoned flour.

Heat the mushrooms in the olive oil, tossing them about until they begin to sweat their juices. (Do not use mushrooms with open black gills as they will darken the sauce too much.) Remove them with a slotted spoon. In the same fat, sauté the kidneys, adding a little more olive oil if necessary. Combine the mushrooms and kidneys, turn up the heat and pour in the sherry or white wine, stirring well for a minute. Lower the heat, add the tomato sauce, stir, cover the pan and leave to simmer for 3–4 minutes. The texture of the dish will depend on the quality of the mushrooms and tomato sauce, but it should not be too dry. If necessary, moisten with a little stock to give plenty of sauce. Serve with plainly cooked rice.

Rabbit sautéed in white wine (serves 4)
Rabbit – like all game – is a very fat-free form of protein, and particularly good in the summer when the bunnies are young and plump. If you do not like rabbit, use a chicken, cut into pieces.

1 rabbit, cut into 6 or 8 pieces	1 wineglass chicken stock
flour	plenty of thyme, savory, oregano
5–6 shallots, finely chopped	
2 tablespoons oil (olive and sunflower mixed)	1 clove garlic
	1 teaspoon Dijon mustard
1 wineglass dry white vermouth	

Sprinkle rabbit pieces very lightly with flour. Soften the shallots in the oil, then add the pieces of rabbit and let them brown. Add the vermouth, chicken stock, herbs, whole clove of garlic, some salt and pepper, and 1 teaspoon mustard.

Simmer uncovered for half an hour, turning the pieces of rabbit from time to time. Add a little more liquid if needed, but there should not be more than half an inch in the bottom of the pan. Simmer until the rabbit is just tender and melting, stir in the remaining mustard and taste the sauce. Serve with potatoes to mop the small amount of delicious sauce, and a green salad.

Jugged hare (serves 6)
Hare has always been considered a very dry meat, needing lots of fatty bacon and butter to lubricate it during cooking. This recipe shows that the use of a marinade and the provision of an accompaniment that is succculent itself, in this case prunes, can provide all the needed juiciness and flavour. Hare, like all game, has a minimum of saturated fat, so eat game rather than other meat whenever you can.

2 wineglasses wine	½ wineglass port
1 tablespoon vinegar	2 tablespoons olive oil
1 hare, cut up	1 lb onions, chopped
1 bay leaf	flour
pinch oregano	¼ pint stock
1 large sprig thyme	1 teaspoon red-current jelly (optional)
6–8 prunes	

Pour the wine and vinegar over the pieces of hare, bury the bay leaf, oregano and thyme in it, and marinate it for 24 hours, turning the meat once. Soak the prunes in the port.

Heat the oil in a wide casserole and stir in the onions. While they are browning, drain the pieces of hare, reserving the marinade; you can pat on a little flour at this stage. Brown the pieces of hare with the onions; when they are nicely browned, pour in the marinade complete with herbs, add the stock, and season with salt and pepper. Simmer covered on top of, or, better, in the oven, until tender – about 2½–3 hours. Retaining the port, drain the prunes and add them about 20 minutes before the end.

Now drain off the juices into a bowl. Skim them, and then if they are very liquid and copious reduce them by about a third. Add the port and, if you like, the red-currant jelly. Bring to the boil and pour the sauce over the pieces of hare, heat through and serve with scalloped potatoes.

Left-over lamb with lentils (serves 6–8)

This dish provides a non-fatty way of stewing lamb, because all the fat is trimmed off before cooking. This trimming actually improves and refines the flavour of the dish, which makes a very good change from shepherd's pie.

1½ lb left-over roast lamb (preferably a leg), cut into 1 by 2 inch pieces	1 lb lentils (the greeny-brown or brown variety)
2 cloves garlic, finely sliced	1 bay leaf
3 tablespoons oil	handful of chopped parsley (preferably the 'flat' type)
1 small onion, finely chopped	3 spring onions, chopped
1 pint stock	handful of chopped marjoram

Pre-heat oven to Reg. 4/350°F. Season the pieces of lamb well with fresh-ground pepper, make incisions here and there in the meat and insert slices of garlic. Fry in hot oil in a saucepan. Drain thoroughly when well browned, and keep on one side. Season with salt.

In the same oil, fry the onion until transparent but not brown. Add the stock and put in lentils, lamb, bay leaf, salt and pepper. Cover the pan and simmer until the lentils are tender and have absorbed the stock. Now stir in the parsley, spring onions and marjoram and, if you like, sprinkle very lightly with olive oil. Serve very hot.

Meat with raisins and almonds (serves 4)

You can use this mixture to stuff green peppers and other vegetables and as an appetizing filling for pancakes.

2 tablespoons olive oil or lard	1 lb tomatoes, skinned and chopped
1½ lb lean minced (ground) beef	2 oz raisins
1 medium onion, chopped	2 oz chopped almonds or walnuts
1 clove garlic, chopped	

Heat the oil in a frying pan and brown the meat. Add the onion and garlic and cook until soft. Add the tomatoes, raisins, and some salt and pepper. Simmer for 20 minutes, stirring occasionally. Stir in the nuts.

As a main course, serve with plain white rice, followed by a mixed salad.

FISH

Fish is a good source of protein and minerals such as iodine, as well as supplying the lightest oil which is kindest to the heart. If we ate fish instead of meat as the Japanese do, then heart disease in this country would fall dramatically.

Baked fish with tomato and green pepper (serves 4)

Fried fish is delicious, but the traditional fried fish and chips is very heavy on fat. More people would bake fish if it did not turn out so tasteless; it is one thing to be healthy, another to eat like an invalid. This recipe is suitable for most white fish, but vary cooking times from short (cod, haddock, hake and soft-fleshed fish) to slightly longer for denser-fleshed fish like mullet and bream; about 20 minutes for the haddock and 30 minutes for bream, in a moderately low oven (Reg. 3/325°F).

about 2 lb white fish	1 large tomato (or 2 medium), skinned and chopped
½ small green pepper finely chopped	thyme, oregano or bay leaf
1 small onion, finely chopped	half a glass of dry white wine
olive oil	

With a sharp knife, slit the belly of the fish and remove innards if the fishmonger has not done so. Wash under cold tap. Chop off head and tail (good for a quick fish stock, so do not throw it away yet). With your most delicate knife, follow the line of the bone down each side, easing the flesh gently away from the bone. Lay the fish out on its back, two white sides lying uppermost. (The bone can go in your stock with a bit of onion-peeling and thyme, the basis of a tasty fish soup.)

Gently fry the green pepper and onion in a little olive oil until they soften. Blend in the tomatoes. Butter an ovenproof dish, lay the fish in it, and smother with mixture. Add a scattering of thyme, oregano or bay leaf. Add a tablespoon of olive oil, dripped on, and the wine.

Cover loosely with foil and bake in moderate to low oven for 20 minutes (haddock, etc.) or about 30 minutes (bream, etc.). The wine keeps the fish moist and preserves the flavours of the green pepper and onion.

Soused herring or mackerel (serves 4)

Herring and mackerel are oily fish and to fry them is to increase the fat level; but if your aim is to push down the fat-intake, this is an easy and delightful way of cooking these fish and they can be cooked the night or even the day before.

4 small herrings or 2 medium mackerel	½ lemon, cut in slices across
1 medium onion, finely sliced in rings	1 bay leaf
	½ pint wine vinegar
12 black peppercorns, coarsely crushed, or 1 chopped fresh green chilli	½ pint water

Ask the fishmonger to clean the fish and open it to make boned fillets – or do it yourself. Cut off heads, removing guts with head. Slice against the side of the backbone with a sharp knife to cut the fish in half. Then lay fish horizontal on a board, place hand flat on top and cut through the other side of the backbone. Peel away the bone. Place the fish flat on an ovenproof or earthenware baking dish so that they fit fairly closely. Scatter the onions over. Add the peppercorns or chilli, lemon and bay leaf. Cover with the vinegar and water.

Bake in a moderate oven, Reg. 4/350°F, for at least 12–15 minutes, when the flesh will be firm; then allow to cool in the juice. Serve next day or after a day or two in the juices, which gradually penetrate and flavour the whole fish, and mop up with plenty of wholemeal bread.

Grilled herring with mustard sauce (serves 2)

By grilling oily fish, you are using its own natural oils to provide the necessary lubrication. Herrings and mustard, a well-tried combination, makes a good simple lunch.

2 plump herrings	2 tablespoons water
a little sunflower oil	2 tablespoons ricotta or curd cheese
For the sauce:	
2 teaspoons Dijon or English made mustard	a handful of freshly chopped parsley, chives, tarragon and chervil

Ask the fishmonger to split and bone the herring, so that they are flat and open like boned kippers. Place on a foil-covered grill pan, skin-side down, and brush very lightly with oil to start them off. Season with salt and pepper. Place under a hot grill for 3 minutes, then turn and cook for 3 minutes more.

While the fish are grilling, mix all the sauce ingredients in a saucepan and heat gently; do not boil. If the sauce is not smooth it can be blended in a liquidizer.

Serve the sauce warm and the herrings piping hot. Scalloped potatoes are good with this dish.

APPENDIX ONE/GOOD FOOD

Kedgeree (serves 4)
As kedgeree is excellent for breakfast as well as making a lovely supper or lunch, the amount of spices to use has been left fairly open. Use a pinch of each for a breakfast dish, at least ¼ teaspoon or more for other meals.

1 smoked haddock	pinch of cinnamon
1 pint milk and water, mixed half and half	pinch of garam masala
	pinch of ginger
parsley stalks	pinch of turmeric
1 bay leaf	½ oz flour
6 oz long-grained rice	2 eggs, hard boiled and chopped
1 oz soft margarine	
pinch of coriander	a handful of chopped parsley
pinch of cumin	

Poach the smoked haddock in a moderate oven, in the milk and water flavoured with a few parsley stalks and a bay leaf. Cook the rice, having first washed it in cold water.

Melt the margarine and fry the spices, using as much or as little as you like – a subtle flavour is obtained by using no more than the tip of a teaspoon of each.

Add the flour and stir, then add enough of the haddock cooking liquid to make a thin creamy sauce.

Flake the fish and remove bones, and mix together with the rice and chopped eggs. Add enough of the sauce to obtain a creamy mixture. Stir in a handful of chopped parsley. Add salt, if needed, and serve very hot.

Prawn and cauliflower salad (serves 3–4)
Instead of eating a whole plateful of prawns, it is just as good to make them into a salad with a vegetable, such as courgettes, potatoes, or in this case cauliflower.

1 cauliflower	pinch of sugar
½–¼ lb prawns in shells	red chilli powder or finely crumbled red chilli
For the dressing:	
3–4 tablespoons sunflower oil	1 tablespoon sprigs of dill weed
1 tablespoon fresh lemon juice	1 tablespoon coarsely chopped spring onions or green onion tops
1 clove garlic, crushed	

Cook and cool the cauliflower, then break into florets. Shell the prawns, leaving two or three whole to decorate the salad. Make a dressing with sunflower oil, lemon juice, crushed garlic, sugar and salt and red chilli powder or finely crumbled red chilli.

Arrange the cauliflower sprigs in a dish. Cover with prawns. Sprinkle the dill over the top, and also the green onion tops or spring onions. Now pour on the dressing and place the whole prawns on the top.

Mussels (serves 4)
Mussels are not only good fat-free protein, but they are also tasty and comparatively inexpensive. Many classic French recipes call for the use of thick cream to carry the flavours of the juices, but the Belgian national dish is a bowl of plainly cooked mussels (accompanied by a heart-rending amount of finely cut crisp chips). The same style of plain cooking, mopping up the juices with the wholemeal bread, is deeply satisfying. For a first course for four (double amounts for a main course) you need:

2 lb of mussels, washed (discarding floaters and broken shells)	1 onion (or two small shallots), finely chopped
	sprig of parsley, chopped
1 tablespoon olive oil	sprig of thyme
1 glass dry white wine	juice of half a lemon
the white of a small leek, chopped	

Put the washed and bearded mussels in a heavy-bottomed pan, and cover with oil, white wine, leek, onion or shallots, parsley and thyme. Squeeze the lemon juice on top.

Put over a steady heat, with the lid on tightly, and cook until mussels open and are cooked (about 7–10 minutes). You can serve them as they are, shells and soup together, with wholemeal bread, and plenty of black pepper (no salt), leaving each person to undo the shells themselves. Dip the bread into the juices.

MIXED DISHES

In these dishes meat or fish is mixed with beans, grains or vegetables to produce a delicious, economical and healthy combination.

Moussaka (serves 4)
Many British cookbooks take dishes like moussaka and bastardize them, enriching the white sauce with cream and eggs, letting the lamb sizzle in its rich fat, even cooking the aubergines in butter. Wrong, all wrong. The secret of our recipe is in its simplicity; no animal fat, all olive oil. It should be cooked in a deep squarish tin, like a bread tin.

1 medium aubergine, thinly sliced, leave skin on	or tomato purée
	sprig of thyme
1 medium onion, finely chopped	*For the white sauce:*
1–2 tablespoons olive oil	1 oz soft margarine
½ lb leg of lamb, cut free of fat and minced or finely chopped	1 oz flour
	½ pint milk
	1 egg yolk (optional)
1 lb cheap tomatoes, chopped	a little grated cheese

If you wish to remove the bitter flavour of the aubergine, sprinkle it with salt, stand the slices in a colander with a weighted plate on top, and let them drain for 30 minutes. Then wash free of salt, and mop dry.

Lightly fry the onion in the oil and remove from the pan. Fry the lamb and finally the aubergine slices, a few at a time.

Make a tomato sauce by simmering the tomatoes for 10 minutes, adding thyme and seasoning, and straining through a sieve.

Make a white sauce, melting soft margarine into a pan, stirring in the flour, and adding as you stir half a pint of boiling milk (skimmed, if you are being rigorous) until it thickens. Leave to cool. If you have not had eggs the same day, add a beaten egg yolk to improve texture – it makes it more custardy.

Line the dish bottom and side with the aubergine slices. Put on the layer of minced lamb. Cover with chicken stock. Smother with the fried onions. Then add a layer of tomato sauce. Finally, pour on the white sauce. Dust with a little grated cheese. Bake in a moderate oven (Reg. 4/350°F) for 30–50 minutes, until top is golden.

Risotto alla rustica (serves 4–6)
How much meat to use for this dish has always depended on the state of the housekeeping money, but in its original Italian days the amount would have been no more than 4 oz or so, just a flavouring for the rice. It is still quite healthy to use ¾ lb beef for four to six people but it is perhaps preferable to use less.

2 tablespoons of oil (olive or sunflower)	1 small glass red wine
	12oz Italian rice, washed thoroughly
1 large or 2 small onions, chopped	14 oz tin tomatoes
1 small slice of ham, chopped	1 dessertspoon tomato purée
2 carrots and 2 sticks of celery, cut into small chunks *or* 4 oz mushrooms, cut in quarters	1–1¼ pints stock
	thyme and oregano
	grated Parmesan
¾ lb minced beef	1 oz dried mushrooms (optional)
2 cloves garlic, chopped	

Heat the oil and fry the onions, chopped ham and the carrots and celery (if you are using these). Add the meat, stir and brown. Add the garlic cloves and the mushrooms (if you are using them). Pour in the wine to scrape up the brown crust from the bottom of the pan. Let it evaporate.

Add the rice to the meat. Let it fry for a minute or two, then add the tin of tomatoes and tomato purée and half the stock. Season and add the herbs. Simmer until the rice is tender, stirring and adding more stock as it is absorbed. Serve with the grated Parmesan.

If you can obtain them, soak 1 oz of dried mushrooms (*ceps* or *porcini*) in warm water for half an hour. Add them, chopped, with the onions and use the soaking liquid with the stock.

Chilli con carne (serves 4)

Here is another example of stretching a small amount of meat a long way; the meat gives body and flavour to the beans, which are the main and really filling part of the dish.

1 lb red kidney beans, soaked overnight	marjoram
2 onions, finely chopped	½ teaspoon dried thyme
1–2 tablespoons sunflower oil	pinch of cumin seeds
½ lb minced beef	14 oz tin tomatoes
2 cloves garlic, crushed	1 tablespoon tomato purée
1 teaspoon dried oregano or	about ¼ pint stock

Put the soaked kidney beans in a pan of cold water, bring to the boil and simmer until just tender. Fry the onions gently in the sunflower oil until they are becoming translucent, then turn up the heat and add the mince. Stir it round, breaking it up with a wooden fork or spoon. When it is frying well, leave it alone so it can start to brown. Add the garlic, herbs and spices, and continue frying. When the meat is browning nicely, add the tomatoes, tomato purée, seasoning and stock. Bring to simmering point, transfer the beans to the meat, and retain their cooking liquid. As the bean and beef mixture becomes somewhat dry, add cooking liquid from the beans in small quantities to keep it just moist. Simmer for 1½ hours. Serve with rice.

Beef stew with beans, peas and rice (serves 4)

A hearty one-dish meal blending a variety of tastes and colours. This recipe, from Trinidad, uses dried beans (or peas) to add vegetable protein to the meats, and the rice absorbs all the flavours.

6 oz dried red kidney beans or dried pigeon peas	2 tomatoes, skinned, deseeded and chopped
small smoked ham hock (shank)	1 green pepper, deseeded and chopped
1 lb stewing beef, cut into 1-in cubes	1 fresh green chilli pepper, deseeded and chopped
1 teaspoon crushed garlic	2 onions, coarsely chopped
½ teaspoon ground cloves	9 oz long grain rice.
2 tablespoons oil	
about 1 pint chicken or beef stock	

Soak the beans and the ham separately overnight in enough cold water to cover.

Next day, drain the ham, cut off the meat and divide it into 1-in pieces. Mix with the beef, and sprinkle on the garlic and cloves and 1 teaspoon of salt.

Heat the oil in a heavy, flameproof casserole and sauté the meats until browned all over. Drain the beans and add to the casserole. Pour on enough hot water to cover, then put on the lid and simmer until tender; this will take 1½–2½ hours depending on the type of beef used. Add a little hot water from time to time if necessary.

Pour off the liquid, measure it and make it up to 1¼ pints with the stock. Pour it back into the casserole and add the tomatoes, green pepper, chilli pepper, onions and rice. Bring to the boil, then reduce the heat, cover and cook very slowly until the rice is tender and all the liquid absorbed.

Serve very hot with mango chutney to make a satisfying lunch.

Pickled gammon with haricots (serves 4)

Haricots are often served with fatty meat like lamb or pork because they mop up the fat. Like most pulses, they are extremely rich in protein, and deserve a better fate. In this modest recipe gammon is used, and the fat removed with the skin after baking in the oven. This dish is nourishing, filling and no threat to the heart.

¾ lb haricot beans	1 lb tomatoes, skinned and chopped, or tin of tomatoes (optional)
½ lb knuckle of gammon or ham bone with some ham on it	

Soak the beans overnight. In separate bowl, soak gammon overnight to draw out some of the saltiness. Strain beans and gammon. Put the gammon in the centre of the beans. Cover with fresh water. Add tomatoes, if desired.

Bake with cover on for 3–4 hours until beans are tender (this depends on the beans' quality) at moderately low heat, about Reg. 4/350°. Remove gammon, which should be tender by now, strip off fat and skin. Return the meat, shredded slightly, to the beans. Serve with fresh vegetables.

Don Luis de Soto's paella (serves 6–8)

This paella is the very complicated and splendid version from the cool kitchen of a Seville olive grower and producer. It should ideally be cooked in a wide, flat paella pan, but an extra-large frying-pan, or even an oven dish would do.

1 lb uncooked pork (blade is best), cut into ¾-inch cubes	4 good pinches of saffron stamens
1 lb uncooked chicken pieces on the bone	1¼ lb long-grain rice
3–4 tablespoons olive oil	4 oz shelled prawns
1 onion, chopped	4 oz shelled peas (frozen will do)
1 bay leaf	12 whole prawns
2 cloves garlic, chopped	1 pint mussels, cooked (use strained liquid for stock)
½ lb raw squid, cut in rings	1 red pepper, cut into chunks
½ lb tomatoes, skinned, seeded and coarsely chopped	12 Spanish stuffed green olives slices of lemon
2 pints of fish or chicken stock	

Brown the pork and chicken in olive oil on all sides in a paella pan, then let the meat cook more gently for about 20 minutes. Add the onion, bay leaf, garlic, squid, tomatoes and the stock in which you have soaked the saffron. Bring to the boil, season with up to 2 level teaspoons salt and ground black pepper, then stir in the rice. Add the peas, cover the pan and let the paella cook in the oven at Reg. 4/350°F for 20 minutes.

Place the prawns and mussels in the half-shell on top, and dot with a few chunks of red pepper and the green olives. Cover the pan again and cook for a further 15–25 minutes until the rice is tender and the stock almost absorbed. Remove the bay leaf. Serve with a slice of lemon on each plate.

PASTA DISHES

In Europe and the Middle East wheat has long been the basic foodstuff. It is of course most familiar to us as bread, but in the form of pasta it is even more versatile. Pasta can be combined with meat, cheese or vegetables in many forms to make a well-balanced dish. It can now be bought ready-made from wholemeal flour – trendy health-conscious Italians have been eating this for some time. Or you can make it yourself, from the recipe that follows.

Classic Noodles (serves 4)

In Italy, most families make their own pasta. British families do not yet know it is quicker – and much more satisfying – to make their own than go out to the shops, buy a packet and bring it home. You do use an egg in making noodles, to bind the flour, but it is a very moderate use of egg. The recipe is brief and to the point: skill in rolling out comes with practice. As for cooking, it is as quick as boiling an egg.

1 lb strong flour	water to moisten
1 egg, beaten	

On a pastry board, make a heap of the flour. Add a little salt. Make a well in the middle, and pour in the beaten egg. Stir with a wooden spoon until it is a pliable mass, then knead it, moistening if necessary with a teaspoon or two of water. Roll into ball. Leave in cool place to settle for half an hour. The fridge will do.

Dust the pastry board with flour, flatten ball, and roll out backwards and forwards, and from side to side. Turn pastry over and continue. Keep on rolling and dusting the pastry board, until dough is thin. If your pastry board is not big enough, you will have to cut the piece in two and carry on rolling.

Cut the rolled-out dough into long thin strips, and loop them over a string 'clothes-line' to dry for 20 minutes or so – longer if you like, but use fresh pasta the same day.

To cook the strips of pasta, drop them, a handful at a time, into a large pan of boiling salted water. They will drop to the bottom. In less than 5 minutes they will rise to the surface, when they are done. Serve with one of the sauces for pasta recommended below, or with olive oil, finely chopped garlic and plain tomato sauce. You should be careful how much cheese you use, but a sprinkling of Parmesan is all right, because 1 oz goes such a long way.

Brown noodles (serves 4)
Noodles can also be made with brown or wholemeal flour; a very good one to use is Prewett's strong brown flour, which contains 90 per cent of the whole wheat.

12 oz strong brown or wholemeal flour	4 tablespoons cold water
2 eggs, beaten	1 teaspoon oil

Mix the ingredients together as in the previous recipe, adding a good pinch of salt, but note that the secret of these noodles is to keep the dough very dry. If it is really too dry to be workable, add more water, but only a teaspoon at a time, and work it in with your hands. You can knead the dough as much as you like, until it binds together smoothly. Work it well, smooth the oil over the surface, and let it rest for 20 minutes wrapped in foil.

Then cut off a piece about the size of a large matchbox and roll it into a long strip as thin as you can make it. Roll it up into a cigar shape, and cut it into strips about ¼-inch wide. These will unroll into nice long noodles. Let them dry for a few minutes, or until you need them, and then drop them into boiling salted water and cook until tender – about 20 minutes. Serve in the usual way.

Spaghetti Bolognese (serves 6)
The amount of sauce to spaghetti is important. In Italy, the sauce would be used just to moisten the pasta, and would be mixed into it in the bowl before being served. The huge dollop of sauce in the middle of a small plate of pasta is a restaurant trick. When less sauce is used, the pasta itself must be very carefully cooked.

2 carrots	1 small glass of red wine
2 sticks of celery	1 lb tin plus 1 small tin (20 oz) tomatoes
2 medium onions	
1 clove of garlic (or more, to taste)	large sprig of thyme
	large pinch of oregano
2 tablespoons olive oil	1 bay leaf
4 oz minced pork	1 tablespoon tomato purée
4 oz minced veal or beef	1 pint of stock
2 chicken livers, finely chopped	

Chop carrots, celery, onions and garlic very finely and soften in oil, stirring occasionally. Turn up heat, add the meats (except for chicken livers), stir and then let the mixture brown over moderate heat. Add chicken livers and wine, and boil until liquid has all but evaporated. Add tomatoes, herbs, salt and pepper, and purée. Simmer 1½ hours, adding stock as necessary. Cover pan for beginning of cooking.

Tomato sauce for pasta (serves 4–6)
This is designed to cut down drastically on the amount of oil and butter, which would usually be added both at the beginning and again at the end. It comes from Padua, where certain people are becoming exceedingly health conscious, mainly to the end of looking youthful on the Sardinian beaches. In fact the traditional tomato sauce comes from southern Italy, where butter would never be used and where there is also very little heart disease. Make this one of your staple meals.

1½ lb tomatoes, skinned	1 stick of celery
1 onion	1 tablespoon olive oil
2 cloves garlic	basil or marjoram (fresh if possible)
1 carrot	

Chop all ingredients, except the basil, and put them into a pan. Add salt and pepper. Stew, until carrots and celery are tender. Purée by putting in the liquidizer or through the blade of a Moulin-légumes. Reheat, adding oil and a handful of basil torn up small.

Gnocchi (serves 4)
This dish, in which the ham is used to flavour the gnocchi rather than to provide sustenance, is meltingly light and surprisingly rich considering the restraint of the ingredients.

¾ pint water mixed with ¼ pint milk	2 oz Parmesan, grated
	2 slices of ham, finely chopped
1 onion, peeled	few sprigs of parsley, finely chopped
1 bay leaf	
nutmeg	1 tablespoon sunflower oil
4 oz semolina	

Bring the pint of water and milk to the boil with the whole onion, bay leaf, nutmeg, salt and pepper. Let it boil for 5 minutes, then remove onion and bay leaf and sprinkle in the semolina, stirring constantly until it thickens. Cook, stirring, over a very low heat, for 5 minutes. Then remove from heat, add half the grated Parmesan and the chopped ham and parsley. Mix in well.

Oil a large flat plate, and spoon the mixture, spreading it out to an even thickness of about ½-inch with oiled hands – it is hot, so do it carefully. Allow to cool, cut into squares, and lay them overlapping in an ovenproof dish. Sprinkle with oil and the remaining cheese, and brown under the grill until heated through and crisp – about 10 minutes. Do not allow the gnocchi to boil or they will disintegrate. Serve hot with tomato sauce (see above) and the remaining Parmesan.

Eat with a mixed green salad – lettuce, endive, fennel and cucumber.

Catalonian macaroni (serves 4)
Pasta, so firmly associated with Italy, is eaten frequently in Spain, too. It is added to soups and stews or combined with mixed vegetables to make a nourishing main dish. You can replace the peas, beans, courgettes and aubergine with any vegetables in season. Grate goat's milk cheese on top for the authentic Spanish dish.

4 oz shelled peas	deseeded and chopped
4 oz shelled broad beans or large lima beans	6 tomatoes, peeled and chopped
2 courgettes, sliced	1 tablespoon almonds, peeled and toasted
1 small aubergine, sliced	
1 lb macaroni	1 tablespoon pine nuts
olive oil for frying	2 tablespoons chopped parsley
2 onions, chopped	3 tablespoons grated cheese
2 cloves garlic, peeled and chopped	
1 red or green pepper,	

Put the peas, beans, courgettes and aubergine (or other chosen mixed vegetables) to boil in a little salted water for 8–10 minutes, or until just tender. Drain and set aside, reserving the liquid. Meanwhile, in another pan, boil the macaroni in plenty of lightly salted water for 10 minutes or until tender, and then drain.

Heat a little olive oil in a flameproof casserole and gently fry the onion, garlic and pepper. When they start to soften, add the tomatoes and the cooked mixed vegetables and stir well. Cook gently for a few minutes, then add the almonds, pine nuts and parsley. Stir in some of the reserved cooking liquid to make a thick sauce.

Put the cooked macaroni into this sauce, stir well and season to taste with salt and ground black pepper. Sprinkle the top with the cheese and a little more black pepper. Brown the top under the grill or in a pre-heated oven at Reg. 6/400°F.

Serve straight from the casserole accompanied by a green salad, bread and wine.

EGG DISHES

The healthy way to eat eggs is with vegetables or as garnishes on other dishes. In this way their taste is enhanced, the heaviness dissipated, and the colour used to good effect. Eggs cooked like this go a long way – a Spanish omelette made from three eggs, will, for example, feed four people.

Spanish omelette (*Tortilla*) (serves 4)

This favourite family dish provides a perfectly balanced meal: the plainness of the potatoes complements the richness of the eggs, and the onion provides flavour.

| 6 tablespoons olive oil | 2 large potatoes, diced |
| 2 large onions, peeled and diced | 3 eggs |

Heat the oil in a frying pan without letting it smoke. Stir in the vegetables, mixing them well together and turning them in the oil with a wooden spatula. Sprinkle on ½ teaspoon salt and cover the pan with a lid. Cook very gently for about 15 minutes, turning often so that they do not brown or stick to the pan.

Beat the eggs in a large bowl. When the vegetables are tender, remove the pan from the heat and lift the vegetables carefully with a slotted spoon into the egg mixture, leaving as much oil as possible in the pan. Stir the mixture quickly.

Make sure there are no bits sticking in the pan and return it to the heat. When the oil starts to smoke, pour in the mixture. Flatten it down evenly right to the edges of the pan and shake to settle the mixture and prevent sticking. Cook over a medium heat for about 5 minutes, shaking often until the mixture sets and begins to shrink from the sides of the pan.

You can cook the top most easily by putting the pan under a hot grill for a few minutes until the *tortilla* is golden brown. Spanish cooks invert a plate over the pan, turn out the *tortilla*, then slide it back from the plate into the pan to cook the other side.

The finished *tortilla* should be like a solid, flat cake. It is good eaten hot or cold. Add other vegetables, such as peas, beans or green peppers, for variation. A tomato and onion salad goes well with a *tortilla*.

Scrambled eggs with sweet peppers (serves 4–6)

This makes a filling lunch dish – as a first course for dinner it would serve six.

2 large onions (preferably Spanish), sliced	1 lb sweet, ripe tomatoes, peeled and chopped
3–4 tablespoons olive oil	pinch of sugar (optional)
2 red peppers, deseeded and sliced thinly	6 eggs

Gently cook the onions in the oil in a heavy pan. After about 15 minutes when they are soft but not browned, add the peppers and simmer until they are tender; it should take about 10 minutes. Add the tomatoes and season with salt and pepper and the sugar if you wish. Let this stew simmer until it thickens.

Now take the pan off the heat. Beat the eggs in a bowl and stir them into the vegetables with a wooden spoon. Put the pan on a gentle heat and keep stirring until the eggs become creamy. Do not overcook or the eggs will separate. Serve at once with plenty of bread.

You can use one red pepper and one green for extra colour, and add two crushed cloves of garlic for a stronger flavour.

SALADS

An imaginative salad eaten with wholemeal bread makes a delicious and satisfying meal in itself – or salad can be served with cold meats or a Spanish omelette (see above).

Green bean salad (serves 4)

Serve this summer salad with ham or cold meats and potato salad for lunch or a light supper.

| 1 lb French (snap) beans | garlic to taste, crushed |
| 3 tablespoons olive oil | 1 tablespoon lemon juice |

Boil the beans in salted water until just tender, then drain and put into a salad bowl. Add the oil mixed with the crushed garlic and stir well before adding the lemon juice and seasoning lightly with salt and pepper.

You can vary the salad by including a little peeled and chopped tomato or finely chopped spring onion or scallions, or both.

Cabbage salad (Serves 8)

This traditional Greek combination of beans with cabbage provides iron in a readily digestible form.

1½ lb white cabbage, shredded	3 tablespoons lemon juice or mild wine vinegar
8 oz haricot beans, cooked or canned	8 black olives
4 tablespoons olive oil	

Put the cabbage and beans into a deep bowl and mix well together. Combine the oil and lemon juice with salt and pepper to taste, blend well and pour it over the vegetables. Turn the salad over and over so that it is well coated with dressing. Garnish with the olives.

Cucumber and yoghurt salad (serves 4)

A light salad, scented and flavoured with mint, which makes a refreshing first course at lunch.

1 large cucumber or 2 small ones peeled and diced	1 tablespoon crushed dried mint, or 2 tablespoons finely chopped fresh mint
2–3 cloves garlic, or more to taste	dried mint for garnish
1 pint yoghurt	

Sprinkle the cucumber lightly with salt and leave in a colander to drain for 30 minutes. Peel the garlic and crush with a little salt. Mix a few tablespoons of the yoghurt with the garlic, then add the mixture to the rest of the yoghurt and mix well. Add more salt and pepper to taste. Finally add the mint, whose aroma and flavour make the salad deliciously refreshing.

Drain the cucumber and mix with the yoghurt dressing. Pour into the serving dish and decorate with more mint.

Tomato and pepper salad (serves 4)

Leave the peppers raw in this salad if you wish, but many people find them more digestible when grilled in this way – and they are certainly deliciously soft and mellow.

2 green peppers	leaves, chopped, or small bunch of parsley, finely chopped
4 firm tomatoes, sliced	
½ Spanish onion, finely chopped, or 6 spring onions (scallions), finely chopped	4 tablespoons olive oil
small bunch of fresh coriander	1–2 tablespoons wine vinegar

Spear the peppers with a fork and turn them over a flame, or turn them under a grill, until they are soft and the skin has blistered all over. Peel off the skin and remove any charred parts under a running tap. Remove the stalks and seeds and cut the flesh into ribbons.

Put them in a serving bowl with the tomatoes, onions and coriander. Season with salt and pepper, pour on the oil and vinegar and toss well. Increase the amounts of oil and vinegar, in the given proportions, if you wish.

Serve as a first course at lunch, with bread to mop up the juices.

APPENDIX ONE/GOOD FOOD

Fresh vegetable salad from Sicily (serves 4)
A simple light lunch for a summer's day. Serve it on its own or with salami.

4 oz freshly cooked green beans	1 cucumber, sliced
2–3 ripe tomatoes, sliced	2–3 oz black olives
2 boiled new potatoes, sliced	5 tablespoons olive oil
	1 tablespoon wine vinegar

Arrange the beans, tomatoes, potatoes, cucumber and black olives in separate piles on a large flat dish. Season with coarse salt and plenty of very coarsely ground black pepper. Sprinkle with the olive oil and vinegar, and serve with bread.

DESSERTS

Desserts do not need to use a lot of sugar and cream to be delicious in flavour. Here we give some recipes which are naturally sweet from the fruit itself. As an exception to the rule we include a recipe for sorbet which does use quite a lot of sugar – but the fruit is all fresh and it is an alternative to that ever-so-unhealthy ice-cream. If you like, use natural yoghurt (see below for recipe) with desserts instead of cream to provide another texture and carry the flavour.

Yoghurt
Since yoghurt can often be used as a substitute for eggs and cream in the thickening of sauces, apart from being an extremely good food in its own right, it is useful to be able to make it at home in quantity. The secret is in nursing the right bacteria at the right temperature, so that they, and they alone, form a culture which sours and thickens the yoghurt to the right flavour and consistency.

To make a pint of yoghurt, the simplest and most primitive method of all is to bring 1 pint of milk to the boil and let it cool until you can keep your finger in it for a count of ten (about 120°F.). If the milk is sterilized, however, then this is not necessary, and you may even use such milk straight from the fridge, although it may then take longer. Mix it in a bowl with 1 tablespoon of plain yoghurt, either from a shop or from a previous batch, and stand the bowl, covered with a folded towel, in a warm place. The place you choose should have a steady temperature – an airing cupboard, warm radiator or over a pilot-light will do perfectly. To get a low-fat yoghurt, use skimmed milk and, if you like, thicken it by stirring in 2–3 tablespoons of dried milk powder per pint before heating it to make the yoghurt. Vary the amount of added powder and make it as thick as you wish. You can make yoghurt from reconstituted powder. A controlled yoghurt-maker may help but it is not really necessary. If you do not want to keep your yoghurt going constantly, you can deep-freeze two tablespoonfuls in a plastic container and use it to start off the next batch whenever you like.

Dried fruit salad with green ginger (serves 4)
Prunes, as we all know, are high on roughage, but what is sometimes overlooked is that they have a really wonderful and luxurious flavour. If you do not want to make custard, mix plain yoghurt with a little honey as an alternative.

1 lb prunes	1 oz fresh ginger (or preserved ginger if fresh unavailable), peeled and sliced
½ lb dried apricots	
2 oz sugar	

Make at least 2 days ahead. Soak the prunes and apricots separately in cold water, for about 12 hours or overnight. When they are soft, put them in a saucepan with sugar and the prune water, strained if necessary. Add the ginger to the fruits, bring to the boil and simmer until the fruit is tender – about 1 hour. Allow to cool, and transfer to a china bowl. Let it sit and steep for at least a day, before serving with or without thin custard.

To make an even more exotic dish, replace the ginger with an inch or two of vanilla pod, and add 2 oz of walnuts after cooking, but while the fruit is still hot. Just before serving, sharpen the juices with lemon juice. Sprinkle pomegranate seeds over the top and serve very chilled.

Prune soufflé (serves 4)

½ pint cider	4 egg whites
2 inch stick of cinnamon	pinch of cream of tartar
½ lb prunes	1 teaspoon poppy seeds

Boil the cider for five minutes with the cinnamon stick. Pour it over the prunes in a bowl and leave to soak overnight. When they are soaked, put them in a pan, cider and all, and simmer until tender. Allow to cool a little, remove the stones from the prunes and put the pulp through the fine blade of a Moulin-légumes, adding enough of the liquid to make a nice thick purée.

Beat the egg whites with the cream of tartar until you have a fairly firm snow. Mix a few tablespoons into the prune purée, then fold the purée into the egg whites with the poppy seeds. Put the mixture into an oiled soufflé dish or charlotte tin and cook in a hot oven, Reg. 7/425°F, for 15–20 minutes. Serve immediately.

Lemon, grapefruit and orange sorbet (serves 4–6)
Any sorbet which uses fresh fruit as a base, and which is free of eggs and cream, makes a clean refreshing ending to a summer meal. This citrus-fruit one can be made in the winter, too. To make a raspberry or blackcurrant sorbet, replace the lemon, grapefruit and orange juice with a pint of fresh fruit purée, having first made the syrup with the lemon peel as before. If the mixture tastes too sweet or bland, sharpen with a little lemon juice.

2 lemons	1 grapefruit
6 oz sugar	2 oranges
1 pint water	1 egg white

Pare the rind from the lemons. Put it in a pan with the sugar and cold water, and bring to the boil. Boil for five minutes, then allow to cool. Strain the cold syrup. Squeeze the juice of the lemons, grapefruit and oranges and mix it with the cold syrup (thus retaining all the vitamins). Pour the mixture into a container, and freeze to a crystalline mush. Break up the crystals thoroughly in the liquidizer, stir in the white of egg, whisked to a soft snow, and refreeze.

Thick rice pudding (serves 6)

2 pints milk	(cornstarch)
5 oz short grain rice	5 oz sugar
2–3 strips lemon rind	ground cinnamon
2 teaspoons cornflour	

Pour the milk into a heavy saucepan with the rice and lemon rind. Stir well and then cook over a gentle heat for about 30 minutes, or until the rice is soft. Mix the cornflour into the sugar, spreading it evenly to avoid lumps when cooking, and stir into the rice. Continue cooking gently for a further 20–30 minutes until the pudding is like very thick cream. Stir from time to time to prevent sticking. Cool slightly, discard the lemon rind and spoon the rice into shallow individual glass bowls. Set aside until cooled to room temperature and covered with a skin. Never serve the pudding hot. Put the cinnamon in a salt shaker and sprinkle over the puddings to make a face or pattern on each.

BAKING

Most cakes are sweeter than need be and commercially produced cakes generally use hard fats for shortening which are bad for the heart. Furthermore they are not made with wholemeal flour. In this section we give recipes for cakes which are much healthier because they use soft margarine, less sugar and wholemeal flour.

There are also many more exciting ways of eating bread – as pizza, or pitta, or with various savoury spreads which you can make yourself. Bread is a good source of protein as well as energy. It is difficult to eat too much of it. If you are putting on too much weight you are probably eating too much of something else. If you get bored with bread sometimes, try making tortillas (see below for recipe) and experiment with delicious fillings.

Good Food / Appendix One

Pastry without butter

Even people who have always liked to use butter in their pastry because of the good flavour it gives, need not be ashamed to offer this pastry to their guests.

- 4 oz plain flour
- 2 oz soft margarine
- 2 tablespoons water

In a bowl, rub the margarine into the flour with a pinch of salt until it resembles cornflakes – that is to say, nowhere near the fine-breadcrumbs stage reached in making ordinary pastry. Add a couple of tablespoons of water and stir it in with the blade of a knife, then use your fingers briefly to make a coherent mass. Use it straightaway, rolling as lightly and quickly as possible, or keep it in the refrigerator, where it will not become too hard to roll.

Banana Bread (makes 1 large loaf)

A light, tasty bread that is quick to mix. Serve at breakfast to spread with margarine and marmalade, jam or honey. It also makes an excellent sweet tea bread.

- 4 oz soft margarine
- 4 oz sugar, refined or muscovado/demerara
- 1 egg
- 8 oz wholemeal flour
- 1 tablespoon baking powder
- ½ teaspoon grated nutmeg
- about 1 lb peeled ripe bananas
- 1 teaspoon vanilla extract
- 3 oz seedless raisins, tossed in a little flour
- 4 tablespoons coarsely chopped pecans or walnuts

Cream the margarine and sugar together in a mixing bowl until light and fluffy. Add the egg and beat thoroughly.

Sift in the flour, baking powder, ½ teaspoon salt, and nutmeg and beat until thoroughly blended. Mash the bananas with the vanilla and beat into the mixture. Add the raisins and nuts and mix well.

Pour into a greased 2 lb loaf tin and bake in a pre-heated oven at Reg. 4/350°F for 1 hour, or until a skewer inserted in the middle comes out clean.

Turn out to cool on a wire rack, then serve sliced.

Carrot Cake (serves 4)

This very moist, spicy cake is a favourite in the wholefood restaurants and bakeries of America. It is an easy cake to mix, with no creaming or rubbing. Be sure to bake it in a deep tin because it rises considerably during baking.

- 10 fl oz honey
- 4 oz carrot, finely grated
- 4 oz raisins
- 3 oz chopped dates
- 1 teaspoon ground cinnamon
- 1 teaspoon grated nutmeg
- ½ teaspoon ground cloves
- 4 oz soft margarine
- 8 fl oz water
- 8 oz wholewheat pastry flour, or fine-ground wholewheat flour
- 2 teaspoons bicarbonate of soda
- 4 oz shelled walnuts, chopped

Mix the honey, carrot, raisins, dates, cinnamon, nutmeg, cloves, margarine and water together in a pan over a gentle heat, then bring to the boil and boil for 5 minutes. Remove the pan from the heat and leave the mixture to cool for about 30 minutes, or until lukewarm.

Mix the flour and a pinch of salt together in a large bowl, then mix in the bicarbonate of soda after first rubbing it in your palm to rid it of any lumps. Add the walnuts to these dry ingredients, then make a well in the middle and pour in the carrot mixture. Mix until they are thoroughly blended.

Pour into a well-buttered and lightly floured cake tin 9-in square, or a round cake tin 10-in across. Bake in a pre-heated oven at Reg. 4/350°F for 55–65 minutes. The cake is ready when it feels firm at the centre if you press it lightly and when a skewer inserted in the centre comes out clean.

Leave the cake to cool in the tin for 10 minutes before turning it out on to a cake rack. It is at its best if eaten while still warm.

Lifespan coffee or chocolate cake

This cake – moist, rich and dark – uses high-fibre flour but does not have a lumpy wholemeal quality. It can be eaten hot as a pudding or cold as a cake and can be coffee- or chocolate-flavoured. For coffee you need:

- 6 oz 100% or 81% wholemeal flour
- 2 oz ground almonds
- 3 rounded teaspoons baking powder
- 6 oz brown sugar
- 6 oz soft margarine
- 2 eggs
- 4 fluid ounces strong black coffee.

For the topping:
- 2 oz walnuts or hazelnuts
- 2 digestive biscuits
- 2 oz brown sugar
- 2 oz soft margarine

Grease an 8½-inch loose-bottomed sandwich-tin and line the base with foil or greaseproof paper. Heat the oven to Reg. 4/350°F. Mix flour, ground almonds and baking powder in a bowl. In another bowl, cream brown sugar and margarine and then add the eggs, one at a time, beating them in well. Fold in the flour, moistening the mixture with the coffee. Put the mixture into the cake-tin.

For chocolate flavour, use 3 oz plain cooking chocolate and 2 tablespoons milk. Where you would add the coffee, instead add milk and chocolate melted over hot water or in a slow oven. Mix thoroughly but lightly before turning the mixture into the tin.

Bake for 15 minutes; then add the topping (see below).

Chop the nuts, crumble the biscuits, mix them lightly with the sugar and soft margarine and sprinkle the mixture evenly over the top of the cake. Bake for a further 35–45 minutes, until set but crumbly.

Walnut cake

Walnuts can be replaced by mixed fruit, poppy seeds, caraway seeds or grated orange peel in this easy basic cake. If you want to eliminate the most branny parts of the flour, sieve it before using or take 81% flour instead of 100% wholemeal flour.

- 5 oz soft margarine
- 5 oz Barbados or brown sugar
- 2 eggs
- ½ lb wholemeal flour
- 2 teaspoons baking powder
- ⅛ pint milk
- 4 oz walnuts (6–8 left whole for decoration, the rest chopped)

Cream together margarine and sugar until light. Beat in whole eggs, again until light. Mix flour and baking powder together and stir lightly into egg mixture. Add milk, stirring until you have a very soft mixture. Finally, add chopped nuts. Grease and dust with flour a deep 7-inch tin. Pour mixture in and decorate top with whole nuts.

Cover top of cake-tin with a piece of foil pierced at approximately ½-inch intervals with a skewer or sharp knife. Bake at Reg. 4/350°F for 1–1¼ hours. After 45 minutes, remove the foil to allow cake to finish rising and to brown. When done, leave cake in pan for 5–10 minutes, then turn it out on a rack to cool.

Malt loaf

- 1 lb stoneground wholemeal flour, ½ lb white, preferably strong, flour
- 2 oz sultanas
- 1 oz yeast
- 2 oz soft margarine
- 2 tablespoons malt extract
- 2 tablespoons black treacle
- 13 fl oz warm water
- 2 tablespoons sugar
- 2 tablespoons milk

Put the flour, sultanas and ½ teaspoon salt in a large bowl and mix thoroughly. Make a well in the centre, pour in the yeast creamed in a little warm water. Add the warm melted margarine, malt, treacle and warm water – enough to make a rather slack, pliable dough. Knead in the bowl until the mixture is even. It thickens up a little and becomes firmer.

Put the bowl in a large polythene bag, oiled lightly inside to prevent it sticking to the dough, and leave to rise for 2 hours, with the mouth of the bag slightly open, or until the dough has doubled in size. Pre-heat the oven to Reg. 5/375°F. Push the mixture down into tins for either two very large 1 lb loaves or three smaller ones, and put back in the bag to prove until puffy and swollen – about 45 minutes.

Bake in the pre-heated oven for 50 minutes, turning halfway through. Five minutes before the end, paint with a glaze made

APPENDIX ONE/GOOD FOOD

with sugar dissolved in milk and boiled for a minute or two until slightly syrupy. Eat, sliced, like ordinary bread, except that this is sticky, gooey and delicious for tea.

Wholewheat bread (makes one 2 lb loaf or two 1 lb loaves)
By using wholewheat flour, and preferably stone-ground wholewheat flour that has had the minimum of processing, all the vitamins, minerals, bran and proteins that are found in wheat are retained in the bread. This recipe is a plain one-rise wholewheat loaf, invented by Doris Grant. Known as the 'Grant loaf', it has a moist texture and good flavour. It will not keep for more than about 2 days, but it freezes well. It is essential to use 100 per cent wholewheat flour for a satisfactory result.

13 fl oz hand-hot water	2 teaspoons dried yeast
4 teaspoons Barbados or dark brown sugar	1 lb wholewheat flour

Grease the bread tin or tins. Put a third of the water into a jug and stir in ½ teaspoon of the sugar and the yeast. Leave on one side for 10 minutes to froth up. Put the flour into a large bowl and mix in the remaining sugar and 2 teaspoons of salt. Add the frothy yeast and the remaining water to the flour and mix well to a dough. It will be rather softer than ordinary bread dough. Squeeze and knead the dough with your hands for a few minutes – it will become smoother and less sticky – and then put the dough into the tin or tins. Cover with a cloth or place the tins in a large plastic bag and leave for 45–60 minutes, until the loaves have doubled in size. When the dough is nearly ready, pre-heat the oven to Reg. 6/400°F. Bake a large loaf for 35–40 minutes, or two small ones for 25–30 minutes. Remove the loaves from the tins and cool on a wire rack.

Bran-plus wholewheat loaf
This recipe was devised by Helen Cleave, wife of T. L. Cleave, whose book, *The Saccharine Disease*, pioneered the fibre story, pointing out the connection between the higher consumption of sugar and modern western diseases. Cleave reasoned that it was important not only to return the bran lost in refining, but to add extra bran to compensate for what has been lost in jams and spreads, where sugar, too, has been refined.

The loaf has a dense texture; simply follow the Grant loaf recipe for wholewheat bread, adding a tablespoon of bran to each pound of flour. You can mix the yeast with two teaspoons of sugar if you want to make the yeast work faster. The bran loaf should be kneaded rather longer than the Grant loaf and given more time to rise.

Raw granola
This makes a very good breakfast cereal. Make it in large quantities and store it in glass jars or tightly closed plastic bags. Seventh Day Adventists, inventors of the first mass-produced breakfast cereals, serve it just as it is with milk – no cooking is needed. Trickle a little thin honey over your bowl of granola if you like your cereal sweet.

1 lb rolled oats or quick oatmeal	4 oz date sugar or brown sugar
4 oz sesame seeds ground	4 oz chopped pecans, raisins or slivered almonds
4 oz sunflower seeds ground	1½ teaspoons finely grated orange rind, or ½ teaspoon ground anise seed
4 oz pumpkin seeds, ground	
4 oz desiccated (shredded) coconut	

Toast the oats for a few minutes in the oven to crisp and brown them lightly, or leave them untoasted if you prefer. Mix them with all the other ingredients and 1½ teaspoons of sea salt, then store in glass jars or plastic bags. Serve with milk.

To add extra vitamins to the granola, you can include 4 oz ground flax seed (linseed); this is also high in polyunsaturated fatty acids.

Pitta bread (makes 8 breads)

1 lb plain white flour	½ pint warm water in a measuring jug
½ oz dried yeast or 1 oz fresh yeast	olive oil
pinch of sugar	

Put the flour in a bowl and make a well in the centre. Put in a warm place to lose its chill. Mix the yeast to a cream with the sugar and 1 fluid ounce of the warm water in the jug. Pour olive oil into the jug until it is back to the ½-pint mark, stir in ½ oz salt and keep it warm. When the yeast starts to froth, pour it into the centre of the flour and then add the water and oil. Knead for 10 minutes. Smooth a little more oil over the outside of the dough and leave it to rise in a warm place for 2 hours, well covered. So far, apart from the addition of olive oil it is very much like making ordinary bread, but from now you treat the dough more like pastry to achieve flat slippers of bread.

Knock the dough down, cut it into 8 pieces and work each piece into a ball. Cover again and leave to prove for half an hour or so. Preheat the oven to Reg. 8/450°F. Knead each ball of dough a little, put plenty of flour on your board and rolling-pin, and roll each ball gently into an oval shape. Put the shapes on greased and floured baking sheets and let them prove for a further 30 minutes, covered with a cloth.

Brush the tops with water and stick as many breads as you can into the hot oven. Bake 8–10 minutes, turning after the first 5 minutes. Take out of the oven while still pale, and wrap in a cloth to keep them soft. Eat after about ten minutes cooling, dip into houmous etc.

Pizza (serves 4)
Borrowed from Southern Italy, the pizza is now almost a national dish in America, and is spreading fast elsewhere. In spite of its rather tarnished image, and like the ubiquitous hamburger, the pizza can be first-rate food, as well as being filling and healthy. This recipe freezes well. Make a plain bread dough as follows:

1 oz yeast or ½ oz dried yeast	garlic to taste, crushed
½ pint warm water	2 dozen small black olives
1 lb plain white flour plus some for kneading	1 tin anchovies
	1 mozzarella cheese
1½ teaspoons salt	plenty of oregano
2 dessertspoons oil	olive oil
2 14 oz tins of tomatoes	

Mix the yeast into a couple of tablespoons of warm water. Put the flour in a bowl, pour in the yeast and leave in a warm place to froth up. When it froths, add just under half a pint of warm water to which you have added the oil and ½ teaspoon of salt. Mix to a dough and knead well, adding more flour if needed. Allow to rise in a warm place, covered with an oiled polythene bag, until it has doubled in size.

While the dough is rising, make a dryish tomato sauce by simmering the tomatoes, flavoured with salt, pepper and garlic, until thick, and allow to cool.

When the dough has doubled in size, cut it into four pieces. Roll each piece into a ball and flatten it into a flat disc, about 8–10 inches across. Spread the dry tomato sauce over the pizza base. Arrange the olives and anchovies on top. Cut the mozzarella cheese into thick slices and arrange on top of this. Sprinkle well with oregano and olive oil. Allow to sit for 10 minutes or thereabouts. Meanwhile preheat the oven to Reg. 8/450°F. Bake fast for 15–20 minutes. Eat immediately.

Wholemeal scones
These scones can be made in a very few minutes and should also be eaten in a few. When they are hot they are like ambrosia; when cold they become plain scones.

8 oz wholemeal flour	2 oz soft margarine
½ teaspoon bicarbonate of soda	¼ pint buttermilk (sour milk will do)

Pre-heat oven to Reg. 7/425°F. Mix together flour, bicarbonate of soda and ½ teaspoon of salt. Rub soft margarine into dry ingredients until finely and evenly distributed. Stir in buttermilk only until all flour is incorporated, and you have a dryish dough. Put on floured board and roll or pat down until ½ inch thick. Cut into circles with 2-inch diameter cutter, or glass. Place on a greased baking sheet. Bake for 10 minutes or until scones are golden brown.

Herb bread

1 French loaf
3 oz soft margarine
1 teaspoon of mixed freshly-chopped herbs – choose from dill, parsley, marjoram, oregano, basil, tarragon, mint
1 clove of garlic, crushed
1 tablespoon grated Parmesan

Cut the bread (not quite right through so that it remains joined together at the base) diagonally into 1-inch slices. Make a paste with the margarine, herbs, garlic, and Parmesan. Spread over the insides of the slices, and press the loaf back together. Make a sort of long-boat out of kitchen foil to enclose the bottom of the loaf, leaving the top open. Bake in a hot oven, Reg. 6/400°F, for 10 minutes.

Tomato toast

This is a lovely, quick, filling outdoor starter for summer, each person making his own toast on the bonfire or over the glowing charcoal. It comes from Spain, where the tomatoes are huge and seem to have a lot of pulp and very few seeds.

Make some thick slices of toast with home-made bread. Cut tomatoes in half. Dribble oil over the toast, then rub the slices with the cut side of half a tomato. Sprinkle with salt and eat straightaway.

Wheat tortillas (serves 4)

4 oz lard
1 lb flour, sifted
8 fl oz water

Rub the fat into the flour with your fingers. Dissolve 2 teaspoons of salt in the water and add to the flour and fat mixture. Mix thoroughly, knead the dough for 5 minutes and set aside covered with a damp cloth for 2 hours.

Knead the dough again briefly. Roll a piece out into a ball about 1½-in across. Place on a floured surface and press with a rolling pin until you have a circle about 7-in across.

Cook over a high heat on a lightly greased frying pan or griddle for about 20 seconds on each side. The surface should be speckled with dark brown.

Serve immediately, or store in a plastic bag and reheat before serving.

Tacos

Tacos are the most common snack in Mexico. A warm tortilla (see above) is filled with meat, fish, fried beans or cheese, moistened with sauce, rolled up and eaten by hand. Tacos are sometimes lightly fried in oil or lard.

Shredded chicken with a little shredded lettuce or a slice of avocado, and freshly grilled meat chopped while it is still hot, make good taco fillings, and most leftovers can be heated up and used. We also give a recipe for a special filling – fresh Mexican tomato sauce – below.

To make tacos with leftover tortillas, first reheat the tortillas by steaming, then roll them around the filling or fold them in half over it. Fry the tacos in very little oil, and serve on a bed of shredded lettuce.

Tacos make excellent barbecue food. Cook thinly cut steaks or lamb and pork chops or a selection of all three over a charcoal grill. Immediately before serving, chop the meat into pieces about 1-inch square on a wooden board. Heat tortillas over the charcoal and place about four overlapping on each plate with the meat on top of them.

Fresh Mexican tomato sauce (makes about ½ pint)

This is a delicious taco filling. You can vary its hotness by adjusting the number of chilli peppers used.

2 tomatoes, skinned and chopped
½ medium onion, chopped
8 sprigs fresh coriander, chopped
3 chilli peppers, seeded and chopped
4 tablespoons water

Combine all the ingredients in a bowl with coarse salt to taste, and mix well. As well as a taco filling, the sauce can be served as an accompaniment to meat, chicken and egg dishes.

BREAKFAST

The good old British breakfast is a health hazard. Certainly, if you are trying to cut out fat intake by a quarter, a breakfast of bacon, egg, fried bread, buttered toast and marmalade, and coffee with cream, is the wrong way to start the day. In fact, many people in this country now eat a cold breakfast, but this usually means cornflakes or one of the proprietary breakfast cereals. These are usually oversweet and over-refined, and the grains may have been cooked in saturated fat.

We recommend you include oats in your breakfast meal. Oats contain a gummy fibre material – also found to a lesser extent in barley. This gummy material, evident when porridge is made, reduces blood cholesterol by a third as well as reducing blood sugar and fats. It is now being recommended for the prevention of diabetes, heart disease and high blood pressure. It appears that oat bran is more effective than wheat bran as a health food. The simplest way of getting it is as porridge or muesli for breakfast. Muesli, invented by Swiss Health pioneer Dr Bircher Benner, has been recommended by health pundits for many years and has become something of a joke – but it really works. Diabetics can obtain much better control of their blood sugar by eating oats. Oats seem to stabilize food absorption in a way beneficial for everyone.

Muesli

Muesli ingredients usually need to be bought from health-food stores. Beware of commercial mueslis: many are far too sweet.

You need a mixture of any or all of these: rolled oat flakes, barley flakes, cracked wheat grains – toasted or not, as you prefer. You can toast your own, tossing them about in a dry frying-pan and being careful not to let them burn. And you can soak the grains in milk or water overnight if you wish, which makes them more digestible but rather pulpy to eat.

Allow a tablespoon of bran per serving.

Dried fruit (dried figs, sultanas and raisins) can be chopped up and a tablespoon per serving added.

Hazelnuts or almonds can be added chopped up, a small sprinkling per serving (these can also be toasted for a few minutes).

Peeled or unpeeled apple, pear, orange, tangerine or banana, may be added before soaking overnight or just before eating.

Honey and wheatgerm are favoured by some but although honey tastes good it does not have magical properties. Wheatgerm oil contains B vitamins, but loses most of its vitamin power in heat-processing, necessary to prevent the oil in the wheatgerm going rancid and bitter. Serve the muesli with semi-skimmed milk (stripey top).

Appendix Two: Your National Health Service Rights

DOCTORS

There are about twenty-five thousand family doctors or general practitioners (GPs) practising in Great Britain. They are organized by the Family Practitioner Committees (FPCs) set up by the Area Health Authorities in England, Wales and the Primary Care Divisions of Scottish Health Boards. There are also private doctors who charge a scale of fees for consultations, and you yourself pay for your drugs, medicines and appliances.

You will find a list of NHS doctors in your district through local FPCs or Health Boards, and at all main post offices, public libraries or citizens' advice bureaux. Some doctors may work on their own, others may be part of a group practice or work in a health centre. Under the National Health Service you are free to choose any general practitioner but they are not obliged to accept you as their patient. This may be because you live too far away or because their number of patients is already high. By law, one of the local doctors must accept you; if you have any problems, get in touch with your local Family Practitioner Committee (or Scottish Health Board), the address of which can be found in the telephone directory, post office or town hall. It is important for patients to give the FPC the names of doctors who have already been approached unsuccessfully.

It is important that you find a doctor in whom you have confidence, although not everyone looks for the same qualities. There are many factors which may influence your choice: the doctor's personality, the look of the surgery and the equipment, the fact he or she has special qualifications in a certain field of medicine or even the fact there is an efficient appointment system. Some doctors do not answer their own emergency calls in the evenings and at night but put these out to a doctor from a deputizing service, which will have no previous knowledge of a patient's problem. It may be an advantage to choose a doctor from a practice which does its own night calls. If you want to check your doctor's qualifications, you can look the doctor's name up in the medical directory in the reference section of the library. The best way of finding a doctor is probably by asking friends, but *always* go and see doctors.

If for some reason you are unhappy with your present doctor, ask him or her for their consent to the transfer. If the doctor agrees, he or she signs part B of your medical card; you then complete part A. Take the card to your new doctor, who also signs part A and then sends the card to the Family Practitioner committee, which sends you a new card.

Should you prefer not to do this, you may write to the local Family Practitioner Committee or Scottish Health Board, enclosing your medical card and telling them that you wish to transfer to the list of another doctor. After fourteen days have elapsed from the time you wrote to them, they will send back your medical card with a slip attached which will enable you within a further month to apply to another doctor for acceptance on his or her list. If you have been unable to secure acceptance within that period you can then apply to the committee for assignment to a doctor.

If you have lost your medical card, ask for an application form for a replacement from the FPC or Scottish Health Board. If you are without a doctor, or your own doctor is unavailable, or you are away from home, you are entitled to any immediately necessary treatment from doctors only if they offer their services under the NHS.

If you are expecting a baby, you can temporarily change doctors to one who specializes in maternity work. You will find names on the local obstetric list. For further information on matters such as home births, induction and health visitors, see page 232. Make sure you are getting all your social security maternity entitlements. A National Council for Civil Liberties booklet, *Maternity Rights for Working Women* (available from NCCL, 186 King's Cross Road, London WC1X 9DE) gives details.

Doctors are required to arrange for medical care to be available at all times. Sometimes other doctors have to cover for your GP when he or she is off duty or on holiday. Some doctors use emergency deputizing services.

If you are genuinely unsure about calling your GP at night or at the weekends, it is best to ring and talk about the problem just to be on the safe side. In an emergency, when you have been unable to contact your GP go to the nearest hospital which has an accident or emergency department open at night and weekends.

If you become ill and want a 'Doctor's Statement' for benefit purposes, it is free; but if you want a private certificate for your employer the British Medical Association recommends various fees for different types of certificate. These are outside the NHS but the usual charge is about 50p. Report your illness immediately to the Department of Health and Social Security or you may lose your benefit. Under new arrangements, people who are off work sick for seven days or less must certify themselves on forms available from hospitals, doctors' surgeries and employers.

If you are abroad or away from home

You can still get medical treatment as an NHS patient if you are travelling in Britain. You can become a temporary patient if your stay is for more than twenty-four hours but less than three months. If you need urgent treatment and you are in an area for less than a day, you can go to any NHS doctor as an 'emergency patient'. In both cases you will have to fill in a form and give your NHS number.

If you are abroad, you do not normally have an automatic right to receive free medical treatment. However, the United Kingdom does have reciprocal health-care arrangements with a number of countries, including all the members of the European Economic Community (EEC). These enable most British visitors to receive immediate treatment on the same terms as the nationals of the various countries. Such treatment is also available to most British visitors to certain other countries outside the EEC.

The arrangements vary from country to country; see DHSS leaflet SA30, available from your local social security office, for details. This leaflet also includes the application form for the certificate of entitlement to treatment (E111) which is needed in most EEC countries. Apply for this form about one month before travelling. But not all countries are covered by reciprocal health-care arrangements with Britain. In countries that are not, you will be expected to pay the full cost of treatment. You are therefore strongly advised to take out private insurance to cover the full cost of medical treatment; this is especially important in the United States.

Some countries require travellers from certain other countries to produce valid international Certificates of Vaccination. Information about vaccinations which are required (or recommended) are contained in the DHSS leaflet SA35 *Notice to travellers* (see also Chapter 9). Your doctor can carry out any vaccinations except yellow fever; for this you will need to go to one of the special centres which are listed in the leaflet.

Prescriptions

There is a standard charge for each item prescribed to a patient, with certain exceptions like wigs and fabric support, which are more expensive. There are also certain exemptions from this charge, notably children under sixteen, women aged sixty and over, men aged sixty-five and over, expectant mothers and mothers who have had a child in the last twelve months. There are other exemptions; for further information get leaflet P11 from the post office. If you find that you were entitled to exemption at the time you paid the charge, you can claim a refund if you obtained an official receipt form (FP57/EC57) when the charge was paid. This tells you how to claim; claims must be made within three months. If you need prescriptions frequently, you may be able to save money by making a single payment in advance, like a season ticket. Leaflet FP95/EC95 from the post office gives details.

Making a complaint against your doctor (or optician or pharmacist)

If you have a complaint it should be made within eight weeks of the date of the incident which caused the complaint. It should be made in writing to the administrator of the local Family Practitioner Committee; if you delay you have to explain why you could not complain earlier. (In Scotland a complaint against a hospital doctor or GP should be made in writing to the Area Health Board. There is no time-limit for complaints against hospital doctors, but for GPs complaints must be made within eight weeks.) Your local Community Health Council can advise and assist you in making your complaint and tell you where you should address it.

If you have a complaint against a dentist, it should be made within six months of completing the treatment or within eight weeks after the matter which gave rise to the complaint came to notice – whichever is sooner.

HOSPITALS

Normally you go to your GP for medical advice and to hospitals in emergencies if you cannot contact your GP or when referred by your GP for special treatment. There are two chief types of cases treated in hospitals: surgical and medical. Your doctor is free to send you to a hospital in another area if he feels you would be treated by consultants with special skills, and depending on your financial circumstances you may be entitled to help with the cost of the fare from the Health Service.

You cannot *demand* hospital treatment: you can only be admitted to hospital if your doctor thinks you need treatment. If you disagree, you can ask for a second opinion. Otherwise you can only change your doctor and try again. Hospital consultants will not always take up cases sent to them by GPs because they may not feel hospital treatment is necessary. The patient has no right to see a particular consultant or doctor under the NHS when in hospital, and you may only see one of his team. If you particularly want to see someone, make an appointment explaining why, or write to the hospital secretary asking for his help.

If your doctor sends you to hospital as an in-patient, he will probably want to be kept informed of your condition. You should encourage contact between your GP and the consultant, especially in cases concerning children or the elderly.

If you are seriously ill and need medical attention or an operation urgently, you will get a bed in a hospital almost immediately. For more routine operations like the removal of tonsils or the treatment of a hernia, patients usually have to go on a waiting list. The situation varies from area to area, and so does the length of the waiting lists. Ask your doctor about this, and see if another hospital could take you in sooner.

You may get a refund of necessary travelling expenses to hospital if you receive supplementary benefits, a pension, family income supplement or you are a dependant of someone who does. You have to produce your allowance book at the medical social worker's office at the hospital. You may also be able to claim the fares of someone who helped or escorted you to hospital if the hospital certifies that it was necessary. The Supplementary Benefits Commission can provide financial help in certain circumstances. See leaflet SB1 from main post offices for details and a claim form, or apply to the local social security office for more detailed advice.

It is up to the hospital whether they provide free accommodation for relatives of a sick adult patient, but hospitals are encouraged to allow mothers to stay in hospital with their children. Mothers (or fathers) should not have to pay for this accommodation if the child is in an ordinary NHS bed. If you need any help or advice on children in hospital, get in touch with the National Association for the Welfare of Children in Hospital (see address below).

If you go into hospital and particularly want privacy although your case may not require it, you can ask for an amenity bed in a single or smaller ward. Charges in the summer of 1982 were £10 a day for a single room and £5 for a bed in a small ward. The charges relate to privacy only; all other services and treatment are provided under the NHS arrangements.

You can refuse treatment, an operation or an examination if you feel strongly about it, but it may not be to your own advantage. A doctor who examines you against your will, or a surgeon who operates without a patient's consent, commits assault; that is why you are asked to sign a consent form when you arrive in hospital. Consent is usually written but it can be verbal. For patients under sixteen, parents or guardians will sign the consent form but the child must also consent to the procedure. Patients can also discharge themselves at any time. However, they may be asked to sign a form declaring they left against medical advice. (This does not apply to mental hospitals.)

You have the right to decline to be available for examination by students at a teaching hospital and not prejudice your treatment. It may mean being seen by a different consultant or a junior doctor. Perhaps if you feel strongly about this you should let the hospital know in advance or not go to a teaching hospital. If you have difficulties over this, get in touch with the Patients' Association (see address below). If you are anxious about delays in hearing the results of hospital tests, your GP may be able to speed things up by ringing the hospital.

Making a complaint about hospital staff
Patients have a legal right to be treated with reasonable care and skill. If a patient suffers as a result of negligence either by a GP or a member of the hospital staff, he or she is entitled to claim compensation or damages by law. However, few people can afford the cost of a lawsuit, and so most people, other than those who qualify for legal aid, are ill-advised to attempt to get legal redress.

If you have a complaint about something which happened to you in hospital which was not settled to your satisfaction at the time, you should write to your district or area administrator (you will get the address from your local citizens' advice bureau, public library or your doctor).

If you have gone through the recognized complaints system and you are still dissatisfied, get in touch with the Health Services Commissioner, the official name for the Health Service ombudsman. He may be able to investigate your complaint, including the way it was dealt with by the AHA, but not if it concerns alleged medical negligence. Otherwise, try your MP.

DENTISTS
You can get a list of dentists contracted to do NHS work in your area from the FPC, post office or library. You are free to approach any dentist on the list, but the dentists are also free to reject you as a patient. Once you are accepted for a course of NHS treatment by a dentist, he or she is obliged under the terms of service to make you 'dentally fit'. If you go to a dental department of a teaching hospital, you may have to be examined by students and the treatment may take longer (see leaflet D11 'NHS dental treatment' available from post offices and citizens' advice bureaux).

Before starting each course of treatment, make sure you are being treated under the NHS. Otherwise your dentist could treat you privately. Adults are entitled to free dental examinations every six months and those under twenty-one to three examinations a year. Expectant mothers are entitled to be examined every four months during pregnancy and for a year after the birth.

Dental treatment is free for all young people under eighteen, or those under nineteen in full-time education, expectant mothers and mothers with a child under one year old. Young people over sixteen and not in full-time education only pay for dentures, alterations and additions. There are exemptions and some reduced charges for some other categories. People on supplementary benefit or family income supplement do not have to pay charges, and anyone with an income at or just above supplementary benefit levels can get form FID from the dentist to claim help towards all or part of the charge.

If you are not satisfied with the dental treatment you have received under the NHS, you should complain in writing to the administrator of the local FPC or Scottish Health Board (see 'Making a complaint . . .', page 230).

OPTICIANS
You can go to one of three different categories of optician under the General Opthalmic Services: (a) the opthalmic optician, who tests sight, prescribes and supplies glasses; (b) the opthalmic medical practitioner, who is a doctor who also tests sight and prescribes glasses; and (c) the dispensing optician who supplies glasses from a prescription. When you need to have your sight tested, simply go along to any optician provided he or she is on the NHS list. If you do not want to have the cheaper NHS frames, you can get more expensive ones which take NHS lenses. Frames and lenses are free to children at school and young people under nineteen in full-time education, provided that they are NHS lenses in NHS frames.

Leaflet G11 from larger post offices gives details of who qualifies for free NHS glasses. If you are not in one of the categories exempted from paying but your income is low, you might still be able to get some help with the cost; ask for form F1 from your optician.

Useful Organizations
The Patients' Association, Suffolk House, Banbury Road, Oxford OX2 7HN (0865-50306); The National Association for the Welfare of Children in Hospital, Exton House, 7 Exton Street, London SE1 8UE (01-261 1738).

GENERAL
Health Education Council, 78 New Oxford Street, London WC1 1AH.
Scottish Health Education Group, 21 Lansdowne Crescent, Edinburgh EH12 5EH.
Department of Health and Social Security, Alexander Fleming House, Elephant and Castle, London SE1 6BY.
Scottish Home and Health Department, Old St Andrews House, Edinburgh EH1 3TD.
Don't forget the many organizations which exist in your own area of the country. Check local libraries or telephone directories for the addresses and numbers of the social services department of the local authority, the social security office, citizens' advice bureau and community health council.

Appendix Three: Further Information

1: PREGNANCY AND CHILDHOOD
Choosing a doctor for ante-natal care
In the UK a woman must sign a form showing her agreement to care from one particular doctor during pregnancy and after the birth. The doctor is paid extra for providing this care. Few women realize that this doctor need not be their usual family doctor. If you want your baby to be delivered at home, ask your GP early in the pregnancy – preferably before you have signed the form agreeing to his care. If you do sign the form and then change your mind, you can still change your doctor by informing the local Family Practitioner Committee. Only certain GPs who are on an official 'obstetric list' (available from main post offices) are trained to deliver babies at home; they would also be a good choice for maternity care generally.

Having your baby at home
If you have difficulty making arrangements to have your baby at home, you may have to write to your local Area Health Authority informing them that you intend to have the baby at home and asking them to help. A woman cannot be compelled to have her baby in hospital, and the AHA has a duty to help a woman who wants to have a home delivery. If you still have difficulty, you may get help from the Society to Support Home Confinements, c/o Margaret Whyte (Secretary), 17 Laburnum Avenue, Durham City.

Childbirth classes
These are run by your local health visitor or local hospital. Private classes are also run by the National Childbirth Trust. For details of these classes, as well as a wide range of NCT leaflets, write to the National Childbirth Trust at 9 Queensborough Terrace, London W2 3TB.

Preconceptual care
More information from Foresight: Mrs Peter Barnes, Woodhurst, Hydestile, Godalming, Surrey GU8 4AY.

Infertility
More information from National Association for the Childless. Dr Jeremy Ward, 318 Summer Lane, Birmingham B19 3RL. Tel: 021-359 2113.

Books about pregnancy
Pregnancy, Gordon Bourne (Pan).
Pregnancy Month by Month, Consumers' Association, Caxton Hill, Hertford, Herts.
New Baby, Health Visitors' Association. Available free from health clinics or health visitors; in case of difficulty, contact Health Visitors' Association, 36 Eccleston Square, London SW1.

Books about childbirth and breast-feeding
Childbirth, William Nixon, revised by Geoffrey Chamberlain (Penguin).
The Experience of Childbirth, Sheila Kitzinger (Penguin).
Birth Without Violence, Frederic Leboyer (Wildwood House/Fontana).
New Life, Janet and Arthur Balaskas. Available from 32 Cholmeley Crescent, London N6.
Active Birth, Janet and Arthur Balaskas (Allen and Unwin).
The Experience of Breast Feeding, Sheila Kitzinger (Pelican).
Reducing the Risks – Safer Pregnancy and Childbirth. Part of DHSS series available from HMSO.

Books about children's early years
First Three Years, Health Visitors' Association. (Free from health visitors).
The Book of Child Care, Hugh Jolly (Allen and Unwin).
Babyhood, Penelope Leach (Penguin).
Baby and Child, Penelope Leach (Michael Joseph/Penguin).
Baby and Child Care, Benjamin Spock (New English Library).
The Newborn Baby, Consumers' Association. Available as above.
You know more than you think you do. Health Education Council leaflet available free from clinics or by post from HEC (address page 231).
Now You're a Family, Health Education Council. Available as above.
The Book of the Child, Scottish Health Education Group (address page 231).

In addition to the more general Health Education Council leaflets mentioned above, there are a number of more specialist publications available in the same manner. These cover topics such as healthy eating, overweight children, feet, bed-wetting, bottle- and breast-feeding, and play.

Childhood accidents
The Health Education Council (address page 231) supplies two helpful booklets: *Play it Safe!* and *Safety in the Home*. And the Royal Society for the Prevention of Accidents (RoSPA) publishes *First Steps to Safety* (Cannon House, The Priory, Queensway, Birmingham B4 6BS).

For general advice about safe equipment, you can consult *What every mum should know about British standards*, available from the British Standards Institution, 2 Park Street, London W1A 2BS. There are several suitable makes of car-safety seats and belts for children but always look for British Standards' kitemark number 3254. First-aid kits can be obtained from your chemist, while fire brigades will advise about suitable fire extinguishers. The Red Cross, St John Ambulance and St Andrew's Ambulance Brigade run courses in first-aid (see page 237 under Emergency for details).

2: EXERCISE
Although it is not necessary to join a club to take exercise, many people prefer company and sometimes competition to spur them on. Most sports have governing bodies which are only too pleased to give details of local clubs; a few such governing bodies for the activities featured in this chapter are given below. One excellent central source of information is The Sports Council, 16 Upper Woburn Place, London WC1H 0QP. Its information centre can provide a leaflet detailing not only its functions but also addresses of regional offshoots – check your local telephone directory for these, if you like. There are also separate Sports Councils for Wales, Scotland and Northern Ireland. These are:
Sports Council for Wales, The National Sports Centre for Wales, Sophia Gardens, Cardiff CF1 9SW.
Sports Council for Scotland, 1 St Colme Street, Edinburgh EH3 6AA.
Sports Council for Northern Ireland, House of Sport, 2A Upper Malone Road, Belfast BT9 5LA.

Your local council should be able to provide details of swimming pools, running tracks, tennis courts and other recreational facilities. Often, clubs have special veteran or novice sections. Many areas now also have multi-purpose sports centres offering everything from yoga to judo, keep-fit classes to weight-training. For people not interested in sports, many local authorities and organizations such as the YMCA run keep-fit sessions and dance classes. Doctors and health visitors may be good sources of information about these. In addition to specialist magazines (e.g. *Running, New Dance, Yoga Today*, etc.), there are also many books devoted to particular types of exercise or sports. These include:
Aerobics, The New Aerobics and *Aerobics for Women*, all by Dr Kenneth Cooper (Bantam).
Look after Yourself. Free booklet from the Health Education Council (address page 231), which details physical exercise and also covers healthy eating.
F/40 – Fitness on Forty Minutes a Week, Malcolm Carruthers and Alistair Murray (Futura, in conjunction with The Sports Council).
Gym and Health Club Guide, Donald Black (Power Books).
Stay Fit in the Office. Health Education Council leaflet.
Physical Fitness. Exercises developed by the Royal Canadian Air Force (Penguin).
The Complete Book of Running, James F. Fixx (Chatto and Windus).
Health and Fitness for Over-40s, B. Watson (Stanley Paul).

Organizations which may be able to give more detailed help beyond that available from The Sports Council and Health Education Council include:
Amateur Athletics Association, Francis House, Francis Street, London SW1P 1DL (01-828 9326).
British Cycling Federation, 16 Upper Woburn Place, London WC1H 0QG (01-387 9320).
Amateur Swimming Association, Harold Fern House, Derby Square, Loughborough LE11 0A1 (0509-30431).
British Sports Association for the Disabled, Stoke Mandeville Stadium, Harvey Road, Aylesbury, Bucks.

Ramblers' Association, 1–5 Wandsworth Road, London SW8 2LJ (01-582 6878).
Keep Fit Association, 16 Upper Woburn Place, London WC1H 0QG (01-387 4349).

Yoga
Most local authorities now offer yoga classes as part of their adult education programmes and many privately organized courses are also available; check local newspapers, health centres, community centres, etc., for details.
Light on Yoga, B. H. S. Iyengar (Allen and Unwin).
Keeping Up with Yoga, Lyn Marshall (Ward Lock).
Bodylife, Arthur Balaskas (Sidgwick and Jackson).

Health checks
Private health screenings for BUPA subscribers cost from £91 for men and £108 for women. Details from:

London: BUPA Medical Centre Men's unit, 210 Pentonville Road, London N1 9TA. (01-837 8641). Women's unit, 300 Gray's Inn Road, London WC1X 8DU (01-837 6484).
Cavendish Medical Centre, 99 New Cavendish Street, London W1 (01-637 8941).
Birmingham: Unicorn House, 29 Smallbrook Queensway, Birmingham B5 4HE (021-632 6738).
Bristol: Stafford Lodge, The Chesterfield Hospital, Clifton Hill, Bristol BS8 1BP (0272-731433).
Glasgow: 295 Fenwick Road, Griffnock, Glasgow G46 6UG (041-638 4445).
Manchester: 9 St John Street, Manchester M3 4DW (061-833 9362).
Nottingham: Clawson Lodge Medical Centre, 403 Mansfield Road, Sherwood, Nottingham NL5 2DP (0602-601826).

3: STRESS AND RELAXATION
For details of relaxation teachers, tape-recorded instruction books, and a correspondence course, send a s.a.e. to Relaxation for Living, 29 Burwood Park Road, Walton-on-Thames, Surrey. Useful books include *Stress and Relaxation*, Jane Madders (Martin Dunitz), and *The Stress Factor*, Donald Norfolk (Hamlyn).

Biofeedback machines are available from Audio Ltd, 26 Wendell Road, London W12, and from Aleph One, The Old Courthouse, High Street, Bottisham, Cambridge, who also stock relaxation tapes.

Details of transcendental meditation centres are obtainable from Roydon Hall, Seven Mile Lane, near Tunbridge Wells, Kent. Details of Siddha meditation from Siddha Yoga Dham, 1 Bonneville Gardens, London SW4.

Insomnia
A useful book is *How To Sleep Better*, Dr Peter Tyrer (Sheldon Press).

Headaches
The Migraine Trust, 45 Great Ormonde Street, London WC1 offers help and advice to sufferers and produces a good booklet, *Understanding Migraine*. Useful books include *Migraine and Headaches*, Dr Marcia Wilkinson (Sheldon Press).

Depression
Useful books include *Overcoming Depression*, Dr Andrew Stanway (Hamlyn), *Depression*, Dr Jack Dominian (Fontana), and *Depression*, Ross Mitchell (Pelican). Two booklets – *What is a Nervous Breakdown?*, A. R. K. Mitchell, and *Anxiety, Nervousness and Depression*, F. R. C. Casson – are available from Family Doctor Publications, BMA House, Tavistock Square, London WC1.

Self-help groups include Depressives Anonymous, 83 Derby Road, Nottingham NG1 9BB, and Cruse, an organization for the widowed, Cruse House, 126 Sheen Road, Richmond, Surrey TW9 1UR (01-940 4818).

Those with post-natal depression may get help from the Association for Post-natal Illness, 7 Gowan Avenue, London SW6 or Mama, 26a Cumnor Hill, Oxford. Books include *Post-natal Depression*, Vivienne Welburn (Fontana).

Suicide
The Samaritans run twenty-four-hour befriending services in most places in Britain. Look in your local phone book. A useful book for those who would like to know more about how they work is *The Samaritans in the 80's*, Chad Varah (Constable).

4: DIET
Recipe books
Cooking for your Heart's Content, D. Wainwright Evans and M. Greenfield (Hutchinson Benham, in association with the British Heart Foundation).
The Anti-Coronary Cookbook, Nathalie Havenstein and Elizabeth Richardson (Lutterworth Press/Richard Smart Publishing).
Measure for Measure Cookery Book, Elizabeth O'Reilly (Heinemann Health Books), for diabetics and weightwatchers.
Bran and High-Fibre Foods – A Simple Way to a Healthier Diet, Neil S. Painter (Pennywise Publishing, Redhill, Surrey).
Taking the Rough with the Smooth: Dietary Fibre and your Health, a Medical Breakthrough, Dr A. Stanway (Pan).
The Sunday Times Guide to the World's Best Food, Michael Bateman, Caroline Conran and Oliver Gillie (Hutchinson).

Diet advice
Eating for Health. Part of DHSS Prevention and Health series available from HMSO.

Slimming
If you have any worries about the advisability of your slimming, then you should check first with your family doctor. We have tried to give you some basic advice on sensible slimming in Chapter 4, but limited space has meant that we cannot go into too much detail. The following publications should prove helpful:
Which? Slimming Guide, Consumers' Association, Caxton Hill, Hertford, Herts.
The Joy of Slimming, Margaret Allan (Coronet). For general advice, calorie-counted recipes, day plans and exercise plans.
Obesity, its Management, Dr D. Craddock (Churchill Livingstone). For an objective yet readable clinical account.
Slimming and Nutrition. Published once every two months; for excellent list of calorie contents of branded goods.

Slimming clubs
The first commercial slimming clubs were introduced into Britain in the late 1960s, and since then the number of organizations running clubs, and the number of clubs within each organization, have increased by leaps and bounds.

The basic principle of group slimming is similar in all the organizations. You pay a membership fee on joining. Then you are weighed and measured and given your recommended weight. On subsequent weeks you pay a weekly fee whether your weight has gone up or down and you must also pay it if you do not actually attend the meeting; the organizations have different rules to allow for sickness and holidays. The dietary advice you will be given will vary with the organization. Weight Watchers will expect you to follow their 'Programme of Balanced Eating' which approximates to a low-fat diet giving about 1200–1500 calories. Slimming Magazine Clubs will analyse a questionnaire that you fill in and will assign you one of their sixteen diets on the basis of your answers. Silhouette Clubs will give you a 1000-calorie diet, called a 40-point diet because they work on the principle that one point equals 25 calories.

If you reach your recommended weight you will be given some token of congratulation (badge, letter from HQ, etc.), but more important, you will be made a free lifetime member. This means that you can attend one meeting a month free of charge provided your weight stays within a specified limit of your recommended weight.

The three major slimming organizations – Weight Watchers, Slimming Magazine and Silhouette – were surveyed independently in 1974. One year after joining, just over a quarter of members had reached their recommended weight with the clubs, although only about half of these had remained with the clubs as free lifetime members. After a year, one in ten of the members was still attending weekly meetings and the rest had left the club at some time during the year. In fact, the average length of membership was just on six months. During this time, the average weight-loss was 9.1 kg (20.3 lb) or, to put it another way, the members had lost 11.3 per cent of their initial weight. By taking into account the average membership and weekly fees charged by the organizations at the time, a cost of £1.91 per kg or 86p per lb was calculated for the weight-loss achieved. A follow-up study to the survey, however, revealed that only 13.1 per cent of the members who had left the group after losing a stone or more had maintained their recommended weight or improved on it. 63 per cent had gained some of their weight-loss, and the rest (23.9 per cent) had regained all their weight-loss and more in some cases. The lessons to be learnt from this survey are:
1. The different methods used by the organizations make very little difference in the long term.
2. If you leave the organization without reaching your recommended weight, your chances of backsliding are great. Those members who reach their recommended weight and can benefit from the free lifetime membership schemes do much better.

If you want to find out more about commercial slimming clubs, here are some names and addresses:
Weight Watchers, 635-637 Ajax Avenue, Slough, Berks. SL1 4DB.

APPENDIX THREE/FURTHER INFORMATION

Slimming Magazine Slimming Clubs, 4 Clareville Grove, London SW7 5AR.
Silhouette Slimming Clubs, 103 Harlestone Road, Northampton.

Private slimming groups
Of course, you do not have to go to a commercial slimming group to benefit from the main advantage of group slimming, i.e., being a part of a group with similar problems. If you have a reliable pair of scales and somewhere you can meet regularly, you can set up your own group. If you decide to collect fees, these can be sent to a charity – a sponsored slim-in; or you could collect a lump sum from each member when they join, perhaps related to the amount of weight they have to lose, and let them have it back bit by bit as a reward for losing the weight.

5: MAINTAINING THE BODYWORK
Back
You and Your Back, David Delvin. Obtainable from the Back Pain Association, Grundy House, 31-33 Park Road, Teddington, Middlesex TW11 0AB. Send a s.a.e. for free leaflet, *Think Back*.
Avoiding Back Trouble, Consumers' Association, Caxton Hill, Hertford, Herts.
Mind Your Back. Free leaflet available from the Health Education Council (address page 231).

Posture
The Alexander Principle, W. Barlow (Arrow). The Society of Teachers of the Alexander Technique, 3b Albert Court, Kensington Gore, London SW7, will give details of local teachers.

Feet
Care of Young Feet, Health Education Council (address page 231).
For a qualified chiropodist in your area, send a s.a.e. to the Society of Chiropodists, 8 Wimpole Street, London W1.
The Disabled Living Foundation, 346 Kensington High Street, London W14, sells notes on footwear, with a list of suppliers and stockists, for those with problem feet.

Skin
If you wish to have any superfluous hair removed, it is important to have it done by a skilled operator or you may be left with scarring. For local addresses write to the Institute of Electrolysis, 251 Seymour Grove, Manchester 16, or to the Association of Electrolysists, 6 Quakers Mede, Haddenham, Bucks, sending a s.a.e.
Send a s.a.e. for further information about eczema or psoriasis to the National Eczema Society, Tavistock House North, Tavistock Square, London WC1 and the Psoriasis Association, 7 Milton Street, Northampton.
Face values, Vernon Coleman with Margaret Coleman (Pan).
Learning to live with skin disorders, Christine Orton (Souvenir Press).
Skin Deep – an introduction to skin camouflage and disfigurement therapy, Doreen Trust (Paul Harris, Edinburgh).
Skin and hair care, edited by Linda Allen Schoen (Penguin).

Joints
See under Chapter 10: A Healthy Old Age, page 237.

Eyes
About your eyes, M. J. Gilkes (Family Doctor Publications).
The Eye Book, John Eden MD.

Ears
Following a programme initiated in July 1980, the range of hearing aids available on free loan through the National Health Service has been extended with the introduction of three new series of high-powered aids. The fully extended range can meet the needs of all but a few patients. Health authorities have the discretion to provide commercial aids in those few cases for which the extended range is still not altogether adequate.

Information on services for hearing-impaired people is included in the Department of Health and Social Security's leaflet, HB1 *Help for handicapped people*, while the Department's booklet HA1 *General guidance for hearing-aid users* gives basic and essential advice to patients wearing hearing aids. These leaflets are available from the DHSS Leaflets Unit, PO Box 21, Stanmore, Middlesex HA7 7AY.

A pamphlet giving information on hearing aids as well as other helpful information is available from the Royal National Institute for the Deaf, 105 Gower Street, London WC1E 6AH. Help with the special problems of deaf children is available from the National Deaf Children's Society, 45 Hereford Road, London W2 5AH.
Deafness – Let's face it, T. H. Sutcliffe. Available from the RNID (address above).
Our Deaf Children, Freddy Bloom. Available from the NDCS (address above).
Noise, Rupert Taylor (Pelican).

Advice about protection from noise in the workplace can be obtained from Wendy Austin, Bilsom Hearing Protection Advisory Service, Bilsom International, Fountain House, Odiham, Basingstoke, Hants; and S. Karmy, Industrial Audiology Services, 9 The High Street, Odiham, Basingstoke, Hants.

Teeth
For free dental treatment (and glasses), leaflet F11 gives details of people entitled to free or reduced charges under the NHS. Available from post offices and local social security offices.
Home Mouth Care Manual. Booklet from British Dental Health Foundation, 3 Harcourt House, 19a Cavendish Square, London W1. The Health Education Council (address page 231) publishes leaflets on dental care.
Caring for teeth, Consumers' Association, 74 Buckingham Street, London WC2.

6: THE MAJOR HAZARDS
Smoking
If any readers want even more information about the risks of smoking, and even more motivation, a very complete survey, full of graphs, statistics and scholarly references, is *Smoking or Health*, which is a report by the Royal College of Physicians, first published in 1971 and revised in 1977 by Pitman Medical and Scientific Books. Free pamphlets and lists of smoking withdrawal clinics are available from Action on Smoking and Health at ASH, Margaret Pyke House, 27–35 Mortimer Street, London W1. There is also an information and advice centre for smokers run by the National Society for Non-Smokers at Latimer House, 40/48 Hanson Street, London W1. See also *Smoker's Guide to Non-Smoking*, published by the Health Education Council (address page 231). The pamphlets are free either from the council (enclose a s.a.e.) or from your local Health Education Officer (your local council offices will tell you where to find them).

The Health Education Officer can also guide you to any local smoking withdrawal clinics in your area. These clinics offer free courses to help you give up smoking. For some people, these clinics are ideal. Whichever method you use to stop, stick with it. The process will take longer if you abandon one method to try another.

Heart disease
See Diet, Smoking, Stress and Fitness for general information about these subjects. The Coronary Prevention Group, Central Middlesex Hospital, London NW10 7NS, can provide information. One way of adopting a lower-fat diet is to eat more vegetarian food, provided eggs and cheese are not used excessively – one egg a day is reasonable on a vegetarian diet. For recipes contact the Vegetarian Society, 53 Marloes Road, Kensington, London W8 6LD, who provide a large selection of cookery books on mail order, and also give cookery demonstrations (send s.a.e. for information). The Vegan Society will provide details of its non-meat and animal-produce diet. This is an extreme diet, but for anyone who is prepared to change eating habits completely it may provide a means of recovery from heart disease caused by atheroma. Write to them at 47 Highlands Road, Leatherhead, Surrey, enclosing s.a.e.
The Heart, D. Longmore (World University Press Library).
How Not to Get a Coronary, A. L. Wingfield (Family Doctor Publications).
Avoiding Heart Attacks. Part of DHSS Prevention and Health series. Available from HMSO.
For recipe books see Chapter 4 in this Appendix.

Cancer
Cancer Information Association, 2nd Floor, Marigold House, Carfax, Oxford OX1 1EF (0865-46654/725223) provides information and advice about cancer. It has leaflets and can arrange talks.
The Health Education Council (address page 231) also provides information on prevention and detection of cancer.

Cancer of the breast
Breast screening for women who have no symptoms is available in some areas on the National Health Service. Ask your GP. Private screening is available as follows:
London: BUPA Medical Centre, 300 Gray's Inn Road, London WC1X 8DU (01-837 6484).
Birmingham: Unicorn House, 29 Smallbrook Queensway, Birmingham B5 4HE (021-632 6738).
Bristol: Stafford Lodge, The Chesterfield Hospital, Clifton Hill, Bristol BS8 1BP (0272-731433).
Glasgow: 295 Fenwick Road, Giffnock, Glasgow G46 6UG (041-638 4445).
Manchester: 9 St John Street, Manchester M3 4DW (061-833 9362).

FURTHER INFORMATION/**APPENDIX THREE**

Nottingham: Clawson Lodge, 403 Mansfield Road, Nottingham NG5 2DP (0602-622826).
Cavendish Medical Centre, 99 New Cavendish Street, London W1 (01-637 8941). Does a general screening including breasts and cervical smear.

Self-help groups for breast-cancer patients: Mrs Alfreda Marter, executive director of the Cancer Information Association, Marigold House, Carfax, Oxford (0865-46654), runs an independent charity which has pioneered cancer education. The association has produced leaflets, film strips, study days and a twenty-four-hour counselling service. A set of leaflets called *What Everybody should Know about Cancer* is available from them, price 50p. The Mastectomy Association, run by Betty Westgate of 25 Brighton Road, South Croydon, Surrey (01-654 8643), puts people who might be going to have the operation (or have had it) in touch with one another. The Tenovus Cancer Information Centre, at 111 Cathedral Road, Cardiff (0222-42851), produced a booklet called *Mastectomy: a Patient's Guide to Coping with Breast Surgery*, Nancy Robinson and Ian Swash.

Useful leaflets on self-examination have been published by the Health Education Council and the Women's National Cancer Control Campaign, 1 South Audley Street, London W1; these are free if you send a s.a.e.

Cancer of the cervix

Cervical cytology screening is available under the NHS from general practitioners, family planning and ante-natal clinics. The priority group for such tests ('smears') consists of all women over thirty-five and those over thirty-five who have been pregnant on three or more occasions. These women should be screened at five-yearly intervals according to current recommendations. The Women's National Cancer Control Campaign, 1 South Audley Street, London W1, runs screening programmes in co-operation with the NHS and some large employers. Their mobile clinics are equipped to provide cervical cytology testing and breast screening.

Alcoholism

Help for alcoholics is offered by a number of bodies including:
Alcoholics Anonymous, 11 Redcliffe Gardens, London SW10 9BG (01-834/8202 for London area; 01-352 9779 for rest of the country).
Accept provides a multi-discipline team community service and treatment centres for problem and dependent drinkers, their families and friends. Contact Accept at Western Hospital, Seagrave Road, London SW6 IR2 (01-381 3155).
Al-Anon family groups help the relatives and friends of problem drinkers c/o 61 Great Dover Street, London SE1 4YF (01-403 0888).
National Council on Alcoholism, 3 Grosvenor Crescent, London SW1X 7EE (01-235 4182) for addresses and telephone numbers of local councils on alcoholism.
Useful publications include two free pamphlets published by the Health Education Council (address page 231): *Good Health* and *Drinking Sensibly*. Other books include:
Alcoholism, Neil Kessel and Henry Walton (Pelican).
Alcoholism – A Social Disease, Max Glatt (Teach Yourself Books).
Countdown on Drinking, D. L. Davies (BMA Family Doctor series).
Alcohol and Alcoholism. A Royal College of Psychiatrists report (Tavistock).
Dealing with Drink: a Handbook, Ian Davis and Duncan Raistrick (BBC).

Drug dependence

The Institute for the Study of Drug Dependence, 3 Blackburn Road, London NW6, sells various pamphlets on drug addiction, including one for parents, *What Every Caring Parent Should Know*. The South Wales Association for the Prevention of Addiction, 111 Cowbridge Road East, Cardiff (0222-26113) provides a twenty-four-hour telephone answering service for counselling on drug abuse and addiction. In London there is now a self-help organization, Narcotics Anonymous, PO Box 246, London SW10, to those who want to stop their drug habit.

Those who mix drugs and alcohol can get help from Alcoholics Anonymous (see above).

7: STAYING HEALTHY AT WORK AND PLAY
Colds and flu
Coughs, Colds and Flu, David Tyrell (Family Doctor Publications).
Flu and colds, Health Education Council (address page 231).
How not to get chronic bronchitis, Professor J. G. Scadding (Family Doctor Publications).

Hazards at work
British workers in this country are now protected by the Health and Safety at Work Act, 1974. This does not replace existing legislation, such as the Factories Act, the Offices, Shops and Railways Premises Act, or the Mines and Quarries Act, which apply to particular places of work. However, the new Act puts the emphasis on all people at work wherever they may be, and places broad duties of care on employers and employees.

Employers are now obliged to provide and maintain safe and healthy places of work. If served with an improvement notice, an employer is required to make that improvement within a specified time. Alternatively, a prohibition notice may be issued stopping the particular operation which gives rise to the hazard, which could apply to a single piece of machinery or a whole factory. The employer can face fines or imprisonment if taken to court.

Employers are also obliged to provide information, instruction, training and supervision to ensure health and safety. This effectively means that employees must, by law, be told of any dangers from their machinery or from the materials they handle, and should be trained to work safely with them.

Detailed advice on the working of the Act can be obtained from your local office of the Health and Safety Executive (see telephone directory for details), or from a trade union.

There are a wide variety of booklets available from the Royal Society for the Prevention of Accidents (RoSPA, Cannon House, The Priory, Queensway, Birmingham B4 6BS) and from the Health & Safety Commission and Executive (available through HMSO bookshops), covering various aspects of industrial safety and the new health and safety legislation. Particularly useful books are: *Hazards at Work: How to Fight Them*, Patrick Kinnersley (Pluto Press), *Noise at Work*, a TUC guide; and *A Guide to the Health and Safety Act*, a leaflet published by the Health and Safety Executive, available from its public enquiry office in Baynards House, Chepstow Place, London W2 4TF.

Allergies
A booklet giving details of exercises is available from the Asthma Research Council, 12 Pembridge Square, London W2 4EM. The National Eczema Society, Tavistock House North, London WC1H 9SR, can offer advice to eczema sufferers. Send a s.a.e. for details.

For more information on allergies, see *Allergies: Questions and Answers*, Dr Doris Rapp and Dr A. W. Frankland (Heinemann Health Books). The Asthma Research Council can supply a free list of books so that you can choose a book which deals most closely with your problem.

For information on air-purifiers and air-conditioning, contact the Air-Conditioning Advisory Bureau, 30 Millbank, London SW1P 4RD (01-834 8827). It is sponsored by the Electricity Council: air-conditioning costs from about £250, electrostatic filters from about £100, humidifiers from about £30.

For Eczema see Chapter 4 in this Appendix.

For more information on diets and the allergy-free home write for booklet to National Society for Research into Allergy, PO Box 45, Hinckley, Leics LE10 1JY.

8: SEX AND HEALTH
The National Marriage Guidance Council has branches all over Britain which offer counselling on any aspect of personal relationships. It is not confined to married people. Look in the phone book under Marriage Guidance. The Brook Advisory Centres will help with birth control and other advice for young people. Write to 233 Tottenham Court Road, London W1. For Catholics, the Catholic Marriage Advisory Council, 15 Landsdowne Road, London W11 gives counselling.

There is a good mail-order book service obtainable from the National Marriage Guidance Council, Herbert Gray College, Little Church Street, Rugby. Send a s.a.e. for booklist on relationships and sex. The Family Planning Association bookshop, 27 Mortimer St, London W1 also sells books on mail order. Send a s.a.e. for their booklist, which includes more about birth control, and VD. Contraceptive help and advice is available to men and women free of charge at family planning clinics (listed under Family Planning Services in local telephone directories) and to women from most GPs.

For those wanting to know more about female masturbation, *The Hite Report*, Shere Hite (Corgi), is useful. Those in sexual difficulties may get help from a do-it-yourself sex therapy book, *Treat Yourself to Sex*, Paul Brown and Carolyn Faulder (Penguin). *The Joy of Sex*, Alex Comfort (Quartet), is undoubtedly the most literate and tasteful sex manual. Ignore the propaganda and enjoy it as a pillow book; it may shock some. *Premenstrual Syndrome and Period Pains*, M. G. Brush, a helpful booklet, is sold by Women's Health Concern, 16 Seymour Street, London W1. *Entitled to Love*, Wendy Greengross (National Marriage Guidance Council), is a book about disablement and sex. The Marie Stopes Clinic, 114 Whitfield Street, London W1 runs a mail-order sex-aids business, where vibrators can be purchased. The catalogue may shock. Ignore its therapeutic claims.

Homosexuality
Gay women and men can get help and advice from the following: Lesbian Line, BM Box 1514, London WC1N 3XX (01-837 1514); Campaign for

APPENDIX THREE/FURTHER INFORMATION

Homosexual Equality, BM Box CHE, London WC1N 3XX; Gay Switchboard on 01-837 7324. *Gay News* has local addresses.

Parents and relatives of gay people can get help and advice from Parents' Inquiry, 16 Honley Road, Catford, London SE6.

Contraception
The Family Planning Association, 27 Mortimer Street, London W1 will advise, and send free leaflets on birth control and VD in return for a s.a.e. For Catholic-approved natural family planning, ring the local Catholic Marriage Advisory Council Centre (see telephone book under Catholic) or write for a list of trained instructors to NFP Department, 15 Lansdowne Road, London W11. They also supply a correspondence course for those not in reach of an instructor. Brook Advisory Centres (see above) specialize in birth control for young people.

Abortion and unwanted pregnancy
More than a hundred and twenty thousand British women have abortions every year. An abortion can be legally performed provided that two doctors certify in good faith that at least two of the criteria laid down in the 1967 Abortion Act are satisfied. Done by skilled doctors, the operation is in theory safer than giving birth. Some doctors, however, are opposed to it on principle and may refuse an abortion on the National Health Service, or just delay until it is too late. If you want an abortion, do not delay. Early abortions are safest. If you need advice, contact one of the following charitable agencies for help: the British Pregnancy Advisory Service, First Floor, Guildhall Buildings, Navigation Street, Birmingham (021-643 1461), or the Pregnancy Advisory Service, 13 Charlotte Street, London W1.

Sexual diseases
Advice and help is available from your local clinic. It is listed under VD in the phone book, but may have some other name such as 'special clinic'. There may also be a number in the phone book which plays a recorded message describing symptoms. Any possibility of sexual infections *must* be checked out.

Free pamphlets are available from the Health Education Council (address page 231), and from the Family Planning Association (see above). Send largish s.a.e. *Sexually Transmitted Diseases*, Dr John Kenyon Oates, a booklet, is available from Women's Health Concern (see above).

The menopause
Books on middle age and the menopause are available from the Family Planning Association bookshop (see above). Family Doctor Booklets include *Women Only*, Philip Rhodes, and *Your Menopause Questions*, Jean Cope. Hormone replacement therapy research is changing so fast that books are quickly out of date. If you want HRT, but have an unsympathetic doctor, you can get a list of menopause clinics from Women's Health Concern (see above). Send a s.a.e. They also produce a booklet *The Menopause*, John McQueen. See also booklist for Depression under Chapter 3 in this Appendix.

9: HOLIDAY HEALTH
Travellers' Health Guide, Anthony Turner (Roger Lascelles, London).
Good Health Abroad, William Jopling (John Wright and Sons, Bristol).

10: A HEALTHY OLD AGE
Retirement
The Pre-Retirement Association, 19 Undine Street, London SW17 (01-767 3225), advises on preparation for retirement, covering health, mental attitude, leisure and finance. It publishes a monthly magazine, *Choice*, as well as books and pamphlets. One such book is *In the Pink*, Dr Deric Wright, a guide to good health in retirement.
A Good Age, Alex Comfort (Mitchell Beazley). Offers an A–Z of positive advice on how to enjoy old age.
Everything You Want to Know About Ageing, Dr Vernon Coleman (Gordon and Cremonesi).
The Care of the Aged, Dennis Hyams (Priory Press).
Health for Old Age, Consumers' Association, Caxton Hill, Hertford, Herts.
Having an Operation, Consumers' Association.
Enjoy Retirement. A booklet published by the Industrial Society, covering mental and physical health among other topics. Available from The Industrial Society, PO Box 1BQ, Robert Hyde House, 48 Bryanston Square, London W1.
Where to Live after Retirement, edited by Edith Rudinger, Consumers' Association.
The Time of Your Life: A Handbook for Retirement. Prepared by Help the Aged in conjunction with the Health Education Council.
Looking after yourself in retirement, Health Education Council.

Old Age (General)
There are a vast number of voluntary organizations offering aid and advice to the elderly. Some specialize in specific problems of accommodation. Some are limited to certain areas of the country. Information about all of them may be given by organizations such as those listed below, or can be found in *The Sunday Times Self-Help Directory*.

Age Concern England (National Old People's Welfare Council), Bernard Sunley House, 60 Pitcairn Road, Mitcham, Surrey CR4 3LL (01-640 5431). A centre of information on all subjects regarding the elderly. It can put you in touch with over a thousand local Age Concern groups.

British Association of Retired Persons, 14 Frederick Street, Edinburgh EH2 2HB (031-255 7334). A quarterly bulletin gives information on how members can help themselves. Telephone calls can only be answered on Mondays, Wednesdays and Friday mornings.

British Red Cross Society, 9 Grosvenor Crescent, London SW1 (01-235 5454). Provides a variety of services for elderly handicapped or disabled people.

Help the Aged, 32 Dover Street, London W1A 2AP (01-499 0972). Publishes a monthly newspaper and promotes day centres, workshops, rehabilitation centres, housing, etc.

National Federation of Old Age Pensions Association, 91 Preston New Road, Blackburn, Lancashire (0254-52606). Monthly paper *Pensioners' Voice* gives information and advice on pensions.

WRVS (Women's Royal Voluntary Service), 17 Old Park Lane, London W1Y 4AJ (01-499 6040). Their 'Good Companions' scheme provides such services as meals-on-wheels, luncheon clubs, transport.

Employment Fellowship, Drayton House, Gordon Street, London WC1H 0BE (01-387 1828). Companionship, useful occupation, and a supplementary income is available through work, adjusted to strength and skill, done at their centres.

St John Ambulance Association, 1 Grosvenor Crescent, London SW1. Helps with home nursing, outings, clubs, day centres, pensions, decorating, gardening, etc.

Shaftesbury Society, 112 Regency Street, London SW1P 4AX (01-834 2656). Housing associations for the elderly and handicapped, and holidays for those in London area only.

Task Force, 1 Thorpe Close, London W10 5XL (01-960 5666). Volunteers to give friendship and practical help such as gardening, decorating and general jobs around the home to the elderly in London.

National Federation of Claimants' Unions, 44 Havelock Road, Handsworth, Birmingham 20. Established to ensure that people get their rights within the welfare state.

Counsel & Care for the Elderly, 131 Middlesex Street, London E1 (01-621 1624). Advice on services and accommodation available to elderly people.

Disabled Living Foundation, 346 Kensington High Street, London W14 8NS (01-602 2491). Advice on aids, clothing and equipment.

Centre for Policy on Ageing, Nuffield Lodge, Regents Park, London NW1 4RS (01-722 8871). General information, particularly on private and voluntary old peoples' homes.

British Pensioners and Trades Unions Action Association, 97 Kings Drive, Gravesend, Kent (0474-61802). Links up pensioners' action groups all over the country.

MIND, 22 Harley Street, London W1N 2ED (01-637 0741). Advisory service and link with 160 local mental health associations.

Abbeyfield Society, 35a High Street, Potters Bar, Herts, runs housing schemes for the elderly in 'homes' of six to ten residents, in which the residents have to participate.

Old Age (Social Services)
Local authorities now have to provide a wide variety of services for elderly and handicapped people. The social services department of your local council will be able to tell you if you qualify. Its address can be found in the telephone directory under 'local authorities' or from the local town hall, library or citizens' advice bureau.

National Association of Citizens' Advice Bureaux, 110 Drury Lane, London WC2B 5SW (01-836 9231). Skilled advice and information, specifically on legislation and state services from almost seven hundred bureaux in Britain.

Your Rights – for Pensioners, Age Concern.

Diet
Easy Cooking for One or Two, Louise Davies (Penguin).
One Plus One, a free recipe book from Age Concern England (address above, send a s.a.e.).

Exercise
For details of keep-fit classes, contact your local education authority; the Keep-Fit Association, 70 Brompton Road, London SW3; or the Women's League of Health and Beauty, Beaumont Cottage, Ditton Close, Thames Ditton, Surrey. Send a s.a.e. and make clear that it is classes for the elderly that interest you.

A good paperback on mental and physical fitness with daily exercise routine, is *Age and Vitality*, Irene Gore, available from Age Concern (address above).

FURTHER INFORMATION/APPENDIX THREE

F/40 – Fitness on Forty Minutes a Week, Malcolm Carruthers and Alistair Murray (Futura).

Hearing
Why do people mumble so much?, free leaflet from Age Concern. Send s.a.e.

Hypothermia
Three useful and free leaflets are *Help with Heating Costs*, available from post offices and social security offices; *Keeping warm in winter*, Health Education Council; and *Heating Fact Sheet*, Age Concern.

Incontinence
The Incontinence Adviser, Disabled Living Foundation (see above, General list) can offer help and advice. Send a largish s.a.e. for notes on how to cope with incontinence and for a list of equipment and suppliers.
Management of incontinence in the home, Charlotte R. Kratz (*Age Concern Today* No.20, Winter 1976–7).
Incontinence, Dorothy Mandelstam (Heinemann Health Books).

Management for Continence, Bob Browne (Age Concern).

Joints
The Royal Association for Disability and Rehabilitation, 25 Mortimer Street, London W1N 8AB (01-637 5400) and the Disabled Living Foundation (see above), can give information on useful gadgets to help arthritis sufferers. Other sources for information are the Arthritis and Rheumatism Council, 41 Eagle Street, London WC1R 4AR, or the British Rheumatism and Arthritis Association, 6 Grosvenor Crescent, London SW1X 7ER.

Mobility
For details of gardening tools and all kinds of other disablement aids, whether walking sticks or wheel-chairs, send a largish s.a.e. to the Disabled Living Foundation (see above). At their London office they will demonstrate aids by appointment. Aids are also to be seen at the Disabled Living Centre, 84 Suffolk Street, Birmingham; the Newcastle Aids Centre, Mea House, Ellison Place, Newcastle; and the Merseyside Aid Centre. Youens Way, East Prescott Road, Liverpool 14.
Your holidays in retirement, Age Concern.

Strokes
Information on physiotherapy for stroke patients, and picture charts which can help them communicate, can be obtained from the Chest, Heart, and Stroke Association, Tavistock House North, Tavistock Square, London WC1H 9JE. The Royal Association for Disability and Rehabilitation (see above) can give information about apparatus to help stroke victims.

11: EMERGENCY!
The Red Cross, St John Ambulance and St Andrew's Ambulance Association run first-aid courses, organized in every county by the local branch of the organization. There are three types of courses: the ordinary first-aid course; the industrial first-aid course; and the emergency first-aid course. There is a small charge made for the courses, which varies from branch to branch.
The First-Aid Manual, published by the Red Cross, St John Ambulance and St Andrew's Ambulance Association is available from W. H. Smith or from Order of St John, Supplies Dept, St Johns Gate, Clerkenwell, London EC1.
Modern First-Aid, A. S. Playfair (Hamlyn).
The Emergency Book, edited by Jane Anthony (Macdonald and Jane's).
First-Aid in Pictures, Dr Robert Andrew (Wolfe).
First Steps in First-Aid, devised, written and produced by E. S. L. Bristol with St John Ambulance Association and Brigade, 1 Grosvenor Crescent, London SW1.

PICTURE ACKNOWLEDGEMENTS
The illustrations in this book are reproduced by kind permission of the following (numbers refer to page numbers):

Candy Amsden: 114, 117; Astral Photo Service: 41; Ian Beck: 159; Barbara Bellingham: 51; Paul Bevitt: 84–5, 87; Liz Butler: 37; David Case: 203; Leslie Chapman: 101; *Daily Telegraph*: 71; Richard Draper: 10, 11, 108, 206–7, 208, 209, 211, 212, 213; Duffy: 44–5; Alain le Garsmeur: 58–9, 193, 201; Lyn Gray: 34, 36, 38; Susan Griggs: 13, 24, 30, 65, 170, 177–8; Brian Grimwood: 95; Fay Godwin: 183; Hargrave Hands: 103, 122, 125; Image Bank: 50, 64, 188, 190, 199; Edwina Keene: 21, 39, 49, 107, 109, 206–7, 210, 212; Ken Lewis: 111, 119, 120, 187; Sarah Midda: 138; Duncan Mill: 128; David Montgomery: 197, 204; David Mostyn: 132–5; Norman Parkinson, Camera Press: 182; Pictorial Press: 26; Picturepoint: 123; Ingram Pinn: 2; QED: 17, 18, 27, 89, 125, 150–1; Ramblers' Association: 43; Ray Rathbone: 83; David Redfern: 182; David Reed: 92, 93; David Rice Evans: 194; Siemens: 22; *Sunday Times*: 46, 47, 52, 53, 61, 62, 143, 155; Suzanne Szasz, Transworld Feature Syndicate: 30; Joan Thompson, Garden Studio: 20, 54–7, 69, 70, 112, 144, 200; Topix; 60; David Watson: 35; James Wedge: 115; Ann Winterbotham: 166; David Worth: 66–7, 152–3, 187, 202.

Index

ASH, 131
abortion, 14, 16, 161, 184
abscesses, teeth, 124
accidents, 206–13; in childhood, 33–9; at work, 157; in old age, 195, 196, 200–1
acne, 117, 118
acupuncture, 110
aerobic exercise, 46–52
aflatoxin, 145
agriculture, occupational hazards, 156
alcohol, 78, 86; alcoholism, 75, 148–53; and cancer, 146; and children, 33, 150; and diet, 148; and driving, 152; and headaches, 72; and hangovers, 152–3; and healthy drinking, 151; and high blood pressure, 141; and heart disease, 148; and liver, 45, 148; in pregnancy, 12, 16, 150; safe amounts, 152; and sex life, 174; and sleep, 71; treatments, 149; withdrawal symptoms, 148–9
allergic rhinitis, 164
allergies, 118, 156, 164–8; and hair dyes, 116; toxic headaches, 72
American Heart Association, 76, 137
amniocentesis, 21, 184
amphetamines, 147
anaemia: and cancer, 144, 145; in pregnancy, 15, 23
anaesthetics: during labour, 25; in pregnancy, 19
anencephaly, 14–15, 21–2
angina, 136
anorexia nervosa, 93
Anstie, Dr Francis, 152
ante-natal care, 12, 22–3;
anthrax, 156
antibiotics, 122, 154, 155, 158, 160, 161, 162, 214
Anti-Coronary Club, 76
antihistamines, 164, 167; and alcohol, 148; in pregnancy, 18
appendicitis, 80
appetite: loss and cancer, 144; appetite-reducing drugs, 104
arsenic, 146
arteriosclerosis, 78
arthritis, 51, 118–19, 203–4
artificial respiration, 208
asbestos, 146, 157
aspirin, 12, 17, 18, 73, 126, 153, 154
asthma, 165
astigmatism, 119
atheroma, 136
atherosclerosis, 138
athlete's foot, 113
Atlas, Charles, 61
autogenic training, 70

babies: care of, 26–9; chest infections, 16; crying, 28; daily routine, 28; diarrhoea, 214; eczema, 167; eyesight, 29; feeding, 25, 26–8; feet, 113; growth, 27, 29; low birth weight, 16, 18; malformations, 12–19; playing, 28; prematurity, 14; sleep, 28; still birth, 18; vaccination, 10; weight gain, 27. See also children; pregnancy
back problems, 51, 106–11
Back Pain Association, 109
bacteria, 154, 155, 158, 160
bagassosis, 156
balance, 123
Balaskas, Janet and Arthur, 19
baldness, 114
bandaging, 207
barbiturates, during pregnancy, 18
bathing, 117
battering, child, 33
Baynham, Sylvia, 46–7, 48
beach, hazards, 191
beans, 85–6; in diet, 81
beds: and back pain, 109–10; bed sores, 196
beer, 148
bereavement, 73, 195
Berg, Dr John, 78
Berry, Dr R. J., 19
bilharzia, 191
Billings, Dr, 179
biofeedback machines, 70
bites, 209
black bryony, 37
bladder, cancer of, 144–5
bleeding, 209
blindness, 14
blood pressure: during pregnancy, 23; health checks, 45; high, 40, 140–1; and smoking, 136
body fat, 103
bonding, mother and baby, 25
bone, cancer of, 145
botulism, 160
bowel: blood in faeces, 214; cancer of, 78; obstruction, 80; and old age, 196, 202–3
brain: cancer of, 145; and sleep, 70–1
bran, 79–80, 145
bread, 79–80; slimmers, 104; wholemeal, 145
breakfast, 32, 86; cereals, 80
breast cancer, 44, 45, 77, 142–4; mastectomy, 143; self-examination, 143, 184
breast feeding, 25, 27
breathing: artificial respiration, 208; exercises for asthma, 165; relaxation, 69–70
British Arthritis and Rheumatism Council, 119
British Cardiac Society, 43
British Dental Association, 30, 127
British Institute of Radiology, 19
British Migraine Trust, 67
brittle bones, 182, 185
bronchitis, 10, 45, 128, 156, 165
brucellosis, 156, 158
Brush, Dr Michael, 175
Burkitt, Dr Denis, 76, 80
burns, 33–4, 209
Butler, Neville, 16
butter, 79
byssinosis, 156

cadmium, 156
Caesarean deliveries, 17
callouses, 113
calories, 90–9; calorie-controlled diet plan, 94–5; calorific content of food, 97–9; empty calories, 93; and exercise, 100–2
cancer, 19, 44, 45, 142–6; and alcohol, 146; avoiding, 145–6; and chemicals and radiation, 156–7; and fats, 77–8, 145; food additives, 146; and hair dyes, 114, 116; risks at work, 146; and smoking, 10, 128, 144, 146; tests for, 44, 45; and vegetables, 80, 145; X-ray detection, 142, 143, 144
candidiasis, 162
cannabis, 12, 18, 147
carbohydrates, 77, 82, 97–9
Carmichael, Dr J. H. E., 19
Carruthers, Dr Malcolm, 68, 69
cars: accidents, 32, 37–8; driving and stress, 68
cat bites, 209
cataracts, 121
Catholic Marriage Advisory Council, 179
Central Public Health Laboratory, Colindale, 78
cereal: breakfast, 80, 145; flour, 79–80; wholemeal, 145
cerebral palsy, 14
cervix, cancer of, 44, 45, 144, 184
chairs, and back pain, 108
chancroid, 181
cheese, 86
chemicals: burns, 209; and poisoning, 36, 157
chest infections, babies', 16
chickenpox, 17, 158
childbirth, 23–5
childcare, 25–39; clinics, 26
children: accidents, 33–9; and alcohol, 33; colds, 154; diet, 29; ears, 214; eczema, 167; eyesight, 30, 120; feet, 31; hearing, 30, 121, 122; ill, 214; school, 32–3; smoking, 33; speech, 30–1; teeth, 29–30, 126, 127; travel sickness, 187–8; vaccination, 10, 25, 32
chiropodists, 113, 195, 201
choking, 33, 209–10
cholera, 186
cholesterol, 76, 77, 78
claudication, 136, 140
Cleave, Surgeon Capt. T. L., 80
clitoris, 169, 171
clothing, sports, 48–9, 51
coal mining, occupational diseases, 155, 156, 157
coconut oil, 78
colds, 154–5
colon, cancer of, 144
coma, dealing with, 213
Common Cold Research Centre, 154
Compound Codeine, 73
concentration, and blood pressure, 141
concussion, 213

consciousness, loss of, 208, 210, 213
constipation, 80; and cancer, 144
construction work, occupational hazards, 155, 156, 157
Consumers' Association, 36, 102
contraception, 12, 175–9; coitus interruptus, 178; diaphragm, 177; IUD, 16, 177–8; pill, 12, 105, 139, 174, 176–7; rhythm method, 179; safe period, 179; sheath, 177, 181; spermicides, 177, 181; sterilization, 178–9; vasectomy, 179
convulsions, 210–11
Cook, Capt. Simon, 54
Cooper, Dr Kenneth, 46, 48, 51
corns, 113
cosmetics, 118, 167
cot deaths, 27
cough, as symptom of cancer, 144
Cruse, 73
cycling, 51, 65; indoor, 63; in pregnancy, 19; skills for children, 38
cyclamates, 104
cystitis, 158, 185
Cytomegalo virus (CMV), 16–17

DDT, 191
Dalton, Dr Katharine, 175
dance, 62
dandruff, 116
De Langen, C. D., 76
deadly nightshade, 37
deafness, 14, 16, 30, 44, 121–3; and flying, 189; and noise, 123, 156; and old age, 121, 195, 196
delirium tremens, 148–9
demolition, occupational hazards, 155, 156, 157
dentists, 126, 127
dentures, badly fitting, 144
depression, 71, 73–4, 75; anti-depressants, 74; menopausal, 183–4; and old age, 195; post-natal, 26, 74
dermatitis, 118, 156, 167
desensitizing injections, 164
desserts, 86
detergents and allergies, 167
diabetes, 12, 45, 88, 120, 180; and foot care, 113
diarrhoea: in babies, 214; and cancer, 144; on holiday, 189–90
diet, 10, 76–105; and allergies, 167–8; balanced, 82, 86; bread and flour, 79–80; calorie-controlled, 94–5; and cancer, 77–8, 145–6; fats and oils, 78–9; heart disease, 76–7, 78, 136, 137, 139; in pregnancy, 12; in old age, 195, 196; and skin, 117; slimming, 88–105
dinner, 86
diphtheria, 32, 158, 186
Disabled Living Foundation, 113
disease, class distinctions, 10
'disclosing' solution, 126
disodium cromoglycate, 164
dizziness, 123
doctor, when to call, 214

INDEX

dog bites, 209
Down's syndrome, *see* Mongolism
driving: and backache, 108; and stress, 68
drowning, 33, 38–9, 311; drown-proofing, 39
drugs: appetite suppressants, 104; allergies, 168; dependence, 75, 147; illegal, 147; and old age, 195, 197; pain killers, 110; in pregnancy, 12, 14, 17–19; and sleep, 71–2; and travel, 188, 189
dust, and allergies, 164
dyspareunia, 174

ears, 121–3; and flying, 189; foreign body in, 211. *See also* deafness
eating habits, 88–91
eczema, 118, 167
eggs, 10, 137; yolks, 79
electric shock, 211
electrocardiogram (ECG), 44; treadmill, 46, 47
electrolysis, 114
elephantiasis, 191
emergencies, 206–73
emphysema, 156
emulsifying ointment, 167
enzymes, 145
epidemiology, 11
epidurals, 25
epilepsy, 14, 18
Epstein-Barr virus, 160
erysipelas, 159
eustachian tubes, 189
exercise, 10, 40–65; aerobic, 40, 42, 46–52; and arthritis, 118–19; in childhood, 31; dynamic, 42; equipment, 61–2; and heart disease, 42, 43, 139, 141; indoor, 53–60; isometric, 42, 61–2, 141; isotonic, 42; keep fit, 54–7; during pregnancy, 19–21; and slimming, 80, 100–2
exhaust fumes, poisoning, 211
eyes, 119–21; abnormalities, 14, 16; accidents, 121; babies', 29; blindness, 121; eye strain, 72; foreign bodies, 211; health checks, 44; infections, 120; injuries, 156, 209; and old age, 195, 200

factory inspectors, 157
faeces, blood in, 214
faints, 211
falls, in old age, 200
Family Planning Association, 177, 178
farmer's lung, 156, 168
fats and oils, 77, 78–9; body fat, 103, 105; and dieting, 93, 137, 139; fat content of foods, 97–9; low-fat cooking, 82–3, 145
feet, 112–13; children's, 31; in old age, 200
fertility, 12, 14
fibre in diet, 79–80
fires, accidents, 33
fitness tests, 48
Fletcher, Charles, 45
fluoride, 30, 124; during pregnancy, 18
flying, and deafness, 123
folic acid, 14, 22
food: additives, 146; allergies, 167–8; mouldy, 145; poisoning, 160, 189
foreign bodies, 211
Foresight, 12

Forfar, John, 17
fractures, bandaging, 206–7
Friedmann, Dr Meyer, 67, 69, 70

gardening: and backache, 109; in old age, 200–1
gas, poisoning, 211
gastro-enteritis, 160
genital warts, 181
German measles, 12, 14, 16, 32, 118, 161–2; and deafness, 121
glandular fever, 160
glaucoma, 44, 120
golf, 65
gonorrhoea, 180
gout, 118
Green Cross Code, 38
gum disease, 124, 126, 127
gymnasiums, 62; home, 60–2

Hadassah University, 16
hair, 114–16; dyes, 19, 114, 116; greying, 114; unwanted, 114
Hanson, Dr James, 150
hare meat, 79
hawthorn, 37
hay fever, 148, 164
head injury, 122, 211
headaches, 72–3
health checks, 44–5
Health and Safety Executive, 156
health clubs, 62
Health Education Council, 26, 28, 31, 131, 132
heart attack, dealing with, 141, 211–12
heart disease, 10, 11, 136–41; as cause of death, 10, 40, 42; and contraception, 139; and diet, 76–7, 81, 137, 139; and drinking, 148; exercise, 42, 43, 139, 141; and old age, 200–1; overweight, 88; prevention, 137, 139; recovery, 139–40; and sex, 185; and smoking, 128, 137; and stress, 67–8, 137, 139; and weight, 88, 139
heart massage, 210, 212
heartburn, 15
heat stroke, 211
heat treatment, 110
Heimlich Manoeuvre, 210
hemlock, 37
hepatitis, 160, 180, 186
herbs, and pregnancy, 18–19
heroin, 18, 143
herpes virus, genital herpes, 180–1; herpes zoster, 162; in pregnancy, 17
Hill, Dr Michael, 78
Hite Report, 173
Hodgkin's disease, 145
hogweed, 37
holiday health, 186–91; diseases, 191; heat and sun, 190–1; hygiene, 189–90; travelling, 187–9; vaccinations, 186–7
home: allergy-free, 166; gymnasium, 61–2; safety in, 33–6
homosexuality, 173–4, 181
hormone replacement therapy, 181–3
housework, and backache, 109
Huxley, Meloma, 19
hydrocephalus, 21–2
hygiene, 158, 163; on holiday, 189–90
hypertension, 40, 140–1
hypothermia, 201–2, 210

Illingworth, R. S., 17

impetigo, 160
incontinence, 195, 202–3
indigestion: during pregnancy, 15; and stomach cancer, 144
industrial injuries, 155–7; cancer risks, 146
infectious diseases, 158–63
infertility, 12, 14, 157
influenza, 154–5, 160; in pregnancy, 17
inhaling: for colds, 155; foreign bodies, 211
insect bites, 158, 209
insomnia, 184; sleeping pills, 71–2, 74
insurance: holiday, 186; life insurance, 88
International Committee on the Standardization of Physical Fitness Tests, 63
International Labour Office, 156
International Union Against Cancer, 142
'intrinsic' allergy, 165
isometric exercise, 42, 61–2
Iyengar, B. K. S., 60–1

jelly fish, 191
jet-lag, 188–9
jaundice, 160, 176
jogging, 43, 46, 48
Johnson, Dr Virginia E., 169, 172, 185
joints: diseases of, 118–19; and old age, 203–4

kala-azar, 191
keep-fit exercises, 54–7, 139
Keys, Ancel, 81
kidney, 197; cancer of, 144–5; disease, 157
Kinsey, Alfred C., 169
Kinsey reports, 169, 173
Kitzinger, Sheila, 16
Koplik's spots, 160
Kuntzleman, Charles, T., 60

LSD, 18, 143
labour, 25
laburnum, 37
larynx, cancer of, 144
lead, tinned food, 12
Leboyer, Dr Frederick, 25
Leitch, Martha, 193
leukaemia, 145, 157
lice, 115–17
life expectancy, 10
lifting, and backache, 108–9, 156
lip reading, 123
liver: and alcohol, 148, 152; disease, 45, 148, 157; health checks, 45; hepatitis, 160
lockjaw, 162
Loma Linda University, California, 78
loneliness, 75; in old age, 195
Longevity Research Institute, 139
Los Angeles Olympics, 1984, 51
'low-fat' produce, 10
lumbago, 107
lunch, 86
lungs, 45; cancer, 10, 128, 144; health checks, 45; occupational hazards, 156–7
lymph glands, 159, 191

Madders, Mrs Jane, 69
malaria, 187, 191
Malta fever, 156, 158
marathons, 48, 51
Marriage Guidance Council, 75, 174, 183

massage, 69, 110
Masters, Dr William H., 169, 172, 185
masturbation, 172, 173
meals: calorie-controlled, 94–5; balanced, 86; light, 86; substitute, 104
measles, 32, 122, 160–1
Medic-Alert bracelet, 168
Medical Research Council, 42, 76, 79
Medicines Code, 34, 36
meditation, 70, 188
memory: and alcoholism, 149; and high blood pressure, 141
meningitis, 161
menopause, 181–4; depression, 183–4; hormone replacement therapy, 181–3; hot flushes, 183
menstruation, 174–5; period pains, 175; pre-menstrual tension, 73, 175; tampons, 175
mental handicap, 14; retardation, 16
Menuhin, Yehudi, 60–1
metabolism, and overweight, 40, 42, 100–1, 105
Michigan Heart Association, 136
microwaves, 157
middle age, 11, 64–5; middle-age spread, 105
migraine, 67, 72–3, 167, 168
Migraine Trust, 72
milk, 10; and allergies, 167
miscarriages, 16, 17
mobility, and old age, 204–5
Mogadon, 71–2
moisturizing cream, 117
Mongolism (Down's syndrome), 14, 21, 184
moniliasis, 162
monkshood, 37
mononucleosis, 160
morbilli, 160–1
Morris, J. N., 42
motherhood, 25–6; mother and toddler groups, 26
mountain fever, 158
mouth, 125; cancer of, 144
mumps, 122, 166; in pregnancy, 17
muscle control, 69–70

nasal polyps, 165
National Association for the Childless, 14
National Childbirth Trust, 19, 26
Naylor Dana Institute for Disease Prevention, New York, 78
National Marriage Guidance Council, 75, 174, 183
neck, cancer of, 144
nettlerash, 165, 167
Nicklaus, Jack, 65
nitrazepam, 71–2
nits, 116–17
noise, 123, 156
non-specific urethritis (NSU), 181
nose: foreign body in, 211; nasal polyps, 165; nose bleed, 211

obesity, 77, 105; in childhood, 105
occupational diseases, 155–7; allergies, 168; protective clothing, 157
oesophagus, cancer of, 144
oestrogen, 182, 183
offal, 79
Ogino and Knaus, 179
oils, cooking with, 79
old age, 10–11, 192–205; and back pain, 107; and exercise, 40,

239

INDEX

198–200, 203; falls, 200–1; and foot care, 113; hearing problems in, 123; heart and blood vessels, 201; hypothermia, 201–2; incontinence, 202–3; joints, 203–4; senile decay, 136; sex life in, 185; and stroke, 205; teeth care in, 205
olive oil, 79
Open University, 194
orgasm, 169; female, 169, 171, 174
ornithosis, 161
osteo-arthritis, 107, 118
osteopath, 110
osteoporosis, 183, 185
ovaries, cancer of, 144

pain-killing drugs, 110
palpitations, 184–5
Paracetamol, 73, 153, 154, 160, 161
paralysis, infantile (polio), 32, 161
parenthood, 25–6, 33
parents, caring for elderly, 195
parrot fever, 161
Patel, Dr Chandra, 69
Pauling, Dr Linus, 154
Pawan, Dr Graston, 153
peanuts, 145
pertussis, 162
Phillips, Dr Roland, 78
physiotherapy, 69–70, 110, 165
piles (haemorroids), 20, 45, 76, 144
pipe smoking, 132
plants, poisonous, 36–7
plaque, 124
playgrounds, safety in, 36
playing, with babies, 28
pneumoconiosis, 155, 156
pneumonia, 161
poisoning, 33, 34, 36–7, 211, 212
poliomyelitis, 32, 161, 186
pollen and hay fever, 164
polyunsaturated fats, 78, 79, 80
post-natal depression, 26
posture, 106–7, 110–12
pre-conceptul care, 12
pregnancy, 12–25, 174; alcohol in, 12, 16, 151; antenatal care, 12, 22–3; diet in, 14–15; drugs in, 12, 14, 17–19; exercise, 19–21; infections during, 16; planning for, 12; relaxation in, 15–16; and sexual intercourse, 16; and smoking, 12, 16, 128–9; tests for, 14; weight, 105
preservatives, food, 12, 14–15
prickly heat, 190
Pritikin, Nathan, 140
prostate enlargement, 145
protein, 77; protein content of foods, 97–9
psoriasis, 118
psittacosis, 161
pubic lice, 181
pulse rate, 46
pyorrhea, 124

rabbit meat, 79
rabies, 161, 187
radiation, 157
radiotherapy, 145
Rahe, Dr Richard, 66, 68
railways, occupational hazards, 156
rambling, 65; in old age, 200
rashes, 165, 167, 214
recovery position, 208, 213
rectum: cancer of, 144; health checks, 45
Reed, Anthony, 109

Reiter's syndrome, 180
relaxation, 69–70; and blood pressure, 141; during pregnancy, 15–16; and sleep, 71
retina, 119, 120
retirement, planning, 192, 194. See also old age
rheumatism, 107
rheumatoid arthritis, 118, 167
ringworm, 161
road safety, children, 33, 37–8
Rosenman, Dr Ray, 67, 69, 70
Ross Institute of Tropical Hygiene, 191
roughage, 76
rowing, 65; indoor, 61
Royal College of Physicians, 43, 76, 77, 93, 129, 137
Royal College of Psychiatrists, 16
Royal National Institute for the Deaf, 123
rubella, 12, 14, 16, 32, 118, 121, 161–2
rubeola, 32, 122, 160–1
running, 10, 48–51

salmonella, 160
salt, 141
Samaritans, 74, 75
Sandels, Dr Stina, 38
Sanders, Col. Harland, 195
scabies, 181
scalds, 33, 209
scarlet fever (scarlatina), 162
Schachter, Dr Stanley, 89
sciatica, 107
scurvy, 117
seat belts, 37–8
sedatives, 147
self-help groups, for depressives, 74
senile decay, 136
Seventh Day Adventists, 78
sex, 169–85, 205; anal intercourse, 172; bisexuality, 173; and guilt, 172–3; homosexuality, 173–4; menopause, 181–4; in pregnancy, 16; sexual difficulties, 174; sexually transmitted disease, 12, 17, 158, 172, 180–1; therapy, 174
shampoos, medicated, 116
shingles, 158, 162
shipping, occupational hazards, 155, 156, 157
shock, dealing with, 213
shoes, choosing, 112–13
silicosis, 156
sitting posture, 111
skin, 117–18; allergies, 165, 167; cancer of, 142, 157; diseases of, 118, 157, 184; and old age, 195; rashes, 214
sleep, 70–2; insomnia, 184; in old age, 205; posture during, 109–10, 112; during pregnancy, 15–16; sleeping pills, 71–2, 74; sleeping sickness, 191
slimming, 88–105; calorie-controlled diet plan, 94–5; cut-down method, 91–9; cut-out method, 100; diet aids, 104; eating habits, 89–91; and exercise, 80, 100–2; recipes, 96; slimming clubs, 102, 104
slipped disc, 106
smallpox, 186
Smith, Joyce, 51
Smithells, R. W., 14
smoking, 10, 33, 78, 105, 128–35;

and asthma, 165; and cancer, 10, 128, 144, 146; giving up, 130–5; and heart disease, 128, 137, 139; during pregnancy, 12, 16, 128–9; reasons for smoking, 129, 130, 132; Smoking or Health, 129
snake bites, 209
spectacles, protective, 119, 120; sunglasses, 121
speech, development of, 30–1
spina bifida, 14–15, 21–2
Spock, Dr Benjamin, 26
sport, 63–5; competitive, 64; family, 65; fitness ratings of sports, 63; team, 64. See also under individual sport
sports centres, 62
Sports Council, 198
squash, 64
squints, 29, 30
Stanford University Heart Disease Prevention Program, 46
staphylococci, 160
sterility, 157
sterilization, 178–9
steroids, 164, 165; corticosteroids, 167
stings, 209
stomach, cancer of, 10, 80, 144; upsets on holiday, 189–90
streptococci, 155, 160
stress, 66, 67–9; coping with, 42; and heart disease, 67, 137, 139; in pregnancy, 15–16
strokes, 10, 77, 136, 205; and diet, 81, 136
stupor, 213
suffocation, 33, 213
sugar: and heart disease, 77; and slimming, 88, 93; and tooth decay, 123–4, 126
suicide, 74–5
sunshine: effect on skin, 117–18; sunburn, 118, 190, 209; sunglasses, 121
swallowed objects, 213
sweating, night sweats, 184
swimming, 52, 65, 198–9; lessons, children, 39; during pregnancy, 19; drown-proofing, 39
syphilis, 17, 180

Taylor, Dr Stanley, 67, 68
teeth, 124–7; babies', 29; brushing, 124, 125; children, 29–30; crowns, 127; decay, 124; dental floss, 126; discoloration, 18; disclosing solution, 126; fillings, 127; fluoride, 30, 124; and old age, 195, 205; pregnancy, 15, 18; toothache, 127
tennis, 64
tetanus, 32, 156, 162, 186
Tetracycline, 18
thorn apple, 37
threshold limit values, 156
throat, cancer of, 144
thrush, 162, 165, 180
Thurgood, Alan, 47, 48
thyroid gland, 144
Time Out, 60
tinea, 161
tinned food, 12
tinnitus, 123
toenails: care of, 113; ingrowing, 113
Tokyo Olympics, 51
Toms, Sgt Tony, 54
toothache, 127
toothbrushes, 126

toxoplasma, 17
tranquillizers, 18, 72, 74, 147
travel sickness, 186–7
trichomoniasis, 180
tuberculosis, 10, 32, 162
typhoid, 186

ulcers, duodenal, 10
ultrasound, in antenatal care, 23
ultra-violet radiation, 157
unconsciousness, dealing with, 208, 210, 213
undulant fever, 156, 158
urine: blood in, 212, 214; health checks, 45; red, 212
urethritis, non-specific, 181
urticaria, 165, 167

vaccination, 10, 16, 32, 154, 158, 161, 162, 186–7
vagina, 169; dryness, 175, 184; episiotomy, 19; thrush, 162, 165, 180; trichomoniasis, 180
varicose veins, 209
Van Keep, Dr P. A., 183
vasectomy, 179
vegetables, 80–1; and cancer, 80–1; oils, 78
vegetarians, 15, 78, 79, 82
veins, varicose, 209
venereal disease, 12, 17, 158, 172, 180–1
venison, 79
verrucae, 113
viruses, 154–5, 158, 160
vitamins, 27, 77, 175; and colds, 154; in pregnancy, 15, 19, 22; and skin, 117
vivonex, 167

walking, 42, 43, 198; posture in, 111–12
warmth, in old age, 195
water, sterilizing on holiday, 189
Wattenburg, Dr Leo, 80–1
Weaver, Mrs Eula, 139–40
weight: health checks, 45; and heart disease, 139; ideal, 89; reduction, 40, 42, 91; weight loss and cancer, 142
weight-training, 61–2
wheelchair, 204
Which?, 36, 102
whisky, 148
Whitehead, Dr Malcolm, 183
wholemeal foods, 80
whooping cough, 162, 186
womb, cancer of, 144
woman, and running, 51
women's liberation groups, 174
Women's Health Concern, 175, 183
work: cancer risks, 146; health hazards, 155–7
Workers' Educational Association, 194
World Health Organization, 148, 186
Wynder, Dr Ernst, 78

X-rays, and cancer detection, 142, 143, 144, 145; during pregnancy, 19

YMCA, 62
yellow fever, 186
yew, 37
yoga, 58–61, 70, 188; during pregnancy, 19–21
Yoga Today, 60